Principles of Pathology for Dental Students

J. B. Walter, T.D.
M.D., M.R.C.P., F.R.C. Path.

Department of Pathology, Banting Institute, University of Toronto, and Departments of Medicine and Pathology, Toronto General Hospital, Toronto, Canada.

Margaret C. Hamilton
F.D.S.R.C.S. (Eng.)

Department of Children's Dentistry and Orthodontics, University of Birmingham, England

M. S. Israel
M.B., M.R.C.P., F.R.C. Path., D.C.P.

Department of Pathology, Institute of Basic Medical Sciences, Royal College of Surgeons of England and Lewisham Group Laboratory, London, England.

Catherine Lappin

Principles of Pathology for Dental Students

J. B. Walter
Margaret C. Hamilton
M. S. Israel

FOURTH EDITION

CHURCHILL LIVINGSTONE
EDINBURGH LONDON MELBOURNE AND NEW YORK 1981

CHURCHILL LIVINGSTONE
Medical Division of Longman Group Limited

Distributed in the United States of America by Churchill Livingstone Inc., 19 West 44th Street, New York, N.Y. 10036, and by associated companies, branches and representatives throughout the world.

First edition 1967
Second edition 1971
Third edition 1974
Fourth edition 1981

ISBN 0 443 02243 7

British Library Cataloguing in Publication Data
Walter, John Brian
Principles of pathology for dental students. —
4th ed.
1. Pathology
I. Title II. Hamilton, Margaret Craig
III. Israel, Martin Spencer
616.07.0246176 RB111 80–41325

Typeset by CCC, printed and bound in Great Britain by William Clowes (Beccles) Limited, Beccles and London

Preface

The student embarking on a career in dentistry must achieve, within a period of five years, sufficient skill to recognize, diagnose correctly, and treat the diseases occurring in the oral cavity. In addition to becoming adept in many complicated practical procedures, the student must also acquire much theoretical knowledge. This knowledge should be based on sound general principles, and Part I of this book is intended to cover the principles of general pathology in a manner suited to the particular needs of the dentist.

The dental surgeon treats not only diseases of the oral cavity but also people—each patient as an individual with problems that may not be confined to the mouth. Dental treatment must be related to other diseases in so far as these may modify the treatment or necessitate the taking of certain precautions. Nowhere is this more pertinent than in a patient with heart disease. Although the dentist need not be medically qualified, there should be sufficient insight into common diseases to afford an appreciation of the patient's general condition, so as to allow an effective co-operation with the medical attendants.

The second part of this book is designed to cover the basic principles of pathology pertaining to some of the special systems. Of necessity this coverage is brief, but it is intended to be adequate, so that when time and opportunity arise, the dentist will be able to consult specialized texts without the feeling of venturing into foreign lands. When the student encounters pathology for the first time, many new words and concepts are met; these we have endeavoured to define when they are first introduced so that the learning may proceed by a series of graded steps. We have appended a list of references to each chapter in the hope of fostering the spirit of enquiry in our students. These references have been rigorously scrutinized in this edition, and most of those over ten years old have been omitted. The old references can easily be obtained from the previous editions and from standard texts of pathology as well as from the current reviews. For the first time the full title of each reference has been included, and it is hoped that this will stimulate the reader to consult the material cited, and to adopt a critical approach.

Six years have elapsed since the third edition was published, and although there have been no striking breakthroughs in medicine, the many advances that have been recorded have necessitated a complete revision. Four new chapters have been added; in Chapter 16, 'Some disorders of metabolism', the section on glucose metabolism is followed by an account of diabetes mellitus and gout. Chapter 17,

'Disorders of nutrition', encompasses the important topics of starvation, the role of vitamins, and the malabsorption syndrome. The topic of calcium metabolism has been expanded and added to the existing section of heterotopic calcification; this now constitutes a new Chapter 18. Chapter 19 is devoted to an account of the collagen vascular diseases. The chapters devoted to immunology have been thoroughly revised, and additions have been made to the chapters on diseases of the heart, gastrointestinal tract, and kidney. Other topics which have either been introduced for the first time or else considerably expanded include the mediators of acute inflammation, the granuloma, the bactericidal mechanisms in polymorphs in relation to immunity, viral diseases (especially the section on the oncogenic viruses and the viruses of hepatitis), axial regeneration in amphibians, the HLA system, the serology of syphilis, leprosy, chlamydial infections, and the clonal origin of tumours. In all, this has necessitated an increase in the size of the book by 153 pages.

One other departure from our previous custom has been the introduction of SI units. These are commonly used in many countries, but the traditional units have been retained alongside the SI units for those readers who are unfamiliar with the new nomenclature.

1981

J B W, Toronto
M C H, Birmingham
M S I, London

Acknowledgements

We wish to thank W B Saunders Company of Philadelphia for generously allowing us to use over 40 illustrations from *An Introduction to the Principles of Disease* (by J B Walter). A number of these figures have previously apppeared in the fifth edition of *General Pathology* by J B Walter and M S Israel and published by Churchill Livingstone. Many of the gross specimens illustrated are from the Wellcome Museum of Pathology, and we are grateful to the president and the council of the Royal College of Surgeons of England for permission to publish them. In accordance with their wishes each is acknowledged at the end of the caption, and their catalogue number is indicated. A number of specimens illustrated are from the Boyd Museum of the University of Toronto, and we thank Dr E Farber of that Institute for permission to use these.

We are indebted to a number of colleagues for providing valuable criticism and for assisting in the realms of their particular expertise: Dr Y Bedard (Toronto) for electron microscopy; Dr G T Simon (Hamilton) for electron microscopy; Dr Leslie P Spence for reviewing the section on virology, and Micheline Fauvel, lately of his Department of Virology at the Toronto General Hospital, for providing many of the new electron micrographs of viruses. We owe special gratitude to those who have given us unpublished material or have allowed us to modify their original work. Each figure is acknowledged separately under its caption.

Our thanks are due to Mrs Sonja Duda, librarian of the Banting Institute, Toronto, for valuable help in obtaining references, and to Mr A A Silcox and Mr J T Manders of the Pathology Department of the Royal College of Surgeons of England, London, for help with photomicrography.

Contents

PART ONE

General pathology

1

Introduction

In the practice of medicine it is soon apparent that the majority of patients who seek help do so because of some abnormality which is causing them distress. Often such *symptoms* can be dispelled by simple remedies—quite often by time and reassurance. Much of medicine is an art which its practitioners, whether doctors, dentists, nurses, or physiotherapists must learn. Nevertheless, there have always been individuals who were not content simply to observe disease and the effects of empirical time-honoured remedies upon it. They have attempted to describe and record the abnormalities in their patients in an objective manner; by introducing measurements they initiated the science which is called pathology.

Disease itself is as difficult to define as is the normal, from which it is a departure. As generally used, the term disease is employed to describe a state in which there is a sufficient departure from the normal for signs or symptoms to be produced. The variations from the normal are called *lesions,* and although generally structural in nature, the term may also be used to describe functional abnormalities, for example *biochemical lesions* (p. 55). The cause of the disease is called its *aetiology* and the development of the lesions its *pathogenesis.* Although aetiology and pathogenesis are generally described as separate entities, in practice it is often difficult to distinguish between them. Indeed, the aetiology of one era may become part of the pathogenesis of the next. An example will suffice. A patient takes a large dose of strychnine, develops convulsions, and dies. Clearly the aetiology of the disease is administration of strychnine. However, a closer consideration may reveal that the drug was self-administered during a phase of depression. The suicidal administration of strychnine would then be part of the pathogenesis of the fatal disease depression.

Although this instance may appear to be an exaggeration of the difficulty in delineating the cause of a disease, many other examples will be encountered. The great advances in bacteriology which started at the end of the nineteenth century fostered the concept that each disease had a single cause. To state that a boil is always caused by the *Staphylococcus aureus* is true, but nevertheless this is an incomplete statement. It is known that patients with diabetes mellitus are prone to develop recurrent boils. Which is the cause of the boils, the staphylococcus or the diabetes? Present doctrine would still favour the organism, but the diabetes would be labelled a major predisposing factor. Multiple causes are probably much more common than we think. The doctrine of one cause for one disease has certainly failed to be a profitable concept in the search for the aetiology of many common diseases such as cancer, arteriosclerosis, emphysema, chronic bronchitis, and dental caries.

An attempt to avoid the difficulty in defining disease has been the introduction of the term *syndrome.* This is a condition in which there occurs a defined collection of lesions, signs, or symptoms which are not necessarily always caused by the same agent. Thus Mikulicz's syndrome is defined as bilateral painless enlargement of the lacrimal and salivary glands from whatever cause. It may be found in leukaemia, but frequently the cause is unknown and it is then said to be *idiopathic.* Clearly the diseases in which the cause is not known are difficult to distinguish from syndromes. Indeed, the two terms are frequently used quite indiscriminately and interchangeably.

Pathology is thus the scientific study of disease. It describes the cause, course, and termination of disease, and the nature of its lesions. In almost all diseases the lesions are of varying nature, and may be morphological, chemical, or functional. Anything which can be measured is within the domain of pathology. The height of the blood pressure, the rate of the heart, and the temperature of the patient are all valid measurements, which if accurately recorded are as scientific as are measurements of the size of a muscle fibre on a section or the amount of fat in a liver.

All good clinicians are thus practising pathologists, and it is for this reason that pathology is such an important part of the curriculum for both dental and medical students.

2

Normal structure

Introduction

The body is composed of innumerable cells which are bound together by a variable amount of intercellular material. Each cell is enclosed by an outer limiting membrane, the *cell* or *plasma membrane,* and contains a nucleus which is bounded by the *nuclear membrane.*

Development from the fertilized ovum is accomplished by two processes:

1. *Division,* whereby more cells are produced and

2. *Maturation,* or *differentiation,* whereby cells develop specific structures which enable them to perform specialized functions, e.g. contraction in the case of muscle fibres. Some highly specialized cells, e.g. neurons, lose their ability to divide as they become differentiated, but others do not, e.g. liver cells. What is lost during the process of maturation is the ability to differentiate along other lines. While the fertilized ovum is *totipotent,* i.e. capable of producing all the tissues of the body, its cellular progeny are not all alike and do not have this ability. Both cytoplasmic and nuclear factors are probably involved in differentiation, but the nature of this process, which may be regarded as a type of ageing, is not understood.

Early evidence of differentiation within the mass of cells composing the developing embryo is the formation of three distinct germ-layers. An outer layer of cells forms the *ectoderm,* while a tube develops within the mass and the cells lining it form the *endoderm.* This tube forms the basis of the future alimentary canal and the organs that bud from it—lungs, liver, pancreas, and others. The *mesoderm* consists of cells lying between the ectoderm and the endoderm. The primitive cells of each germ-layer can differentiate along two separate lines to form either epithelium or connective tissue. These are described later (see p. 31). It is evident that the cells of the body show a considerable diversity of structure and function, yet each is in fact remarkably independent. Each receives a supply of oxygen and foodstuff from the blood stream with which it must produce its own structural components and secretions, and from which it must release the energy required for mechanical, chemical, or electrical work. It is therefore not surprising that all cells are built upon a similar basic plan.

The number of chemical reactions known to occur inside the cell is so great that it would be difficult to understand how these could proceed in a structure as simple as the cell appears to be under the light microscope. The electron microscope has changed all this—from a barren wilderness, the internal structure

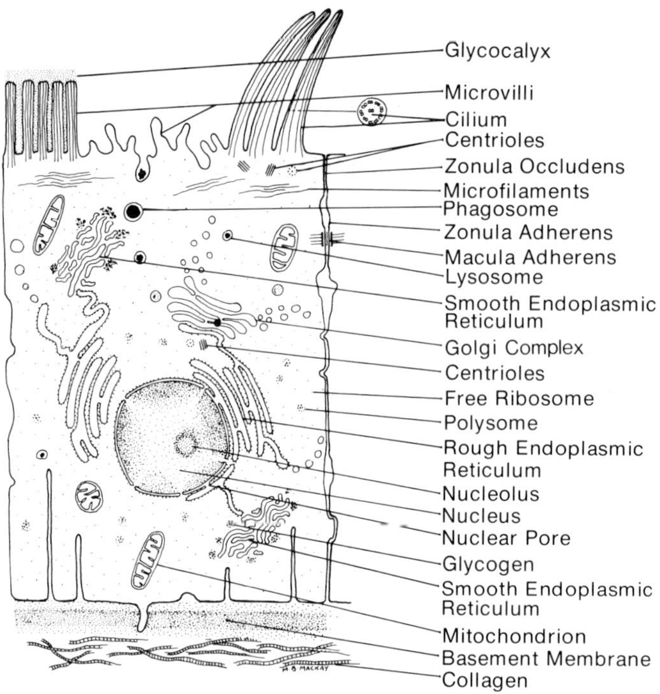

Fig. 2.1 Diagrammatic representation of a hypothetical typical epithelial cell. The free surface of the cell has projecting microvilli, which on the left are arranged regularly to form a brush border. In the centre the villi are irregular, and micropinocytotic-vacuole formation is depicted. On the right cilia are shown. The cell adjoins its neighbours with some interdigitation of their plasma membranes; one junctional complex is shown. The nucleus contains one nucleolus, and is surrounded by a double-layered membrane. Between the nucleus and the free border is the cell centre, or centrosome, and adjacent to this is one Golgi complex. There are two centrioles lying at right angles to each other. The base of the cell rests on a basement membrane, and adjacent to this collagen fibres are shown. The plasma membrane, like the other membranes of the cell, has a trilaminar structure. Ribosomes are scattered free in the cell cytoplasm, and are also attached to the rough endoplasmic reticulum and the outer nuclear envelope. (*Drawn by Margot Mackay, Department of Art as Applied to Medicine, University of Toronto*).

of the cell is now seen to resemble a large industrial city with its factories, warehouses, streets, power-stations, etc. (Fig. 2.1 and Fig. 2.6).

CELLS

STRUCTURE OF CELLS

Each cell possesses an outer limiting membrane (the cell or plasma membrane) and within its protoplasm there is another limiting membrane which encloses the nuclear material. Most cells possess a single nucleus which is centrally placed; the basal nuclei of some columnar epithelial cells and the eccentric nuclei of plasma cells are obvious exceptions to this rule. Cells with more than one nucleus are called *giant*, or *multinucleate cells.* The osteoclast is an example of such a cell normally found in the body. Giant cells that are formed under pathological conditions are described later.

The cell membrane[1,2]

The cell membrane is an extremely important structure, since it forms the interface between the cell cytoplasm and the interstitial tissue fluids, or in the lower forms of life, the exterior. Its functions may be listed as movement, cell recognition, adhesion, control of cell growth, and transfer function.

Cell movement[3]

Examination of living cells reveals that the plasma membrane is not a rigid structure, but is in constant motion. This motility is particularly well developed in certain cells, and permits them to move bodily through the tissues. The white blood cells—polymorphonuclear leucocytes, lymphocytes, and monocytes—behave in this way. The undulating surface of the macrophage is particularly characteristic. Folds of the membrane have been observed to entrap a droplet of fluid by a process known as *pinocytosis.*

Apart from locomotion, the surface movement of monocytes and polymorphonuclear leucocytes produces another effect. By pushing out projections, or *pseudopodia,* around particles, they are able to surround and finally engulf them. This process of ingestion is called *phagocytosis.*

Cell recognition

The membranes of the cell, including the plasma membrane, are associated with the antigens by which the body is able to recognize its own cells and tolerate them. Cells from another individual are regarded as aliens, and are attacked by the immune response which they provoke.

Receptor function. Many agents act on cells at specific points, or *cell receptors.* Thus influenza viruses attach themselves to specific receptors on the red-cell envelope (p. 260). Likewise drugs and hormones act on their own receptors. The presence of these specific receptors on particular cells is indeed the explanation of how hormones act only on their target cells and not on other cells. The mechanism of action of many non-steroid hormones is of great interest. The attachment of the hormone to its receptor activates the enzyme adenylate cyclase, which is situated in the cell membrane. This enzymatic activation causes ATP, which is present in abundance on the inner side of the cell membrane, to be converted into adenosine 3′,5′-cyclic phosphate—a nucleotide known more widely as *cyclic AMP* or simply *cAMP.*[4] This important compound has many actions. Thus in a liver cell acted upon by adrenaline, the formation of cAMP leads to the activiation of a phosphorylase that converts glycogen to glucose: this is then released from the cell. In other instances cAMP acts on the nucleus and stimulates the expression of some particular genetic information (Fig. 2.2). In this way cAMP acts as a *second messenger* for the action of glucagon, thyrotrophic hormone, ACTH, and other hormones. Insulin also acts *via* a specific cell membrane receptor, but another nucleoside, guanosine 3′,5′-cyclic phosphate or cGMP, is its second messenger. With the steroid hormones the specific cell receptors are in the cytoplasm (see Ch. 39).

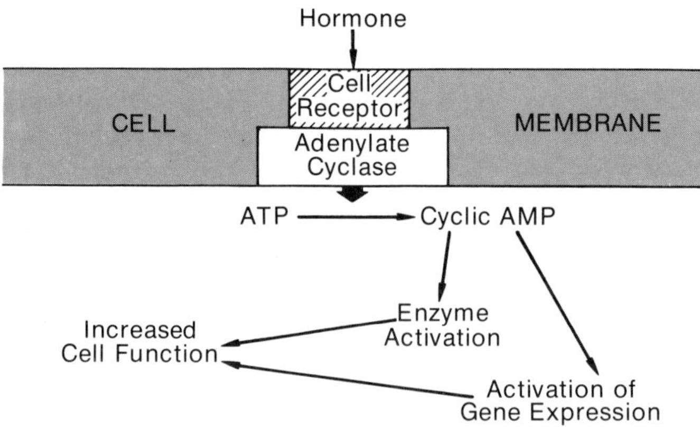

Fig. 2.2 The second-messenger concept. Many hormones act first by becoming attached to specific receptor sites on the membranes of target cells. Thus, adrenal cells have receptors that 'recognize' adrenocorticotrophin. The enzyme adenylate cyclase is activated in the cell membrane and passes into the cytoplasm where it catalyzes the formation of cyclic AMP, which acts as a second messenger. It may therefore be regarded as a type of chemical switch that turns on the cell to perform specific functions. (*Drawn by Anthony J. Walter.*)

Cell adhesiveness

The cell membrane is concerned with adhesiveness, which is a factor that induces cells of like constitution to stick together. If the cells of an embryo are separated from each other and are then allowed to come together again, they aggregate to form organs and tissues. This affinity which cells have for their own kind must be an important mechanism in the development and maintenance of the architecture of multicellular animals. But not all cells behave in this manner. The cells of the blood do not exhibit adhesiveness, nor to some extent do cancer cells, for they are able to infiltrate freely into the surrounding tissues.

Cell growth

The mitotic activity in epidermis is greatly increased in an area of skin adjacent to a wound. The increased production of cells continues until epidermal cells from one side of the wound meet those migrating from the other side. Contact of like cells with like then inhibits cell division; the phenomenon is called *contact inhibition* (p. 121). It appears to be a function of the cell membrane. Malignant transformation, infection of a cell by a virus, and treatment with proteolytic enzymes all appear to alter the cell membrane and release cells from this inhibition.

Transfer function

All substances which enter or leave the cell protoplasm must cross the cell membrane, and the properties of this membrane are responsible for the peculiar chemical composition of the cytoplasm.

Chemicals soluble in organic solvents enter cells much more readily than do those which are water soluble. The absorption of some substances is related to enzymatic activity occurring at or near the cell surface. How chemicals cross the membrane and the factors which regulate their passage can be understood only in relationship to the structure of the membrane itself, for as in other realms of pathology, structure and function are interdependent.

Membrane structure in relation to function.[3] Electron microscopy has shown an intact membrane some 7.5 nm* in width, which at high magnification of suitably prepared material can be resolved into two electron-dense laminae with an intervening clear space. This trilaminar structure, as first described by Robertson, is known as a *unit membrane,* and it appears to have no pores such as have been postulated to explain the observed permeability of the cell membrane.

Substances are transported across the cell membrane either by bulk transfer or by diffusion. *Bulk transfer* involves the processes of phagocytosis, pinocytosis (previously described), and micropinocytosis. In *micropinocytosis* small invaginations of the cell membrane (Fig. 2.1), the *caveolae intracellulares,* become nipped off to form vesicles; in this way small quantities of fluid or particulate matter may be imbibed by a process that resembles pinocytosis but on a small scale. Indeed, the processes of phagocytosis, pinocytosis, and micropinocytosis are commonly grouped together as *endocytosis,* in contrast to *exocytosis,* in which the contents of membrane-bound vacuoles (e.g. secretions) are liberated at the cell surface by fusion of the cell membrane with the vacuolar membrane. The contents of endocytotic vacuoles are still membrane bound and not in the cytoplasmic ground substance proper. The fusion of the vacuole with a primary lysosome containing lytic enzyes results in the formation of a *secondary lysosome, phagosome,* or *heterophagosome,* and by the digestion of its contents may result in their being released by diffusion into the substance of the cell.

The formation of micropinocytotic vesicles on one side of a cell and their discharge from another surface by exocytosis, is one postulated mechanism whereby substances may cross a cellular barrier, e.g. blood-vessel endothelium. The process is known as *cytopempsis.*

The *passive diffusion* of small ions across the cell membrane and the sodium pump are described on page 60.

In *active transport* there is the passage of chemicals across the cell membrane against a physico-chemical gradient, and the mechanism requires the expenditure of energy (Fig. 2.3). Amino-acid transport is a good example, and is of great importance in the intestine and the renal tubules. Thus there is a failure to reabsorb cystine, lysine, ornithine, and arginine in the kidney in the classical type of *cystinuria.*

It is generally accepted that the cell membrane is made up of a lipid–protein combination but the details of its construction are not known. Davson and Danielli introduced the concept of a bimolecular lipid leaflet with two layers of lipid molecules having their polar (hydrophilic) ends turned outwards, and being covered by protein. This concept of a lamellar structure fits well with the observed electron microscope appearance of an approximately 7.5 nm thick trilaminated membrane.

The current concept of the cell membrane is that it is composed of two layers of structurally asymmetrical lipid molecules with their hydrophilic polar heads turned outwards (Fig. 2.4). Globular proteins form an integral part of the

* 1 mm = 1000 μm. 1 μm = 1000 nm. The Ångström unit (Å) is a tenth of 1 nm, and is no longer used in measurement.

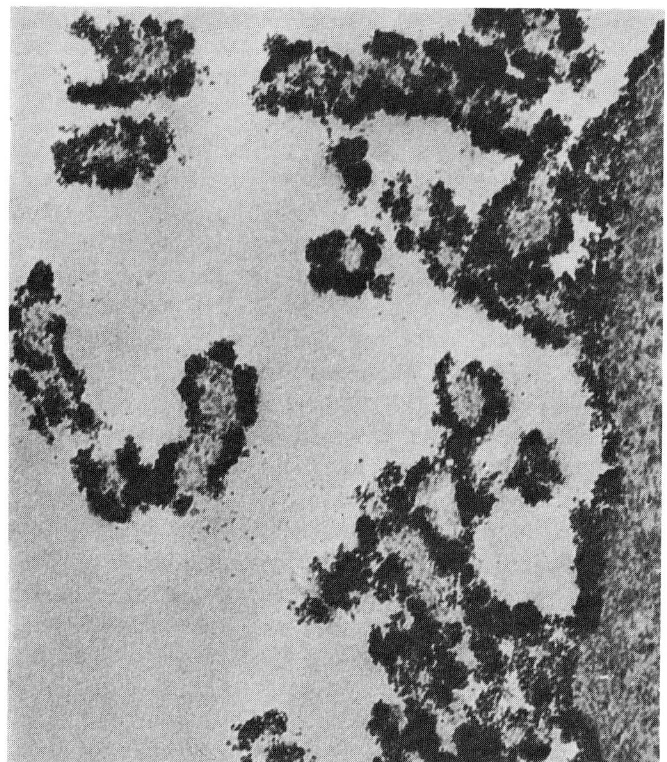

Fig. 2.3 Detail of the plasma membrane of a HeLa cell with much surface activity in the form of profuse filamentous microvilli. After staining for enzymes splitting adenosine triphosphate, dense reaction-product had been deposited with close precision at the cell membrane, indicating that the enzymes are localized there, presumably for the supply of energy requirements. ×55 000. (*Electron micrograph by courtesy of Professor M A Epstein and Dr S J Holt*).

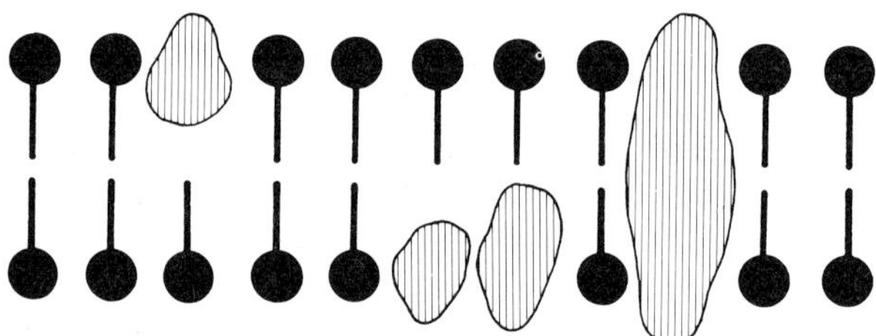

Fig. 2.4 Diagrammatic representation of the plasma membrane. The membrane is shown as a double layer of phospholipid molecules with their hydrophilic (water-loving) ends pointing outwards and their hydrophobic (water-hating) ends facing inward. Globular proteins are partially or completely embedded in the lipid. This concept of a fluid lipid bilayer with embedded protein was described by Singer and Nicolson (Science, 1972, *175*: 720). It is believed that the carbohydrate side-chains of the protein molecules form the glycocalyx, which is illustrated in Fig. 2.5. (*Drawn by Margot Mackay, Department of Art as Applied to Medicine, University of Toronto.*)

membrane and are bonded by hydrophobic interaction with lipid. These proteins are thus floating in a sea of lipid, thereby forming a fluid mosaic.[5] The proteins can move laterally, and while some are exposed only on one side of the membrane, others traverse it completely.

The proteins of the cell membrane are heterogeneous—some act as antigens, while others are specific receptors for hormones, lectins, viruses, etc. Others have transport or enzymatic functions (Fig. 2.3). The cell receptors are probably linked to the microtubules and microfilaments of the underlying cytoplasm. The microtubules connecting one receptor with the next could be regarded as forming a cytoskeleton anchoring respective receptors. The microfilaments, on the other hand, could act as contractile elements, so that the receptors could move within the cell membrane. That such movement can occur is well known, for the attachment of an antibody to its specific receptor in the cell membrane can result in movement of the complexes to form groups, or caps, which subsequently enter the cell by endocytosis. In this way receptors can be removed from the cell surface and the corresponding antigen can enter the cell.

In summary, the structure of the plasma membrane is very complex and contains lipid and protein. It can consume energy and change its shape in response to stimuli. Its protein molecules are heterogeneous, some being responsible for the receptor sites, others for antigenicity, enzyme activity, etc.

Relationship of cells to each other

Epithelial cells are generally closely applied to each other, but even then there is an electron-lucent area of 15 to 20 nm between their adjacent cell membranes. This is probably due to a covering of mucopolysaccharide. The free surface of epithelial cells is also covered by an additional coat, the *glycocalyx*, which on high-resolution electron microscopy can be seen to be filamentous (Fig. 2.5).

Cell junctions.[6] Adjacent cells exhibit specialized junctional areas that subserve two functions:

1. They enable cells to adhere to their neighbours, and can be adapted to form a seal to prevent substances passing between them. This is particularly important in the intestinal epithelium (Figs 2.5 and 2.6) and in the endothelial lining of blood vessels.
2. They form areas of close contact through which cells can *communicate* with each others. Most cells do not live in isolation; they co-operate, and co-ordinate their activities with those of their neighbours. How this is brought about is poorly understood, but the phenomena of peristalsis, contact inhibition (p. 121), and tissue induction may well be regulated by mechanisms that involve cell junctions. One might speculate that these structures are also important in the organized processes of embryogenesis, repair, and regeneration, as well in the disorganized proliferation of neoplasia.

THE CYTOPLASM

Chemical composition

The cytoplasm is that part of the protoplasm not included in the nucleus, and is composed largely of water. There is also about 8 per cent of protein. The contents

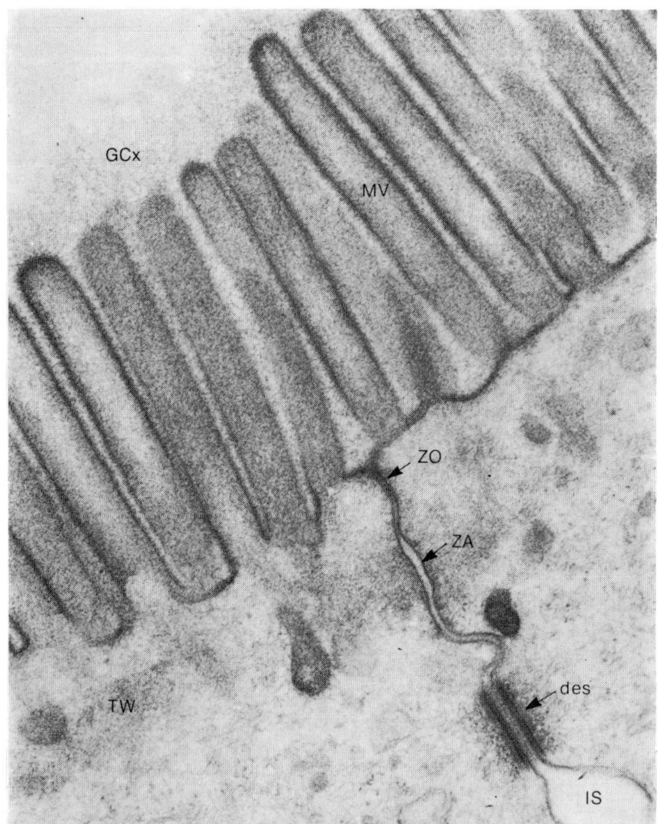

Fig. 2.5 Details of the luminal surface of an absorptive cell of the human small intestine. The apical cell membrane is thrown into regular microvilli (MV). There is a fuzzy covering, which is termed a *glycocalyx* (GCx). One junctional complex is shown. It consists of three parts: (1) The tight junction, or *zonula occludens* (ZO), which is an area where the plasma membranes of the two adjacent cells appear to fuse. 'Zonule' means an encircled band or girdle; the zone forms an effective seal between adjacent cells. It is an area where one cell can communicate with adjacent ones. (2) The *zonula adherens* (ZA), which is an area where the cell membranes are closely applied to each other but are not fused. Filaments of the terminal web are concentrated at this area. (3) The desmosomes or maculae adherentes (des), which are complex structures and are button-shaped. Numerous microfilaments converge on the desmosomes. Where junctional complexes are not present there is often a space between adjacent cells (IS = intercellular space). (× 112 000). (*Photograph by courtesy of Dr Y C Bedard.*)

differ from the extracellular fluid in several important respects. There is a high concentration of potassium, magnesium, and phosphate which contrasts with the sodium, chloride, and bicarbonate found in the extracellular fluids. The osmotic pressure within the cells (exerted principally by protein, potassium, magnesium, and phosphate) is equal to that of the extracellular fluid (exerted by sodium, chloride, and bicarbonate).

Water and chloride diffuse readily across the cell membrane, but potassium and sodium do so comparatively slowly, potassium diffusing about one hundred times faster than sodium. Others, phosphate and protein, do not diffuse at all. The net negative charge of protein and phosphate within the cell is balanced by potassium.

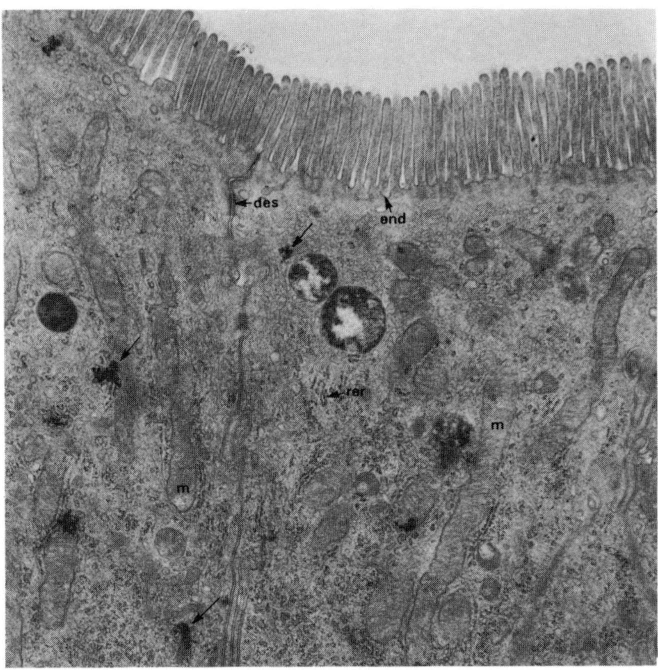

Fig. 2.6 Radioautograph of mouse jejunum. The mouse was killed one hour after the instillation of radioactive iron in its stomach. The silver grains (arrows) represent radioactive iron that has been absorbed into the cell. The course of this radioactive material can be followed by examining animals killed at different times after being fed with labelled iron. Note the regular arrangement of the microvilli, which form the brush border of light microscopy. This arrangement appears to be adapted for absorption. An endocytotic vesicle is clearly shown (end). A junctional complex with its desmosome (des) is seen near the free border of the two epithelial cells depicted in this illustration. Figure 2.5 shows details of this complex. Mitochondria (m) and rough endoplasmic reticulum (rer) can be identified but are shown more clearly in other figures. (*From Bedard, Y C: Ultrastructural and Radiographic Studies on Iron Absorption in the Mouse. University of Toronto Ph.D. Thesis, 1972.*)

In a passive diffusion system the result would be a greater concentration of ions within the cell than outside it, and the cell would swell. However, there is a mechanism in the cell membrane which actively excludes sodium. This is the '*sodium pump*', which requires ATP for its operation. The ultimate source of energy is mitochondrial cell respiration; it follows that damage to these organelles is characterized by cell swelling. In severe illnesses, such as heart failure and hepatic failure, there is an increase in the cell-membrane permeability. Potassium leaves the cells and sodium enters them. This has been called the '*sick-cell syndrome*', and is evident biochemically as hyponatraemia.

Formed structures

Electron microscopy has revealed that the structure of the cytoplasm is very complex indeed. It is subdivided into many compartments by membranes which closely resemble the plasma membrane in structure. The most extensive subdivision is effected by the *endoplasmic reticulum*, but the cytoplasm contains

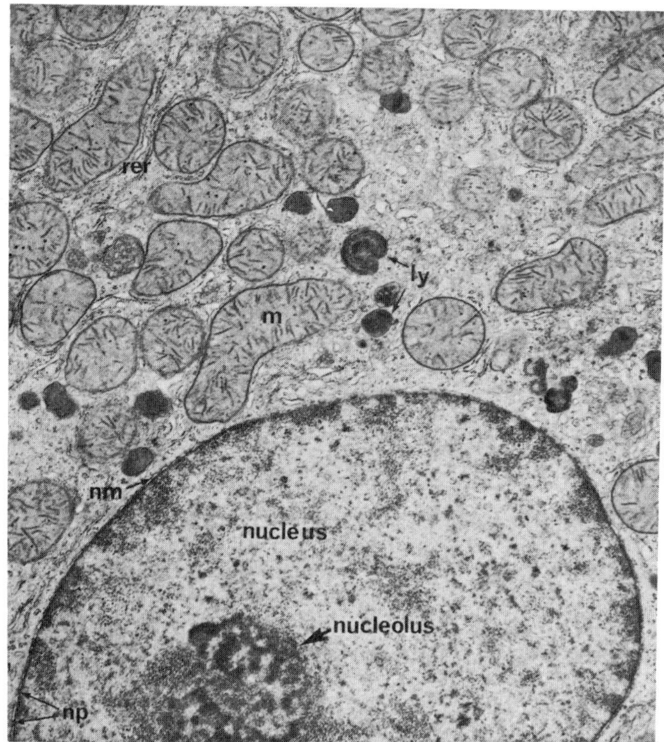

Fig. 2.7 Rat liver cell showing the main features of a cell as revealed by electron microscopy. The nucleus is bounded by the nuclear membrane (nm) in which there is a nuclear pore (np). A nucleolus is present in the part of the nucleus which is included. In the cytoplasm there are mitochondria (m) with cristae, lysosomes (ly), and rough endoplasmic reticulum (rer). The tissue was fixed in osmic acid and embedded in epon-araldite mixture. × 10 000. (*Photograph by courtesy of Dr Y le Beux*).

many membrane-bound structures, or *organelles*—mitochondria, lysosomes, etc. (Fig. 2.7).

Endoplasmic reticulum

Rough endoplasmic reticulum. This consists of a series of membranes which are formed into an inter-communicating series of tubes, vesicles, and cisterns (Figs. 2.1, 2.7, and 2.8). It is in these spaces that the secretion of some glands first appears. Situated on the outer surface of the endoplasmic reticulum there are granules, about 15 nm in diameter, which are rich in *ribonucleic acid (RNA)*. These are called *ribosomes,* and give the endoplasmic reticulum a rough appearance. Similar granules lie free in the cytoplasm and are not attached to the endoplasmic reticulum. The ribosomes play a very important part in cellular metabolism because it is in relation to them that *protein synthesis* occurs (p. 24). When the ribosomes are lying free the protein is for the cell's own internal requirements. Protein for export is synthetized in relation to the endoplasmic reticulum. Sometimes ribosomes are grouped together to form polysomes (Fig. 2.8).

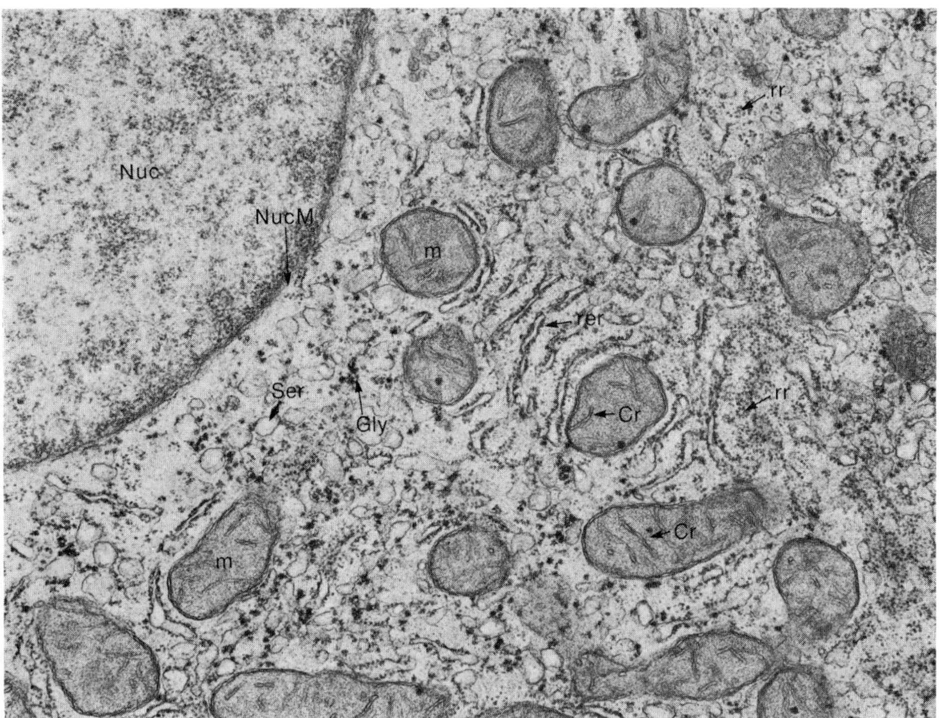

Fig. 2.8 Liver cell showing part of its nucleus (Nuc) and cytoplasmic organelles. Mitochondria (m) with their cristae (Cr) are shown along with rough endoplasmic reticulum (rer) to which are attached ribosomes (r). Smooth endoplasmic reticulum (Ser) is associated with glycogen granules (Gly). Some ribosomes appear free in the cytoplasm and are forming rosettes (rr). Note also the nuclear membrane (NucM) surrounding the nucleus (× 24 000). (*Photograph by courtesy of Dr Y C Bedard.*)

The endoplasmic reticulum and its associated ribosomal granules cannot be distinguished in the 'paraffin' sections used in routine pathology. The RNA content, however, is distinguishable by its red staining with pyronin and its blue staining (*basophilia*) with haematoxylin—the latter, being a basic substance, combines with acids, e.g. the nucleic acids. It follows that the cytoplasm of cells actively engaged in protein synthesis appears blue or mauve in haematoxylin and eosin stained (H. & E.) sections. Plasma cells are an excellent example of this, for immunoglobulin (a glycoprotein) is formed in the rough endoplasmic reticulum. Sometimes the accumulation of glycoprotein is so excessive that the cisterns of the rough endoplasmic reticulum become greatly dilated and contain masses that are visible in light microscopy. These take the appearance of refractile, eosinophilic, PAS-positive, spherical masses either solitary or else forming grape-like structures in the cell cytoplasm. They are called *Russell bodies,* and must not be mistaken for fungi in sections of chronic inflammatory tissue (Fig. 2.9). They are particularly frequent in chronic inflammation of the oral tissues.

Smooth endoplasmic reticulum. In some cells the endoplasmic reticulum also forms a complex lattice of tubules which has no attached ribosomes and therefore appears *smooth.* The smooth and rough elements of the endoplasmic

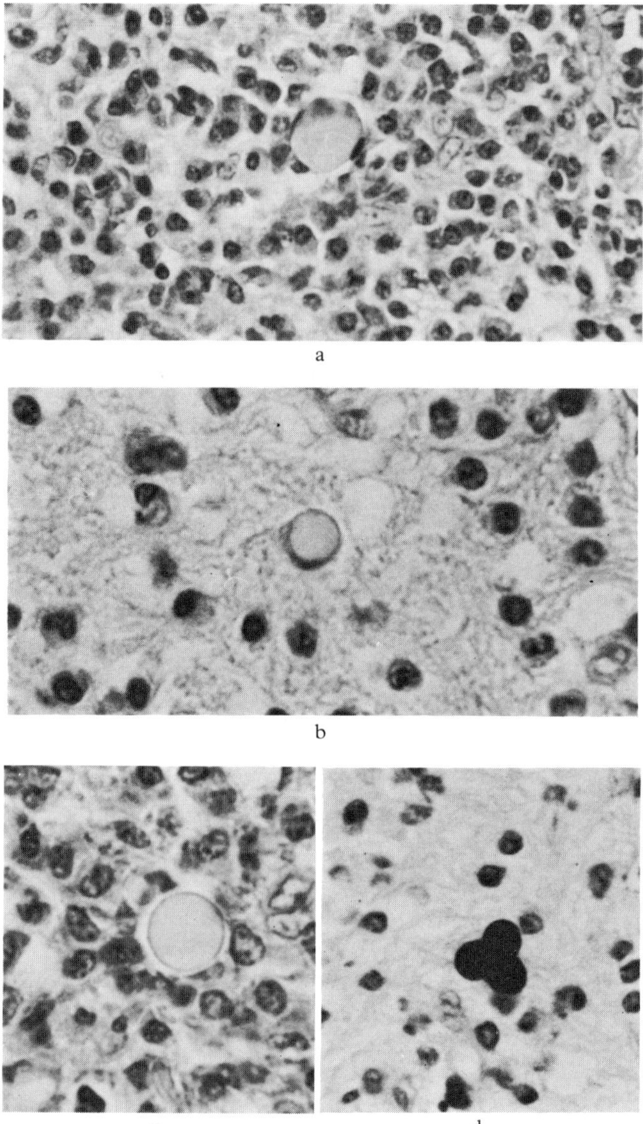

Fig. 2.9 Russell bodies. (*a*) Nasal biopsy from patient with rhinoscleroma showing many plasma cells and one Russell body. (*b*) Chronic inflammatory granulation tissue showing one Russell body in the cytoplasm of a plasma cell. The nucleus of the cell is compressed to one side. (*c*) Russell body lying free in tissue; same case as (*a*). (*d*) Russell bodies stained with Giemsa's stain. These structures are stained strongly with the PAS method and must not be mistaken for fungi. ×600.

reticulum are continuous with each other, with the outer lamina of the nuclear membrane, and perhaps also with the plasma membrane. The smooth endoplasmic reticulum has been related to the following functions:

Drug metabolism. Following the administration of barbiturates and other toxins there is an increase in the smooth endoplasmic reticulum of the liver cells. This appears to be an adaptive response to ensure detoxification

Steroid and cholesterol metabolism

Carbohydrate metabolism. In the liver glycogen synthesis occurs in close relationship to smooth endoplasmic reticulum (Fig. 2.8)

Muscle contraction. In striated muscle specialized smooth endoplasmic reticulum is important in the release and recapture of calcium ions during the contraction and relaxation of fibres.

Mitochondria

These rod-shaped bodies have a smooth outer limiting membrane and an inner, electron-dense membrane which is folded into incomplete septa, or *cristae*, that subdivide the mitochondria into compartments (Fig. 2.8 and Fig. 2.10).

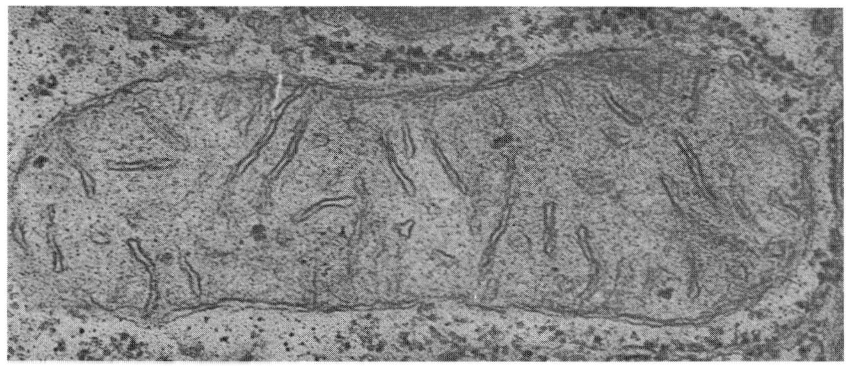

Fig. 2.10 Liver cell mitochondrion. The organelle is surrounded by an outer membrane with a second, inner membrane close within it; the inner membrane is folded into shelf-like cristae which protrude into the interior. × 52 000. (*Photograph by courtesy of Professor M A Epstein.*)

This complex structure of the mitochondria is a reflection of their function. They contain all the enzymes of the Krebs cycle and of the terminal electron transport system (cytochrome system). The *Krebs cycle* is a system whereby products of carbohydrate, fat, and protein metabolism are oxidized to produce energy (Fig. 2.11). The latter is stored in the form of the high energy bonds of adenosine triphosphate (ATP), and is utilized whenever the cell performs any kind of work. The mitochondria are the power-stations of the cell, and are among the first structures to be affected when adverse conditions prevail. Mitochondria are capable of enlargement, and replicate by transverse division. Mitochondrial DNA may play a role in this process (see p. 29).

Golgi complex

The *Golgi complex,* or *apparatus,* consists of a series of flattened sacs and small vesicles (often arranged in curved stacks), much smaller than those of the endoplasmic reticulum. They are usually adjacent to the *centrosome,* a clear area near the centre of the cell and which contains one or more *centrioles.* The Golgi complex is best developed in glandular cells, and is usually situated close to the nucleus on the side nearest the lumen.

The main function of the Golgi complex is the modification and packaging of material synthetized in the rough endoplasmic reticulum. The material in the

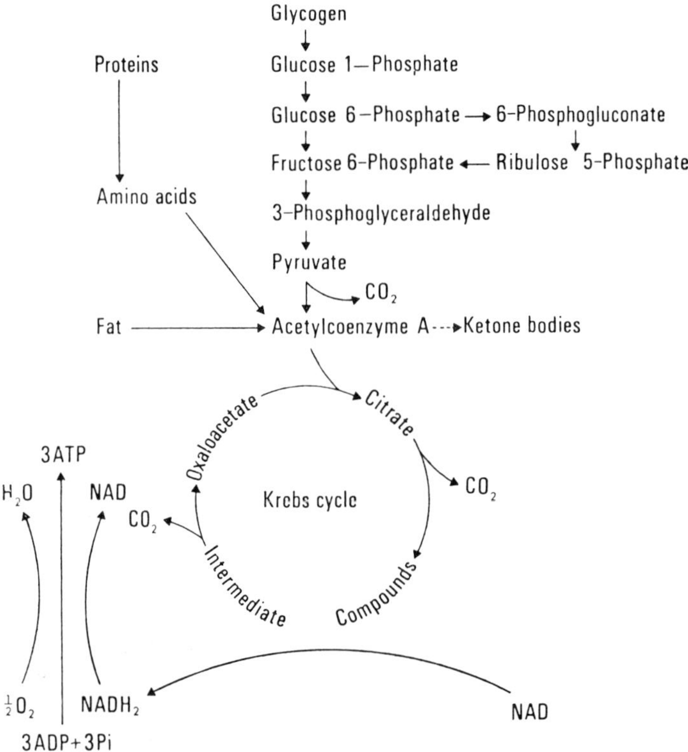

Fig. 2.11 Outline of the metabolic pathways concerned in energy production. The whole process in the oxidation of glycogen to CO_2 and water can be considered as occurring in two phases. The first, or anaerobic, phase results in the formation of pyruvate, and is known as glycolysis. The second, or aerobic, phase is the Krebs cycle. Products of carbohydrate, fat, and protein metabolism are fed into the Krebs cycle *via* acetylcoenzyme A. Several enzymic reactions of the Krebs cycle involve the reduction of NAD to $NADH_2$. Reoxidation of $NADH_2$ by the cytochrome system is coupled with phosphorylation of ADP to ATP, viz.

$$NADH_2 + \tfrac{1}{2}O_2 + 3ADP + 3Pi \rightarrow NAD + H_2O + 3ATP.$$

The hexose monophosphate shunt, or pentose-phosphate pathway, leads to the formation of ribulose phosphate and is an alternative pathway in certain cells. It is an aerobic process, and in addition to its products re-entering the glycolytic sequence, sugars of 4–7 carbon atoms are formed and utilised in various synthetic process.
Key: NAD—Nicotinamide adenine dinucleotide. $NADH_2$—Dihydronicotinamide adenine dinucleotide. Pi—Inorganic phosphate. ADP—Adenosine diphosphate. ATP—Adenosine triphosphate.

rough endoplasmic reticulum is pinched off in smooth covered vacuoles (*transport vesicles*) which pass to the forming face of the Golgi complex (this is generally the convex surface). The membrane of the vesicle fuses with that of the Golgi complex, and its contents pass through the stacks, being finally released from the maturing face of the Golgi complex as membrane-bound vacuoles. During its passage through the stacks the material may be condensed, sulphated (e.g. the glycoproteins of ground substance), or combined with carbohydrate. The vacuoles leaving the maturing face of the Golgi complex can be of many varieties, according to the cell type. Some are secretary vacuoles, others contain mucopolysaccharide

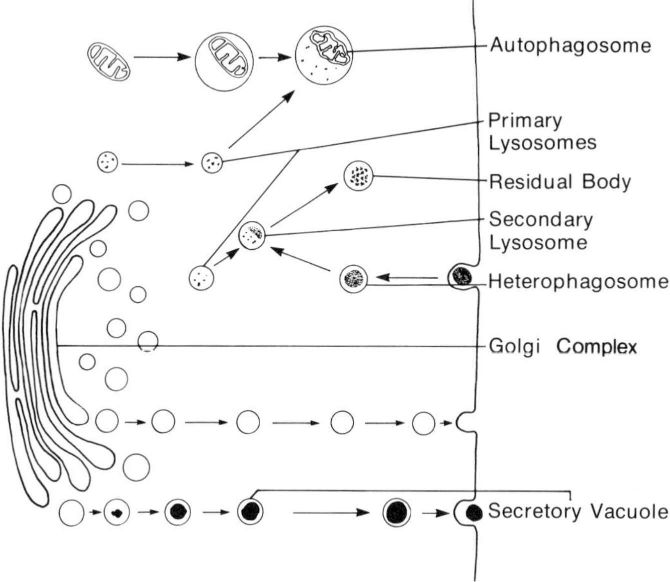

Fig. 2.12 The Golgi complex (Golgi apparatus) and its possible functions. This diagram depicts the Golgi complex as a series of flattened sacs from which numerous vacuoles arise. Some vacuoles contain secretory material that has been synthetized in the endoplasmic reticulum. Some vacuoles appear to be empty and travel to the cell surface where their membranes fuse with the cell membrane. Other vacuoles contain lytic enzymes and become primary lysosomes. These fuse with autophagosomes or heterophagosomes to form secondary lysosomes. Undigested material remains in residual bodies. (*Drawn by Margot Mackay, Department of Art as Applied to Medicine, University of Toronto.*)

or tropocollagen, others are primary lysosomes, while others pass to the cell surface and by fusing with the cell membrane, contribute material to it (Fig. 2.12).

Lysosomes

Lysosomes are rounded, membrane-bound organelles that contain lytic* enzymes active at a low pH, i.e. acid phosphatase, deoxyribonuclease, and cathepsins. The lysosomal enzymes are formed in the rough endoplasmic reticulum, and pass into the Golgi complex where they are packaged. They are released from the maturing face of the Golgi complex as *primary lysosomes.* Membrane-bound material in the form of *heterophagosomes* formed as a result of endocytosis, or as *autophagosomes* (or *cytolysomes*) containing damaged or worn-out cell components, fuse with the primary lysosomes to form *secondary lysosomes.* These bodies present a variety of appearances. They contain foreign ingested material or fragments of recognizable cell components—mitochondria, endoplasmic reticulum, etc. (Fig. 2.13). Sometimes they contain lipid which assumes the form of a concentric lamination of myelin figures (Fig. 2.14). Eventually the lysosomes contain only indigestible material, and they remain as *residual bodies* containing lipofuscin. These are the wear-and-tear pigments of light microscopy.

* Lyse—to render soluble.

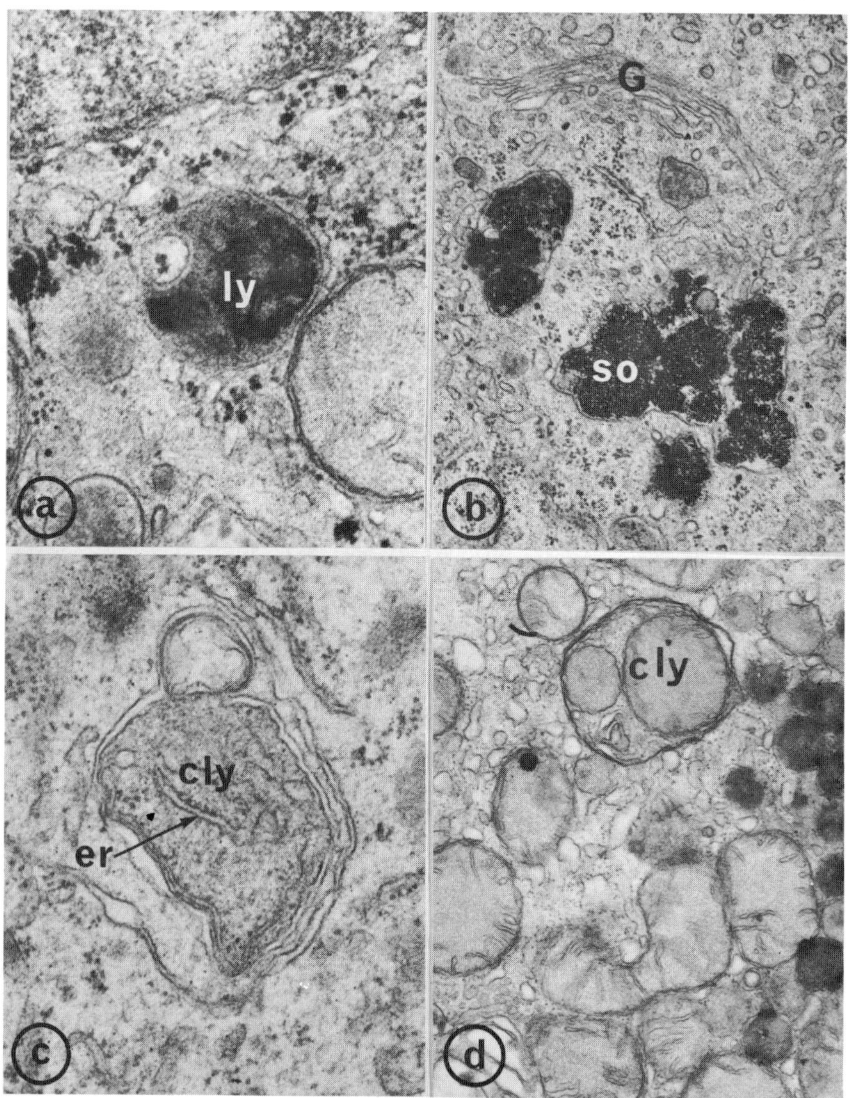

Fig. 2.13 Various types of lysosome. (*a*) A lysosome (ly) in a normal parenchymal liver cell. Lead hydroxide. × 43 750. (*b*) Membrane-bound structures containing ferritin granules. These are sometimes called siderosomes (so). G—Golgi complex. Lead hydroxide. × 22 400. (*c*) A cytolysome (cly) in a normal rat hepatocyte containing small fragments of the rough-surfaced endoplasmic reticulum (er). Lead hydroxide. × 46 200. (*d*) A cytolysome (cly) containing structures which are probably degraded mitochondria. Lead hydroxide. × 17 900. (*Photographs by courtesy of Dr Katsumi Miyai.*)

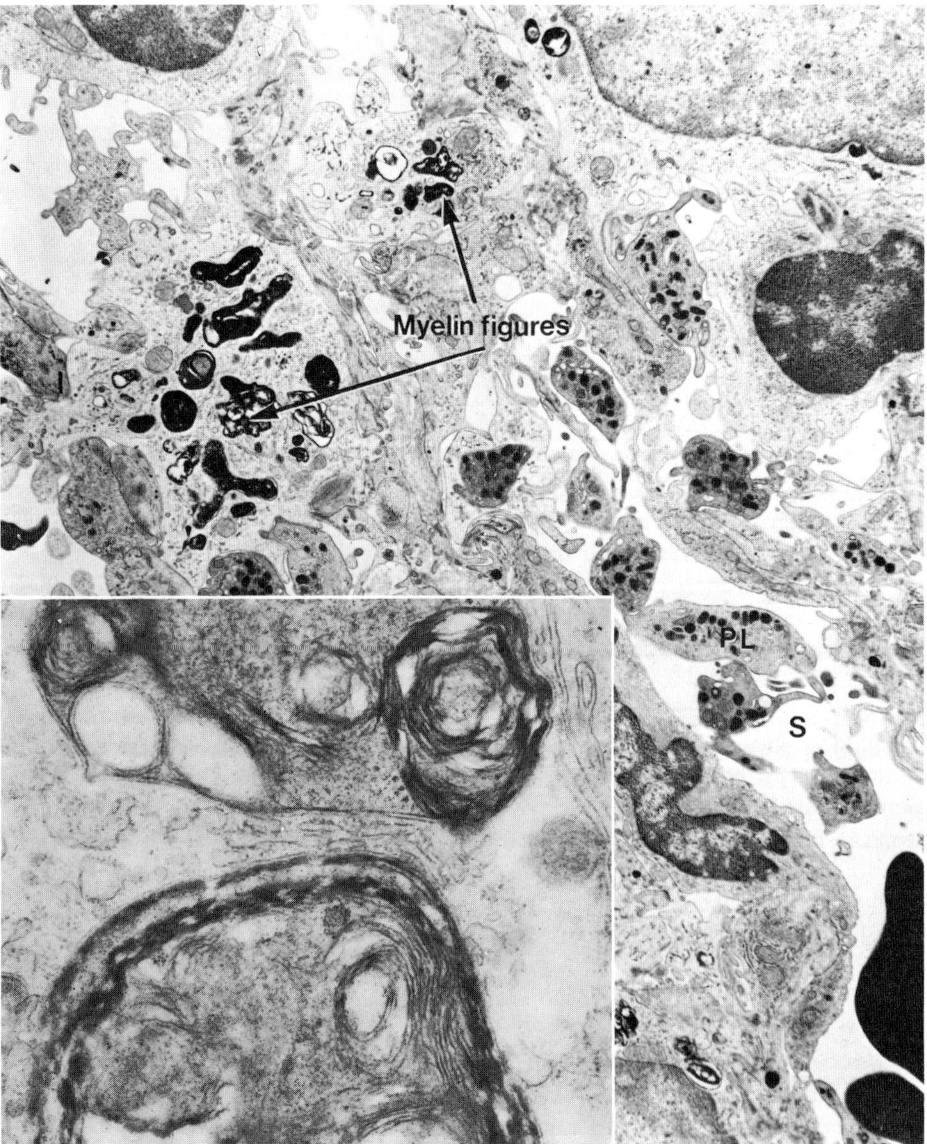

Fig. 2.14 Myelin figures in spleen. Many platelets (PL) are seen lying free in a splenic sinusoid (S). One platelet has been engulfed by a phagocytic cell. Note the numerous myelin figures in some reticulo-endothelial cells. The insert shows the typical laminated appearance as seen under higher magnification. The spleen was from a patient with thrombotic thrombocytopenic purpura. (*Photographs by courtesy of Dr G T Simon.*)

The stability of the lysosomal membrane can be increased by the action of glucocorticoids; this may be a factor in their protective action against the damaging effects produced by ultraviolet light, bacterial endotoxin, etc.

Lysosomal digestion plays a part in the removal of unwanted cells during embryonic development. Thus, after cell death the lysosomal enzymes are probably responsible for the cell's digestion and ultimate dissolution. Lysosomal enzymes also play a part as mediators of acute inflammation (p. 86), and their release from polymorphs can cause local tissue damage. This is particularly prominent in immune-complex reactions (p. 185).

Microbodies

Microbodies are membrane-bound, rounded organelles characterized by their content of oxidases, such as urate oxidase and catalase, an enzyme which acts on hydrogen peroxide and liberates oxygen. This enzyme is of some importance in the oral cavity (p. 94).

Microtubules and Microfilaments

High-resolution electron microscopy has revealed that most cells contain fibrillar material which is composed of either thin filaments or tubules. Their composition, structure, and function probably vary from one cell type to another and only a brief description will be given here.

Microtubules. These are tubular structures about 25 nm in diameter. Their centres are composed of material of low electron density, and they therefore appear as hollow tubes. Microtubules are composed of protein subunits called tubulin, and can undergo rapid break-down and re-assembly. This re-assembly is inhibited by the alkaloid colchicine. In some cells, e.g. diatoms, the microtubules appear to provide rigidity, acting as a cytoskeleton, and they may be responsible for the relatively fixed shape of some cells, e.g. blood platelets and podocytes. Another function of the microtubules is that of assisting the transport of material within the cell; they serve to direct secretory granules, e.g. those containing insulin, to the cell surface prior to exocytosis. Their function in relationship to cell receptors has already been described (p. 11). The filaments of the spindle at mitosis are composed of microtubules, therefore colchicine inhibits mitosis at the metaphase.

Microfilaments. Most cells also contain long filamentous structures about 6 to 8 nm in diameter. Bundles of these are clearly seen in squamous epithelial cells, and are known as tonofibrils. Actin, myosin, and tropomyosin have been identified in microfilaments, and it is believed that these structures are contractile, performing important functions in cell movement, as well as in the movement of structures, such as granules, within the cell itself.

Centriole

The centriole is a cylindrical body about 15 nm long, which is concerned with the orientation of the spindle (p. 31). Each cell has two centrioles (at least) which are situated in the centrosome and which divide before the onset of mitosis. (Fig. 2.1).

Other cytoplasmic components include glycogen granules, fat globules, etc. Some cells contain specialized structures, e.g. granules in eosinophils. Furthermore, as the resolution of the electron microscope is being increased, so further structures are being described. In many instances their function is not known, but there is little doubt that in due course the ultrastructure of cells will turn out to be very complex—as complex indeed as life itself.

THE NUCLEUS

Situated within the cell and enclosed by a membrane is the *nucleus,* an important structure because it contains, in chemical form, the coded information which is handed down from one cell to its progeny and from one generation to the next. The chemical which performs this vital function is a nucleoprotein consisting of a histone combined with *deoxyribonucleic acid* (DNA). The acidic components of the nuclear material, since they combine with basic dyes like haematoxylin, are responsible for the basophilia with H. & E. The basophilic material in the nucleus is often called *chromatin,* a name coined before the discovery of DNA.

Chemical structure of DNA

DNA is a polymer of high molecular weight (6 to 10 million daltons*) composed of a long chain of monounits, or nucleotides (Base–Deoxyribose sugar–Phosphate). The deoxyribose molecules are linked together by a phosphate, and a base is attached to each sugar (Fig. 2.15). The common bases are either purines (adenine and guanine) or pyrimidines (thymine and cytosine). As a result of x-ray diffraction studies, Watson and Crick proposed a structure which fits remarkably well with our concept of DNA as a self-reduplicating genetic material. They postulated that the molecule is composed of two polynucleotide chains spiralled around a common axis. The bases are directed towards the axis, and the two chains are linked by hydrogen bonds between a purine and a pyrimidine. They showed that only adenine could pair with thymine, and guanine with cytosine.

Role of the nucleic acids as genetic material[7]

It is believed that the DNA in the nucleus contains genetic information which is passed *via* RNA into the cytoplasm, where it is utilized in the manufacture of proteins (often enzymes) of exact composition. The word *gene* is used to describe the hypothetical unit of heredity for any single characteristic. Genes are present in the DNA, and are an expression of its contained genetic information.

The order of the bases in DNA constitutes the genetic code, a sequence of three bases corresponding to a single amino acid. A type of RNA (*messenger RNA,* or *mRNA*) is made in the nucleus in the presence of DNA-dependent RNA polymerase. The process is called *transcription,* and the mRNA is modelled on one of the polynucleotide chains of DNA which acts as a template. The base sequence of the RNA is thus complementary to that of DNA, i.e. cytosine corresponds with guanine, etc. This mRNA passes into the cytoplasm and becomes associated with

* A dalton is the weight of one hydrogen atom.

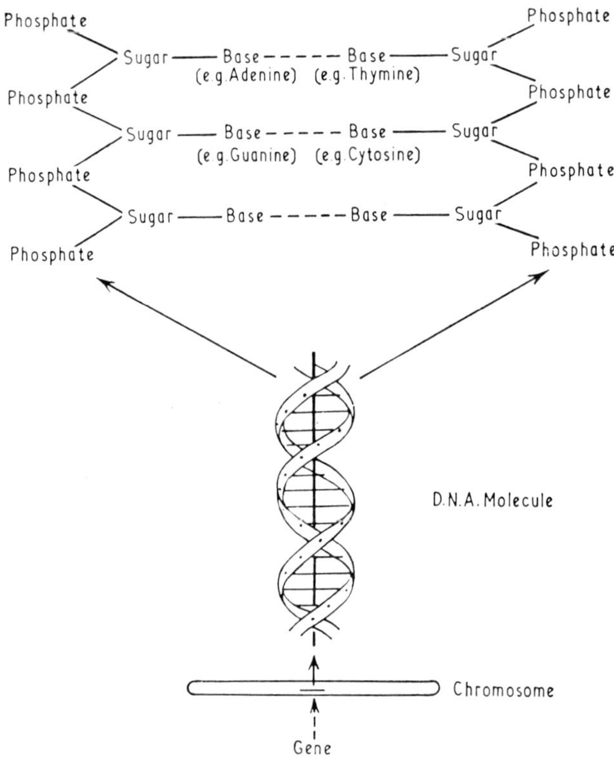

Fig. 2.15 Suggested chemical structure of DNA. The two polynucleotide chains are united by their bases, the order of which constitutes the genetic code. (*After Watson J D, Crick F H C 1953 Nature (Lond) 171:737.*)

a group of ribosomes (*a polysome*). Here protein synthesis occurs. Each triplet, or *codon,* of the RNA base order is responsible for one amino acid.* As the ribosomes 'read along' the RNA molecule, successive amino acids are added to an ever increasing polypeptide chain. In this way a protein of exact composition is built up; secondary and tertiary structure are presumably a consequence of this. The actual addition of each amino acid is effected by another type of RNA (*transfer RNA,* or *tRNA*), a separate form of which exists for each of the amino acids. The process is complex and is described as *translation,* for the code of the DNA finally appears legible in the form of a polypeptide chain (Fig. 2.16).

Thus the genetic code of DNA consists of codons which determine the insertion of particular amino acids in the peptide chain. The sequence of the codons is colinear with the sequence of amino acids. The codons responsible for a whole peptide chain form a group called a *cistron.* It is believed that a number of cistrons are grouped together to form a larger unit, the *operon,*[8] which is described below. The actual code has been investigated by various means. Synthetic polyribonucleotides have been prepared and can act as mRNA in cell-free preparations

* With 4 bases, 64 triplets are possible, but as only about 20 amino acids have to be coded, some duplication occurs. The code is therefore said to be degenerate. Thus UUU and UUC both correspond to phenylalanine. The code is written in terms of the order of bases in the mRNA. It is thought that the code is universal, i.e. the same for all organisms.

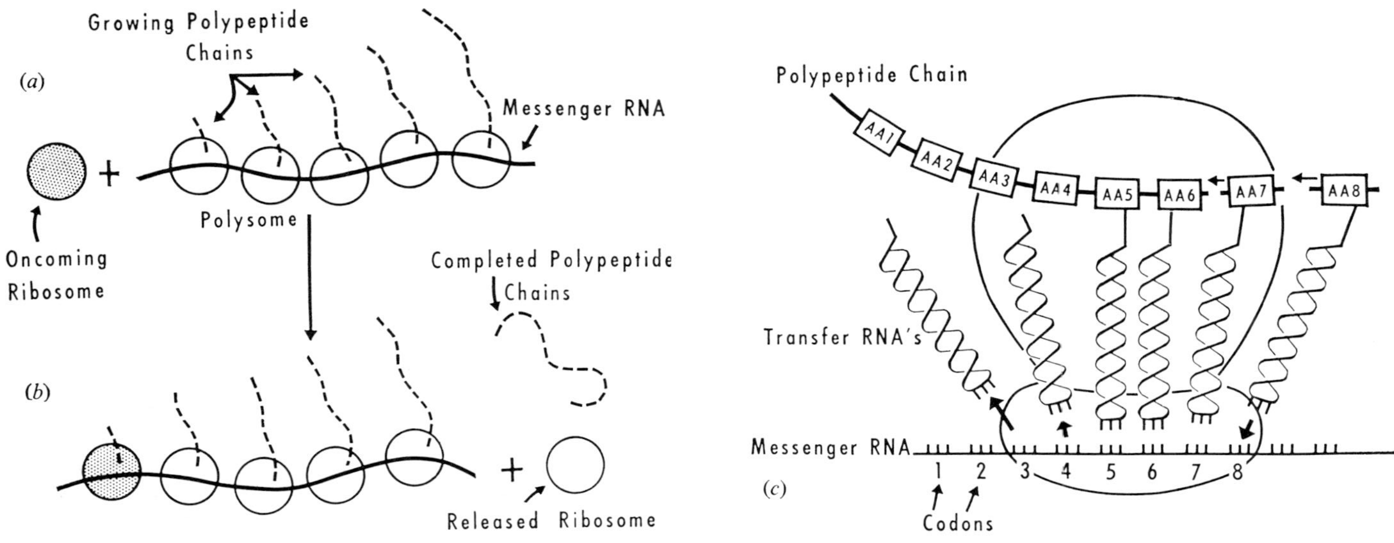

Fig. 2.16 Schematic model of protein synthesis. In (*a*) and (*b*) a long single-stranded molecule of messenger RNA (mRNA) is seen associated with a group of ribosomes to form a polysome. As each ribosome moves along the mRNA, an ever-growing polypeptide chain is produced. In (*c*) a single ribosome is depicted as a combination of two particles of unequal size. The sequence of bases of the mRNA forms triplets, or codons, which for the sake of clarity are drawn as groups of three upright lines. Each molecule of transfer RNA (tRNA) is composed of a long thread bent on itself to form a helical structure. At one end of the molecule there is a particular amino acid (AA1, AA2, etc.), and at the other end, where it is bent on itself, there are three unpaired bases which form an anticodon. Each codon of the mRNA is 'recognized' by a corresponding anticodon of a tRNA. In this way specific amino acids are added to the polypeptide chain in a specific linear sequence determined by the mRNA which is itself modelled on the nuclear DNA. (*Drawn by the Department of Art as applied to Medicine, University of Toronto, after Warner J R, Soeiro J 1967 New England Journal of Medicine 276:613 and Nirenberg MW 1963 in The living cell. Freeman, San Francisco.*)

containing ribosomes, suitable substrates, and a source of energy. Thus a polynucleotide containing uridine only (poly U) leads to the formation of phenylalanine. Hence the code for this amino acid is UUU.

Control of gene action

It is evident that each nucleated cell of the body contains the necessary information for the manufacture of every protein of which the body is composed. That they do not do so all the time is evidence that there is some very adequate control mechanism. Thus erythroid cells manufacture haemoglobin, plasma cells immunoglobulin, etc. Nevertheless, it is not surprising that under abnormal circumstances cells produce substances which are alien to their accustomed products. This occurs in metaplasia, and an excellent example is the secretion by

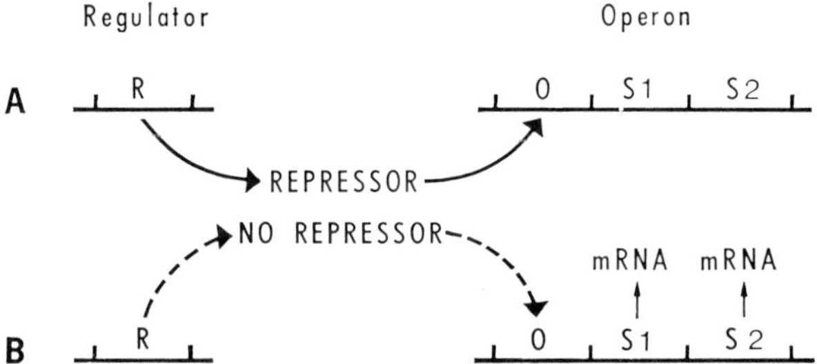

Fig. 2.17 The regulator-operator hypothesis.
A. The regulator gene (R) forms a repressor substance which acts through the cytoplasm to repress the operator gene (O). When O is thus inhibited, the structural genes (S1 and S2) in its operon cannot form mRNA.
B. If the regulator gene cannot form repressor substance, or if the repressor does not reach the operator gene, the operator is *derepressed* and S1 and S2 are then able to produce mRNA. (*Diagram redrawn from Fig. 3.10 in Thompson J S, Thompson M W 1966 Genetics in medicine, Saunders, Philadelphia. The hypothesis is that of Jacob F, Monod J 1961 Journal of Molecular Biology 3:318.*)

certain cancer cells of hormones which normally are produced only in the very specialized cells of the endocrine glands (p. 333).

The control of gene action is poorly understood, but is being actively investigated at the present time. Some genes lead to the production of proteins which are enzymes, or which are used in the metabolism of the cell. These are termed *structural genes.* In certain bacteria it has been found that a group of genes are closely linked, and either function together or are completely repressed, i.e. no mRNA is produced. The mechanism of control is also under genetic influence, and Fig. 2.17 illustrates a scheme of this based on that proposed by Jacob and Monod. Each group of genes, or *operon,* is controlled by a closely associated gene called the *operator gene.* This itself is regulated by another gene, the *regulator gene,* which through its own mRNA leads to the production in the cytoplasm of a protein (*repressor substance*) which suppresses the operator gene. The regulator gene may itself be inhibited, and in that event the operator is derepressed and the genes of the operon are allowed to act; mRNA is produced and protein synthesis proceeds (Fig. 2.17). The complexity of the subject is apparent when it is appreciated that in every cell, every gene is under continuous control and so regulated that the requirements of the body are met. This applies not only during adult life but also during the complex process of development. The ovum provides an excellent example of how protein synthesis can be inhibited, only to be switched on suddenly by the event of fertilization.

It should be noted that each resting somatic cell nucleus contains a constant amount of nucleic acid. This is termed the 2n amount (see below). Certain exceptions are found. In normal liver with increasing age some cells are found with nuclei containing abnormal, multiple amounts of DNA, i.e. 4n, 8n, or 16n amounts. These are called *polyploid* nuclei, and are formed as the result of cells replicating their genetic material but having been blocked in the G_2 phase of the cell cycle. Polyploidy is also a feature of hypertrophied muscle, and is encountered in megaloblasts (Ch. 30). Cells may contain an amount of DNA that is not an exact multiple of the normal amount, a condition called *aneuploidy,* which is a feature of malignant cells.

Chromosomes

The DNA molecules are not lying free in the nuclear sap, but are contained in long threads called *chromosomes.* Each resting somatic cell contains a definite number of chromosomes, the *diploid,* or 2n, number. This corresponds to a definite amount of DNA, the 2n amount. In humans the diploid number is 46, and of these 23 are derived from each parent. Two chromosomes are related specifically to sex, and these are called the *sex chromosomes.* One is considerably larger than the other and is called an X chromosome, while the smaller one is called a Y chromosome. Females have two X chromosomes whereas males have an X and a Y chromosome. The remaining 22 pairs are identical in appearance in both sexes and are called *autosomes.*

During the period between cell division (interphase) the chromosomes are present in the nucleus as long drawn-out threads. These are not visible as such using the light microscope, but in some areas along the thread there is sufficient coiling for the condensation of material to render these areas recognizable as chromatin dots of the nucleus. Such chromatin (*heterochromatin*) appears as areas of deep staining, and is thought to represent regions of the chromosomes which are condensed and relatively inert metabolically. The remainder of the nucleus is lightly stained, and the dispersed chromatin material (*euchromatin*) is in an active form. It follows that the actual morphology of the nucleus varies considerably from one cell to another, and that an assessment of function can be made from nuclear structure. In active cells, e.g. neurons, the nucleus is vesicular and very little heterochromatin is present. Heterochromatin is more abundant in epithelial cells and gives the nucleus a stippled appearance. In inactive cells, e.g. small lymphocytes, late normoblasts, and spermatozoa, the heterochromatin occupies most of the nucleus which therefore appears deeply basophilic. In the mature plasma cells the heterochromatin is disposed close to the nuclear membrane in clumps to produce the cartwheel, or clock-faced, appearance so typical of this cell (Fig. 10.4).

Some cells which are very large, e.g. the osteoclasts of the bone marrow, contain many nuclei and are called *multinucleate giant cells.* Some of the RNA component of the nucleus may appear as a separate structure called the *nucleolus*. This is particularly prominent in cells which are actively metabolizing—e.g. cancer cells.

The Barr body. A feature which has assumed great importance is a discrete mass of chromatin, first noted by Murray Barr in the nerve cells of the cat. He noted that this was present in the cells of the female but not in those of the male. It is therefore called the *sex chromatin*, or *Barr body*. It is easily demonstrated in the human by examining suitably stained cells scraped from the buccal mucosa, and appears as a demilune on the nuclear membrane (Fig. 2.18). The Barr body is

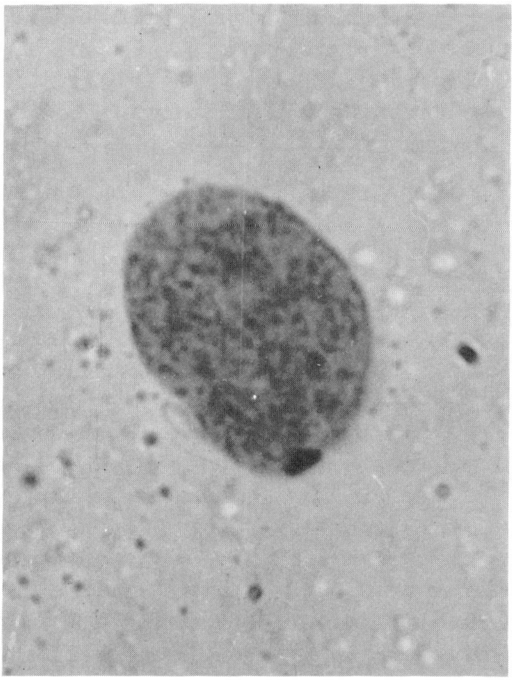

Fig. 2.18 The Barr body. Nucleus of a cell from buccal mucosal smear of a female, showing the sex chromatin mass on the nuclear membrane. Stained by acetic orecin. (*Photograph by courtesy of Dr Nigel H Kemp.*)

derived from a single X chromosome, and the number of Barr bodies seen in a cell is one less than the number of X chromosomes present. One X chromosome in each nucleus behaves like the autosomes. It becomes uncoiled between each cell division and therefore is not seen. If another X chromosome is present it remains inactive and appears as a Barr body. It follows that the normal male, having only one X chromosome, is chromatin negative while the normal female is chromatin positive, i.e. has sex chromatin.

The Y body. The Y chromosome selectively takes up the dye quinacrine hydrochloride ('atebrin'), which has the property of fluorescing strongly under ultraviolet light. If a smear of buccal mucosal scraping or peripheral blood is stained with the dye, a bright fluorescent dot in the nucleus indicates the presence of a Y chromosome (Fig. 2.19).

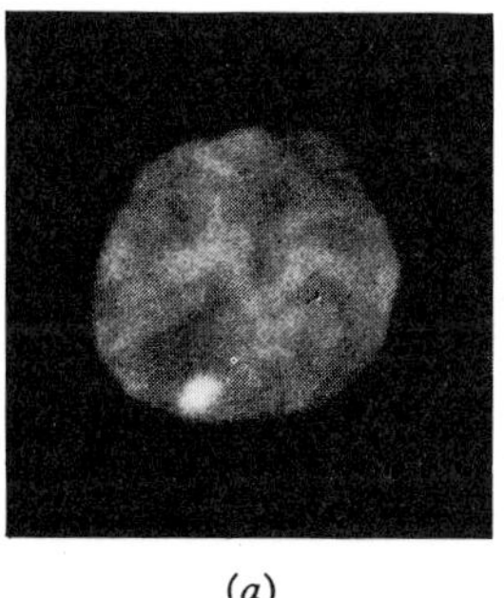

(*a*)

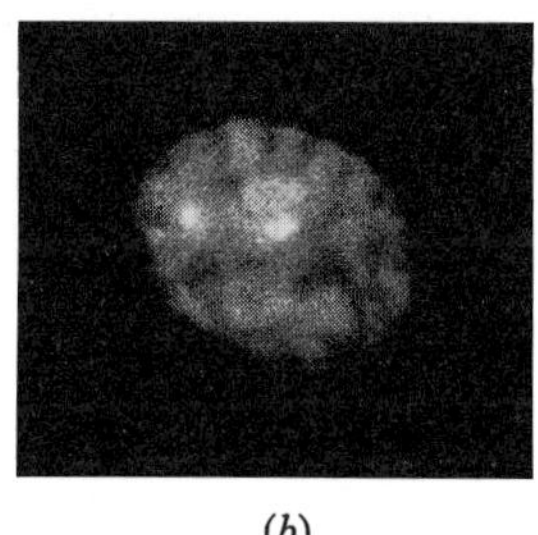

(*b*)

Fig. 2.19 The fluorescent Y chromosome. Blood smears were aid-dried, fixed in methanol, and after staining in 0.5 per cent quinacrine dihydrochloride (atebrin) and washing, were examined in ultraviolet light. The Y chromsome shows a characteristic point of fluorescence in the nuclei of the two cells shown. In (*a*) the blood was taken from a normal male, whilst in (*b*) the blood was from an individual with the karyotype 47/XYY. (*Photographs by courtesy of Dr Peter K Lewin. From Lewin P K, Conen PE 1971 Nature 233:334.*)

Cytoplasmic DNA[9, 10]

The presence of DNA in the cytoplasm is now well established. Some is present in the mitochondria, and appears to direct protein synthesis *via* specific mRNA. Many other forms of cytoplasmic DNA are known, and have been most extensively studied in bacteria. Some can act as infectious agents (e.g. bacteriophage), or may replicate in unison with cell division and therefore act as cytoplasmic genetic material. These agents are called *episomes,* or *plasmids,* and their presence can greatly alter the function of a cell. Thus the production of toxin by the diphtheria bacillus is related to the presence of one of these agents, as is also the development of antibiotic resistance. Their role in mammalian cells is at present speculative, but it may well be related to the inheritance of certain diseases, viral infections (for instance slow viruses), and the development of cancer.

Individual chromosome identification. New staining techniques involving Giemsa stain and also quinacrine mustard in conjunction with ultraviolet microscopy have revealed that the chromosomes have a characteristic banded appearance. Many individual chromosomes can now be identified and abnormalities in them detected.

THE CELL CYCLE

The cell cycle is reckoned to begin at the completion of one cell division (mitosis) and to end at the completion of the next division. The time taken for one cell cycle is the *generation time.*

Immediately following cell division the cell enters the first resting, or G_1 phase. The length of this phase is the most variable component of the cell cycle. Sometimes a cell may remain in this state for a long period; it is then described as having entered the G_0 phase. It may later return to the cell cycle, or else become so fully differentiated as to become incapable of further mitosis. There are some cells, notably the neuron, which cannot undergo mitosis.

Thc G_1 phase is followed by a synthesis, or S, phase, during which the DNA of the nucleus replicates. There then follows a short gap, the G_2 phase, before the beginning of mitosis.

Mitosis

The mechanism whereby somatic cells divide is a complicated process in which the nuclear material is reduplicated, and then carefully divided into two equal parts, which reform the nuclei of the two daughter cells (Fig. 2.20).

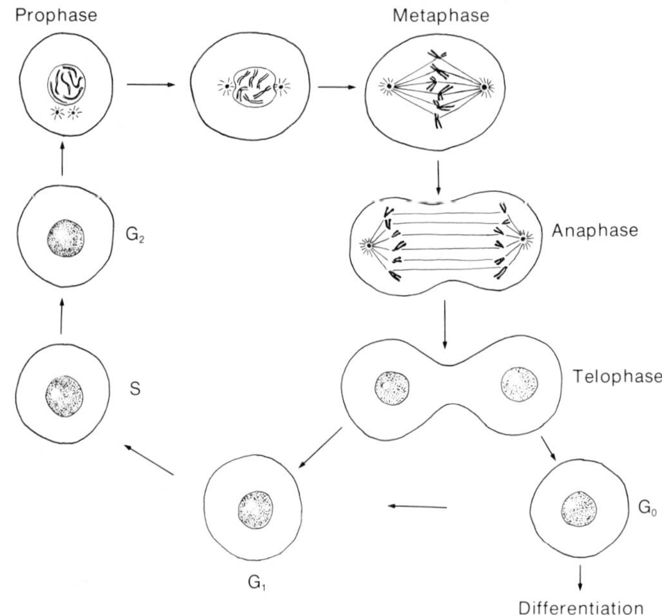

Fig. 2.20 The cell cycle. DNA reduplication occurs during the synthesis stage (S). This is followed by a short resting stage (G_2) before the cell enters mitosis. Following division the daughter cells may enter the second resting stage (G_1) before recommencing DNA synthesis. Other daughter cells can pass into a resting phase (G_0), and after a period can either re-enter the cell cycle or become differentiated and cease to be capable of mitosis. In prophase the individual chromosomes become visible—for the sake of clarity only six are shown, but the normal human cell contains 46. Each chromosome has already split into two chromatids. In metaphase the chromosomes are arranged along the equatorial plate, and the spindle is fully formed. In anaphase, the chromatids, now called chromosomes, move apart. In telophase the daughter nuclei reform, and the cytoplasm divides to produce two cells each with the amount of DNA corresponding to the normal number of chromosomes.

During the period between mitoses (*interphase*) the chromosomes are present in the nucleus as long drawn-out threads. These are not visible as such using the light microscope, but in areas along the thread there is sufficient coiling for the condensation of material to render these areas recognizable as the heterochromatin of the nucleus. Each chromosome is thought to contain many DNA molecules rather than a single long one.

Following the G_2 phase, each chromosome is seen to have divided longitudinally into two *chromatids* which are held together by a *centromere.* The chromosomes show coiling along their length; in this way they become shorter and thicker, and therefore visible. The cell has now entered into the first phase of mitosis—the *prophase*. Meanwhile in the centrosome the microtubules become arranged so as to form the spindle fibres which converge on a dense body adjacent to the centrioles. The centrioles move away from each other to opposite poles of the cell, and in this way the *spindle* is formed; its microtubules are attached to the centromeres, and each centriole looks like a star, or *aster*.

Concurrently the nucleoli and nuclear membrane disappear. The cell is now in *metaphase* with the split chromosomes being arranged along a plane which bisects the cell (the 'equatorial plate').

During the next phase (*anaphase*) the centromeres divide, and each set of chromatids (now called chromosomes) is guided by the fibrils of the spindle to either pole of the cell.

The final stage (*telophase*) involves division of the cytoplasm of the cells, and the reconstitution of the nucleoli and nuclear membrane of each daughter cell.

It can be readily understood how during mitosis each chromosome reduplicates itself exactly, and each daughter cell contains an identical quota of nuclear material. It is presumed that each DNA molecule (and gene) is also reduplicated exactly. Should an error occur during mitosis such that an abnormal gene is produced, the process is called a *somatic mutation*. It is possible that cancer develops in this way.

Meiosis

In the testis and ovary the process of cell division is more complex, and is called *meiosis*. The process results in cells which contain only half the number of chromosomes (the n, or *haploid*, number, i.e. 23 in the human), and half the amount of DNA. These cells develop into gametes, either sperms or ova. With fertilization the diploid number of chromosomes, 46, is restored. It sometimes happens that during meiosis a pair of chromosomes fail to separate, and both are drawn into the one daughter cell. This is called *non-disjunction*. Sometimes fragments of a chromosome are lost (*deletion*), or become attached to another chromosome (*translocation*). If these abnormal gametes are fertilized, it is evident that an abnormal offspring may result. This is considered in Chapter 3.

ARRANGEMENT OF CELLS

The majority of cells in the human body do not occur separately, but are grouped together to form tissues. Traditionally, two main types of cells are distinguished—those of the epithelia and those of the connective tissues.

Epithelial cells

Epithelial cells cover surfaces, e.g. the skin, or line cavities, e.g. the mouth, and in these situations they are essentially protective in function. Covering epithelium may also perform a secretory function; the respiratory epithelium, for instance, secretes mucus.

In addition to covering extensive surfaces, the secretory type of epithelial cell may be arranged to form glands. These may be simple, like the mucous glands of the colon, or more elaborate, like those of the breast and salivary glands. A feature common to all epithelial cells is that they are closely contiguous to one another. This is evident on light microscopy, and even under the electron microscope these cells appear to be separated by only a thin layer of low electron density, about 15 nm in width.

Connective tissue cells

Connective tissue cells are the other type of cell present in the body. They are usually separated widely from each other by a gelatinous material (*ground substance*) in which are embedded fibres (usually *collagenous*). This type of connective tissue, typified by bone, cartilage, tendon, and fibrous tissue, is primarily supportive in function. Other connective tissue cells have been endowed with specialized cytoplasm, e.g. for contraction (muscle fibres), conduction (neurons), phagocytosis (monocytes), and oxygen carriage (red cells).*

It is generally assumed that connective tissue contains primitive multipotential cells which when suitably stimulated can differentiate into reticuloendothelial cells, haematopoietic cells, and probably other connective tissue cells as well. These *stem cells* are poorly defined morphologically, and indeed may differ in appearance in different organs. In the bone marrow they may resemble small lymphocytes. In the lymphoreticular tissues they are difficult to distinguish from *reticular cells,* which form the reticulin-fibre framework of such tissues as spleen and lymph nodes—tissues where stem cells are believed to be plentiful.

The division of the cells of the body into two groups is convenient for some purposes, as will be seen when the classification of tumours is described. Nevertheless, the division is arbitrary and in some ways unsatisfactory. Thus, the flattened cells which line the blood vessels are usually considered to be connective tissue, although they are, in fact, performing a covering function. The same may be said of the mesothelial cells lining the pleura and peritoneum, and those of the synovium.

THE RETICULO-ENDOTHELIAL SYSTEM

Among the most important cells of the connective tissue are those that constitute the reticulo-endothelial (RE) system. This system of cells is widely scattered throughout the body, and all share in common an ability to phagocytose coarse particles and to abstract highly diluted dyes from the blood. As these cells are the main phagocytes (scavengers) of the body, they play a part in many of the pathological processes mentioned later. The RE cells are closely associated with lymphocytes, and they are sometimes considered together as the *lymphoreticular system.*

There are two groups of RE cells:

1. Fixed—these comprise the cells that line the sinuses of certain organs, notably the liver, spleen, bone marrow, and lymph nodes (*sinus-lining,* or *littoral*

* Some authorities prefer to restrict the connective tissues to bone, cartilage, etc., and regard the specialized elements as belonging to separate systems, e.g. haematopoietic, nervous, etc.

cells), and also the resting *histiocytes* that lie in the various connective tissues of the body; those in the central nervous system are called *microglia.*

2. Mobile or wandering—these are the blood *monocytes.*

When there is a local pathological process in a tissue, such as infection or haemorrhage, RE cells migrate to the area, become phagocytic, and are then called *macrophages.* They are mobilized both from the blood monocytes and the local histiocytes. It should be noted that the other phagocytic cells of the body, the neutrophil granulocytes of the blood, are not included in the RE system, because they cannot perform the same type of phagocytosis as has been defined for the RE system. The name reticulo-endothelial system derives from the situation of the sinus-lining cells of liver, spleen, etc. which are found in close relationship to the reticulin framework of the organs (p. 34), and which superficially resemble flattened endothelial cells, such as are found in the blood vessels. As the cells differ from vascular endothelial cells and reticular cells both morphologically and functionally, the name reticulo-endothelial is unfortunate and has been deprecated. An alternate name for this highly phagocytic cell system, the *mononuclear phagocytic system,* has therefore been suggested.[11]

Apart from their essential function of phagocytosis of organisms and debris (Chs. 5, 7, and 10), these cells also play an important part in the immune response (Ch. 11), and in the breakdown of ageing red cells (Ch. 30). They become distended with abnormal lipids in the lipidoses (Ch. 37).

THE INTERCELLULAR SPACE

The Ground Substance[12]

The ground substance varies in consistency from an amorphous gel forming the translucent material of hyaline cartilage to the glairy fluid found in the synovial joint cavities. It is in the molecular meshes of the ground substance that the extracellular interstitial fluid is contained. This extracellular interstitial fluid constitutes about one third of the total body water, and lies between the blood vessels and the cells. It contains various electrolytes in a concentration similar to that of the plasma and also small uncharged solute material, such as oxygen, CO_2, glucose, and urea, which is conveyed either for cellular metabolism or for excretion. In addition the ground substance contains:

Glycoproteins. These are proteins which contain a firmly-bound moiety of carbohydrate. They stain red with the PAS* method.

Mucoproteins are loose combinations of protein with acid mucopolysaccharides. The latter have attracted much attention: they consist of polymers of hexose sugars, some of which possess amino groups, e.g. hexosamines like D-glucosamine and D-galactosamine. The amino groups are presumably responsible in part for the mucoid properties of the polymers. Meyer[13] has subdivided the acid

* *The Periodic Acid-Schiff Reaction.* When periodic acid is applied to a section many carbohydrate components are oxidized to aldehydes. Aldehydes produce a red colour with Schiff's reagent (a solution of basic fuchsin decolorized by sulphurous acid). Therefore if Schiff's reagent is applied to a treated section, the parts containing carbohydrate are stained red. The PAS reaction is useful for the demonstration of glycogen, ground substance, and epithelial mucus.

mucopolysaccharides as listed below. The alternative names in brackets are those proposed by Jeanloz.[14]

Non-sulphated Group
Hyaluronic acid
Chondroitin

In these the acid grouping is due to uronic acid, e.g. glucuronic acid.

Sulphated Group
Chondroitin sulphate A (chondroitin 4-sulphate)
Chondroitin sulphate B (dermatan sulphate)
Chondroitin sulphate C (chondroitin 6-sulphate)
Heparitin sulphate (heparan sulphate)
Keratosulphate (keratan sulphate)

The physical (e.g. optical) and presumably chemical properties of each connective tissue depend upon the nature of the ground substances as well as upon the physical arrangement of the fibres themselves. For example, keratosulphate forms 50 per cent of the total acid mucopolysaccharide in the cornea, but is present only in small quantities in osteoid. It is generally agreed that fibroblasts (and osteoblasts) form acid mucopolysaccharides

Collagen[15-18]

Collagen constitutes about one third of the body's protein; it forms a scaffold in all tissues and is the chief component of fascia, dermis (including gingiva), cornea, dentine, and tendon, and gives these structures tensile strength. Isotope studies indicate that although much of the body's collagen is metabolically stable, some of it is rapidly synthetized and degraded; the excretion of hydroxyproline in the urine gives some indication of the amount of collagen which is being degraded. Thus the excretion is high in hyperparathyroidism. Collagen comprises almost 90 per cent of the organic matrix of bone, and its particular composition is adapted for the deposition of the bone salts.

The collagen of connective tissue is synthetized by fibroblasts or similar cells such as are found in tendon, cornea, bone, and cartilage. An exception to this is the collagen component of basement membrane, which is formed by the adjacent epithelial or endothelial cells and differs in several respects from other collagens. Indeed, as more research is carried out on the composition of collagen, it is evident that many forms exist and it is misleading to talk of collagen as if it were a single entity of fixed composition and structure.

Light microscopic appearance of collagen

The first formed collagen consists of fine branching fibres called *reticulin.* These are demonstrated by silver impregnation methods. In many organs of the body collagen formation stops at this stage, and the reticulin forms a scaffold for the parenchyma (e.g. liver, spleen, and lymph nodes). There is good evidence that this reticulin differs chemically and antigenically from the reticulin formed in the granulation tissue of the repair process.[19] In the connective tissues proper the fibres become further enlarged, and then are called *collagen fibres.* They lose their affinity for silver, but readily take up eosin, or aniline blue combined with phosphotungstic acid (Mallory's stain). They also stain red with picrofuchsin (Van Gieson's stain).

Electron Microscopic Appearance of Collagen

The electron microscope reveals that the collagen and reticulin *fibres* are made up of *fibrils*, which show a cross banding with a periodicity of about 64 nm (Figs. 2.21a and b). It is thought that these fibrils are made up of tropocollagen molecules each of which is about 280 nm long and 1.4 nm wide. It was at first thought that the molecules were joined together with a quarter-length overlap with their lateral neighbours. It is now known that there is a gap of about 41 nm between the head of one molecule and the tail of the next as shown in Fig. 2.22. In osteoid tissue these gaps serve as a nidus for the deposition of bone salts. The thickness of the collagen fibrils varies from tissue to tissue. In cartilage they measure 15 to 25 nm, while in tendon they reach 130 nm in thickness. It is evident that different lateral

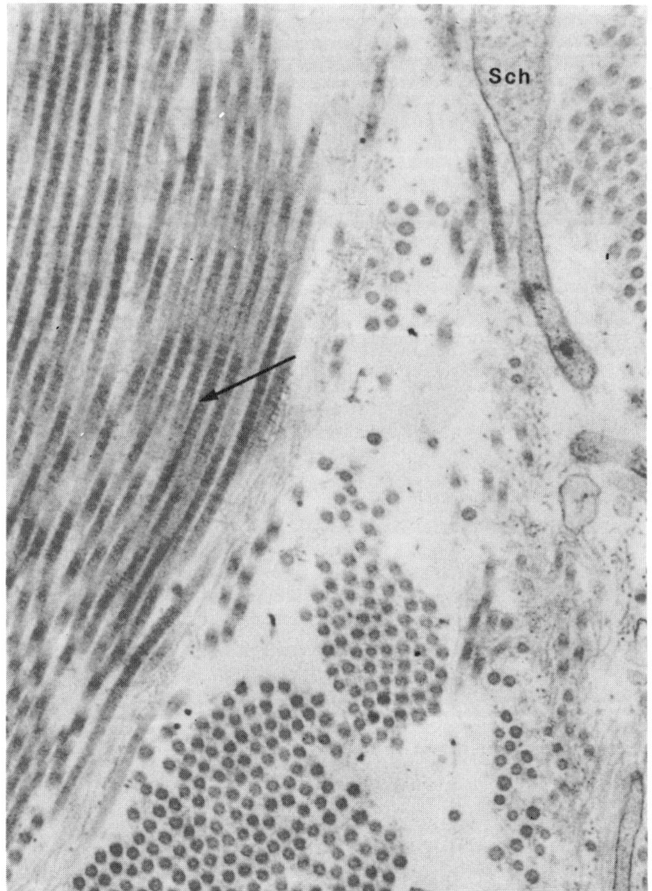

Fig. 2.21a Section of collagen fibrils in a peripheral nerve. The fibrils show the characteristic cross-banding (arrow), which is best seen where the fibrils are cut longitudinally. Part of the cytoplasm of a Schwann cell (Sch) is also shown (× 12 000). (*Photograph by courtesy of Dr N B Rewcastle.*)

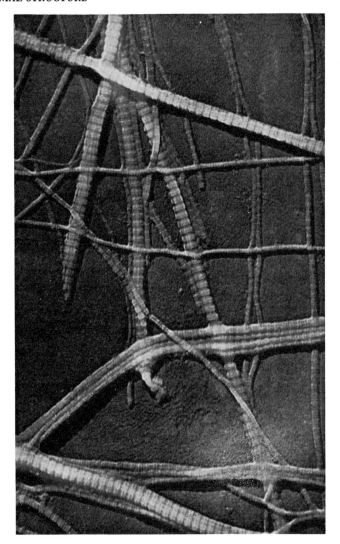

Fig. 2.21b Teased preparation of collagen from the *tendo achilles*. The specimen has been shadowed to accentuate the characteristic 64 nm banding. This process involves the throwing of a vaporised heavy metal such as palladium or gold on to the specimen at a small angle. Now that ultra-thin sections can be cut, this technique is not often used. × 34 000. (*Photograph by courtesy of Dr C I Levene.*)

arrangements of the tropocollagen could form fibrils with different periodicity, and such have in fact been found to exist.

Solubility of collagen

Adult fully-matured collagen is very insoluble, and only denaturation by strong acids or heat can render it soluble. The final product is then gelatin. In young collagen a fraction can be extracted by cold neutral buffers. This probably contains tropocollagen, and on warming the solution, typical banded fibrils are reformed. An additional fraction can be extracted by dilute acid solutions, and this

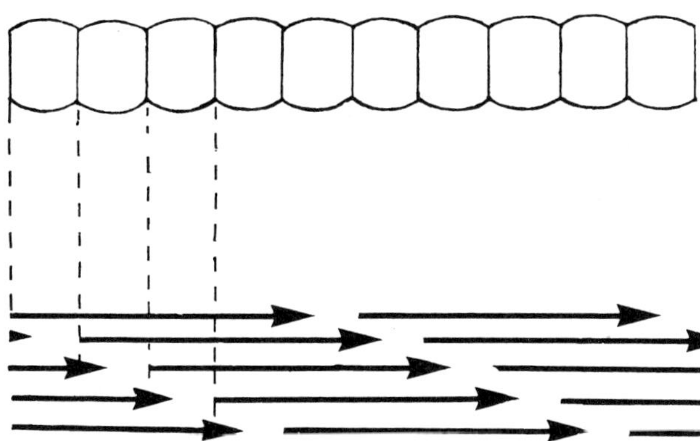

Fig. 2.22 Diagram to illustrate how the lateral arrangement of tropocollagen molecules, depicted as arrows, results in the formation of a banded collagen fibril.

component persists as maturation proceeds. Ultimately the collagen becomes insoluble due to the increasing numbers of cross-linkages which are formed (p. 39).

Chemical composition of collagen

Collagen has a characteristic X-ray diffraction pattern, and from this its structure has been surmised. The basic unit of collagen is called *tropocollagen*, a molecule 280 nm long and 1.4 nm wide, with a molecular weight of about 340 000 daltons. Tropocollagen consists of three polypeptide chains. Each of the polypeptide chains is coiled, and the three molecules are wound around a common axis like a three-stranded rope. It is thus a 'coiled coil'.

Five types of chain are known, and are designated: $\alpha(I)$, $\alpha 1(II)$, $\alpha 1(III)$, $\alpha 1(IV)$, and $\alpha 2$. Various combinations of these polypeptide chains are known to combine to form four types of collagen:

Type I: $[\alpha 1(I)]_2\alpha 2$. This type of collagen is widely distributed, and is the major component of dermis, tendon, bone, and dentine. It consists of two $\alpha 1(I)$ chains and one $\alpha 2$ chain. Its molecular form is therefore recorded as $[\alpha 1(I)]_2\alpha 2$.

Type II: $[\alpha 1\ (II)]_3$. This type of collagen consists of three $\alpha 1(II)$ chains and is chiefly found in cartilage.

Type III: $[\alpha 1(III)]_3$. This type of collagen comprises approximately 50 per cent of the collagen of the heart valves and the major arteries.

Type IV: $[\alpha 1(IV)]_3$. Collagen composed of three $\alpha 1(IV)$ chains is found only in basement membranes.

Each polypeptide chain consists of about 1000 amino-acid residues and has a molecular weight of about 95 000 daltons. It is coiled to form a helix in which, unlike the usual protein α-helix, there are no hydrogen bonds between adjacent amino acids on the same chain. Each helix is stabilized by hydrogen bonds with adjacent polypeptide chains. Throughout most of the chain every third amino acid is glycine, and a common sequence is glycine—proline—hydroxyproline. Collagen is indeed characterized by its high content of glycine (33 per cent) and proline and hydroxyproline which together constitute about 22 per cent. Hydroxyproline is an amino acid which is not found to any great extent in other proteins, and an estimation of its amount in hydrolysates of tissue may therefore be used to measure the amount of collagen present. It is also noteworthy that collagen contains hydroxylysine, and it is to this amino acid that carbohydrate is attached (either galactose or glucogalactose).

Biosynthesis of collagen

The primary polypeptide chains are formed in the rough endoplasmic reticulum under the influence of specific mRNA (Fig. 2.23). The three polypeptide chains

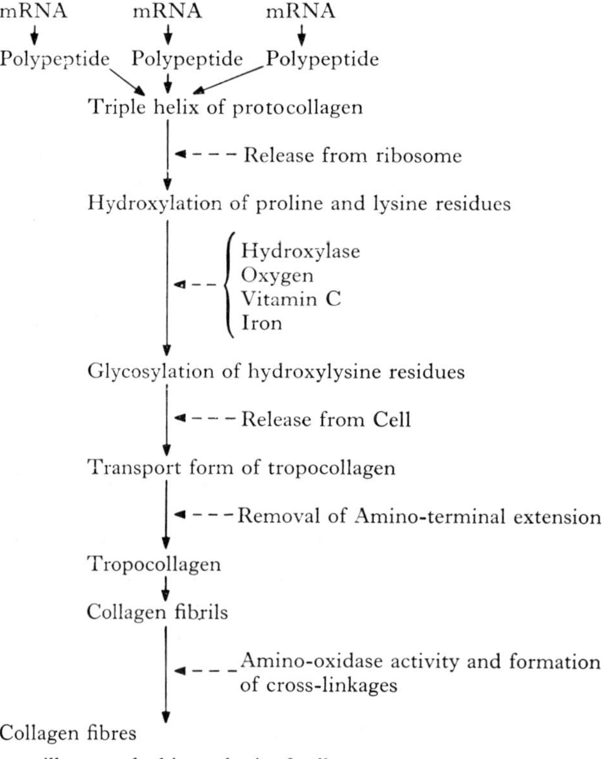

Fig. 2.23 Diagram to illustrate the biosynthesis of collagen.

are probably formed simultaneously and immediately unite to form a triple helix. The molecule first formed is called protocollagen; it differs from tropocollagen in not containing hydroxyproline, hydroxylysine, or glycosylated hydroxylysine. The next step in the formation of collagen is the *hydroxylation of proline and lysine*; for this specific enzymes, free oxygen, and *ascorbic acid* are required.

Thus hydroxyproline and hydroxylysine in collagen are formed in the polypeptide chains by hydroxylation of the parent amino acids. They are not directly encoded by specific mRNA, and this raises another problem. What factors determine which proline or lysine is hydroxylated? No definite answer can be given, but it is not surprising that the degree of hydroxylation varies somewhat from one collagen to another even within the same individual.

Glycosylation of hydroxylysine. Glycosylation occurs at some of the hydroxylysine residues; to some of these sites glucose is further added to the galactose. It has been postulated that in diabetes mellitus excessive glycosylation could lead to the deposition of an abnormal collagen in basement membranes.

Formation of tropocollagen. The manner by which the three polypeptide chains are formed simultaneously and united is not known. There is some evidence that the first formed polypeptide chains have an extension at the amino terminal end (see below), and that this contains cysteine. Hence disulphide bonds could be formed, and initiate the formation of the triple helix. This sulphur-containing component probably persists until the tropocollagen molecules finally polymerize into mature collagen. These findings help to explain why sulphur-containing amino acids are necessary for normal wound healing (p. 125).

Extrusion of collagen from the cell. Tropocollagen is released from the ribosomes into the cisternae of the endoplasmic reticulum. It may then leave the cell *via* the Golgi complex as does secretion in exocrine glands, or else pass by a more direct route. A failure in hydroxylation or glycosylation inhibits this extrusion. Protein synthesis is not immediately inhibited, but the defective collagen is not extruded, and extracellular deposition therefore ceases. This occurs in scurvy.

Extracellular incorporation of tropocollagen into collagen fibrils. Newly synthetized collagen consists of a molecule larger than tropocollagen, due to the presence of the cysteine-containing extension. This is called *procollagen*, or *transport form.* When the extension is removed, aggregation occurs. Fibres are formed by the lateral alignment of the molecules with a quarter overlap as shown in Fig. 2.22. This quarter-stagger arrangement presents problems if one tries to construct a three-dimensional model with match-sticks. Perhaps four or five polymer chains are arranged so that in cross-section they form a square or pentagon. In this way there is limitation of the points of contact between the chains. Whatever the precise arrangement, the carbohydrate content of the collagen and the mucopolysaccharide composition of the ground substance seem to play a part in the determination of the size of the fibres produced.

Cross-linkage of fibrils to form fibres. The fibrils which are formed when tropocollagen aggregates have little strength. It is by the formation of cross-linkages that tensile strength is produced. Aldehyde groups are produced under the catalytic action of an amino-oxidase. These groups form cross-linkages, but the process is slow, and it can readily be understood that tensile strength of collagen in a wound can steadily increase over several months (p. 120).

The first-formed collagen fibres are coated with much ground substance and it is in this that silver is deposited with suitable staining techniques. The maturation of collagen and the formation of cross-linkages has been suggested as a possible mechanism of tooth eruption.[20].

Catabolism of collagen

Although collagen appears to be metabolically very stable, it is evident that under some circumstances it can be formed very rapidly and equally rapidly degraded and removed. The denaturation of collagen involves the actions of proteolytic enzymes, either specific collagenases or non-specific proteases.[21]. Both play a part under some circumstances.

Non-specific proteases. Proteolytic enzymes are present in the lysosomes of neutrophils and macrophages. In inflammatory lesions these enzymes play a part in collagen degradation. Thus in suppuration the collagenous framework of a tissue is removed and an abscess formed. In other inflammatory lesions macrophages are seen to ingest collagen fibres. A good example is found in necrobiotic lesions.

Collagenases. It is now well established that specific collagenases are formed by many tissues. Thus, during *post-partum* involution of the uterus, and in the early stages of the regeneration of an amputated newt's arm, there is a rapid dissolution of the collagenous framework of the tissues. Likewise, in the maturation of scar tissue it is evident that collagen is removed at the same time as new collagen is laid down, so that the scar steadily becomes stronger as its tissues are remodelled. It seems likely that collagenases are important and that their function is to degrade collagen. This action is balanced by collagen synthesis, so that under normal conditions the proper amount of collagen is present in the tissue. Increased collagen synthesis or decreased collagenase activity results in fibrosis.

Collagenase inhibitors are known to exist in plasma, but their role in collagen homeostasis is not known.

Elastic fibres

The elastic fibres of the aorta and its large branches, the ligamentum nuchae, lung, etc., appear very different from collagen on light microscopy; they stain *deep red with eosin, dark brown with orcein,* and *black with the resorcinol fuchsin stain of Weigert.* Early electron-microscopic studies of elastic fibres showed them to be amorphous and quite unlike collagen. More recent investigations have shown that elastic tissue consists of two components: one is the microfibril and the other is a homogeneous material of variable electron density. The microfibrils are obvious during the formation of elastic, but with ageing are more difficult to detect. Elastic tissue is very resistant to digestion by acids and alkalis, but is readily attacked by the enzyme elastase produced by some organisms.

Chemically elastic fibres consist of a protein, *elastin,* with polysaccharide. Although some authorities regard elastic fibres as being derived from collagen, most maintain that this is unlikely in view of the great difference in amino-acid composition between elastin and collagen. Elastin contains two amino acids, desmosine and isodesmosine, which are thought to be important in forming the cross-linkages which give to elastic tissue the resilience which is its characteristic physical property. With age there is an increase in the content of desmosine and isodesmosine, and this is accompanied by a loss of resilience. Calcification of elastic fibres is another feature of the ageing process; it also occurs in metastatic calcification (see p. 301).

Elastic fibres are formed by the activity of smooth muscle cells in some situations, e.g. in the aortic wall and in atheromatous plaques. In other tissues, cells which resemble fibroblasts appear to be involved. No specific 'elastoblasts' have been identified. There is little doubt that new elastic fibres can be formed in adult life. Thus degeneration of elastic tissue is sometimes accompanied by new elastic fibre formation, so as to give an appearance of fraying or reduplication.

GENERAL READING

Ham A W 1974 Histology, 7th edn. Lippincott, Philadelphia, 1006 pp. An excellent reference book that co-ordinates structure with function.

Leeson C R, Leeson TS 1976 Histology, 3rd edn. Saunders, Philadelphia, 605 pp.

Ross L M 1974 The cell. In: Clinical Symposia (Ciba) 26: 4–35.

REFERENCES

1. Berlin R D, Oliver J N, Ukena T E, Yin H H 1975 The cell surface. New England Journal of Medicine 292:515
2. Nicolson, G L, Poste, G (1976) The cancer cell: dynamic aspects and modifications in cell-surface organization. New England Journal of Medicine 295: 197 & 253
3. Various Authors: Cell movement and cell contact. 1961. Experiment Cell Research, Supplement 8:
4. Pastan I 1972 Cyclic AMP. Scientific American, 227 No 2, 97
5. Singer, S J, Nicolson, G L 1972 The fluid mosaic model of the structure of cell membranes. Science, 175: 720
6. Weinstein, R S, McNutt, N S 1972 Cell junctions. New England Journal of Medicine, 286: 521
7. Ycas M 1969 The Biological Code North Holland Publishing Co, Amsterdam
8. Stent G S 1964 The operon: on its third anniversary. Science, 144: 816
9. Preer J R 1971 Extrachromosomal inheritance hereditary symbionts, mitochondria, chloroplasts In Annual Review of Genetics, ed Roman H L Vol 5, Annual Reviews Inc: Palo Alto, p 361
10. Wolstenholme, G E W, O'Connor, M. (eds) 1969 Bacterial Episomes and Plasmids, Ciba Foundation Symposium, Churchill, London
11. van Furth R et al 1972 The mononuclear phagocyte system: a new classification of macrophages, monocytes, and their precursor cells. Bulletin of the World Health Organisation, 46: 845
12. Lehninger A L 1975 Biochemistry, 2nd edn, Worth Publishers Inc, New York, p 271
13. Meyer K 1959 In Wound Healing and Tissue Repair, ed. Patterson, W B, University of Chicago Press, Chicago, p 25
14. Jeanloz R W 1960 The nature of mucopolysaccharides. Arthritis and Rheumatism, 3: 233
15. Miller E J, Matukas, V J 1974 Biosynthesis of collagen. Federation Proceedings, 33: 1197
16. Grant, M E, Prockop, D J 1972 The biosynthesis of collagen. New England Journal of Medicine, 286: 194, 242, and 291
17. Ramachandran G N (ed) 1967 Treatise on Collagen, Vol 1 Academic Press, London, p 556
18. Gould B S (ed) 1968 Treatise on Collagen, Vol. 2, Academic Press, London, Part A p 434, Part B p 488
19. Holborow, E J Faulk W P, Beard H K, Conochie L B 1977 Antibodies against reticulin and collagen. Annals of the Rheumatic Diseases, 36: Supplement No 2 p 51
20. Thomas N R 1965 The effect of inhibition of collagen maturation on eruption in rats. Journal of Dental Research, 44:1159
21. Gross J, Lapière C M 1962 Collagenolytic activity in amphibian tissue: a tissue culture assay. Proceedings of the National Academy of Sciences of the United State of America 48:1014

3

The cause of disease

The abnormalities in structure or function which are the hallmark of disease are due to the effects of an interplay between two basic factors—these are the *inherited genetic constitution* of the individual on the one hand and the *environment* on the other.

THE GENETIC BASIS OF DISEASE[1,2]

Introduction

Traditionally much of pathology is concerned with the effects of adverse factors such as heat, trauma, and bacteria acting on a normal individual. Many diseases are regarded as being caused by particular agents—thus tuberculosis may be said to be caused by the tubercle bacillus. Such a one-sided approach to medicine is no longer tenable. If a hundred people were to be exposed to a particular dose of tubercle bacilli, only a few would develop the disease. No two people are the same, nor do they react in exactly the same way. Each individual is different, and the difference is thought to lie in the coded information (or genetic material) that is handed down to that person from his or her parents. This information is very precise, and is capable of exact analysis. Today we think of inheritance in terms of the structure of the DNA molecule and the sequence of its bases. However, the science of inheritance is not new; it started a century ago when the Austrian monk Gregor Mendel, by observing the mode of inheritance of particular characteristics in the garden pea, noted that the characteristics behaved as if they were determined by units which were passed unchanged from one generation to the next. To these units the name *genes* was given, and it is postulated that a pair of them is present in every somatic cell. Each gene is situated at a specific site, or *locus*, on one of a pair of chromosomes, and the genes forming a pair are called *alleles*, or *allelomorphs*. If they are alike the individual is called a *homozygote* for that particular gene, while if dissimilar the word *heterozygote* is used. The genetic makeup of an individual is called his *genotype*, and the effects which these genes produce is the *phenotype*.

Mode of inheritance

In order to explain Mendelian inheritance several assumptions have been made:

1. Genes occur in pairs

2. One gene of each pair is received from each parent
3. Genes remain unchanged through many generations
4. Some genes may be considered as dominant and some as recessive. A *dominant gene* produces its effect both in the heterozygote and in the homozygote. *Recessive genes*, on the other hand, produce their effects only in the homozygous condition. Genes which occupy an intermediate position are described later. Sometimes a particular *locus* can be occupied by one of many possible genes. A simple example of this type is illustrated below in respect of the ABO blood groups.

Dominant genes. The pattern of inheritance of a dominant gene may be illustrated by reference to the ABO blood group. The allelic genes concerned occupy one *locus*, and may be *A*, *B*, or *O*.

A homozygous individual who has two *A* genes (genotype *AA*) has in the red cells the blood group substance A (phenotype group A). Likewise the heterozygote *AO* is also phenotypically blood group A, because the *A* gene is dominant and the *O* is recessive. The *B* gene, like *A*, is dominant, and both are described as *co-dominants*. The possible blood groups in this system are shown below*:

Genotype	*Phenotype*
AA	A
AO	A
OO	O
BB	B
BO	B
AB	AB

Thus the six genotypes produce only four recognizable blood groups. The occurrence of two or more genetically different classes of individuals with respect to a single trait is known as *polymorphism*†.[3] The blood groups provide an excellent example, but many others are also known. Thus there are genetically determined variants of haemoglobin and of many of the plasma proteins.

Some diseases are inherited as dominant characteristics, e.g. achondroplasia and dentinogenesis imperfecta. The mode of inheritance is shown in Fig. 3.1, and it should be noted that:

1. The disease appears in every generation, or else it dies out. The occasional instance of poor penetrance (p. 46) and the occurrence of a new mutant provide exceptions to this rule. If the disease greatly reduces the breeding potential of the sufferer, it follows that most cases encountered will be sporadic and due to new mutations
2. Unaffected members do not pass on the disease (but see penetrance, p. 46)
3. The affected members are usually heterozygous, and if the breeding partner is normal, the chances of the offspring being affected are 50 per cent
4. Males and females are equally liable to be affected.

* It will be appreciated that the ABO blood group is much more complex than is described in this book.

† The frequency should be greater than 1 per cent, since very rare traits can arise by mutation and their occurrence in a population does not constitute polymorphism.

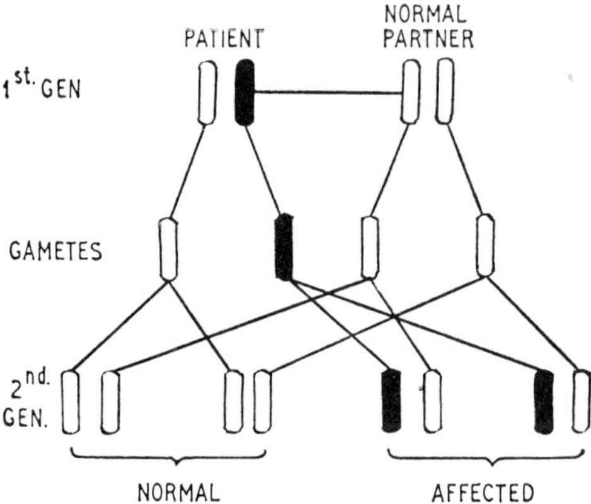

Fig. 3.1 Diagram illustrating the transmission of a disease inherited as a dominant factor. One pair of chromosomes is shown for each individual, the black chromosome being the one carrying the defective gene. It will be seen that half the children of an affected patient are themselves diseased.

Recessive genes. Diseases inherited as recessive traits are frequently severe and reduce the breeding chances of the sufferer, e.g. galactosaemia (p. 47) and xeroderma pigmentosum (p. 364). The birth of an abnormal individual is often the first indication that an abnormal gene is present in the family. Fig. 3.2 shows the mode of transmission, and it can be seen that both parents of the affected individual are themselves heterozygous carriers. Most individuals are heterozygous for several harmful genes, and since some members of one family are likely to have the same recessive gene, the dangers of close interbreeding are apparent.

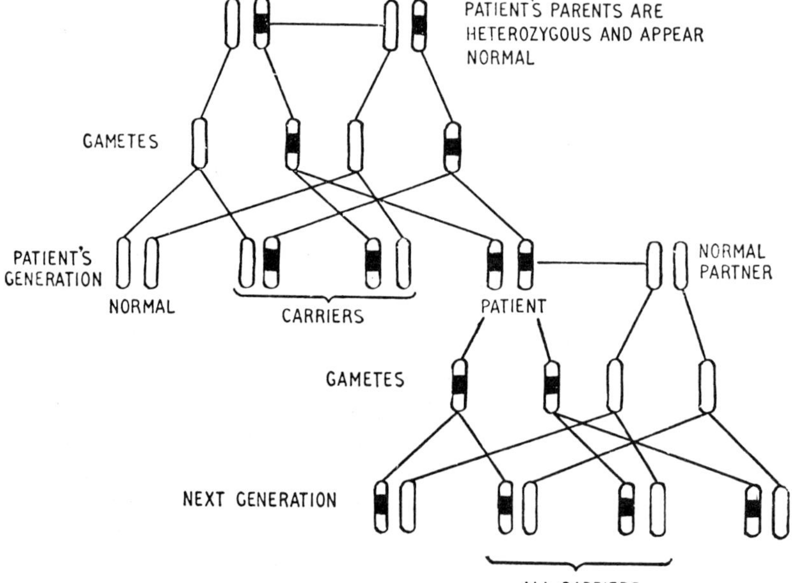

Fig. 3.2 Diagram to illustrate the transmission of a disease inherited as a recessive factor. It will be seen that the patient's parents are both unaffected heterozygotes, and that all the patient's children are likewise carriers.

Sex-linked genes. A gene is said to be sex-linked when it is localized on an X or Y chromosome. Usually the gene is recessive, and is situated on the X chromosome. The bleeding diseases haemophilia and Christmas disease are inherited in this way (Fig. 3.3). Female heterozygotes are protected by the normal gene on their other X chromosome; half the carrier's sons, however, have the disease.

Sex-linked dominant traits are recognized but are rare. Affected females convey the gene to half their sons and daughters, whereas affected males transmit it only

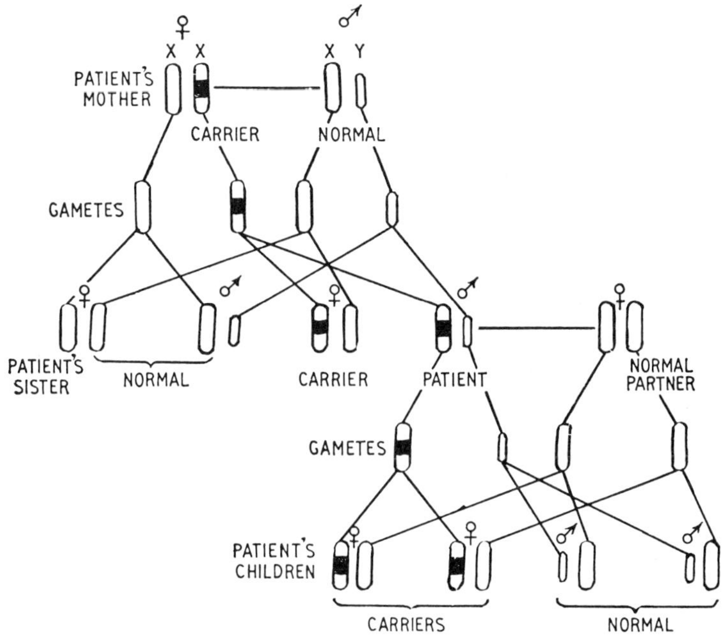

Fig. 3.3 Mode of transmission of a disease like haemophilia, which is inherited as a sex-linked recessive factor. The abnormal gene is situated on the X chromosome, and therefore produces its effect in the male but not in the female except in the rare event of her being homozygous. All the patient's daughters are carriers, but all his sons are normal.

to their daughters. Since there can be no male-to-male transmission, there is an excess of female victims. Haemolytic anaemia due to glucose 6-phosphate dehydrogenase deficiency is an example of this type of inheritance.

Intermediate inheritance. When the heterozygote differs from either homozygote, the inheritance is described as intermediate. A good example is sickle-cell anaemia, in which the heterozygote has the sickle-cell trait and differs both from the normal individual and the patient with sickle-cell anaemia (see p. 46).

Concept of expressivity. So far genes have been considered as behaving either as dominant or recessive. In fact the position is much more complex. A gene may produce a severe disease in one individual but only a minor deformity in another. The concept of *expressivity* has been introduced to explain this. If a gene which usually produces a severe effect is found to cause a minor one in a particular individual, it is said to show poor expressivity. In some instances it produces no detectable effect at all, and a dominant trait may then miss a generation. This is an example of *reduced penetrance*, a term used when some individuals with the appropriate genotype fail to express it. Another complication is the failure of a trait, in other respects behaving as a dominant, to be manifest in one sex. This is called *sex limitation*. Baldness is said to behave in this way since it affects males much more frequently than females.

Multifactorial or polygenic inheritance. Multifactorial inheritance, where several genes each influence one particular function, is a further complication. Variation in stature is an example of this. With some diseases the mode of inheritance defies exact analysis.

Molecular diseases[4, 5]

With the discovery of chromosomes and DNA, it was not unnatural that attempts should be made to equate genes with segments of the DNA molecule. This translation of the mysterious gene action into concrete chemical terms was first achieved successfully with a group of diseases in humans known as the *haemoglobinopathies*, in which an abnormal form of haemoglobin is manufactured.

Many other diseases are now known in which the body synthetizes an abnormal form of protein, either a structural protein or an enzyme. These diseases are grouped together as the *molecular diseases*.

Haemoglobinopathies. The globin of the molecule haemoglobin is a protein of known amino-acid sequence. In certain individuals, usually of African stock, the haemoglobin contains an abnormal globin in which valine replaces the usual glutamic acid in one of the peptide chains in the globin molecule. Presumably this is due to an error in one codon of the DNA molecule. Homozygous individuals manufacture the abnormal haemoglobin Hb-S, and this has the effect of rendering their red blood cells liable to become distorted to a sickle shape at low oxygen tensions. They are more easily removed from the circulation and destroyed, with the result that the patients become severely ill with *sickle-cell anaemia*. Heterozygous individuals suffer from a mild anaemia, and are said to have the *sickle-cell trait*. Their red cells contain both normal adult haemoglobin Hb-A and Hb-S. It might be wondered why the sickle-cell gene, being so harmful, should not have killed off all its carriers and died out. It appears that those with the trait, although at a slight disadvantage in a temperate climate, are at a distinct advantage in the tropics, because they have greater resistance to malaria than do normal individuals. Through natural selection this apparently harmful gene has become widely distributed in tropical climates and has reached a high frequency. The haemoglobin molecule has been the object of intense study, and a large number of variants are now known. This is an example of the *genetic heterogeneity*[5] in the population, and other instances are noted below in respect of certain enzymes.

Other molecular diseases. Sometimes a particular protein is completely absent, and this is most noticeable when the protein concerned can easily be detected. Thus in the rare analbuminaemia the plasma lacks albumin. Commonly the gene product is an enzyme, and an abnormal gene gives rise to a protein with defective enzymatic activity. As examples there are at least 78 known variants of glucose 6-phosphate dehydrogenase deficiency and three of galactosaemia (described below). This particular subdivision of the molecular diseases falls into the group of genetically determined biochemical defects, or **inborn errors of metabolism**, a term coined by Archibald Garrod over 50 years ago.[6] These are uncommon diseases, but they point a finger in the direction which should be followed by those who would unravel the mode of gene action. As noted by William Harvey over 300 years ago, 'nature is nowhere accustomed more openly to display her secret mysteries than in cases where she shows traces of her workings apart from the beaten path'.*

A representative example of such a disease is *galactosaemia*.[7] Babies with this defect lack an enzyme which converts galactose to glucose. The galactose, or its metabolites, derived from the lactose in milk, accumulates in the blood and interferes with the development of the brain, the eye, and the liver. Mental defect, cataracts, and cirrhosis of the liver are the results of this simple biochemical defect. The effects can be ameliorated by avoiding lactose and galactose in the diet. The ethics of condemning a child to a lifelong artificial diet might, however, be questioned.

A second example of this type of disease is *phenylketonuria*, which affects between 3 and 5 persons per 100 000 of the population and is characterized by retardation of mental development. The disease is due to the absence of an enzyme that converts the amino acid phenylalanine to tyrosine. Hence, with a normal diet an affected baby develops a high blood level of phenylalanine and its keto derivatives. These are the cause of brain damage, which can be largely averted by the administration of a diet low in phenylalanine. Early diagnosis, by finding phenylalanine or its derivatives in the urine, is therefore very important. The condition is inherited as a Mendelian autosomal recessive trait; 1 per cent of the population are heterozygotes, and can be detected by the administration of a test dose of phenylalanine, when the blood level rises. This does not occur in a normal individual. This detection of heterozygotes has a practical value. If a married couple are both carriers, their chance of producing an affected child is 25 per cent: they can be warned of this risk. This is a good example of the kind of information offered in genetic counselling.

Many other inborn errors of metabolism have been discovered. Some result in severe disease, while in other instances they are of no importance save for their anthropological interest. Deficiency or abnormality of an enzyme may induce in the individual an intolerance to a particular drug. For example, those who have a defective *pseudocholinesterase*[8] are very susceptible to the drug suxamethonium used in anaesthesia. This drug is used to produce relaxation or paralysis of muscles, and is inactivated by the enzyme pseudocholinesterase. Patients with this enzyme defect are unable to metabolize the drug quickly, and if given it, are liable to develop prolonged paralysis with cessation of breathing and death. Enzyme-deficient red cells are considered on page 453.

Disease associated with genetic constitution

In spite of the great advances in biochemical genetics, there are many diseases in

* The Works of William Harvey, M.D. translated by Robert Willis, p. 616, Sydenham Society, London, 1847. (Cited by Garrod A E 1928 Lancet 1: 1055.)

which the mechanisms involved are not understood. They appear to be more common in certain families, and are spoken of as *familial diseases*, but their occurrence and distribution cannot be predicted. High blood pressure, obesity, and heart disease seem to fall into this group.

Sometimes particular characteristics are associated with certain diseases, though they themselves are not the obvious cause. The association of a particular disease with race, e.g. diabetes mellitus and Gaucher's disease in Jews, or with sex, e.g. goitres in women and cancer of the lung in men, is an example of this. In addition, innate immunity to infection (see p. 175) is an inherited characteristic, and so is the inherited liability to develop hypersensitivity (p. 184). The association of blood groups with disease has also been recognized: cancer of the stomach is more frequent in group-A subjects, while duodenal ulceration is more common in those of group O. There is a relationship between certain histocompatibility genes and disease, e.g. HLA-B27 and ankylosing spondylitis.[9] We are quite ignorant of the mechanisms involved, but undoubtedly this type of association was noted by the great clinicians of the past, who often referred to a characteristic disease diathesis.

Diseases associated with gross chromosomal abnormalities[10]

As mentioned on p. 27, the human being has 46 chromosomes in each cell, of which two are sex chromosomes and the remainder autosomes. Certain individuals

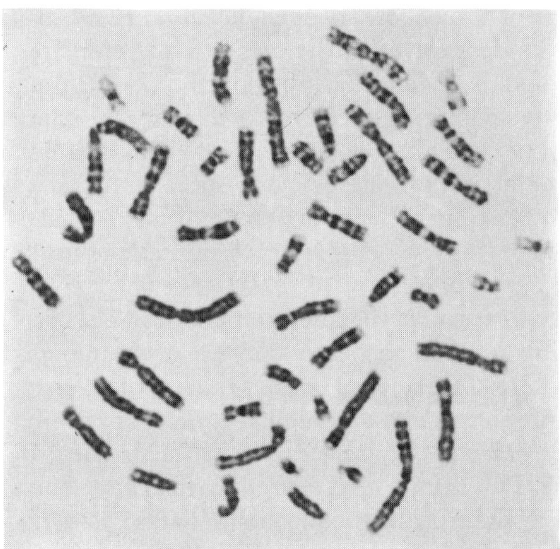

Fig. 3.4a Human chromosomes at metaphase. Lymphocytes from the blood of a normal woman were grown in culture for 72 hours before colcemid (a colchicine derivative) was added. This chemical inhibits spindle formation so that mitoses are halted at metaphase. Two hours later a hypotonic solution was added to make the cells swell. The dispersed chromosomes were then stained with Giemsa after they had been pretreated with trypsin. This technique brings out the banding of the chromosomes.

The mitosis shown contains 46 chromosomes, each of which is a divided structure joined by a centromere. The individual chromosomes can be cut out with scissors and arranged in pairs as shown in Fig. 3.4b. Such an arrangement is called a karyotype. (*Photograph by courtesy of Dr H A Gardner, Division of Cytogenetics, Toronto General Hospital.*)

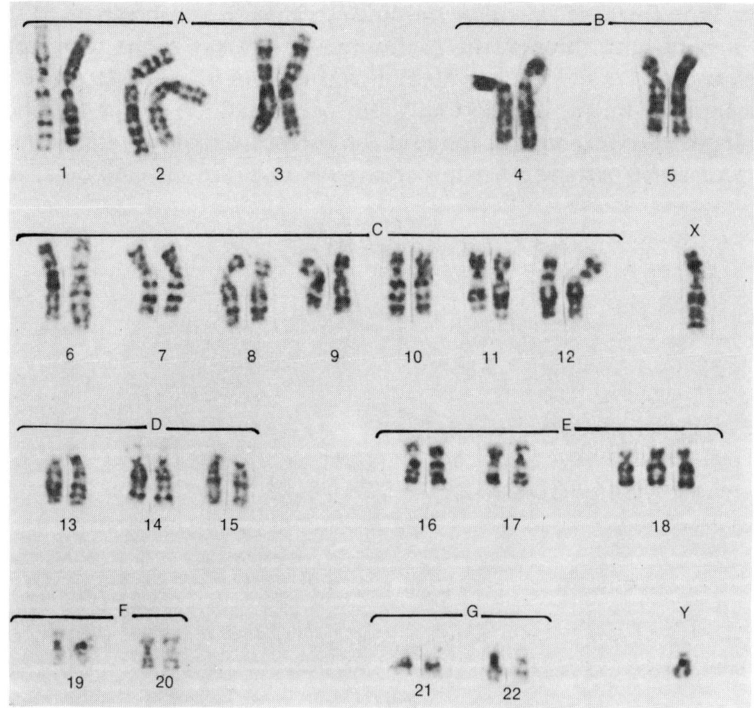

Fig. 3.4b Karyotype showing trisomy 18 from a stillborn male with cyclopia. The karyotype is that of a cell with 47 chromosomes. It is evidently from a male, since there is a Y chromosome. The anomaly must therefore be of fetal origin, since the mother had a normal 46, XX karyotype. The additional chromosome No. 18 arose by nondisjunction; its manifestations were incompatible with postuterine life. (*From Lang A P, Schlager M, Gardner H A 1976 Trisomy 18 and cyclopia. Teratology 14: 195.*)

have been found to have more than 46 chromosomes, while others have less (Figs. 3.4a, and 3.4b). Finally, abnormalities in the shape or form of individual chromosomes have also been noted. These abnormalities may be considered under two headings:

1. *Alteration in number of chromosomes*
2. *Alteration in structure of chromosomes.*

Although the finding of a chromosomal abnormality is regarded as uncommon, it is now apparent that those cases detected in post-natal life represent only the residue of a much larger group of abnormal zygotes. About half the spontaneous abortions in the first 3 months of pregnancy have chromosomal anomalies, one of the commonest being triploidy (the cells having 69 chromosomes). About 30 per cent of zygotes are aborted spontaneously, and gross genetic errors are clearly a major cause.

Alteration in number of chromosomes

Additional chromosomes. The commonest example is where there is one extra chromosome.

Trisomy. The presence of three chromosomes of a kind instead of two is called trisomy. An example is Down's syndrome (trisomy 21, or mongolism) in which a child is born with three of the 21 chromosome. Usually the total number of chromosomes is 47, and the karyotype is recorded as 47, XX, 21+ (or 47, XY, 21+ according to the child's sex). In occasional cases the additional 21 chromosomes is translocated to the 15 chromosome, so that the total number is 46. This *translocation mongolism* is important because the chromosomal defect is

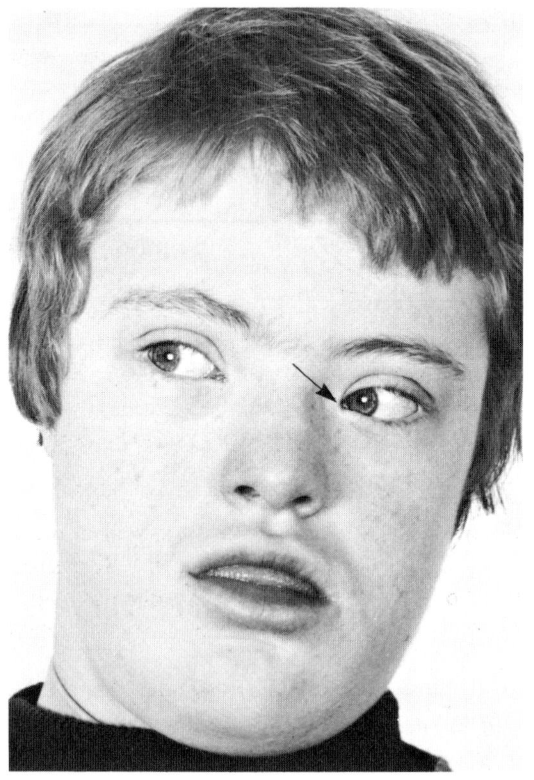

Fig. 3.5 Down's syndrome. Note the oval, slanting palpebral fissures with the prominent epicanthic folds (arrow) at the inner aspects of both upper eyelids. It is this appearance that is reminiscent of the Mongolian race, and has given rise to the name mongolism. Other typical features are the short nose with depressed bridge, the large tongue, and the rounded upper jaw. (*Photograph by courtesy of the Department of Clinical Illustration, Birmingham Dental School, Birmingham, England*)

frequently present in one of the parents without producing clinical effects. In these circumstances the chromosomal defect is transmitted to many of the offspring.

The characteristic manifestations of Down's syndrome, the mongoloid facial features and the mental defect, are all too familiar, since such children are produced with an incidence of approximately 1 in every 600 live births (Fig. 3.5).

Several other syndromes are recognized in which other autosomes are trisomic, but they are rare.

The presence of additional sex chromosomes is not uncommon. Certain individuals are found to have an extra X. Some are apparent males, have the genetic constitution 47, XXY, and their cells are chromatin positive. They have small testes which fail to develop at puberty, there is little facial hair, they may have a female type of breast development (*gynaecomastia*), and are sterile. These features become evident at puberty, and the condition is known as *Klinefelter's syndrome*. Another group of patients are the *poly-X females*, 47, XXX, who are females having an extra X.

In the 47, *XYY syndrome* there is normal male development, but some individuals are abnormally tall and exhibit a criminally aggressive temperament.

Reduction in number of chromosomes. The loss of an autosome appears to be incompatible with postuterine life. In those cases where such a state has been described, a small chromosome is involved, and it seems likely that the chromosome is in fact present but has become attached to another chromosome (i.e. it has been translocated).

The sex chromosomes appear to be less vital, and deletion of one is compatible with life. About 1 in every 3000 births produces a female with 45 chromosomes, having the normal number of autosomes but with only one X. This 45, X, or *ovarian dysgenesis syndrome*, becomes obvious at adolescence, when ovulation and menstruation fail to occur. Such individuals are short, stunted, and sterile. When accompanied by two or more of a number of somatic abnormalities, e.g. webbing of the neck, a shield-like chest with widely-spaced nipples, short fourth metacarpal bone, coarctation of the aorta, or hypoplastic nails, the eponym *Turner's syndrome* is applied. Their cells are chromatin negative, since only one X is present.

Abnormalities of chromosome structure

Many abnormalities in the size, shape, or banding of chromosomes have been described. These will not be considered in detail. Sometimes a portion of a chromosome is deleted, and the remaining portions join together to form a *ring chromosome*. Translocation results in abnormal chromosomes (see translocation mongolism).

Although certain syndromes, many of them very uncommon, are now recognized as being accompanied by chromosomal abnormality, the actual pathogenesis is obscure. In a number of tumours the affected neoplastic cells have been found to have a constant chromosomal abnormality. The best known example of this is *chronic myeloid leukaemia*, in which the abnormal white cells and red-cell precursors, in some cases, lack one arm of chromosome 22. This small chromosome is called the *Philadelphia, or Ph′, chromosome*. Again, the significance of this finding is not understood, but the deletion is a useful diagnostic marker for this type of leukaemia.

Avoidance of genetic defects

Genetic counselling may serve to persuade some high-risk couples from procreation, but when once conception has occurred, the only course open may be the induction of an abortion. Amniocentesis (the removal of a sample of amniotic fluid from the amniotic cavity surrounding the fetus) allows the testing of the amniotic fluid for the prenatal detection of fetal abnormality.[11] The supernatant fluid can be examined biochemically and checked for the presence of virus, while the amniotic cells, which are of fetal origin, can be examined for the presence of the X and Y chromatin. These cells can also be cultured for biochemical investigation and chromosomal analysis. These investigations can generally be completed between the sixteenth and twentieth weeks of gestation. If a defect is found, an abortion can be performed in relative safety at this time, but whether such a course is pursued depends on legal and moral factors.

Environmental factors causing disease

Much of human pathology is concerned with those diseases which are acquired in postnatal life as a result of the action of external factors. The effects of physical and chemical agents, living organisms, and dietary deficiencies are the common causes of these *acquired diseases.* It must not be forgotten, however, that the developing fetus is also sensitive to environmental influences—in some instances much more so than is the adult. Intrauterine events may produce defects which are present at birth (*congenital*), but which are not inherited, since no genetic mechanism is involved. Some congenital lesions of acquired aetiology may copy abnormalities of genetic cause; these are therefore called *phenocopies.* For example, the condition of small brain (microcephaly) may be inherited, or may result from intrauterine irradiation, or infection with toxoplasmosis. The other causes of congenital defects—infection, ionizing radiation, drugs, etc.—are considered in greater detail in Chapter 24.

A final point deserves consideration: hereditary diseases may be congenital, e.g. achondroplasia, but they may also appear later on in life, e.g. polyposis coli (p. 364). The time of onset of a disease gives no indication as to whether the cause is environmental or genetic.

GENERAL READING

Emery A E H 1975 Elements of medical genetics, 4th edn. University of California Press, Berkeley
Nora J J, Fraser F C 1974 Medical genetics: principles and practice, 399 pp. Lea and Febiger, Philadelphia
Thompson J S, Thompson M W 1973 Genetics in medicine, 2nd edn. Saunders, Philadelphia
Valentine G H 1975 The chromosome disorders, 3rd edn. Heinemann, London
Yunis J J, Chandler M E 1977 The chromosomes of man—clinical and biologic significance. American Journal of Pathology 88: 466

REFERENCES

1. Erbe R W 1976 Principles of medical genetics. New England Journal of Medicine 294: 381 and 480
2. Carter C O 1969 An ABC of medical genetics. Lancet 1: 1014, 1041, 1087, 1139, 1203, 1252, and 1303
3. Townes P L 1969 Human polymorphism. Medical Clinics of North America 53: 886
4. Harris H 1968 Molecular basis of hereditary disease. British Medical Journal 2: 135
5. Childs B, Der Kaloustian V M 1968 Genetic heterogeneity. New England Journal of Medicine 279: 1205 and 1267
6. Childs B 1970 Sir Archibald Garrod's conception of chemical individuality: a modern appreciation. New England Journal of Medicine 282: 71
7. Stanbury J B, Wyngaarden J B, Fredrickson D S Eds 1972 The metabolic basis of inherited disease, 3rd edn. McGraw-Hill, New York

8. La Du B N 1969 Pharmacogenetics. Medical Clinics of North America 53: 839
9. Leading Article 1975 HL-A antigens and rheumatic diseases. British Medical Journal 2: 238
10. Gerald P S 1976 Sex chromosome disorders. New England Journal of Medicine 294: 706
11. Milunsky A 1973 The prenatal diagnosis of hereditary disorders. C C Thomas, Springfield, 253 pp

4

Cell and tissue damage

CELL DAMAGE

Since the tissues of the body are all ultimately derived from a single cell, the fertilized ovum, it is reasonable to assume that all the complex functions of the body and all the intricacies of disease will ultimately be explicable in terms of the function and disorders of individual cells. The concept of *pathology as a cellular study* stems from the invention of the compound microscope by Van Leeuwenhoek in the seventeenth century, and blossomed in the nineteenth century with its application to disease by the German school of pathology headed by Virchow. Recent advances in technology have extended this approach. Electron microscopy, with its resolution several hundred times greater than that of the light microscope, has enabled pathology to enter a subcellular phase. The damaged cells in disease can now be described at a subcellular, or even a molecular, level. This study has been augmented by applying chemistry to the examination of cells, using the techniques of *histochemistry*. A simple example of this is the identification of haemosiderin, an iron-containing pigment which occurs in the tissues after haemorrhage. If acid is added to a section of tissue, haemosiderin granules release Fe^{3+} ions, and these are detected by the addition of potassium ferrocyanide. The intense colour of Prussian blue indicates the previous location of the haemosiderin. Analogous methods are available for the identification of glycogen, polysaccharides, nucleic acids, and many enzymes.

Chemists have, however, exerted a quite different influence on the study of disease by adopting another approach. Instead of concentrating on the individual cell or its organelles, they have turned their attention to specific chemical reactions. Thus, in respect of the metabolism of galactose, most cells can be regarded as behaving in a standard way. One important feature in the metabolism of galactose is the enzyme galactose 1-phosphate uridyl transferase, which converts galactose 1-phosphate to glucose 1-phosphate. Deficiency of this enzyme produces the disease *galactosaemia*, which can therefore be explained without recourse to a microscope or the study of individual cells. This second approach to pathology has been of immense value both in the delineation of disease processes and in the treatment of individual patients. Ultimately this broad concept of biochemical disorder must be reduced to a cellular level. In some instances this has already happened, and it is convenient therefore to consider first some examples of cellular damage caused by lesions of known chemical mechanism.

Biochemical lesions

The concept of a biochemical lesion was first put forward by Rudolph Peters,[1] and was based upon the observation that pigeons subjected to a thiamine-deficient diet developed severe neurological symptoms (e.g. convulsions) and died. In spite of the severity of the disease no abnormality could be found by histological examination of the brain. The cells looked normal, but they were not functioning correctly. Peters found that thiamine was one of the factors necessary for the conversion of pyruvate to acetylcoenzyme A (Fig. 2.11). This substance is the fuel, derived from glucose, protein, and fat metabolism, with which the Krebs cycle is fed. Hence in thiamine deficiency Krebs cycle activity is reduced, and with it so also is energy production. Nerve cells, with their high metabolic requirements, are among the first to be affected, and this explains the nervous manifestations of thiamine deficiency. It should be noted that although pyruvate accumulates in the brain and in the blood, it is an effect of the biochemical lesion and not the cause of the symptoms. In other biochemical lesions the unused metabolite does produce a harmful effect. For example, in galactosaemia galactose 1-phosphate accumulates and interferes with other essential metabolic processes. There is no shortage of glucose 1-phosphate, since this can be derived from sources other than galactose.

Biochemical lesions can be deliberately induced in cells by feeding them with agents that closely resemble metabolities. For example, cells fed with 5-fluorouracil respond to the agent as if it were uracil, but the abnormal end-product blocks other essential processes. This deliberate sabotage of cellular metabolism has been called *lethal synthesis* by Peters, and has been used with some success in the treatment of malignant disease. Thus local applications of 5-fluorouracil destroy the abnormal cells in actinic keratosis and actinic cheilitis. Another example of lethal synthesis is the action of chemotherapeutic agents on bacteria. Thus, sulphonamides are treated as para-aminobenzoic acid by some bacteria. This ultimately blocks cellular metabolism. Likewise, penicillin blocks cell-wall synthesis, thus rendering the bacteria extremely fragile and easily destroyed by osmotic effects.

There are relatively few examples of biochemical lesions in which the detailed changes are known. Certain poisons act by blocking a particular metabolic pathway, and there are the group of inborn errors of metabolism in which a specific enzyme is defective or absent (p. 46). Nevertheless, it is presumed that many bacterial toxins and other damaging agents act in this way. The chemical lesions which they induce are not known, and only the morphological changes in the affected cells are visible. These changes, if severe or prolonged, are liable to lead to the death of the cell—for this reason the changes are generally classified as degenerative, and the group of conditions is spoken of as the *degenerations*.

The degenerations

The various morphological types of cellular degeneration may result from the cells being submitted to a wide variety of adverse circumstances which may be either internal or external events. These may be summarized:

Causes

Internal events: *genetic error*—enzyme defects
deprivation of essential chemicals—e.g. hormones, vitamins, oxygen, etc.
hypersensitivity
loss of blood supply.

External agents: *physical*—heat, cold, trauma, radiation
chemical—poisons, lack of oxygen
microbial—microbial invasion and the effects of toxins.

The names attached to the degenerative processes in the cells are mainly descriptive; while some are appropriate, others are frankly misleading. Two main groups are described. Firstly, there is a group associated with an *excessive accumulation of water* in the cell: these are *cloudy swelling, vacuolar degeneration,* and *hydropic degeneration.* Secondly, there is *fatty change*, which in the past has been subdivided into fatty degeneration and fatty infiltration (Fig. 4.1).

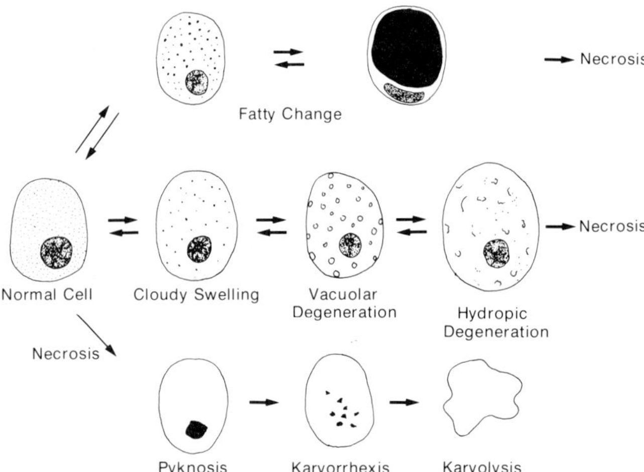

Fig. 4.1 Diagram to illustrate the cellular changes which are generally described as the 'degenerations'. A damaged cell may exhibit progressive waterlogging, and pass through the stages of cloudy swelling, vacuolar degeneration, and hydropic degeneration. Alternatively, fat may accumulate, firstly as fine droplets, but later as the condition advances, a large globule is formed. In the bottom row the changes accompanying necrosis are depicted; these are pyknosis, karyorrhexis, and karyolysis (see p. 63). These changes become evident about 12 hours after cell death and are not reversible. (*Drawing by Margot Mackay, Department of Art as Applied to Medicine, University of Toronto.*)

Changes associated with accumulation of water

Cloudy swelling. This is generally described in specialized cells, e.g. those of the heart, liver, and kidney. The affected organ is swollen, and its cut surface bulges. It has a grey, parboiled appearance, and the consistency is soft. Microscopically the cells are swollen and the cytoplasm is granular. From being a common descriptive term, cloudy swelling has now largely fallen into disuse.

This is partly because the changes are ill-defined, and partly because they are very easily confused with those of post-mortem autolysis (p. 63).[2]

Vacuolar degeneration. The naked-eye appearances described as typical of cloudy swelling are sometimes associated with swollen cells containing vacuoles rather than granules. This is vacuolar degeneration, and its causes and distribution are similar to those of cloudy swelling.

Hydropic degeneration. The cells show great swelling (ballooning) due to an accumulation of fluid. This is the most severe form of this group of degenerative changes, and, although it is reversible, the affected cells frequently rupture and die. Examples of this are to be seen in the liver cells in acute viral hepatitis and in the basal cells of the epidermis in lupus erythematosus.

Changes associated with the accumulation of fat

An accumulation of excess stainable fat is a frequent finding in parenchymal cells; it is especially common in the liver, and its causes are the same as those of cloudy swelling. In this organ alcohol, carbon tetrachloride, and phosphorus are particularly liable to cause such a change. A fatty liver is enlarged, and is soft in consistency. On section its cut surface bulges and appears greasy. Its colour is pale and in severe cases yellow.

Fatty change is common in the kidneys, where it produces pallor and swelling of the cortex.

An accumulation of fat in the heart muscle, as in severe anaemia, produces yellow flecks on the endocardial surface ('tabby-cat heart').

Microscopically the cells are swollen and contain small droplets of neutral fat (glycerol triesters). In the liver the fat accumulation may proceed until the cell contains one large vacuole of fat and its appearance bears some resemblance to a normal fat cell (Fig. 4.2).

Nature of the changes[3]

It is often assumed that the cellular changes of cloudy swelling or hydropic degeneration are the same regardless of the organ affected, be it liver, kidney, or islet of Langerhans. Such is not the case. Using the electron microscope, it has been possible to probe more deeply into the nature of these changes. Whereas the light microscope can give a vague impression of intracellular events and detect the changes when they are severe enough to affect the cell as a whole, electron microscopy can reveal which parts of the cell are affected and indicate the sequence of events and metabolic changes which are occurring. The structure of the cell now appears more complex than did the anatomy of the whole body a hundred years ago. Just as 'coma' ceased to be an intellectually satisfying ultimate diagnosis when specific conditions affecting the brain were recognized, so cloudy swelling is equally unsatisfactory now that organelles are known to exist. The first steps in the recognition of the cell's response to injury have been taken, and cellular pathology promises to become as complex as organ pathology. At this stage one must expect newly described lesions to prove as useful—and at times as misleading—as were those used initially in organ pathology.

It is not easy to give a clear generalized account of the cell's response to injury, since relatively few cell-types have been investigated to any extent. Most work has been carried out on liver and kidney subjected to a variety of chemical poisons, e.g. carbon tetrachloride, ethionine, barbiturates, ethanol, etc. Some of the changes in the cell's components will be described:

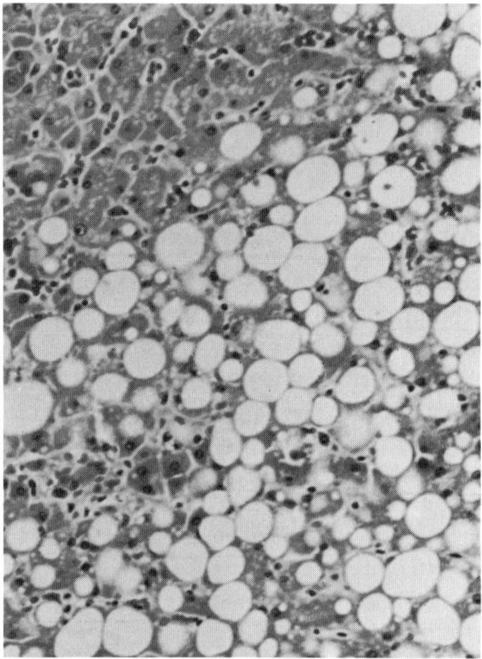

Fig. 4.2 Fatty change of liver. Many of the liver cells are distended with fat globules to the extent that their nuclei are pushed to the cell wall. In other cells the fat is present as small droplets in the cytoplasm. The material was taken at the necropsy of an elderly woman who died of septicaemia. ×100.

Nuclear changes

A variety of nuclear changes have been described in poisoned cells. One of the earliest is clumping of the chromatin along the nuclear membrane and around the nucleolus. The nucleoli show loss of their granular component, and the fibrillar material is sometimes dispersed into separate fragments. Nucleoli are therefore smaller but more numerous. The loss of granular material may indicate impaired synthesis of ribosomal material and messenger RNA. Reduced RNA synthesis is found in damaged cells, and this is reflected in the cytoplasm as reduced protein synthesis. It should be stressed that by light microscopy nuclear changes are not obvious or characteristic in cells showing degeneration.

Cytoplasmic changes: morphological considerations

These may be considered under five headings.

Evidence of increased cell function. Cellular components may proliferate or reorganize in a manner which suggests a state of *hyperfunction.* In response to certain poisons, e.g. phenobarbitone, the smooth endoplasmic reticulum becomes more abundant and forms complex whorls or gyrations (Fig. 4.3); this is regarded as an adaptive mechanism and indicates an attempt to increase the cell's ability to detoxify the substance.

It may also be the morphological expression of a drug-induced enzyme induction. Thus phenobarbitone causes an increase in smooth endoplasmic reticulum as well as leading to enzyme induction. The latter has the effect of

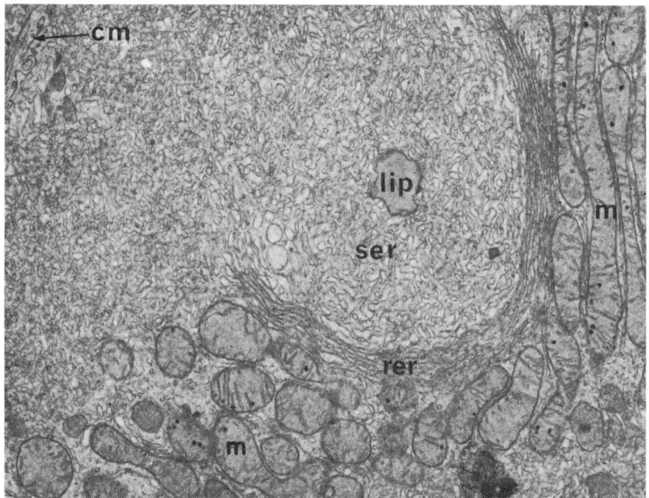

Fig. 4.3 Advanced proliferation of the smooth endoplasmic reticulum (ser) in the periphery of a rat hepatocyte following ethionine administration. The proliferated vesicles of the agranular reticulum are tightly packed and well demarcated from the rough endoplasmic reticulum (rer), which can be identified by the ribosomes studded on the membranes. Mitochondria (m) are elongated. cm—cell membrane; lip—lipid droplet. Lead hydroxide. × 5500. (*Photograph by courtesy of Dr Katsumi Miyai*)

increasing the metabolism of coumarin anticoagulants, a fact that must be borne in mind if the two drugs are given simultaneously. There is also increased enzymatic glucuronidation of bilirubin, an effect of therapeutic value. However, some agents, including carcinogens, cause a proliferation of smooth endoplasmic reticulum that is accompanied by decreased enzymatic activity. Likewise free ribosomes, rough endoplasmic reticulum, and the Golgi complex may proliferate; the number of lysosomes may increase, and mitochondria become more abundant, enlarge, and exhibit an increase in their internal complexity. Evidently the cell's metabolism is increased, for protein synthesis, ATP production, and catabolic activity may all be stimulated as may sometimes glycogen synthesis.

Micropinocytotic activity may increase, and this results in the appearance of numerous vacuoles in the cytoplasm.

Evidence of decreased function. Cellular components may become less numerous and show evidence of *hypofunction.* In damaged liver cells the rough endoplasmic reticulum shows dilatation of its sacs and loss of attached ribosomes. Polysomes are reduced in number. These changes are particularly associated with hydropic degeneration, and indicate *impaired protein synthesis.* As noted above, hypofunction may be accompanied by proliferation of cell components. Thus 'hypoactive hyperplastic endoplasmic reticulum' is a feature of liver cells infected with hepatitis B virus, and is responsible for the abundant ground-glass cytoplasm that is a feature of virus-infected cells.

Mitochondrial changes are frequent. These organelles may show swelling and a loss of cristae. An increase in calcium content has also been described. Impaired function results in reduced oxidative phosphorylation, and ATP production is reduced. Since this substance forms the main immediately available source of energy for cellular metabolism, it is not surprising that many cell functions are impaired. Thus ATP is required for the operation of the mechanism, or pump, regulating the concentration of ions in the cell. The sodium pump is impeded, and sodium and water accumulate in the cell, which in this way becomes progressively enlarged and waterlogged. The electrolytes can pass freely across the cell membrane, but the proteins within the cell cannot escape. When the sodium pump breaks down, there is therefore a *tendency* for the cell to become hypertonic. This is counteracted by the entry of water into the cell which thereupon swells. The breakdown of proteins into smaller molecules may further increase this tendency to hypertonicity. Mitochondrial swelling is commonly found in cells showing cloudy swelling.

Evidence of altered function. Changes may occur which indicate that the cell has acquired a new function; thus the endothelial cells of the glomerular tuft can become actively phagocytic for fibrin.

Abnormal accumulation of substances in the cell. Lipid is an example, and is described later.

Degenerative changes. Localized areas of the cell may appear to become degenerate, and the term *focal cytoplasmic degeneration* has been applied. Sometimes cytoplasmic components, e.g. endoplasmic reticulum and mitochondria, are seen within vacuoles containing lysosomal enzymes. These are called *autophagocytic vacuoles, autophagosomes*, or *cytolysomes*, and an increase in their number is an indication of cell injury. Sometimes an area of cytoplasm degenerates and is actually cast off: damaged renal tubular cells can show loss of the brush border, which together with an area of the underlying cytoplasm is desquamated into the lumen. Such changes have been called necrosis of part of a cell.

Myelin figures.[4] It is not uncommon to find intracellular whorls of laminated lipid material resembling the myelin of nerves. These are called *myelin figures*, and may either be artefacts or else represent real structures. It is well known that if hydrated lipid is allowed to remain undisturbed *in vitro*, myelin figures can form. Likewise, the prolonged fixation of lipid-containing tissue with glutaraldehyde (which fixes lipid slowly) will lead to the formation of myelin figures both within cells and in the extracellular spaces. Sometimes, however, myelin figures are present in membrane-bound structures containing lysosomal enzymes. These are called *myeloid bodies*, or *myelinoid bodies*, and are present whenever the secondary lysosomes are overloaded with lipid.

It should be appreciated that these various changes indicating hyperfunction, hypofunction, altered function, and focal degeneration can all occur within a single cell either simultaneously or sequentially. A damaged cell is not an inactive cell, and its reaction to injury may end in recovery. Parts injured beyond recovery are lysed or extruded, and the remaining structures reform the lost components.

The cell may return to normal but some alterations may persist. Thus the retention of an abnormal function is seen in metaplasia and perhaps also neoplasia. The reaction of damaged cells is a highly complex and varied affair, but so far as routine human pathology is concerned it is rarely possible to obtain tissue fresh enough to detect these intracellular events even if time and equipment were available.

Not all the changes described above occur under any single circumstance. Cells subjected to adverse conditions show a complex reaction: some changes may be regarded as degenerative, while others are adaptive. A liver cell showing cloudy swelling due to carbon tetrachloride poisoning would therefore not be expected to show the same changes as one infected with a virus, or a kidney cell damaged by hypoxia.

Chemical considerations of cell damage

Experimentally the liver cell has been most extensively investigated in respect of its reaction to chemicals. Several patterns of response have been delineated.

Pattern I. *Harmless Reaction.* The majority of chemicals are metabolized to harmless products, often by conjugation with glucuronic acid and subsequent excretion.

Pattern II. *Metabolic Imbalance.* A few chemicals produce an imbalance in the cells during their metabolism. Thus the methionine analogue ethionine induces ATP deficiency by excessive trapping of adenine.[5] A similar mechanism may explain the liver damage produced by ethanol. A knowledge of this mechanism is potentially very useful because, if the deficiency can be identified, it may also be remedied and cell damage averted.

Pattern III. *Activation to Toxic Metabolites.* Some chemicals are metabolized to highly reactive derivatives which then cause cellular damage. Carbon tetrachloride acts in this way. Often the active derivative of a drug can be trapped by sulphydryl-containing compounds such as glutathione. A depletion of glutathione may thus predispose to liver damage. The administration of methionine, by increasing the glutathione concentration, may protect the liver against toxic compounds. This has found practical application. Patients who take an overdose of acetaminophen (an analgesic sold as paracetamol, tylenol, campain, exdol, etc) may develop severe fatal liver damage. The administration of N-acetylcysteine, a glutathione substitute which combines with the hepatotoxic acetaminophen metabolite, is an effective antidote.[6]

Pattern IV. *Induction of Enzymes.* This has been described previously.

Pattern V. *Carcinogenesis.* Many carcinogens, e.g. the nitrosamines, are thought to be converted into active products which then lead to the poorly-understood changes that result in tumour initiation.

Nature of fatty change[5]

Electron microscopy has revealed that many normal cells contain small droplets of lipid, but (with the obvious exception of adipose cells) these are not visible on light microscopy. The lipid is found within the endoplasmic reticulum; this is well shown in the intestinal epithelial cells during fat absorption. Excessive accumulations of fat are found in response to many adverse conditions, e.g. hypoxia and poisoning. This occurs readily in the liver, and the lipid accumulations appear in the rough endoplasmic reticulum and sacs of the Golgi complex. Such membrane-bound lipid droplets are termed *liposomes*. Later, if the adverse conditions persist, much larger, non-membrane-bound lipid droplets appear and gradually fuse together until one droplet comes to occupy much of the cytoplasm. Precisely how the liposomes evolve into these droplets is not known, but the process may be related to a defect in the synthesis of components needed to package lipid in the Golgi complex. The excess fat that appears in damaged cells is derived from the fat depots in adipose tissue.

Depot fat is composed mostly of neutral fat, and when it is mobilized it is transported in the blood as free fatty acid bound to albumin. This is removed by the tissues and utilized for metabolic purposes. If the cells are damaged by hypoxia, poisoned, etc., their metabolic activity is impaired and the fat normally brought to them is inadequately utilized; it accumulates as droplets which are at first small, but later fuse into larger globules.

In the past the appearance of fine droplets was labelled *fatty degeneration*, while cells showing a large globule were said to show *fatty infiltration*. Clearly the pathogenesis is the same in each condition, and to avoid confusion both these terms have now been dropped, and *fatty change*, or *fatty metamorphosis*, substituted. It should not be confused with the accumulation of true fat cells in the tissues such as commonly occurs in the heart and pancreas of obese people. Similar local deposits of fat are also sometimes found accompanying chronic inflammation and following atrophy, e.g. of lymph nodes and thymus. These conditions are sometimes called fatty infiltration, but confusion is most easily avoided if the term *adiposity* is used. *Interstitial fatty infiltration* is an alternative name, but it must be clearly understood that the condition bears no relationship to the lesion depicted in Fig. 4.2, in which the excess neutral fat is in parenchymal cells.

Fatty change in the liver due to inadequate diet. The liver occupies a central position in fat metabolism. Non-esterified fatty acid derived from the adipose tissue is brought to it, metabolized, e.g. by conversion into phospholipids such as lecithin (phosphatidyl choline), and finally passed into the blood in the form of lipoproteins. If because of an inadequate diet there is a deficiency of choline, conversion cannot take place and neutral fat accumulates in the cells. This mechanism is the most probable cause of the fatty liver seen in starvation, and is particularly severe in kwashiorkor (p. 281). Paradoxically, overfed animals may also show fatty livers; this may be due to a relative deficiency of lipotropic substances. The fatty liver of chronic alcoholism may in part be due to malnutrition, but in addition there is the factor of a direct action on the liver of large amounts of ethanol, and cirrhosis is an important complication.

DAMAGE TO DNA[7]

Damage to DNA can occur in a variety of ways. An alteration in the sequence of nucleotides can occur as a result of a *mutation*. New nucleotides can be inserted as a result of *viral infection*. *Ultraviolet light* has the specific effect of causing damage to the bases without leading to a breakage of the polynucleotide chains. Dimers are formed between adjacent bases, especially thymine. This damage can be repaired by enzymatic action. First the chain is broken and the damaged segment is excised. A new section is then synthetized on the template provided by the undamaged chain. This is finally inserted into the chain by the action of a polynucleotide ligase. It follows that after the application of ultraviolet light to a tissue there is a burst of DNA synthesis which is not related to mitosis. This is termed *unscheduled DNA synthesis.* A defect in this repair mechanism occurs in xeroderma pigmentosum, and is related to the development of carcinoma.

Ionising radiations also cause DNA damage. Both chains of the molecule can be broken and this may lead to chromosomal breaks. If only one strand of the double helix is broken, the lesion can be repaired by a process similar to that described for ultraviolet-light damage.

CELL DEATH AND NECROSIS

Cell death is difficult to define in precise terms, but in practice may be regarded as having occurred whenever a cell is incapable of further division or of continuing its normal synthetic functions.

The appearance of the dead cells varies according to the cause of the injury. If the cells are killed suddenly as the result of physical or chemical trauma, initially they show no changes other than those directly attributable to the agent concerned, e.g. disruption in electrical injuries, effects of freezing, burning, etc.

Cells less severely damaged, e.g. by poisons, may develop biochemical lesions which first result in changes previously described as degenerative, e.g. cloudy swelling and fatty change. It will be recalled that the changes detectable by light microscopy are cytoplasmic, and in themselves do not indicate cell death.

In the dead cell respiration ceases, but glycolysis proceeds for a while and results in the production of lactic acid and therefore a drop in the pH. The synthetic activities of the cell stop, but the lytic destructive enzymes continue their work. These enzymes derived from lysosomes are most active at a low pH, and include a wide range of proteases, lipases, esterases, deoxyribonuclease, ribonuclease, etc. The cell undergoes a process of *self-digestion*, or *autolysis*, and within a few hours shows certain morphological changes (see below) by which cell death can be recognized. This is called *necrosis* and it may be defined as the *circumscribed death of cells or tissues with structural evidence of their death.* Necrosis and cell death are therefore not synonymous.

The microscopic changes of necrosis that occur affect the whole cell. The *cytoplasm* becomes homogeneous and often brightly eosinophilic; these early autolytic changes may resemble those seen in the degenerative lesions of living cells. Following cell death, however, the nucleus also shows autolytic changes, and it is these which are to be regarded as pathognomonic (absolutely diagnostic) of necrosis.

Nuclear changes of necrosis. The nucleus becomes smaller, while the chromatin loses its fine reticular pattern, becomes clumped, and stains intensely. This is termed *pyknosis.* The pyknotic nucleus either breaks up into fragments (*karyorrhexis*), or becomes indistinct as the nuclear material is digested (*karyolysis*).

Diagnosis of necrosis by biochemical means

A diagnosis of the occurrence of necrosis is frequently of great clinical importance. When areas of heart muscle, pancreas, liver, or brain are dying the patient's life is often in jeopardy. As necrosis occurs, various soluble substances, e.g. enzymes, diffuse out of the cells and are absorbed into the blood stream, and their detection is an aid to clinical diagnosis. Some examples may be cited. A raised plasma level of creatine phosphokinase (CPK) is found after skeletal-muscle necrosis, and is also elevated in some types of myopathy (see also p. 415). Plasma glutamate oxaloacetate transaminase (SGOT), hydroxybutyrate dehydrogenase (HBD), CPK, and lactate dehydrogenase (LHD) are all raised after myocardial infarction. Increased plasma glutamate pyruvate transaminase (SGPT) and LDH are found after liver-cell necrosis. Some enzymes can be separated into separate fractions by electrophoresis. In the case of LDH these *isoenzymes* are of different origin: LDH_1 and LDH_2 are released from heart muscle, while LDH_5 is of hepatic origin.

Types of necrosis

Coagulative necrosis

Necrotic tissue usually becomes firm and slightly swollen. It seems likely that the proteins are denatured. This process involves an unfolding of the three-dimensional arrangement of the molecule without necessarily changing its empirical formula. This causes the tissue to become opaque and firm, as does the white of an egg on boiling. It also becomes more reactive chemically, and side-chains previously saturated become exposed and are available for binding. This explains why the tissue initially binds dyes, e.g. eosin, more avidly than does normal tissue. Thus an increased eosinophilia of heart muscle fibres is a useful *post-mortem* indication of a recent myocardial infarct, and the magnitude of hypoxic brain damage can be judged by the extent and degree of the eosinophilia of the cortical neurons in patients who have died shortly after an episode of cerebral ischaemia, e.g. following cardiac arrest. The increased binding capacity of necrotic tissue might also be a factor in causing *dystrophic calcification* (p. 300).

A common cause of necrosis is sudden deprivation of the blood supply to a part. This is called *infarction*, and is quite common in the heart and kidney when their supplying arteries are occluded. These infarcts show the typical changes of coagulative necrosis. Microscopically, in addition to the nuclear changes, another feature is noteworthy: the general architecture of the tissue is still recognizable, even though its constituent cells are all dead. This is therefore called *structured necrosis*. In other examples of coagulative necrosis microscopic examination of the dead tissue fails to reveal any structure—this is *structureless necrosis*. The caseous necrosis of tuberculosis is an example of this (p. 215).

Necrosis in certain tissues presents special features. In adipose tissue fat is liberated from the damaged cells, and is phagocytosed by macrophages. These cells, distended with fat, are called *foam cells*. Deposition of cholesterol crystals, giant-cell formation, and fibrosis complete the microscopic picture of *traumatic fat necrosis* (Fig. 4.4). The condition is seen in the breast following injury, and may resemble tuberculosis histologically. Another type of fat necrosis occurs in the peritoneum whenever lipase escapes from the pancreas, as after its injury or inflammation (acute pancreatitis). Necrosis of collagen is decribed on p. 69.

Colliquative necrosis

This is necrosis with softening, and rarely occurs as a primary event except in infarcts of the brain. Liquefaction is seen as a secondary event in suppuration (p. 81), and following caseation (p. 217).

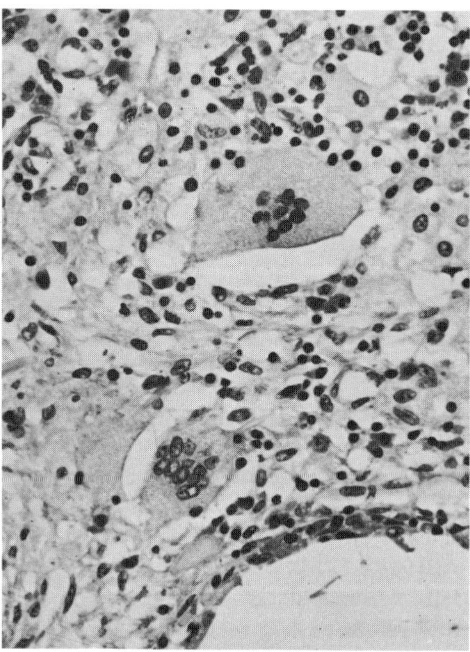

Fig. 4.4 Traumatic fat necrosis of breast. The adipose tissue cells have an opaque, granular cytoplasm due to the breakdown of neutral fat and the production of fatty acid. Two large foreign body giant cells with a foamy, fat-filled cytoplasm are present. × 180.

FURTHER CHANGES IN NECROTIC TISSUE

Necrotic tissue usually excites an *acute inflammatory reaction* followed by a phase of *healing* (Fig. 4.5): these events are considered in later chapters. An occasional complication is gangrene.

Gangrene

Sometimes the dead tissue is invaded by saprophytic protein-splitting anaerobic bacteria, which cause its decomposition with the production of hydrogen sulphide and other foul-smelling substances. There is blackening of the area due to the formation of iron sulphide from the iron of decomposed haemoglobin. This *necrosis with superadded putrefaction* is called *gangrene*, an old clinical term which was applied to any black, foul-smelling area in continuity with the living.

Clostridial gangrene

The putrefactive bacteria are usually the clostridia of intestinal origin, and therefore necrosis of the bowel is often followed by gangrene. These putrefactive bacteria are of little importance in themselves, because they live on dead tissue and do not invade or harm the living tissue; nevertheless, gangrenous lesions always contain other bacteria which can cause futher tissue destruction. It follows that gangrene is a very serious condition, and *unless treated expeditiously is fatal.*

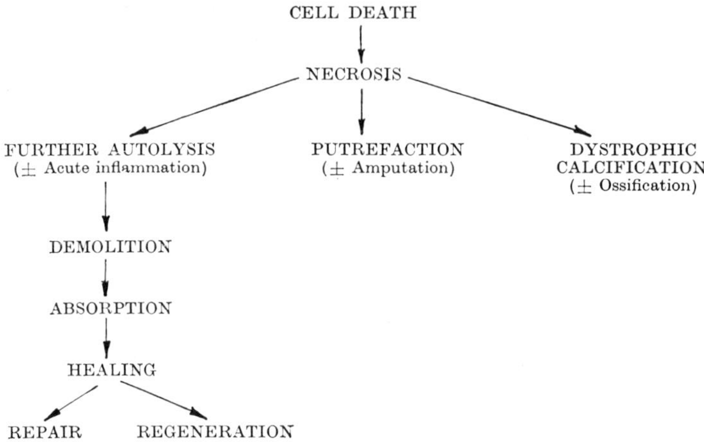

Fig. 4.5 The sequelae of cell death.

Gangrene of the limbs. This is usually seen in the legs following arterial obstruction (p. 502). It is particularly common in diabetic patients. The limb becomes swollen and black ('wet gangrene'), and in addition to the putrefactive bacteria there are also pathogenic organisms present, which invade the adjacent living tissue. Gangrene of this type therefore steadily spreads.

If the blood supply to a limb is *slowly* obstructed, the tips of the digits become black and necrotic, and at the same time undergo desiccation. This greatly impedes bacterial growth, and infection with pathogenic organisms is not a feature. The condition slowly extends until a point is reached where the blood supply to the tissue is adequate. A line of demarcation develops, and the dead tissue is discarded by a process of spontaneous amputation. This condition is called '*dry gangrene*', but since the amount of putrefaction is minimal, the term is somewhat of a misnomer. The process is in fact mummification of an infarcted portion of a limb.

Gangrene due to other organisms. Some putrefactive bacteria are also pathogenic, e.g. certain strains of anaerobic streptococci (p. 205) and members of the family *Bacteroidaceae.* The latter includes the well-known member *Fusobacterium fusiforme*, which is often found in the company of *Borrelia vincenti* ('Vincent's organisms').

The putrefactive organisms mentioned are frequently associated with the common type of ulcerative gingivitis (Vincent's infection, or 'trench mouth'). It affects the free gingiva and the interdental papillae, and may be either acute or run a chronic relapsing course. A more severe gangrenous lesion which affects the soft tissues of the face, and may involve the bone is called *cancrum oris*, or *noma*, and occurs in malnourished debilitated children following an infectious disease, particularly measles.[8] Extensive tissue destruction occurs. This condition is almost unknown in Britain and North America, but is not uncommon in developing countries.

Gangrene of the lung. A putrid lung abscess is an occasional complication of dental extraction under general anaesthesia, when the root of a tooth is inhaled and lodges in a bronchus. Once again organisms belonging to the family *Bacteroidaceae* are responsible for the putrefaction.

DAMAGE TO CONNECTIVE TISSUE

Abnormalities of collagen

The amount of collagen in a tissue is determined by a balance between collagen catabolism (presumably effected by collagenases) and the rate of collagen formation. Excessive catabolism, diminished synthesis, or a combination of the two lead to atrophy. The converse situation leads to fibrosis. It is unfortunate that in many human pathological conditions we are ignorant of the precise mechanisms involved and can only describe the end-results—either *atrophy* or *fibrosis.*

Collagen atrophy

There are many conditions in which collagen degradation exceeds collagen synthesis. *Glucocorticoids* inhibit collagen synthesis, and if administered in large doses over a prolonged period lead to generalized collagen atrophy. Thus the skin becomes paper-thin, and bleeding follows mild injury. Osteoporosis (p. 585) poses a major threat. Local injections of glucocorticoids into the skin lead to dermal atrophy: this action is utilized in the treatment of keloids (p. 126), but the results are indifferent.[9]

Excessive production of collagenase is thought to be important in the pathogenesis of several diseases. In *rheumatoid arthritis* the destruction of the joint cartilage has been ascribed to the presence of collagenase produced by the synovium. The destruction of alveolar bone that leads to loss of teeth in *chronic periodontal disease* has likewise been attributed to collagenase activity.

In old age there is a generalized atrophy of collagen and there is an increased cross-linkage between adjacent fibrils. Hence the amount of extractable soluble collagen decreases with age.

Fibrosis

An increase in the amount of collagen, or *fibrosis*, is a common finding in chronic inflammation (see p. 139), and is a feature of any condition in which granulation tissue is formed. Thus myocardial fibrosis is the end-result of myocardial ischaemia as areas of necrotic muscle fibres are replaced by scar tissue.

In those organs where collagen fibril development is incomplete, the fibrils may mature to form histological collagen. This may explain fibrosis in organs like the spleen and lung.

Hyalinization

The term hyaline is used in a purely descriptive capacity—it literally means glassy and is employed to describe any homogeneous eosinophilic material. Necrotic cells may take on this appearance, and under particular circumstances they have by tradition been described as hyalinized. Sometimes homogeneous areas in cells have been called hyaline. Thus eosinophilic areas in degenerating liver cells in the alcoholic patient have been called 'alcoholic hyaline'.

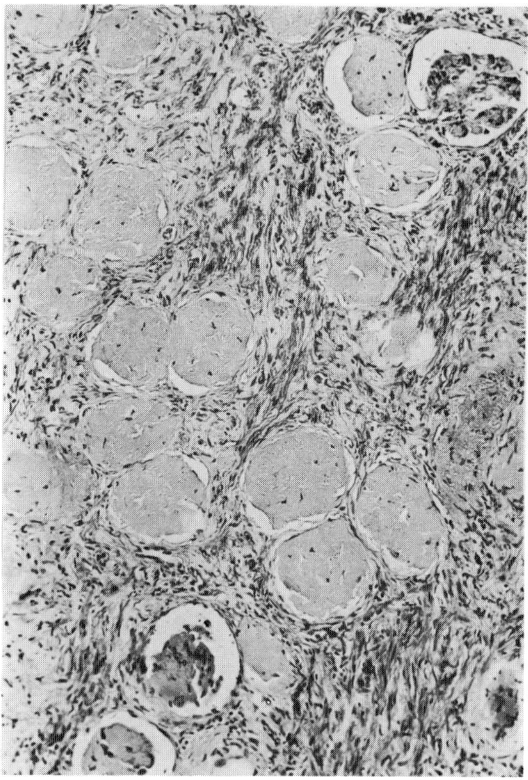

Fig. 4.6 Hyalinized glomerular tufts. Most of the glomeruli have been converted into dense, solid masses of hyalinized material, virtually devoid of cellular components. The section is from a case of chronic pyelonephritis. ×65.

Hyaline can also be used to describe extracellular material, and it is in relation to the connective tissues that the term is most commonly used. In collagen, with the passage of time, the fibres appear to fuse together to form a glassy, eosinophilic material. This hyalinization is very common in fibrous tissue which has been laid down as a replacement for lost parenchyma. Therefore it is very common in scars of any type (Fig. 4.6) and in chronic inflammatory lesions. Hyaline material is also seen in the intima of small blood vessels ('vascular hyaline'); it is a normal ageing process in the spleen, but in other organs, especially the kidneys, it is associated with hypertension. Amyloid may also be described as hyaline material (p. 436).

Necrosis of collagen

Sometimes when connective tissue is damaged, its associated fibrocytes undergo necrosis and its fibres appear to degenerate. They break up, and are removed in the course of an inflammatory reaction. This necrosis of collagen differs from hyalinization in several important respects.

1. Hyaline material is extremely stable. Necrotic collagen, on the other hand, is either removed or organized.

2. Hyalinized collagen retains the staining characteristics of normal collagen. Necrotic collagen, on the other hand, stains brightly with eosin and in fact takes on many of the staining characteristics of fibrin, e.g. it is PAS positive. The term *fibrinoid necrosis* is therefore often used. Fibrinoid necrosis is seen in the *walls of small blood vessels* in a variety of conditions: malignant hypertension (p. 478), the Arthus phenomenon (p. 185), and the generalized Shwartzman reaction (p. 105). The necrotic material may be degenerating collagen, damaged muscle, fibrin, or antigen-antibody complexes. Fibrinoid necrosis, like hyalinization, describes a particular microscopic appearance and does not imply a single morphological change or aetiological agent.

Fibrinoid necrosis occurs in collagen following severe injury, e.g. burning and exposure to ionizing radiation, and is also a feature of some collagen diseases (p. 303). It is particularly prominent in rheumatoid arthritis, and the fibrinoid material, which appears to be altered collagen, excites a chronic inflammatory reaction. The necrosis is sometimes called necrobiosis, which is unfortunate because this same term is also used to describe the physiological death of cells (p. 317).

Changes in elastic tissue

An increase in the number of fibres which stain black with orcein like elastic is a common finding in the dermis, and is a reaction to prolonged exposure to the ultraviolet light of sunshine. While there is little doubt that new elastic fibres can be formed in the adult, in *elastosis* of the skin the fibres are probably altered or damaged collagen.

Changes in the ground substance

Sometimes the connective tissue shows an excessive accumulation of ground substance, which appears as a basophilic pool of structureless material. This overhydration of the ground substance is sometimes a physiological event and appears to be under hormonal control: thus the colourful swelling of the sexual skin of the baboon is in large part due to this change. However, sometimes the associated connective tissue fibres undergo degeneration, and the condition is called *myxomatous degeneration.* A good example of this is seen in the aorta, where owing to the resulting weakness in the vessel its wall may rupture with dramatic effects (p. 491).

There is a group of genetically determined diseases involving an abnormality in the metabolism of mucopolysaccharide (*the mucopolysaccharidoses*). They are usually accompanied by skeletal deformities. The best known member of this uncommon group of diseases is *Hurler's syndrome*, which because of the grotesque appearance of the head is also known as *gargoylism*. Specialized texts should be consulted for details.[10]

In this chapter some of the effects of cellular damage have been considered. Local injury is usually the prelude to inflammation and healing, and these are described in the chapters that follow. They are all local events, but it must not be forgotten that any injury, except the most trivial, is accompanied by a generalized response. This is considered in Chapter 8. Injury initiates changes which involve the whole individual, and it is a mistake to think of the reaction to injury solely in terms of local cellular degeneration or necrosis. Likewise at a clinical level, not only must the injuries be treated, but also the patient.

REFERENCES

1. Peters R A 1963 Biochemical lesions and lethal synthesis. Pergamon Press, Oxford
2. Trump B F, Goldblatt P J, Stowell R E 1965 Studies on necrosis of mouse liver *in vitro*; ultrastructural alterations in the mitochondria of hepatic parenchymal cells. Laboratory Investigation 14: 343
3. Magee P N 1966 Toxic liver necrosis. Laboratory Investigation 15: 111
4. Hruban Z, Slesers A, Hopkins E 1972 Drug-induced and naturally occurring myeloid bodies. Laboratory Investigation 27: 62
5. Farber E, Lombardi B, Castillo A E 1963 The prevention by adenosine triphosphate of the fatty liver induced by ethionine. Laboratory Investigation 12: 873
6. Rumack B H, Matthew H 1975 Acetaminophen poisoning and toxicity. Pediatrics 55: 871
7. Baserga R 1972 Pathology of DNA. In: Farber E (ed) The pathology of transcription and translation, Marcel Dekker, New York, p 2
8. Linenberg W B, Schmitt J, Harpole H J 1961 Noma, report of a case. Oral Surgery, Oral Medicine and Oral Pathology 14: 1138
9. Calnan J 1977 Keloid and Dupuytren's contracture. Annals of the Rheumatic Diseases 36: Supplement No 2, 18
10. McKusick V A 1972 Heritable disorders of connective tissue, 4th edn. Mosby, St Louis, 878 pp

5

The acute inflammatory reaction

Acute inflammation is one of the fundamental reactions of the body to injury, and although its pathogenesis is complex, the main features of the response are relatively simple and familiar to anyone who has ever experienced a boil. The area is *red, swollen, warmer* than the surrounding skin, and is *painful*. These four, *rubor, tumor, calor,* and *dolor*, are the *cardinal signs of inflammation* as described by Celsus (first century A.D.). Loss of function has been added subsequently but its origin is obscure. To attribute it to Galen is to perpetuate a misconception which has been handed down by many authors. Its Latin version *functio laesa* gives this origin an air of respectability but not truth.[1]

The suffix -itis is used to denote an inflammatory lesion, e.g. appendicitis or pulpitis. Unfortunately tradition sometimes demands that this rule be broken—e.g. osteitis fibrosa cystica is not an inflammatory lesion.

Causes of acute inflammation

Since the inflammatory reaction is a response to injury, its causes are those of cell damage. These may be enumerated briefly:

Physical agents. Trauma, e.g. mechanical injury such as cutting and crushing, heat, cold, and ionizing radiation.

Chemical agents. There are innumerable chemicals which injure cells. Many, like corrosive acids, alkalis, and phenol, are fairly non-specific in their action, while others affect particular cells, e.g. mercuric chloride causes renal tubular necrosis.

Deprivation of blood supply. Infarction is described in Chapter 31.

Living organisms. Inflammation is often a feature of infection.

Antigen-antibody reactions. Damage mediated by sensitizing immunoglobulins, immune complexes, and sensitized lymphocytes is described in Chapter 13.

CHANGES IN ACUTE INFLAMMATION

The vascular response

Hyperaemia. Changes in the blood vessels are the most obvious manifestation of acute inflammation. Following trauma there may be an initial constriction of the blood vessels, but this is soon followed by a prolonged period of vasodilatation. It affects the arterioles, so that more blood passes into the area. Tissues near the skin surface are normally cooler than the arterial blood which supplies them, and, as the blood flow increases, so the area becomes warmer. This explains the *calor* of inflammation. The first result of arteriolar dilatation is that the blood flows by the most direct route to the veins through the *central*, or *thoroughfare, channels.* Subsequent opening of the precapillary sphincters allows blood to pass into the capillary bed, and vessels which were temporarily shut down become functional. The inflamed part therefore appears to contain an increased number of vessels. In addition, their calibre is increased. The whole area shows *hyperaemia*, i.e. it contains more blood and appears red (*rubor*). If incised it bleeds profusely.

Inflammation can be studied by examining fixed sections of tissue, but it is in the living animal that a truer picture of its ever-changing manifestations can be appreciated. Cohnheim based much of his classical description of inflammation on his observations on the tongue of the frog. The mesentery of the rat and the rabbit ear-chamber (p. 116) can also be used. Using these methods *changes in the blood flow* are particularly prominent.

Changes in blood flow. In the arterioles of normal tissue the blood flow is so fast that the individual cells cannot be identified other than by the use of high-speed photography. In the venules the flow is considerably slower but it is still difficult to identify individual cells. However, they can be seen to travel in the central, or axial, part of the stream and leave a clear, cell-free *plasmatic zone* adjacent to the endothelium. In acutely inflamed tissue the velocity of the blood increases at first, but it soon diminishes. *Stasis* ensues, and coincidentally the clear plasmatic zone becomes occupied by innumerable colourless, glistening white blood cells. This is called *margination of the white cells*, and very soon the endothelium becomes covered, or *pavemented*, by them. This phenomenon is very characteristic of acute inflammation, and is due to changes in the vascular endothelium—the cells become swollen and *sticky*. White cells which strike the endothelium by chance, instead of bouncing off and passing on their way, are dragged back and retained. The white cells, for the most part polymorphs, soon push pseudopodia between adjacent endothelial cells, penetrate the basement membrane, and emerge on the external surface of the venule. This remarkable process is called *emigration of the white cells*, and eventually large numbers of them accumulate in the extravascular space. The gap in the vessel wall closes up behind the emigrating white cells; a few red cells may, however, be forced out passively by the hydrostatic pressure of the blood. This is called *diapedesis of the red cells*, and must be distinguished from frank haemorrhage due to destruction of the vessel wall.

The inflammatory exudate

The most important feature of acute inflammation is the formation of the *inflammatory exudate*, This is a collection of fluid in the extravascular tissues and consists of:

The fluid exudate
The cellular exudate.

The fluid exudate

The really crucial factor in the formation of an inflammatory exudate is an *increased permeability of the vessel walls to plasma proteins.* If trypan blue is injected intravenously into an animal (a 'blued animal'), the dye becomes bound to the plasma albumin and does not readily leave the circulation. When an inflammatory response is elicited, the tagged albumin can be seen to pass into the inflamed area as the exudate forms. This experimental method is often used to demonstrate an increase in permeability to plasma proteins. A similar type of labelling may be done with radioactive iodine. In experimentally produced acute inflammation, it has been found that exudation of fluid occurs in several phases. Two phases were originally recognized—an *early transient phase,* mediated by histamine and due to leakage from venules, and a *prolonged delayed phase,* which required several hours

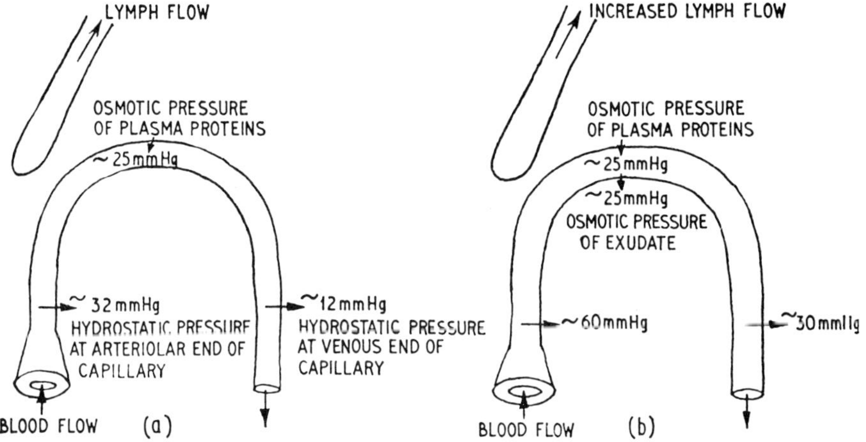

Fig. 5.1 Fluid exchange between blood and tissue spaces: (a) under normal conditions, (b) in acute inflammation.

to develop and was attributed to capillary damage. The situation is more complex than this, and other patterns of reaction have been described:

Immediate-transient phase. This lasts about 30 minutes, affects venules, and is largely mediated by histamine.

Immediate-prolonged phase. The exudation starts immediately but persists for days. It appears to be due to direct damage to vessels.

Delayed-prolonged phase. Capillaries and venules are affected both by direct injury of the agent (e.g. heat) and by chemical mediators.

Mechanism of formation of the fluid exudate. As is described in detail in Chapter 28, the exchange of fluid between the blood vessel lumen and the interstitial tissues is related to the hydrostatic blood pressure within the vessel which drives the fluid out, and the effective, or colloidal, plasma osmotic pressure, also called the *plasma oncotic pressure,* which draws it into the blood vessel (Fig. 5.1). The effective osmotic pressure is due to the plasma proteins which are too large to pass through the vessel walls. Smaller molecules exchange with ease. In acute inflammation four mechanisms operate to cause fluid to leave the blood vessels and form the interstitial exudate.

1. There is an *increased vascular permeability* to plasma proteins. In this way the restraining colloidal osmotic pressure of the plasma is removed, and the hydrostatic pressure is free to drive a protein-rich fluid into the tissues. An exudate has virtually the same protein composition as plasma.

2. There is an *increase in the capillary blood pressure* due to arteriolar dilatation.

3. There is *breakdown of large-molecule tissue proteins* into many small, osmotically-active fragments.

4. There is an *increase in the fluidity of the tissue ground substance.* This has the effect of allowing exudate to diffuse more readily, thereby preventing an immediate rise in tissue tension. A rise in tissue tension is probably the important limiting factor in stopping the accumulation of tissue fluids both under normal conditions and those of acute inflammation. For this reason inflammatory oedema is a prominent feature of inflammation involving, or adjacent to, very lax tissues such as the eyelids and the scrotum. Swelling is not a feature of an infection involving a tissue under tension such as the pulp of a finger.

Since by far the most important factor leading to the formation of the fluid exudate is the increase in vascular permeability, it is not surprising that this has been intensively studied. Two phases of exudation occur after many kinds of injury. The *immediate phase* is obvious in a minute or so and is over within an hour. Then follows a *delayed phase*, which may itself have several components, and this lasts for many hours. In mild thermal injury to the rat cremaster muscle, the immediate phase is accompanied by venular damage while the delayed response is related to capillary damage. However, in turpentine injury to the rat pleura, both phases are due to venular damage and there is an additional capillary component to the delayed phase. With severe damage the various phases so overlap each other that only one prolonged phase is apparent. The precise response therefore depends upon the tissue involved, the irritant used, and the species of animal. There is evidence that the two phases are mediated by different agents, and this is described later in the section on chemical mediators.

Vascular permeability in normal tissues. Normally the walls of the capillaries and venules are freely permeable to water and electrolytes but not to proteins and other large molecules. Rapid exchange takes place between intravascular and extravascular water, and in fact about 70 per cent of the water in the blood crosses the vessel wall every minute and is replaced by water from the interstitial space. The mechanism whereby this exchange takes place has been much debated. In most tissues the barriers which must be considered are:

1. The endothelial cell
2. The basement membrane, which forms a complete sheath
3. Pericytes, which form a discontinuous outer coat together with connective tissue fibres.

The following possiblities have been suggested:

Direct transport through the cell by simple diffusion. The lipid (and presumably waterproof) nature of the cell membrane has led many authorities to regard this as an unlikely mechanism.

Transport across the endothelial cell by cytopempsis (p. 9). This process does probably take place, but it seems unlikely that it could explain the large volume of fluid which is known to leave the vessels. Furthermore, the vesicles formed by micropinocytosis would be expected to contain protein, but the fluid which escapes from the blood vessels has a low plasma protein content.

Passage through pores in the endothelial cells. Pores are present in the sinusoids of the liver; in certain other sites, e.g. kidney and intestine, there are fenestrations which are covered by a very thin membrane. In other areas no pores or fenestrations can be seen on electron microscopy.

Passage through spaces between the endothelial cells. The endothelial cells closely adjoin each other and the gap between them is about 15 nm wide. Junctional complexes are present, and in the zonula adherens (Fig. 2.4) the central fused membrane is about 4 nm thick.

The relative importance of these possible methods of transport is not clear at the present time.

A final consideration concerns the basement membrane, since all substances leaving or entering the vessel must cross it. The membrane appears to have no holes nor does it seem to be a barrier to the passage of water or electrolytes. Cells, large particles, and perhaps the plasma proteins are held back and their passage delayed.

Vascular permeability in inflamed tissue. Examination of the endothelial cells of capillaries in acutely inflamed tissue has revealed several changes—increase in the number and size of the micropinocytotic vesicles, blebs under the luminal cell membrane, and projections or spikes arising from the membrane. The changes are, however, inconstant and seem inadequate to explain the great increase in vascular permeability. On the other hand, it has been shown that when 5-hydroxytryptamine or histamine is applied to rat cremaster muscle important changes occur in the venules. Gaps (0.1 to 0.4 μm in diameter) appear in the endothelial lining due to the separation of adjacent endothelial cells.

If the animal is first given an intravenous injection of mercuric sulphide suspension, the particles, which are 10 to 15 nm in diameter, are found to be situated between the endothelial cell and the basement membrane. It appears therefore that in acute inflammation the gap between endothelial cells widens, thereby allowing plasma to reach the basement membrane and escape to the extravascular spaces. The particles of mercuric sulphide being unable to penetrate the intact basement membrane accumulate between it and the endothelial cell (Fig. 5.2).

Similar results are obtained if India ink is used and trauma applied to produce an acute inflammation. Thus, both the early exudation of acute inflammation and the application of histamine are associated with a separation of the endothelial cells and an escape of plasma. Whether other changes occur, for instance in the basement membrane, and whether the prolonged phase of exudation is associated with other features, is not yet clear.

As plasma escapes from the vessels, the plasmatic zone becomes reduced in size. This zone has great functional importance, for the viscosity of plasma is much lower than that of whole blood, and therefore the peripheral resistance is lower than it would be if the blood components were intimately mixed. In inflammation the lubricating action of this zone is impaired or lost and the blood stream slows. This is the explanation of the *statis* of inflammation, and it may be so marked that thrombosis sometimes supervenes. This may cause further tissue damage.

Function of the fluid exudate. All the constituents of the plasma are poured into the area of inflammation. These include natural antibacterial substances, like complement, as well as specific antibodies. Drugs and antibiotics, if present in the plasma, will also appear in the exudate. The importance of the early administation of therapeutic agents is obvious when it is remembered that they are merely carried to the inflamed area in the exudate, and are in no way concentrated there. The fluid of the exudate (*inflammatory oedema*) has the effect of diluting any

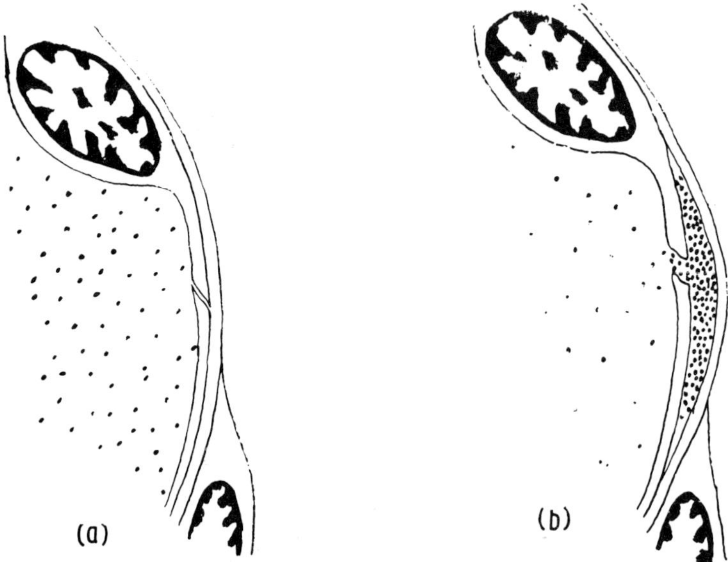

Figure 5.2 Diagrammatic representation of the changes in a venule following the intravenous injection of a suspension of mercuric sulphide (particle size 10–15 nm). (*a*) Shows the wall of normal venule with the particles distributed in the plasma. (*b*) After the local application of histamine. The appearances suggest that the plasma has leaked through the gap between the endothelial cells, and that the basement membrane has held back the particles but allowed the fluid exudate to pass through.

irritant substance causing the inflammation. The fibrinogen in it is converted into fibrin by the action of prothrombinase (p. 464) and a *fibrin clot* forms.

This fibrin has three main functions:

1. It forms a *union between severed tissues*, as in a cut
2. It may form a *barrier against bacterial invasion* (p. 108)
3. It aids phagocytosis (p. 79).

The exudate accounts for the remaining cardinal signs of inflammation. It causes swelling (*tumor*), and the increased tissue tension is an important factor in the causation of pain (*dolor*), which is particularly severe in tissues that cannot swell readily, e.g. the pulp space of a finger, the pulp of a tooth (where pain is the only symptom), and the medullary cavity of a bone. Pain limits activity, and this explains the loss of function.

Changes in the lymphatics. The small lymphatics of a tissue form a blind-ended system of vessels, which closely resemble the vascular capillaries except that a basement membrane is incomplete or absent and their walls are permeable to proteins. One of their main functions is to allow any plasma protein which has escaped from the blood vessels to drain away and ultimately reach the blood stream again. In acute inflammation the lymph vessels are held widely open, the permeability of the wall is increased, and the flow of fluid, containing excess protein, is augmented.

The cellular exudate

The emigration of the white cells and their accumulation in the extravascular space has already been described (p. 72). These cells accumulate at the same time

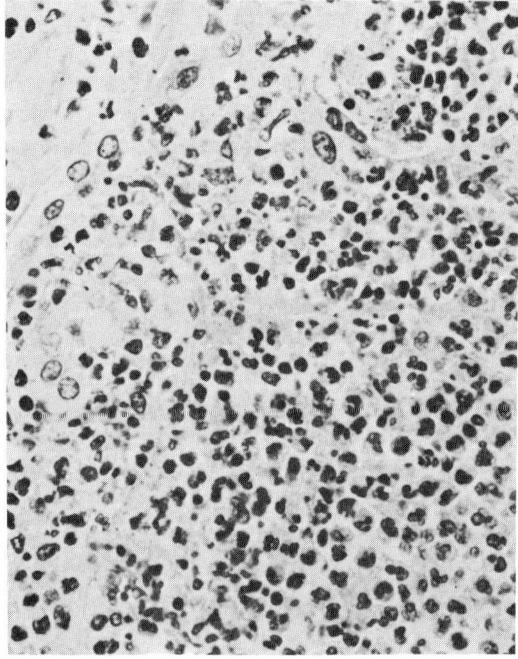

Figure 5.3 Suppurative pyelonephritis. The structure of the kidney is almost completely destroyed except for some degenerated tubular elements at the top of the figure. There is a very heavy infiltration of polymorphs, most of which show disintegration (pus cells). × 165

as the fluid exudate forms; they constitute the cellular component of the exudate (Fig. 5.3). At first the majority of the cells are neutrophil polymorphonuclear leucocytes, but later monocytes predominate. Within a few days the polymorphs undergo necrosis but the mononuclears remain. It therefore follows that *the cellular exudate changes from polymorphonuclear initially to mononuclear at a later stage.*

Mechanism of formation of the cellular exudate. The stimulus which impels the white cells to force their way through the vascular wall and move to the area of tissue damage is generally thought to be the attraction of some chemical substance. Such directional movement in response to a chemical gradient is well known in biology, and is called *chemotaxis*. The *Boyden chamber* has facilitated the study of the possible mediators. Polymorphs are placed in the upper of a double tissue-culture chamber; the chambers are separated by a membrane of 3 μm pore size. Test substances are placed in the lower chamber, and the number of cells migrating to the lower side of the filter is a measure of the chemotactic effect.

Both neutrophil polymorphs and monocytes have been shown to be attracted *in vitro* to a number of agents; these include starch and certain bacteria. Antigen-antibody complexes and dead tissue are chemotactic, but only if complement is activated. The activated trimolecular complex $C\overline{576}$ and the anaphylatoxins C3a and C5a are also chemotactic agents. Kallikrein and some fibrinopeptides have also been claimed as chemotactic agents.

With monocytes chemotaxis has also been demonstrated, and they appear to react to many of the substances which attract polymorphs. The change in the cell population of the exudate from neutrophils in the early stages of acute inflammation to monocytes later on has been the topic of frequent speculation. One explanation is that the polymorphs which have short life-span (3 to 4 days at most), soon die and disappear. The long-lived monocytes remain, an effect that could be accentuated by the presence of the migration-inhibition factor (p. 189). The relative number of monocytes would steadily increase. Another possibility is that the monocytes undergo division before assuming macrophage activity.

A number of observations now suggest that some chemotactic agents are selective in their action. Thus, when sensitized lymphocytes react with antigen, factors called lymphokines are released (p. 157). Some of these are chemotactic agents, and separate agents affect neutrophils, monocytes, and eosinophils. The reaction of antigen with mast cells sensitized by IgE causes the release of an agent that is chemotactic for eosinophils (see ECF-A, p. 183). This could well explain why these cells are prominent in some of the inflammatory lesions associated with atopy and also in many parasitic infections.

The varied and changing population of inflammatory cells found in inflammatory disease would be more easily understood if selective chemotaxis were the mechanism. Precisely how the phagocytes sense the presence of a chemical gradient and respond to it is not known. Movement is presumed to involve the actin-myosin contractile elements associated with the microfilaments of the cell. The energy needed is derived from the hexose monophosphate shunt. One final point deserves consideration: so far no substance has been found to be chemotactic for lymphocytes. How they traverse the vessel wall and why, are questions that remain unanswered. Lymphocytes are found in certain inflammations, particularly viral infections and acute dermatitis.

Function of the cellular exudate: Phagocytosis. The major function of neutrophils and macrophages is phagocytosis. They ingest foreign particles as well as bacteria. Phagocytosis is aided by two mechanisms:

1. *Opsonins.* These are proteins present in the plasma which coat organisms and cause them to be more easily phagocytosed. It is believed that they cover up noxious surface antigens. Two types are recognized:

(a) *Non-specific opsonins*, which are present in all normal individuals.

(b) *Immune opsonins*, which are a type of antibacterial antibody, and are therefore specific for each organism. It follows that phagocytosis is more marked in the individual who has been immunized against the particular infecting organism.

2. *Surface phagocytosis.* Phagocytes can ingest organisms even in the absence of

opsonins, if a suitable framework is provided in which they can trap the organism. Fibrin provides such a surface, and the process is called surface phagocytosis.

Both polymorphs and monocytes have surface receptors for the Fc component of immunoglobulin as well as for C3. Hence these cells adhere to particles coated with antibody or complement, and this is soon followed by phagocytosis. It will be readily appreciated therefore that activation of complement is an important process in the mediation of phagocytosis, since membrane-bound C3b is recognized by cell receptors of the phagocytes. Opsonization also aids the phagocytosis of bacteria by the RE system.

The energy for phagocytosis both by polymorphs and macrophages is derived mainly from anaerobic glycolysis. Phagocytosis of a particle is accompanied by the production of lactic acid (p. 107). Following phagocytosis a series of metabolic events occur that have been called the 'respiratory burst', since they result in a dramatic increase in glucose utilization through the hexose monophosphate shunt. This burst of oxidative metabolism results in the formation of powerful oxidizing agents, such as H_2O_2, which are essential for the intracellular destruction of bacteria (p. 107).

Fate of ingested particles. Material ingested by neutrophils is enclosed in phagocytic vacuoles, the membrane of which fuses with that of the granules—both the specific ones and the azurophil granules. The lysosomal enzymes thus enter the phagosomes, and as digestion vacuoles are formed the neutrophils undergo degranulation. It is not difficult to envisage how lysosomal enzymes could escape from the cell as lysosomal membranes fuse with those of the phagosomes as they are formed. The cells also release *pyrogen*, which is a major factor in the pathogenesis of the fever that accompanies acute inflammation.

Fate of ingested bacteria. The mechanisms whereby intracellular organisms are destroyed are described on pages 106 to 107.

Macrophages. These cells are highly phagocytic and play an important role in the destruction of micro-organisms and in the demolition phase of the inflammatory reaction. This is considered below. In addition to this they have a *secretor function.*[2] Factors which they are thought to release, particularly when engaged in phagocytosis, include: *endogenous pyrogen, lysosomal enzymes, lysozyme, plasminogen activator, collagenase, elastase,* and *complement components* particularly C4 and C2. Some other factors appear to stimulate adjacent cells. Thus there is the *colony stimulating factor* (p. 458) and a fibroblast stimulating factor (p. 139). Other factors act on lymphocytes, either functioning as mitogens or else stimulating them to activity, e.g. Ig production in the case of B cells, or helper function in the case of T cells. Finally the macrophages play a part in the initiation of the immune response, probably by processing antigen. In turn their activity as effector cells is modified and stimulated by lymphokines released by sensitized lymphocytes.

Eosinophils.[3,4] These cells are found instead of the usual neutrophil leucocytes in inflammation produced by helminthic parasites, e.g. ascariasis and schistosomiasis, and also in some allergic conditions (asthma and hay fever) which are accompanied by a high plasma level of IgE. Eosinophils are motile, but unlike neutrophils are poorly phagocytic. Their role in inflammation is poorly understood, but they may play a moderating part in allergic processes. Thus several of their granule constituents may alter the hypersensitivity reaction by inhibiting or promoting the action of mediators of inflammation, and arylsulphatase, preferentially present in eosinophils, inactivates slow-reacting substance of anaphylaxis (SRS-A). Stimulated eosinophils produce an inhibitor of histamine release which acts through the cyclic-AMP system; it seems to be a mixture of E_1 and E_2 prostaglandins.[5]

Lymphocytes. The lymphocyte is a key cell in the immune response; this is considered in later chapters.

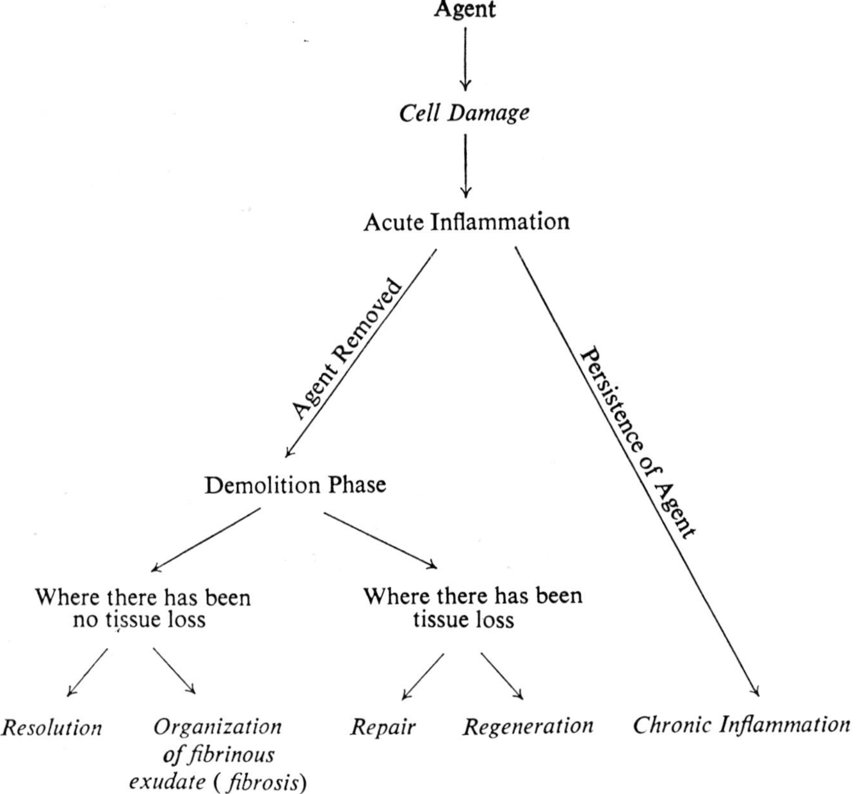

Fig. 5.4 The sequence of events following tissue damage.

Local sequelae of acute inflammation

The changes which follow the formation of an acute inflammatory exudate depend upon two major factors (Fig. 5.4):

1 The amount of tissue damage sustained
2 Whether or not the causative agent remains.

Assuming that the causative agent is removed or destroyed, the initial polymorphonuclear exudate is replaced by a mononuclear one. Their appearance heralds the onset of the demolition phase. The mononuclear cells are phagocytic, and regardless of their origin are called *macrophages*.

Origin of macrophages. The macrophages which accumulate in areas subjected to injury in lower forms of life appear to be derived from histiocytes, which are resting tissue representatives of the RE system. In mammals tissue histiocytes may also perform a similar function, but the current evidence suggests that the majority of macrophages present in the stage of demolition are the progeny of monocytes that emigrated from the blood stream.

Monocytes originate in the bone marrow where they have a generation time of about 24 hours. They circulate in the blood for 1 to 3 days and then randomly leave the circulation to become tissue macrophages.[6] In inflammation they accumulate selectively, presumably in response to chemotaxis. Labelling experiments indicate that monocytes can divide and assume the morphology of lymphocytes and macrophages. Reports that lymphocytes can change into macrophages may be misleading. The cellular events in small experimental wounds in human skin have been studied by placing glass cover-slips over the wound and examining the cells adhering to the glass. All stages in the transformation of small lymphocytes to macrophages have been described, but it seems unlikely that the cells described as small lymphocytes are the same as those present in the blood and thoracic-duct lymph. Lymphocytes do not readily adhere to glass, and it may well be that the small cells observed in these experiments are derived from monocytes.

Demolition phase

Macrophages engulf fibrin, red cells, degenerate polymorphs, bacteria, etc., and thereby perform a scavenger function. They therefore contain a variety of intracellular structures—fat, haemosiderin, cholesterol, and foreign material. Sometimes they fuse together to form giant cells. If the macrophages ingest large quantities of fat they become swollen and are called *foam cells.*

Resolution

In acutely inflamed tissue in which cellular damage has been relatively slight, the cellular and tissue changes are reversible, and necrosis does not occur. The demolition phase results in the removal of the exudate, and the organ returns to normal. To this process the term *resolution* is applied, and one of the best examples is found in lobar pneumonia (p. 531). *Resolution thus means the complete return to normal following acute inflammation.*

It should be noted that while demolition is proceeding there is a reversed flow of exudate back into the blood vessels. Most of the exudate, however, is carried away by the lymphatics.

Sometimes removal of the exudate appears to be delayed, and then the fibrin is invaded by granulation tissue. In this way fibrous adhesions, e.g. pleural and peritoneal, are produced.

Suppuration

When the noxious agent produces much necrosis, resolution is impossible and the process frequently proceeds to *suppuration.* This is typical of pyogenic infection, e.g. boils, but can also occur when the agent is a chemical substance, e.g. turpentine.

The first reaction is circumscribed necrosis accompanied by a profuse polymorph infiltration. The agent kills many of these leucocytes—which are often called 'pus cells'. The necrotic material undergoes softening by virtue of the proteolytic enzymes released from the granules (lysosomes) of the dead leucocytes as well as through the autolysis mediated by the tissue's own lysosomal enzymes. The resulting creamy fluid material is called *pus*, and is contained within a cavity to form an *abscess*. This is lined by a *pyogenic membrane*, which at this stage consists of inflamed and necrotic tissue with much fibrinous exudate and polymorphs. This soon undergoes organization into granulation tissue.

The pus itself is made up of:

1. *Leucocytes*, some of which are dead
2. *Other components of the inflammatory exudate*—oedema fluid and fibrin
3. *Organisms*, many of which are living and can therefore be cultured; if the pus is chemically induced it is sterile
4. *Tissue debris*, e.g. nucleic acids and lipids.

The pus tends to track in the line of least resistance until a free surface is reached. Then the abscess bursts and discharges its contents spontaneously—in clinical practice this is usually anticipated by surgical drainage. An abscess when drained heals by granulation tissue, but sometimes chronic inflammation ensues.

If, as occasionally happens, the abscess is not drained but remains isolated, or sequestered, in the tissues, its walls become further organized and converted into dense fibrous tissue and the pus undergoes thickening, or *inspissation*, as its fluid component is gradually absorbed. In due course it develops a porridge-like consistency, and may eventually become *calcified.*

When an acute suppurative inflammation involves an epithelial surface, the covering is destroyed, and an *ulcer** is formed. The floor is composed of necrotic tissue and acute inflammatory exudate; this layer of dead tissue forms the *slough*, and is at first adherent because the dead material has not been liquefied. Eventually, however, the slough becomes detached, and the ulcer heals by the processes of repair and regeneration, as described in Chapters 8 and 9.

Chronic inflammation

The other sequel of acute inflammation is progression to a state of chronic inflammation in which the inflammatory and healing processes proceed side by side. This is described in Chapter 10.

Conclusion

Inflammation may be defined as *the reaction of the vascular and supporting elements of a tissue to injury, and results in the formation of a protein-rich exudate provided the injury has not been so severe as to destroy the area.* Acute inflammation is thus essentially a vascular phenomenon, and cannot occur in an avascular tissue like the cornea or cartilage. The reaction is usually beneficial, but this is not necessarily so under all conditions. The inflammatory cells may themselves spread infection

* An *ulcer* is a localized defect of a covering or lining epithelium. Occasionally the term is applied to a similar defect of mesothelium or endothelium e.g. atheromatous ulcer (p. 489). Dead tissue still adherent to the floor of an ulcer is called a *slough*.

(see tuberculosis, p. 217) and the inflammatory oedema may, in a situation like the larynx, actually endanger life. The relationship between inflammation and infection is further considered in Chapter 7.

The term *subacute inflammation* is used by some authorities; it appears to mean a mild acute inflammation, but since no exact definition is possible, there seems no good reason for retaining the term.

THE CHEMICAL MEDIATORS OF ACUTE INFLAMMATION[7]

The apparent uniformity of the inflammatory response irrespective of its cause has led many investigators to presume that the changes are mediated by chemical agents which are formed when tissue is damaged, rather than being caused directly by the damage itself. The search for these mediators has a practical as well as a theoretical objective. If they could be identified, antagonistic drugs might be designed and administered to prevent or modify the acute inflammatory response.

Many mediators have been identified and the list seems to be never-ending; only a brief account will be given with emphasis on these agents that seem to be of importance in human pathology. The mediators may be classified as follows:

I. Amines
   (a) histamine
   (b) 5-hydroxytryptamine (5-HT)
II. The kinins.
III. Kinin-forming enzymes
   (a) kallikrein
   (b) plasmin
IV. Biologically active products of the complement system
V. Biologically active components of polymorphs
VI. Prostaglandins
VII. Others.

The amines

Histamine. The classical experiments of Lewis on the triple response showed that injury to the skin produced a type of inflammation which had many features in common with the effect of an injection of histamine. Lewis showed that injured skin released some substance ('H' substance) which behaved like histamine.

There is good evidence that histamine is liberated in acute inflammation, and that it can mimic some of the vascular events. It seems likely that it is important during the early phase and in certain hypersensitivity responses (see p. 182).

Histamine, bound to heparin, is contained in the granules of mast cells. It can be released by injury, by the action of various histamine-releasing agents (including the anaphylatoxins C3a and C5a), and by antigen if the cells have been previously sensitised by IgE (see later).

5-Hydroxytryptamine (5-HT, or serotonin). A smooth muscle contracting substance is found in the early inflammatory exudate of experimentally produced turpentine pleurisy in the rat. In this species 5-HT rather than histamine is liberated during the early phase of acute inflammation; it is liberated from mast cells or platelets.

The kinins

The name kinin has been applied to a variety of physiologically-active polypeptides which cause contraction of smooth muscle. *Bradykinin* is the most important, and was so named because of the slow contraction which it induces *in vitro* in the muscle of the guinea-pig ileum; it appears to be the active agent in producing the effects of poisoning due to certain snakebites. It may also be concerned in the regulation of blood flow in the salivary glands. This same kinin is formed when human saliva acts upon blood proteins, thereby revealing an unexpected relationship between human saliva and snake venom.

Bradykinin, a nonapeptide, has been synthetized, and is ten times more active as a vasodilator than is histamine (on a molar basis). It produces pain when applied to tissue. Bradykinin causes an increase in vascular permeability and stimulates the contraction of smooth muscle, but is not chemotactic to white cells. *Kallidin* is a decapeptide, lysyl-bradykinin, and is formed when pancreatic and other tissue kallikreins act on plasma kininogen. It is rapidly converted into bradykinin by plasma aminopeptidase.

The kinins are formed from precursor *kininogens* by the action of the enzymes *kallikrein* or *plasmin* (Fig. 5.5). Two groups of kininogens are known. The *low-molecular-weight kininogens* are acted upon by plasmin only, while the *high-molecular-weight kininogens* are the substrate for both kallikrein and plasmin. The part played by the kinins in inflammation is not yet known. Since they are capable of producing vasodilatation, increasing venular permeability, and causing pain, it has been suggested that they act as mediators during the early phases of inflammation.

Kallikrein*

Kallikrein is an enzyme that can form bradykinin from high-molecular-weight kininogen of the blood. It can also activate Hageman factor (Factor XII) to Factor XIIa, and is chemotactic to white cells. The enzyme exists as an inactive precursor (*prekallikrein*), which can itself be activated by Factor XIIf (also called prekallikrein activator before its relationship to Factor XII was known). Plasma kallikrein is one member of a group of enzymes that can form kinins from plasma. Others occur in urine, pancreas, and snake venom.

Plasmin

Plasminogen is a normal component of the plasma proteins. It can be converted into plasmin by the action of kallikrein (previously called plasminogen activator). Plasmin itself is a proteolytic enzyme, and digests fibrin as well as other plasma proteins. The breakdown of fibrin leads to the formation of a variety of polypeptides (*fibrinopeptides*) that have a number of properties, including anticoagulant activity, the ability to increase vascular permeability, and being chemotactic to white cells.

Plasmin can increase vascular permeability in many ways. It can act directly on kininogen to liberate kinin; this action is slow compared with that of kallikrein.

* Kallikrein is so called because it is found in high concentrations in pancreas. *Kallikreas* is Greek for pancreas.

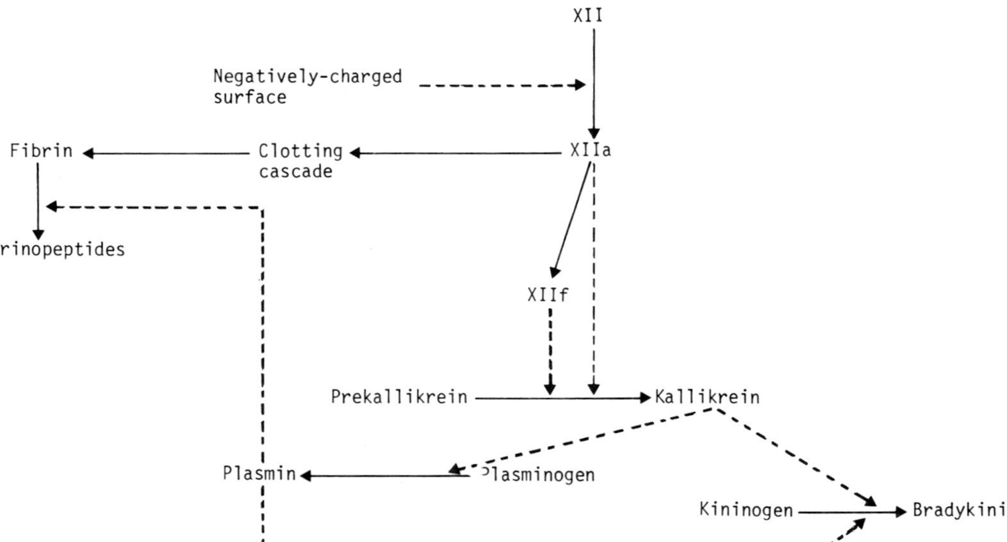

Figure 5.5 The current hypothesis for the activation of the kinin system. Note the central role of Hageman-factor (factor XII) activation which initiates clotting, fibrinolysis, and kinin formation. Factor XIIa has a major role in initiating the clotting cascade but a minor one in activating prekallikrein. Factor XIIf, on the other hand, has as its major action the activation of prekallikrein to kallikrein. The separate types of kininogen are not shown (see text). Transformations are depicted as solid lines, while enzymatic actions are shown as interrupted lines.

Secondly, it can activate prekallikrein to kallikrein. Finally, it can act on the third component of complement to produce C3a and on Factor XIIa to produce Factor XIIf.

Other proteolytic enzymes have been described. One is present in skin, and another, present in white blood cells, leads to the formation of leucokinin.

Biologically active cleavage products of complement

Activation of the complement system leads to the formation of two anaphylatoxins, C3a and C5a, which cause the release of histamine from mast cells. They also exert a chemotactic influence, as does $C\overline{567}$ (p. 175). These components are important in the pathogenesis of aggregate anaphylaxis and in the inflammation present in some lesions of immune-complex disease (p. 185). The alternate pathway of complement activation explains how vasoactive complement components can be formed following tissue damage which is not immunologically mediated. Necrotic tissue, e.g. heart muscle,[8] can release enzymes capable of activating C3, and so also can the lysosomal enzymes released from polymorphs. What part they play in inflammation in the non-immune animal and that due to trauma is not known.

Biologically active components of polymorphs

Neutrophils release a variety of agents in acute inflammation. The following agents have been described:

Cationic proteins. These have various actions, including direct action on blood vessels to increase permeability, histamine-releasing factors, neutrophil-immobilising factor, and a chemotactic factor for monocytes.

Acid proteases. These act on a kininogen to produce a kinin (leucokinin).

Neutral proteases. These have been credited with many activities: they degrade collagen, basement-membrane material, fibrin, etc., they cleave C3 and C5 to form active products, they activate kininogen to kinin, and they have a direct effect on blood vessels to increase their permeability. These actions are inhibited by α_1-antitrypsin.

Prostaglandins. See below.

Pyrogens. See Chapter 27.

The release of these various neutrophil substances may occur by a type of secretion, as the contents of granules are discharged by exocytosis—particularly during phagocytosis. They are also released when the cell dies and undergoes autolysis.

It is evident that the role of polymorphs in acute inflammation is very complex. Under some circumstances they provide protection against micro-organisms, since infection introduced into animals rendered leucopenic can be spreading and lethal, while a similar infection in a normal animal would lead merely to a local acute inflammation. On the other hand, the damage seen in the lesions of the Shwartzman reaction and in the vasculitis of immune-complex disease appears to be produced by agents released by the polymorphs.

Vasoactive acidic lipids

The prostaglandins.[9] The name prostaglandin was given to a substance found in human seminal fluid by von Euler. Prostaglandins have been isolated from virtually every tissue of the body, and have been grouped on the basis of their chemical structure. They are derivatives of prostanoic acid, the 20-carbon parent substance. They are credited with many diverse functions—from acting as chemical transmitters in the nervous system to playing an important role in conception and parturition. Their role in thrombosis is described on page 481. They have been isolated in the tissues of human skin in allergic contact dermatitis,[10] and are released from polymorphs during phagocytosis.

Some, e.g. PGE_1 and PGE_2, produce vasodilatation, increase vascular permeability, and cause pain; others have converse effects, protecting tissues from these actions. An effect of some prostaglandins that may be of importance is their potentiation of the action of kinins in increasing vascular permeability. The prostaglandins may therefore be significant mediators of acute inflammation either by a direct action or, more likely, by regulating or *modulating* the action of other mediators.[11]

One important source of prostaglandin is the platelet, which contains prostaglandin-forming enzymes. It is significant that aspirin and indomethacin both inhibit the formation of prostaglandins from the substrate arachidonic acid;[12] this may well account for the hitherto unexplained anti-inflammatory action of aspirin. The release of prostaglandins from platelets is inhibited by glucocorticoids.

Slow-reacting substance of anaphylaxis (SRS-A). This vasoactive lipid is released from mast cells, and is described on page 182. It is not chemotactic to white cells. SRS-A is broken down by aryl sulphatase B, an enzyme found in eosinophils.

Other possible mediators of the inflammatory response

Many other possible mediators of acute inflammation have been described. *Lactic acid* is present in inflamed tissue, and may play a part in the vasodilatation and change in vascular permeability. The *lymphokines*, which are described in Chapter 12, are undoubtedly liberated in certain types of inflammation in which immune mechanisms are involved.

It is possible that some *bacterial toxins* are capable of directly initiating or modifying the inflammatory response. The gas-gangrene organisms, in particular *Cl. oedematiens*, produce toxins which appear to act directly upon blood vessels and increase their permeability.

It is instructive to summarize the role of the mast cells and platelets at this point.

Role of the mast cell in inflammation

The mast cells can release the contents of their granules when directly injured, and also in response to a number of other stimuli. C5a is a cleavage product of C5 (p. 175), and has such an action; it is the classical anaphylatoxin, so named because its formation, by causing the release of histamine, can produce a state resembling acute anaphylactic shock. C3a is another anaphylatoxin, but is less potent. Another agent is one of the cationic proteins of polymorphs. Mast-cell degranulation can be mediated immunologically; if the cells are coated with IgE, contact with antigen causes degranulation.

Mast cells release the following agents:

1. Histamine
2. Slow-reacting substance of anaphylaxis—SRS-A
3. Eosinophil-chemotactic factor of anaphylaxis—ECF-A
4. Platelet-activating factor—this causes platelets to undergo the release reaction.

Role of the platelets in inflammation

Platelets become adherent to areas of vascular damage, and undergo a release reaction whereby the contents of their granules are liberated. The dense granules contain vasoactive amines (histamine or 5-HT according to species), while the α granules contain lysosomal enzymes.

Summary

The number of chemicals that have been suggested as mediators of acute inflammation is now so large, and their inter-relationship is so complex, that it is not possible to give any clear account of their role in acute inflammation. Indeed, as noted by Ryan and Majno, the inflammatory 'soup' is so complicated that no single individual can claim to know how the dozens of components relate to each other or how they change during the evolution of an inflammatory response.

It is generally agreed that the exudation of acute inflammation involves both capillaries and venules. The capillaries are so narrow that any marked increase in their permeability would bring about their blockage; the resulting ischaemia would lead to a cessation of the inflammatory process and necrosis of the area involved. It is doubtful whether any such mechanism would be evolved. In support of this contention is the observation that capillaries do not respond to the action of vasoactive drugs. Hence it is unlikely that any mediator acts directly on the capillaries. On the other hand, capillaries do appear to respond to direct injury.[13]

The present evidence suggests that the capillary changes in acute inflammation are due to a direct effect of the injuring agent—trauma or chemical or microbial toxin.

The venules, on the other hand, react to vasoactive drugs and mediators. Histamine is an accepted mediator of the early exudation of acute inflammation, and the kinins are probably important also. The prostaglandins probably modulate their actions. The mediators of the late and prolonged phases of inflammation remain enigmatic; every mediator mentioned in this chapter has at some time or another been proposed as a candidate.

The accumulation of inflammatory cells in inflammation is believed to be due to chemotaxis, and the most likely agents are the activated components of complement. The change in cell population from polymorph to macrophage, and the appearance of eosinophils in some inflammations, are related largely to the actions of different chemotactic agents that attract the particular cell in question.

Although much stress has been placed upon the uniformity of the inflammatory reaction regardless of its cause, it must not be forgotten that there is, in fact, also very considerable individual diversity, both in the amount of exudate and in the type of cell involved. This was stressed by Kettle, who recognised that the individuality of an inflammatory reaction was a reflection of the individuality of the agent causing it. It would be hard to deny the importance of many bacterial products; the leucocidins, haemolysins, kinases, permeability factors, etc., must all influence the final outcome. Products of tissue damage and mediators generated from plasma constituents are not the only agents present in the inflammation of infection. So far, much research has been done on the vasodilatation and increased vascular permeability of acute inflammation caused by trauma or chemical agents. The complex cellular changes and the intricacies of infection have been largely neglected. Until we have much more reliable information, the role of the individual chemical mediators in acute inflammation will remain ambiguous.

GENERAL READING

Cohnheim J 1889 In Lectures on general pathology, London, New Sydenham Society, p 248. (This is a translation of the second edition of Cohnheim's book published in 1882)

Ryan G B, Majno G 1977 Acute inflammation. American Journal of Pathology **86:** 183

Movat H Z (ed) 1971 Inflammation, immunity and hypersensitivity. Harper and Row, New York

Zweifach B W, Grant L, McCluskey R T (eds) 1974 The Inflammatory Process. 2nd edn Vols 1–3 Academic Press, New York

REFERENCES

1. Rather L J 1971 Disturbance of function (functio laesa): the legendary fifth cardinal sign of inflammation, added by Galen to the four cardinal signs of Celsus. Bulletin of the New York Academy of Medicine **47:** 303
2. Unanue E R 1976 Secretory function of mononuclear phagocytes. American Journal of Pathology **83:** 396
3. Cohen, S G 1974 The eosinophil and eosinophilia. New England Journal of Medicine **290:** 457
4. Leading article 1971 Mechanisms of eosinophilia. Lancet **2:** 1187
5. Leading Article 1977 What eosinophils do. Lancet **2:** 388
6. Territo M C, Cline M J 1975 Mononuclear phagocyte proliferation, maturation and function. Clinics in Haematology **4:** 685
7. Hersh E M, Bodey G P, 1970 Leukocytic mechanisms in inflammation. Annual Review of Medicine **21:** 105
8. Hill J H, Ward P A 1971 The phlogistic role of C3 leukotactic fragments in myocardial infarcts in rats. Journal of Experimental Medicine **133:** 885
9. Leading Article: New light on inflammation 1971. British Medical Journal **3:** 61
10. Greaves M W, Sondergaard J, McDonald-Gibson W 1971 Recovery of prostaglandins in human cutaneous inflammation. British Medical Journal **2:** 258
11. Marx J L 1972 Prostaglandins: mediators of inflammation? Science **177:** 780
12. Vane J R 1971 Inhibition of prostaglandin synthesis as a mechanism of action for aspirin-like drugs. Nature New Biology **231:** 232
13. Hurley J V 1972 Acute inflammation. Churchill Livingstone, Edinburgh

6

The body's defences against infection

Introduction

Micro-organisms can cause disease in two ways. Either they gain access to the tissues of the host, multiply, and cause *infection*, or they manufacture powerful toxins which are subsequently introduced into the body and produce an *intoxication.*

Staphylococcal enterotoxic food-poisoning and botulism provide typical examples of an intoxication.

By far the most important method whereby micro-organisms cause disease is by their *invasion of and multiplication in the living tissues of the host.* This is the definition of *infection*, and organisms capable of producing it are termed *pathogens.*

TRANSMISSION OF ORGANISMS TO THE BODY

With the exception of certain rare congenital infections, all infection is derived from the external environment. The organisms may be injected directly into the host, but more usually they are first *transmitted* to the surface of the body which thereby becomes *contaminated.*

Usually, when a body surface is involved, the organisms are destroyed, but occasionally they penetrate into the living tissues and cause infection.

The following modes of transmission are important:

Transplacental spread

During the early stages of pregnancy the fetus is particularly susceptible to the damaging effect of infection transmitted by the mother. Rubella (German measles) may give rise to fetal infection and deformities. The protozoal disease toxoplasmosis may result in hydrocephalus, mental defect, and blindness when transmitted across the placenta.

Ingestion of contaminated food

Food may be contaminated directly by a human carrier or indirectly by flies. These insects carry many pathogenic organisms on their hairy legs. Diseases transmitted by food include typhoid fever, bacillary dysentery, and amoebiasis. Poliomyelitis is acquired by ingestion. Milk and eggs may contain bacteria because the animal itself is diseased, e.g. bovine tuberculosis and brucellosis, and *Salmonella* infections of fowls.

Inoculation

The agent may be an insect whose bite transmits pathogenic organisms, e.g. arboviruses, *Yersinia pestis*, and rickettsiae. The iatrogenic disease* virus B hepatitis is caused by the introduction of the virus by means of a contaminated needle or instrument (p. 260).

Direct skin contact

Wound infection may result from contact with a staphylococcal carrier or by contamination with soil containing clostridia. Contaminated air is important in causing wound infection in hospitals. The venereal diseases, e.g. syphilis and gonorrhoea, are also transmitted by direct contact.

Spread by droplets and dust[1]

Droplets are produced when air, passing rapidly over a mucous membrane, causes atomization of the secretion which covers it. A few of these droplets are large, and due to the effect of gravity have a limited range. The vast majority are smaller than 100 μm in diameter, and dry up almost instantaneously to form *droplet nuclei* which stay suspended in the air for many hours.

Droplet formation occurs during talking, coughing, and particularly sneezing; the main source is from the *saliva in the front of the mouth.* Only during snorting is the nose an important source of droplets. It is possible for aerosols from high-speed dental handpieces to spread infection from the patient to the dentist; precautionary measures, such as wearing a mask and spectacles, or goggles, are recommended. The viruses of mumps, measles, smallpox, and chickenpox are found in the saliva, and these diseases may well be spread in this way.

Bacteria residing in the nose (*Staph. aureus*), nasopharynx (*Strept pyogenes*), or lung (tubercle bacilli) do not commonly reach the front of the mouth, and it is very unlikely that droplets are an important vehicle of their spread. Some may be spat out as sputum, but the most important means of dissemination is by the fingers and handkerchief. Using fluorescein or test organisms as markers, it has been found that normal human beings frequently dispense nasal secretions and saliva to their hands, face, and clothing, and to every object that is touched. After desiccation the organisms are readily disseminated in the form of dust particles, and it is these which are important in the transmission of many infections.

HOSPITAL INFECTION[2,3]

Whenever human beings live together in confined quarters, there is always the danger that in the group there will be carriers of pathogenic organisms. Although not suffering from clinical illness themselves, they may pass on the organisms to others who, having little resistance, succumb to the infection. In turn they further transmit the disease. This is called *cross-infection.* In the past there have been many examples of epidemics of meningococcal meningitis and dysentery occurring in nurses' homes, army camps, and other places housing large numbers of people. In

* Iatrogenic from the Greek *iatros*, meaning physician, and *genein* to produce. The term is applied to a disease produced by the physician as a consequence of his treatment. Drug reactions are the commonest example.

hospitals it is not uncommon for patients to acquire severe infections from their environment; this is hardly surprising, because many patients are debilitated and their resistance to infection is lowered. Furthermore, surgical incisions provide a ready avenue for the invading bacteria.

A particular feature in hospitals is that the staff acquire pathogenic organisms from their patients, become carriers, and further disseminate the bacteria. Often the strain is one that is resistant to the antibiotics which are in common use in that particular hospital. The infection is therefore all the more serious.

In the past *streptococcal infections* were serious, particularly in labour wards. Identification of the strain of organism involved, using the Griffith method of typing (p. 203), and a subsequent search for the source of infection has usually incriminated the throats of a few members of staff. The exclusion and treatment of such carriers and general measures designed to improve aseptic techniques have usually brought such an epidemic to a halt. Penicillin therapy is very effective in streptococcal infections, since resistant organisms do not occur. It follows that outbreaks of streptococcal hospital infection are not a problem at the present time.

The staphylococcus has, on the other hand, attained a much more prominent position. Outbreaks of postoperative wound infection are not uncommon, and the methods of control which proved effective with streptococcal outbreaks are quite inadequate. Often the majority of the staff are found to be carriers, and in addition the hospital itself—the floors, air-conditioning plant, bedclothes, etc.—is also contaminated with a virulent strain of staphylococcus. Although human carriers provide the reservoir, the hardy staphylococcus often infects patients by indirect means, for instance in airborne dust particles. The problem of control is not easy; indeed there is no simple answer to an outbreak of staphylococcal wound infection.

Other organisms which sometimes cause hospital infection are the coliform group, *Proteus* species, and *Pseudomonas aeruginosa*. As with the staphylococcus, the transfer of these organisms is usually indirect, *via* dust, contaminated articles, and fomites*. The source of organisms is often a patient with urinary tract infection who contaminates the immediate environment—bedclothing, urine bottle, and other articles with which contact can be made.

DEFENCES OF INDIVIDUAL BODY SURFACES

It is evident that there may be contamination of the body, both externally on the skin and internally in the intestinal, respiratory, and other tracts. Many of these surfaces are habitually colonized by organisms of low-grade pathogenicity, e.g. *Staph. albus* in the skin and *Strept. viridans* in the mouth and throat. Such organisms are called *commensals*, or 'resident flora', and as will be shown later, play an important role in the decontamination of these surfaces against pathogenic organisms. Contamination with virulent organisms is a common event, but infection is rare. Whether contamination is followed by infection is dependent upon:

* Fomites are articles, such as bedding or clothing, capable of acting as a medium for the transmission of organisms which may give rise to infection.

1. *The mechanical integrity of the body surface*
2. *Its powers of decontamination*, i.e. its ability to remove organisms.

These protective mechanisms vary greatly from one tissue to another, and each will therefore be considered separately.

The skin

The skin is frequently contaminated, and its exposed position renders it liable to both major and minor physical trauma. Its protective function is carried out mainly by the epithelial cells, and indeed the inability of the subepithelial tissues to resist infection was one of the limiting factors in pre-Listerian surgery. Its defences are:

Mechanical strength. The many layers of epithelial cells, the tough outer layer of keratin, and the distinct basement membrane all play a part in the formation of a mechanical barrier, which if impaired, may result in infection. For example, excessive sweating softens the keratin layer; for this reason skin infections are very common in the tropics, and boils are frequently seen in moist areas like the axillae and groins.

The skin when intact appears to be completely impervious to invasion by organisms, but following trauma it becomes the portal of entry for staphylococci, streptococci, and the clostridia. In the tropics insect bites penetrate the skin barrier, and serve to introduce the causative agents of plague, typhus, yellow fever, malaria, dengue fever, etc.

Decontamination.[4] The powers of decontamination of the skin may be demonstrated by deliberately contaminating the hands with haemolytic streptococci, and subsequently estimating their rate of disappearance by taking swabs at regular intervals. The organisms are often removed or destroyed within 2 to 3 hours. The mechanisms involved may be considered under three headings—mechanical, biological, and chemical:

Mechanical. The *desquamation* of surface squames removes some of the superficial organisms. *Desiccation* is probably of some importance in destroying organisms on the surface of the skin.

Biological. It is probable that the resident flora plays an important part in the decontamination mechanism both by producing antibiotic substances* and by competing with other organisms for essential foodstuffs. The *resident flora* includes *Staph. albus*, diphtheroids, sarcinae, and aerobic sporing bacilli. In addition about 25 per cent of people harbour *Staph. aureus* particularly on the hands, face, and perineum. It is impossible to remove all the resident organisms from the skin; they survive in the gland ducts, and though the surface may be disinfected, the organisms are soon replaced. It is for this reason that sterile rubber gloves must always be worn while performing any surgical procedure.

Chemical. The sweat is normally acid and is unsuitable for the growth of most pathogens. This bactericidal activity is probably due to its lactic acid content. There are certain gaps in this acid coat; these are the alkaline areas where infection

* An antibiotic is a substance produced by one organism which is inimical to the growth of another. Thus *penicillin* is produced by the mould *Penicillium notatum*.

is quite common, e.g. axillae, groins, and interdigital clefts of the toes. *Unsaturated fatty acids* are present in the sebaceous secretion and are bactericidal; it is interesting that some of the diphtheroids grow only in the presence of these fatty acids, so well are they adapted to their environment.

There is no doubt that the mechanical strength together with the decontaminating mechanisms are of great importance in maintaining the integrity of the skin. When one remembers how often it must be contaminated with all types of organisms, and, apart from staphylococci how rarely it is invaded, one appreciates its efficiency as a protective coat.

The alimentary tract

The mouth and throat

As in the case of the skin the defence mechanism is twofold:

Mechanical strength. The toughness and integrity of the mucous membrane is important; this mechanical barrier is weakest at two points:

The *gingival margin* has only a thin epithelium, and is therefore easily traumatized. This is particularly so in the interdental region, where it is believed that a covering epithelium is present only in young healthy adults.

The *tonsillar crypts.* Here the epithelium is very thin; it has been shown that carmine powder dusted on to the tonsils appears in the underlying cells and connective tissue within 20 minutes. Probably the dye is transported there by phagocytes which are normally resident on the surface. Organisms may similarly reach the subepithelial tissue. It is therefore no wonder that these two sites, the tonsils and the gingivae, are the places where infection occurs when the general body defences are impaired, e.g. in acute leukaemia and agranulocytosis. Nevertheless, it is remarkable how the tissues of the mouth, including the bone, can resist infection even with the contamination that follows injuries or dental extraction. On the other hand, skin wounds caused by human bites often become infected, and they heal very badly. Some form of 'tissue immunity' in the oral cavity must be postulated, but its nature is obscure.

Decontamination.

Mechanical. A regular flow of saliva is of importance for its mechanical action in keeping the mouth clean.

The continual backward flow of saliva traps organisms, which are then swallowed. Carbon particles placed on the mucosa are removed from the mouth in 15 to 30 minutes.[4]

Biological. As in the skin the resident flora is important. These organisms are α-haemolytic streptococci (*Strept. viridans*), *Neisseria pharyngis*, diphtheroids, lactobacilli, pneumococci, *Borrelia vincenti*, actinomyces organisms, *Candida albicans*, and various *Bacteroidaceae*. Many strains of α-haemolytic streptococci produce hydrogen peroxide, and this has been thought to play some part in the decontaminating mechanism*.

Chemical. The saliva inhibits many pathogens: this may be due to its mucin,

* In this connexion the rare Japanese hereditary disorder of *acatalasia* is of interest. The enzyme catalase which normally breaks down H_2O_2 is absent from the blood, and peroxide formed in the mouth produces sufficient damage to cause ulcerating gangrenous lesions in the mouth.

lysozyme, or IgA content. As with other secretions, saliva contains antibodies of the IgA class; these are produced locally and passed into the secretions as a dimer linked to a distinct secretory polypeptide. The secretion of saliva is therefore of importance, as can be appreciated when its secretion is suppressed for example in shock, dehydration, and fever, or as a result of infective processes, neoplasia, or irradiation.

Under these circumstances the lips, tongue, teeth, and remainder of the mouth become coated with a mixture of food particles and dead epithelial cells, which if not actively removed, become the site of bacterial colonisation and a source of infection. Thus there may be an ascending infection of the salivary glands terminating in suppurative sialadenitis.

In spite of the defence mechanisms of the mouth potent pathogens can adapt themselves to the mouth and throat, e.g. meningococci, diphtheria bacilli, *Haemophilus influenzae*, and *Strept. pyogenes*. These may lead to infection, but if the person has considerable immunity, they may remain as 'transients' for a period of time. Such carriers are of great importance in the spread of streptococcal infections, diphtheria, and meningococcal meningitis.

The stomach

The stomach stands guard over the intestines and deals not only with food, but also with the secretions of the mouth and swallowed sputum. Its defence mechanisms are:

Mechanical strength. The continuity of the epithelium is probably not important. Acute ulcers are common, and neither these nor the more serious chronic ulcers appear to provide points of entry for organisms.

Decontamination. *Mechanical.* Vomiting removes chemical and bacterial irritants, but is of little value in combating infection.

Biological. Under normal conditions the gastric juice is sterile.

Chemical. Without doubt the bactericidal activity of gastric juice is due to its hydrochloric acid content, and not to its enzymes. Gastric juice loses its bactericidal activity when neutralized.

Coliform organisms and tubercle bacilli can withstand the acidity of the stomach, and are able to reach, and occasionally infect, the lower intestinal tract.

Staphylococci and *Salmonella* organisms will pass through the stomach if ingested with food or large quantities of fluid; likewise enteroviruses can withstand moderate acidity. Milk with its potent antacid properties is a particularly favourable vehicle for organisms, e.g. *Brucella abortus*, though in fact any food is liable to have a protective action.

Strept. pyogenes and pneumococci are very easily killed by acid, and these organisms almost never reach the intestine nor cause infection there.

The intestine

The intestine undoubtedly relies upon the stomach's protective action. The minor intestinal upsets of infancy may in part be related to the low gastric acidity in this age-group. The intestine has, however, its own defence mechanism.

Mechanical barrier. As in the stomach this is probably not important. It is interesting that some organisms, e.g. *Salmonella typhi* and the tubercle bacillus, can penetrate the mucosa without causing obvious damage. Probably phagocytes are normally present on the surface of the gut ready to ingest passing organisms. These are carried into the tissues, so that infection follows.

Decontamination. *Mechanical.* Irritation of the intestine, whether it affects the small intestine (e.g. typhoid fever) or large gut (e.g. bacillary dysentery) usually causes diarrhoea. This mechanism expels organisms during an established infection, but it seems doubtful whether it plays any part in the prevention of infection.

Biological. The small intestine generally contains few organisms, while the colon is heavily contaminated with coliforms, *Bacteroides* organisms, *Streptococcus faecalis*, and clostridia. Although the importance of the flora is well known, the exact mechanisms involved are not established. However, when the flora is altered by the ingestion of broad-spectrum antibiotics, infection with *Staph. aureus* may be a fatal complication (p. 202). *Candida albicans* can likewise cause a troublesome stomatitis and pruritus ani.

Chemical. It has been shown that intestinal as well as other secretions, e.g. milk, contain specific IgA antibodies. They are secreted locally by plasma cells, and are important in providing the mucous membranes with local immunity (p. 154). It should also be noted that the lymphoid tissue of the intestine is thought to act as the central organ responsible for the development of the peripheral lymphoid tissues destined to produce all classes of immunoglobulins (p. 159).

The appendix is one of the weakest links in the alimentary tract, the reason for which is not known. Possibly damage by hard concretions and the ease with which its lumen can be obstructed play a part, but it is humiliating to admit how little we know about the cause of such a common disease as acute appendicitis.

The conjunctival sac of the eye

Large particles are prevented from contaminating the eye by the action of blinking. This also is important as it ensures that the conjunctiva and cornea are always covered by a thin protective layer of lacrimal secretion.

In the absence of the *blink reflex* the cornea desiccates, and repeated trauma leads to its ulceration and infection. Impairment of this reflex occurs under two circumstances:

1. Motor loss—in facial nerve paralysis, e.g. Bell's palsy
2. Sensory loss—with trigeminal nerve lesions, e.g. following zoster.

In order to prevent corneal ulceration and ocular infection, the eye should either be covered with a pad or else the lids should be sutured together.

The lacrimal secretions have other important functions, for if the cornea is irritated the volume of secretion is increased. The tears so produced mechanically wash away the irritant. The other important protective function of tears is due to their content of *lysozyme* (*muramidase*);[5,6] they contain the highest concentration of lysozyme of any body fluid. First described by Fleming, this bactericidal enzyme, a polysaccharidase, is capable of lysing some organisms and inhibiting the growth of others. It acts on the muramic acid of bacterial cell walls, but with many organisms the outer coat must first be damaged by other means, e.g. complement activation or the action of peroxide, before the organism is killed.

The respiratory tract

The respiratory tract acts as a whole, the upper part functioning as an air-conditioner for the lungs. The vibrissae filter off large particles, but the main filter is the nasal mucosa itself, covering as it does the complicated ramification of the turbinates. Not only is the inspired air warmed and humidified, but the mucus-covered surface traps organisms and particles just as flies are trapped on fly-paper. The anterior nares are distinct from the remainder of the respiratory tract, because their epithelium and bacterial flora resemble that of the skin. Their great importance lies in their frequent colonization by *Staph. aureus.*

The nose and nasopharynx

Mechanical barrier. The epithelium of the respiratory tract does not provide an adequate barrier against local infection. This is well demonstrated by the ease with which rhinoviruses and adenoviruses cause acute upper respiratory tract infection. Meningococci are apparently able to penetrate the mucosa of the nasopharynx without much difficulty.

Decontamination. Irritants are expelled by the act of sneezing. If organisms are deliberately implanted in the nose, they disappear within 15 minutes. One of the main mechanisms involved is the continuous flow of mucus backwards to the nasopharynx. The nasal secretion is both bactericidal and virucidal: some antibodies have been demonstrated in it against influenza and poliomyelitis viruses. Lysozyme and lactoferrin are also present. Nevertheless, pathogens like meningococci and diphtheria bacilli can colonize the nose, and carriers of these constitute an important reservoir of human infection. The fact that the olfactory mucosa is non-ciliated and has beneath it much lymphoid tissue has been held to explain why some organisms gain entry through this area. Experimentally dye, proteins, and viruses can be shown to penetrate the olfactory mucosa and enter the underlying lymphoid tissue.

The nasopharynx has a resident bacterial flora similar to that of the throat (especially *Strept. viridans* and *Neisseria pharyngis*), and this has a biological decontaminating function.

The trachea and lower respiratory tract

Mechanical barrier. Below the larynx the respiratory tract should normally be sterile. The mucosa itself forms a poor mechanical barrier as in the nose, and is easily infected by a number of viruses, e.g. the influenza virus.

Decontamination.[7,8] The cough reflex initiated by stimulating the larynx or upper trachea expels irritants, but may also disseminate organisms within the lung. Although the diameter of the air passages decreases steadily with each division from the trachea downwards, the total cross-sectional area of all the respiratory bronchioles is over a hundred times that of the trachea. It follows that the velocity of the inspired air steadily decreases as it passes down the air passages, and this allows particles to fall out of the stream and adhere to the mucus-covered walls. The film of fluid which covers the mucosa is derived partly by transudation and partly from the secretions of surface goblet cells and the underlying mucous glands. By its chemical composition it protects the epithelial cells from dangerous gases, e.g. SO_2, and its proper consistency allows the cilia to move it on as a continuous sheet. The sheet of mucus ever moving upwards by ciliary activity is an important decontaminating mechanism, and any obstruction to it impairs the defences of the respiratory tract. This frequently leads to infection, and is well seen in the bronchopneumonia which follows the obstruction caused by carcinoma or a foreign body, e.g. an inhaled tooth or root.

In the respiratory bronchioles and alveoli, mucociliary streams play little part in the defence of the lung, and it is here that the macrophages, or *septal cells*, are important. Bacteria are phagocytosed by these RE cells and killed in their cytoplasm.

The bronchial mucus contains lactoferrin, lysozyme, and antibodies. Although IgA is regarded as an important protective antibody, patients with a low IgA do not seem, curiously enough, to be particularly prone to respiratory infections.[9]

Summary

An important aspect of the defence mechanism against infection is the manner whereby the various body surfaces are able to rid themselves of contaminating bacteria. But apart from this it appears that each surface has an intrinsic ability to resist infection which cannot easily be explained. Thus the skin is frequently colonized by *Staph. aureus*, and yet infection is relatively uncommon. These organisms when introduced into the subcutaneous tissues readily cause infection. The skin itself is able to resist infection, and therefore exhibits some type of local tissue immunity. The nature of this is unknown. Nowhere is this type of immunity more important than in the mouth. Subepithelial tissues, muscle, and bone may be exposed and contaminated, and yet no infection ensues. Were it not for this defence mechanism dental extraction and oral surgery would be impossible.

REFERENCES

1. Hare R 1964 The transmission of respiratory infections. Proceedings of the Royal Society of Medicine 57: 221
2. Williams R E O, Blowers R, Garrod L P & Shooter R A 1966 Hospital Infection, 2nd edn, 386 pp. London: Lloyd-Luke
3. Lowbury E J L, Ayliffe G A J, Geddes A M & Williams J D 1975 Control of Hospital Infection. London: Chapman and Hall
4. Wilson G S & Miles A A 1975 In Topley and Wilson's Principles of Bacteriology, Virology and Immunity, 6th edn, p 1303. London: Arnold
5. Chipman D M & Sharon N 1969 Mechanism of lysosome action. Science 165, 454
6. Glynn A A 1968 Lysozyme: antigen, enzyme and antibacterial agent. The Scientific Basis of Medicine: Annual Reviews London 31
7. Newhouse M, Sanchis J & Bienenstock J 1976 Lung defense mechanisms. New England Journal of Medicine 295: 990 and 1045
8. Leading Article 1976 In defence of the lungs. British Medical Journal 1: 733
9. Leading Article 1975 Selective IgA deficiency. Lancet 2: 1291

7

The body's response to infection

Patterns of infectious disease

When organisms gain access to the tissues of the body, their fate depends on the resultant of two factors: the *immunity* of the host and the *virulence* of the organism. Immunity and virulence are in effect two descriptive approaches to the encounter between an organism and its host. The possible end-results of such an encounter are:

1. Rapid destruction of the organisms, e.g. non-pathogens
2. The organisms grow for a time, but are soon destroyed, e.g. minor or subclinical infection
3. The organisms enter into a symbiotic state with their host, e.g. herpes simplex virus and adenovirus
4. There is a local proliferation of organisms to produce tissue damage, but there is little spread of the infection, e.g. a boil due to *Staph. aureus*
5. Organisms may proliferate locally and produce severe damage to distant tissues by means of a soluble exotoxin. The local lesion may be insignificant, as in tetanus, or severe as in diphtheria
6. A local lesion is produced, but rapid spread of organisms follows, so that a diffuse, ill-defined inflammation results. This is called *cellulitis*, and is most commonly caused by *Strept. pyogenes*
7. No local lesion forms but the organism spreads rapidly, e.g. European typhus due to *Rickettsia prowazeki*
8. No local lesion forms initially, but the organisms spread rapidly and later a lesion develops at the portal of entry, e.g. syphilis. typhoid fever, and scrub typhus due to *Rickettsia tsutsugamushi*
9. The organisms induce cellular proliferation, e.g. Rous's sarcoma. Proliferation may occur and be followed later by necrosis, e.g. smallpox.

This list is by no means complete. Thus, the slow viruses produce a type of infection which appears to be unique, but is not well understood (p. 267). Cholera is peculiar in that the organisms multiply in the gut, produce a toxin which damages the epithelium, but yet never penetrate beyond the basement membrane.[1] It is obvious in this example how difficult it is to separate true infection from intoxication. Some of these possibilities must now be examined in more detail.

Pathogenicity of organisms—virulence

An organism is described as *non-pathogenic* if it is unable to multiply in the tissues and produce disease. Such an organism is usually phagocytosed by the polymorphonuclear leucocytes and macrophages, and destroyed in the cytoplasm of these cells. Specific receptors are required for cells to be susceptible to certain infections. Thus the Duffy blood-group antigens are necessary for the parasitization of human red cells by the protozoon (*Plasmodium vivax*) that causes benign tertian malaria.[2] A factor is present on chromosome 19 that determines human susceptibility to poliovirus.[3]

Pathogens. Some organisms, on the other hand, are capable of causing disease (i.e. are *pathogenic*) and have the ability to grow in the tissues where they produce *infection.* Disregarding for the moment the immune state of the host, the severity of this infection depends on the intrinsic nature of the organism, and the factor concerned is generally described as its *virulence.* This may be manifest in two ways:

1. The ability of the organism to spread throughout the tissue
2. The ability of the organism to cause tissue damage, for instance by the production of toxins.

The ability to spread, in respect of many organisms, is inversely proportional to the tendency to produce initial local damage and a subsequent inflammatory reaction. Thus an organism like *Staph. aureus* produces severe tissue damage, a marked inflammatory response, and usually has little tendency to spread. On the other hand, some organisms, e.g. many viruses, *Mycobacterium leprae*, etc., excite little immediate inflammatory reaction, and are able to spread widely without leaving any trace of the site of entry. Other organisms, although behaving essentially in the same manner, produce diseases in which a lesion develops later at the site of entry. Syphilis is an excellent example of this, and it should be noted that the local lesion (chancre) occurs *long after the organisms have spread throughout the body.*

Sometimes an organism may live in a symbiotic state with its host and produce no damage. Such a relationship exists between humans and the virus of herpes simplex. The virus lives harmlessly in the sensory nerve cells until the subject develops a 'cold'. Then it multiplies and produces the familiar 'cold sores', or herpes febrilis. Such latent virus infections are probably quite common—probably many tumour-producing viruses behave in a similar manner. This is considered in Chapter 16.

The existence of L-forms (p. 242) raises many possibilities. They are generally considered to be non-pathogenic, but following an overt infection they might remain in the tissues in a dormant form and provide sufficient antigen to sustain an immunological response. Rheumatic carditis and chronic post-streptococcal glomerulonephritis are obvious candidates for such a pathogenesis. L-forms might also revert to type; this could explain recurrent infections, e.g. chronic pyelonephritis and infective endocarditis.

From this brief review it is evident that micro-organisms are capable of initiating a great number of disease patterns, and that no simple generalization will suffice to describe the types of host response that occur with infection.

Manner by which organisms produce damage[4]

In the early days of bacteriology it seemed reasonable to suppose that organisms produced damage by elaborating potent chemical substances which were termed toxins. The *exotoxins* were the first bacterial products to be identified. They are freely diffusible and therefore found in the medium of a bacterial culture. They can be purified, identified, and estimated with relative ease. Their mode of action is known in many cases, and it is very specific. On a quantitative basis exotoxins are very potent; thus botulinum toxin is the most poisonous substance known. Bacteria whose main offensive weapon is an exotoxin are called *toxic organisms*. Examples of these are the causative organisms of *diphtheria*, *tetanus*, *gas-gangrene*, and *scarlet fever*. Although the infection which they produce remains localized, distant tissues of the host are damaged as a result of circulating toxins.

With most other organisms no such powerful toxins have been demonstrated. Cultures may be toxic to animals, but the responsible substances seem to be derived from the bodies of the organisms. These have been called *endotoxins*, but it is probable that in reality they are the complex constituents of the bacterial body. They are of protein—lipopolysaccharide constitution, and, on the whole, of low potency and their action on the tissues is non-specific.

Further investigations of the endotoxic group of organisms have shown that some substances do indeed diffuse out of the living cell body. The coagulase of *Staph. aureus* and hyaluronidase of *Strept. pyogenes* are two such substances. Some microbiologists call these exotoxins, but this is probably an error of judgment. It is even debatable whether coagulase and hyaluronidase are toxins at all. Therefore whatever theoretical argument, in practice the term exotoxin should be restricted to those substances which diffuse easily out of the organism, are highly toxic, and cause some or many of the lesions of the disease. Organisms which do not produce exotoxins as described above are called *invasive*. They are characterized by the tendency to spread widely throughout the body and enter the circulation. The pyogenic organisms, *Salmonella typhi*, and *Bacillus anthracis* are good examples. This term serves a useful purpose, because it emphasizes that lesions can be produced only in the actual presence of the organism.*

The manner whereby the invasive organisms produce damage is not clearly understood. Some seem to have a direct action on the tissues, and produce necrosis and acute inflammation. The pyogenic organisms fall into this group. In infections with some organisms it seems that damage is caused by the interaction of the organism or its products with sensitizing immunoglobulins or sensitized T cells.[5] Tuberculosis provides a good example of this situation. It is also well-documented in measles and respiratory-syncytial-virus infections that the disease can be more severe in the partially immunized individual than in the non-immune. In infection with other organisms the situation is much more complicated. *Typhoid fever* illustrates this particularly well.

Typhoid fever

The pathogenesis of mouse typhoid (infection with *Salmonella typhimurium*) has

* There are certain exceptions to this, as when invasive organisms produce lesions by some hypersensitivity mechanism, e.g. acute rheumatic fever.

been studied in considerable detail, and by analogy the sequence of events in humans is probably as follows:

Typhoid fever is contracted by the ingestion of food contaminated with *Salmonella typhi.* The organisms reach the lumen of the small intestine, and on its mucosal surface they are taken up by phagocytes. They are carried into the mucosa itself and thence to the local lymphoid tissue (Peyer's patches). Scarcely

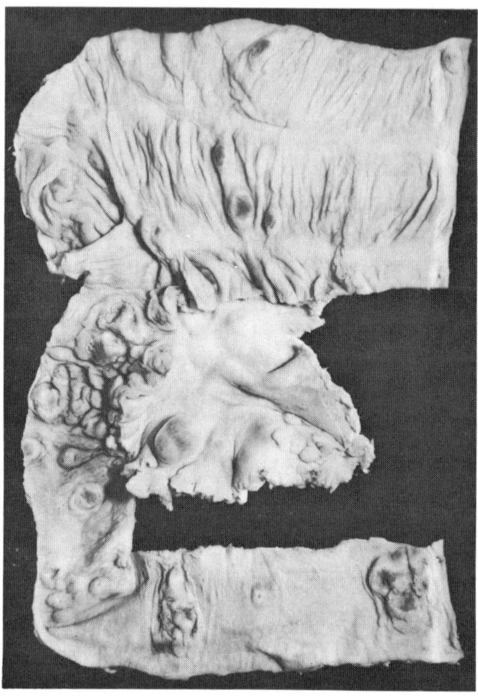

Fig. 7.1 Typhoid ulceration of the bowel. The ileum and ascending colon contain many ulcers which have retained the shape and size of the Peyer's patches and lymphoid follicles from which they have arisen. The walls are punched-out, and the bases are darkly staining due to the bile-pigmented necrotic debris in them. In the mesentery there is an enlarged lymph node. (A 50.3, *reproduced by permission of the President and Council of the Royal College of Surgeons of England.*)

any local damage occurs, and little or no inflammation results. The organisms multiply, and some pass on through the lymphatics to the mesenteric nodes and finally reach the blood stream *via* the thoracic duct. In this way there develops a *bacteraemia, which is defined as the transient presence of organisms in the blood stream.* The phagocytic cells of the RE system are well able to deal with this, and the organisms are engulfed by them. However, the organisms are able to live and multiply in these cells. By about the tenth day the parasitized cells undergo necrosis, and the blood stream is flooded with large numbers of bacilli. This is the end of the incubation period (usually 10 to 14 days), and the patient becomes seriously ill with *septicaemia, which is defined as the presence of organisms in the blood stream (proven by a positive blood culture) which are causally associated with severe constitutional upset.* This differs from *bacteraemia* in the following ways:

1. It is associated with severe clinical symptoms
2. There are more organisms in the blood
3. It indicates that the host's resistance to the organism is very inadequate.

The septicaemic phase lasts about one week and is characterized clinically by a progressive rise in temperature (step-ladder pattern) and severe constitutional symptoms. Death may occur at this stage.

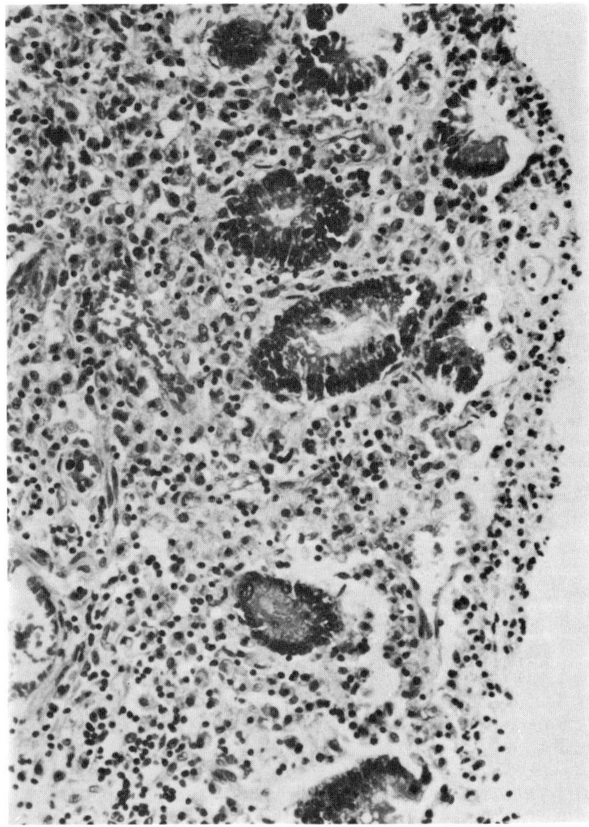

Fig 7.2 Typhoid ulceration of the small bowel. The mucosa is ulcerated, and an inflammatory infiltration consisting of lymphocytes and swollen macrophages is present around the remaining glands. Polymorphs are not present. × 200.

The next phase of the disease is marked by the onset of diarrhoea, ulceration of the small intestine, and the appearance of organisms in the faeces. The bacilli reach the gut *via* the bile, which is heavily contaminated as a result of the passage of the bacteria from the RE cells of the liver. The ulceration occurs over the inflamed Peyer's patches, and is associated with mesenteric adenitis (Fig. 7.1). In both the ulcers and the lymph nodes there is an accumulation of macrophages, while polymorphs are not present (Fig. 7.2). The most likely explanation of these events is that the local lymphoid tissue of the gut has become sensitized to the organism, and that subsequent contact with it produces damage. The local production of sensitizing antibodies must be postulated, because the blood level of detectable antibodies (agglutinins) does not rise till later in the course of the disease. During the second week diagnosis depends upon finding the organism in the faeces. By the third week the level of antibodies in the serum rises (Widal reaction), and the patient gradually recovers (Fig. 7.3).

Many viruses, e.g. smallpox, behave in a way similar to the typhoid bacillus. They produce no lesion on entry, but after dissemination and multiplication in the body cause extensive tissue damage as a result of some type of tissue hypersensitivity (see also syphilis, p. 229). Such a mechanism should always be suspected in an infective disease that has an incubation period exceeding 7 to 10 days.

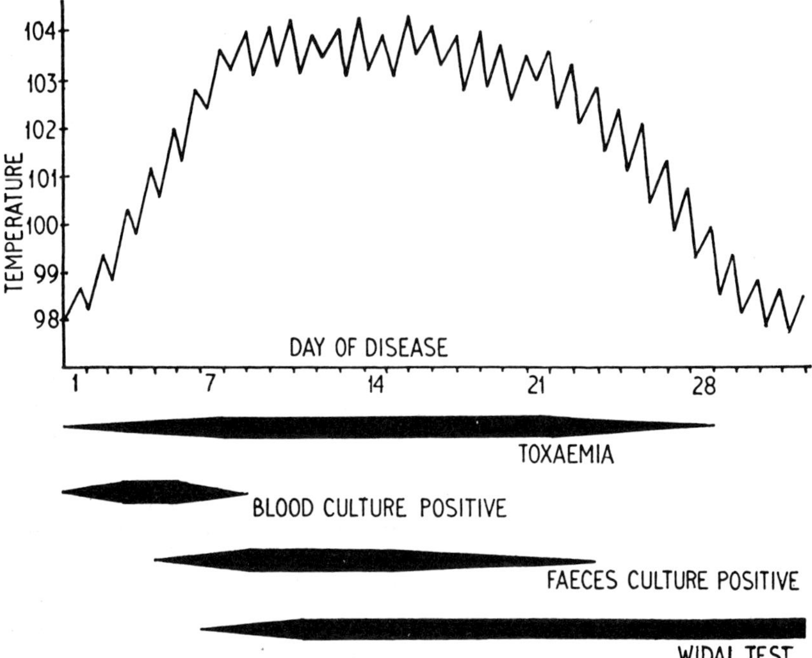

Fig. 7.3 Chart correlating the clinical course of a typical case of typhoid fever with the principal methods of bacteriological diagnosis. (*After Harries E H R, Mitman M 1947 Clinical practice in infectious disease, 3rd edn. Livingstone, Edinburgh, p 464*)

Septicaemia

The cause of death in septicaemia is poorly understood. It has been most extensively studied in anthrax.[6] *Bacillus anthracis* infection in animals leads to a fatal septicaemia, and the animals die with vast numbers of organisms in the blood. The organism, although a typically invasive one, has been found to produce a number of factors (anthrax toxic complex) both *in vitro* and *in vivo* that act to increase the permeability of blood vessels. A state of hypovolaemic shock develops. Early treatment with antibiotics will save infected animals, but there is a critical time after which treatment is of no avail. Although the organisms may be destroyed, the animal still dies as shock passes into an irreversible phase.

In septicaemia due to streptococci and staphylococci, death can reasonably be attributed to intense toxaemia consequent on the release of endotoxins. However, with other organisms, e.g. pneumococci, the symptoms are less easily explicable, because these organisms do not appear to produce toxic substances.

The generalized Shwartzman phenomenon

Gram-negative bacilli, e.g. *Salmonella typhi* and coliform organisms, produce an ill-defined endotoxin of lipoprotein nature. Experimentally it has been shown that this substance can produce shock if injected intravenously, especially if the dose is repeated *twenty-four hours later*. This enhancing effect of a previous dose is known as the *generalized Shwartzman phenomenon*,* and may be the experimental counterpart of the shock which is seen in some human cases of coliform septicaemia. The mechanism of the Shwartzman phenomenon is not well understood. It is probable that the endotoxin causes endothelial cell damage and that this initiates intravascular clotting. The occlusion of the vessels in the kidney leads to cortical necrosis with subsequent acute renal failure. The effect of the first injection of endotoxin is probably to block the reticulo-endothelial system so that the second injection of endotoxin is less quickly removed. The generalized Shwartzman reaction is not an immunologically mediated hypersensitivity reaction.

Types of acute inflammation

Although all examples of acute inflammation have many features in common, certain types have been categorized, depending upon some particular feature. The terms are useful for descriptive purposes but are of no fundamental significance.

Suppurative inflammation. Certain organisms, termed the pyogenic organisms, as well as some chemicals, produce considerable tissue destruction. This is associated with a marked neutrophil infiltration, and the disintegrating phagocytes liberate proteolytic enzymes which cause liquefaction of the dead area. The fluid produced is *pus*, and the inflammation is called *suppurative*. Suppuration occurring in infection generally indicates that localization is becoming established, and therefore in the days before chemotherapy it was regarded as a favourable sign; hence the origin of the term 'laudable pus'. The presence of pus in a natural cavity is called an *empyema*, and this occurs most frequently in the pleural cavity.

While suppuration is usually localized, pus formation may occasionally occur in a spreading cellulitis. Such a diffuse suppurative process is generally caused by *Strept. pyogenes*, and this type of inflammation is called *phlegmonous*.

Serous inflammation. In inflammation of loose tissues and in serous sacs the fluid component of the inflammatory exudate exceeds the cellular one, because the limiting factor of increased tissue tension (p. 74) is absent. There results a large accumulation of inflammatory oedema, and this is termed *serous inflammation*. Gas-gangrene provides another example. The invading organisms (particularly

* This should not be confused with the *localized Shwartzman phenomenon*. To demonstrate this, a quantity of Gram-negative bacterial endotoxin is injected into the skin of an animal and 24 hours later an intravenous dose is given. The site of the skin injected then undergoes necrosis. The pathogenesis is not understood, and there is little evidence that a similar reaction ever occurs in any human disease.

Clostridium oedematiens) produce toxins that directly act on blood vessels to increase their permeability.

Fibrinous inflammation. Fibrin formation is a feature of inflammation in serous sacs and in the lungs. It is well marked in most forms of pericarditis and peritonitis. It is also frequent in pneumococcal and staphylococcal infections. Often there is considerable serous exudate, and the inflammation is then termed *sero-fibrinous.*

Haemorrhagic inflammation. A blood-stained exudate indicates that the irritant has caused severe vascular damage. It is seen in the lungs in phosgene poisoning and acute influenzal pneumonia.

Catarrhal inflammation. This type is seen when a mucous membrane is involved in an acute inflammatory reaction. There is some destruction of the epithelial cells, and a profuse mucus secretion from those that remain as well as from the underlying glands. The common cold provides an excellent example.

Membranous inflammation. A membrane of mucus and fibrinous exudate covering an inflamed area of mucosa is seen in *membranous bronchitis.* It may be coughed up as a cast.

Pseudomembranous inflammation. This type differs from membranous inflammation in that the membrane contains necrotic epithelium as well as fibrin and inflammatory cells. It is seen typically in diphtheria and in pseudomembranous enterocolitis.

Gangrenous inflammation. Gangrene occurs in inflammation when the dead tissue is invaded by putrefactive organisms (p. 65).

Variability of the cellular exudate. Certain inflammations do not show the usual neutrophil polymorph response. In typhoid the inflammatory reaction has virtually no polymorphs, but instead is characterized by macrophages. Why this is so is not at all clear, but it may well be that the development of a delayed type of hypersensitivity is involved, since the mononuclear response is characteristically seen in this condition. Eosinophils are usually plentiful in inflammations produced by parasitic worms, and also in some allergic conditions (see p. 184). Lymphocytic infiltration is frequent in inflammatory lesions produced by viruses, even in the early stages. It is also a feature of acute inflammation in many skin diseases. This variation in cellular response is presumably related to the nature of the causative irritant which, in a variety of ways, leads to the release of specific chemotactic factors. This is discussed in greater detail in Chapter 5.

Mode of destruction of organisms in the inflammatory exudate

Although a completely teleological view of the inflammatory reaction is unjustifiable, it is generally accepted that the reaction is an adaptive response having survival value for the species. It creates around the invading organisms a micro-environment unfavourable for their multiplication and survival. *Local inflammation is therefore the first line of defence against the spread of infection.* An inhibition of the inflammatory reaction generally decreases the resistance to infection.

The manner in which organisms are killed in the exudate must now be considered:

Part played by phagocytes. *The polymorphonuclear leucocytes.* Although many pathogenic organisms can multiply in the cytoplasm of the polymorphonuclear leucocytes and even be spread by them, the ultimate destruction of the organism often takes place within these cells. The precise mechanism involved probably varies from one organism to another. The following intracellular antimicrobial agents may be involved:

1. *Lysosomal enzymes.* Although these acid-hydrolytic enzymes digest dead bacteria, it is unlikely that they can kill living organisms.
2. *Lysozyme.* This enzyme is released by both the specific and the azurophil granules of the polymorphs.
3. *Acidity.* The low pH may destroy some organisms. Lactic acid is bactericidal, and is produced as a consequence of the glycolysis that accompanies phagocytosis.
4. *Lactoferrin.* This protein inhibits bacterial growth by binding iron which is an essential growth requirement for micro-organisms.
5. *Cationic lysosomal proteins.* At least 7 antimicrobial proteins of this type are found in neutrophils. One of these is called *phagocytin.*
6. *Oxidizing agents.*[7] A number of bactericidal oxidizing agents are formed as a result of the hexose-monophosphate-shunt-activity that follows phagocytosis. The *superoxide anion* O_2^- and *singlet oxygen* are thought to be important. Also important is H_2O_2 which acts on bacteria in the presence of a halide and the enzyme myeloperoxidase that granulocytes contain.

The mononuclears. These phagocytic members of the RE system are particularly important in providing a defence against acid-fast bacilli, fungi, and viruses. General conditions, like shock and haemorrhage, impair the RE system's phagocytic activity. This may well explain the lowered resistance under these circumstances.

Part played by the fluid exudate. The inflammatory oedema contains complement and other antibacterial substances present normally in the plasma. It contains lactic acid in considerable quantities. This may be a factor in the destruction of invading organisms. Indeed, the conditions may be so unfavourable that some of the host cells as well as the bacteria are destroyed. To some extent this may actually be beneficial, because necrotic tissue has been shown to contain bactericidal substances.

Part played by acquired immunity. Antibodies, e.g. opsonins, are present in the inflammatory exudate and aid phagocytosis. Antibody-dependent cell-mediated cytotoxicity is further described on page 156. Activation of complement is another important mechanism whereby antibodies assist in the destruction of organisms.

It is also probable that the immune response affords protection by producing some degree of tissue hypersensitivity, such that there is acceleration of the inflammatory reaction and with it the normal mechanism of destruction.

The macrophages of an immune animal are more adept at destroying organisms, but the mechanism is poorly understood (p. 157).

Spread of infection

Local spread. The natural cohesion of tissues tends to prevent the spread of organisms. The tissue fluids are, however, in constant motion under normal conditions. Organisms are carried in any stream of fluid which may be present.

The activity of muscles causes considerable movement of tissue fluids, and it is for this reason that the time-honoured treatment of inflammation is to rest the part. It should be noted that the motility of the organism itself appears to play no part in its spread. There is no correlation between the motility of the organism and the rapidity with which it spreads. Thus, *Clostridium tetani* is a motile organism but tetanus is a localized infection, whereas *Clostridium welchii* is non-motile and yet produces the rapidly spreading gas-gangrene.

Local spread may also occur in an entirely different way. Organisms ingested by phagocytes may be transported by these cells. This is an important means of spread in tuberculosis, and almost certainly occurs in many other infections.

The local defence mechanism. The acute inflammatory reaction must be regarded as a defence mechanism, although as we have seen, it is called forth only in the case of certain infections. With these infections the acute inflammatory reaction, including the laying-down of fibrin, plays an important part in the destruction of the organism. It has been thought that the fibrin forms a barrier and is important in limiting the spread of infection. However, it seems much more likely that it is the whole inflammatory response which is important rather than the fibrin itself. The presence of a fibrin barrier around the zone of infection is thus indicative of a severe inflammatory response which causes destruction of the organism, and is probably not the prime mover in the destruction itself.

Spread by natural channels. If local spread implicates a natural passage, infection may spread by this route. The following examples are important: *peritoneum*—Infection may spread rapidly throughout the peritoneal space from localized lesions; it is for this reason that acute appendicitis is serious. Following perforation of the organ, the whole peritoneal cavity becomes infected, and as a large surface is involved, there is a rapid absorption of toxic substances. Infection may likewise spread through the *pleura*, *subarachnoid space*, *pericardium*, and *joint spaces.*

Infection may also spread along tubes, like the *bronchi* (in bronchopneumonia and pulmonary tuberculosis), the *ureter*, and the *gut.*

Spread by lymphatics. In acute inflammation lymphatic vessels are held open by the increase in tissue tension. The permeability of their walls is increased, as is also the flow of lymph. Invading organisms frequently gain access to the lymphatics, and are carried to the nearest lymph node. Phagocytes which have ingested the organisms but which are unable to destroy them, also travel by the same route. Here the RE cells lining the sinuses phagocytose the organisms and prevent their further spread. The lymph nodes may be regarded as the *second line of defence* against the spread of infection. Toxins may also be absorbed by the lymphatics. *Lymphangitis* is therefore a common event in spreading lesions, and when the vessels are superficial, as in the forearm, they appear as bright red streaks. Organisms may become arrested in the lymph nodes and yet not be destroyed. In this way *lymphadenitis* arises; the filter will have protected the individual, but at the expense of the node. If organisms pass through the lymphatic barrier, they then enter the blood stream.

Spread by the blood stream. The blood stream forms the *third and last line of defence* against the spread of infection. It has two main defence mechanisms.

1. The circulating blood itself contains a wide array of antibacterial substances.

These include complement, properdin, and opsonins, as well as antibodies of specific acquired immunity.

2. The RE system, especially the sinus-lining cells of the liver (Kupffer cells), bone marrow, and spleen, forms the main defence against generalized infection. Organisms injected experimentally into the blood stream are rapidly removed. In natural infections with highly invasive organisms like the typhoid bacillus early invasion of the blood stream occurs, and the circulating organisms are rapidly taken up by the RE system. This is the first step in the afferent limb of the general immune response (p. 164).

Mode of entry of organisms into the blood stream

The presence of organisms in the blood stream is a common event. It occurs under several conditions.

Direct invasion of blood vessels. A few organisms may invade blood vessels in the course of any local infection, e.g. a boil. The infection is often quite trivial, but the adjacent blood vessels may be ruptured by trauma, thereby allowing organisms to enter. Gingival infection or abscesses related to the apices of the roots of teeth are common lesions in which this is thought to occur, e.g. following dental extraction, scaling of teeth, or even chewing hard food. When small numbers of organisms enter the blood stream in this way, they are rapidly removed by the phagocytes of the RE system and are destroyed. Bacteraemia usually causes few symptoms, but rigors may occur in the bacteraemia which follows catheterization. Its real importance, however, is that under certain conditions it may lead to serious sequelae.

Metastatic lesions. Experimentally it has been shown that when an animal has a bacteraemia, histamine injected at any site will precipitate a local infection with the organism concerned. Trauma has a similar effect. Staphylococci may be localized in a bone in this way and set up osteomyelitis (p. 143). Another danger is that the organisms are filtered off by the kidneys, and if there is a coincidental obstruction to the outflow of urine, pyelonephritis may result. A further hazard of bacteraemia is that the organisms may colonize a damaged heart valve and cause endocarditis (p. 515).

Transplacental spread. If the patient is pregnant, organisms may cross the placenta and reach the fetus (p. 90).

Septic thrombophlebitis. When infection spreads to a vein, its wall becomes inflamed and thrombosis may occur, a condition called thrombophlebitis. If the thrombus is invaded by pyogenic organisms, it may soften and parts of it become detached, leading to the condition of *pyaemia.*

Pyaemia is the presence in the circulation of infected thrombi which are carried to various organs where they produce metastatic abscesses or septic infarcts. Which of these occurs depends on the vascular arrangements of the organ in which the emboli become lodged (p. 499). Pyaemia was a common complication of the staphylococcal osteomyelitis before the days of chemotherapy. It is now much less frequent. It sometimes follows suppuration of the gastrointestinal tract, e.g. acute appendicitis and infected piles, and the *portal pyaemia* produces multiple abscesses in the liver.

Spread from the lymphatic system. Organisms which are not held up in the tissues at the site of entry or in the lymph nodes, reach the venous circulation *via* the lymphatic ducts. Bacteraemia produced in this way is a common event with many invasive organisms, e.g. *S. typhi.* If the cells of the RE system, having phagocytosed the organisms, are unable to destroy them, the bacteria proliferate and are subsequently liberated into the circulation which is flooded with them. The patient becomes gravely ill with septicaemia.

Spread along nerves. Some viruses, e.g. rabies virus, are believed to travel up the nerves to reach the central nervous system. Whether they pass up the axoplasm or in the periaxonal space is uncertain.

Factors determining the localization or spread of infection

It is convenient at this point to summarize the factors which determine whether a particular organism is likely to spread from the site of infection or remain localized.

Factors involving the organisms

Virulence. It should be appreciated that within each species of organism there are many strains, each with differing degrees of virulence. Thus certain staphylococci produce severe infection, while others produce trivial skin lesions.

Dose. With many organisms a large dose produces a severe spreading lesion while a small one produces a minor lesion which heals. This is seen in tuberculosis produced experimentally in animals. It is probably not true of viral infections.

Portal of entry. Some organisms will cause infection only if administered by a particular route, e. g. *Vibrio cholerae* is non-pathogenic if injected, but may cause cholera if swallowed.

Synergism. The combined effect of two infecting organisms may be greater than either one alone. The best known example is Vincent's infection, which is a common cause of gingivitis and in which two organisms, the *Fusobacterium fusiforme* and the *Borrelia vincenti*, are in association. (See also clostridial infections, p. 207).

Products of the organisms. Certain organisms produce factors which may aid their spread; streptococci produce an enzyme *hyaluronidase* which acts by depolymerizing the ground substance, and probably aids in spreading the infection. *Strept. pyogenes* also produces the enzyme *streptokinase* which aids in the lysis of the fibrin barrier by activating the plasmin system (p. 467).

Factors involving the host

General factors. *The general state of health* of the host is important. Starvation and haemorrhagic shock have been shown experimentally to render animals more liable to infection. It is frequently observed that patients with chronic debilitating diseases, like chronic nephritis and diabetes mellitus, are less capable of resisting infection. The factors involved are complex, and probably involve both humoral factors, e.g. a low complement level, and an impaired activity of the phagocytes.

The immune state. This involves both non-specific factors like complement and the specific antibodies of acquired immunity. Primary infections tend to spread much more widely than do subsequent ones due to the absence of active immunity (see tuberculosis, p. 188).

Low white-cell count. Infections tend to spread whenever the neutrophil polymorphonuclear leucocytes count is low, e.g. in agranulocytosis or acute leukaemia. Functional defects of neutrophil activity are described on page 170.

Local factors. The local blood supply is important. Ischaemia from whatever cause, e.g. injection of adrenaline, peripheral vascular disease, etc., adversely affects the inflammatory response designed to destroy the organism. Similarly, foreign bodies and chemicals which cause necrosis are harmful. Thus silica potentiates the pathogenic action of the tubercle bacillus, and ionic calcium aids the inception of anaerobic infections in wounds (p. 209).

It is evident from this account of the various patterns of infection that the relationship between the host and the infecting organism is extremely complex. This is well illustrated in the case of the human subject and the *Brucella* organism. The infection can vary from an acute illness to a chronic disease, or even a symptomless carrier state in which a symbiotic relationship has been established. Only in the case of the exotoxin-producing organisms is the pathogenesis of the disease which they cause at all clearly understood. It is not surprising therefore that it is in this group of infections that our understanding of immunity is also most complete.

REFERENCES

1. Carpenter C C J 1972. Cholera and other enterotoxin-related diarrheal diseases. Journal of Infectious Diseases 126 : 551
2. Gerald P S 1976 A new frontier for infectious disease research? New England Journal of Medicine 295 : 337
3. Miller D A 1974 Human chromosome 19 carries a poliovirus receptor gene. *Cell* 1 : 167
4. Wilson G S, Miles A A 1975 In Topley and Wilson's Principles of Bacteriology, Virology, and Immunity, 6th edn, p 1273 Arnold : London
5. Webb H E 1968 Factors in the host-virus relationship which may affect the course of an infection. British Medical Journal 4 : 684
6. Green D M 1973 In Medical Microbiology, ed Cruickshank R, Duguid J P, Marmion B P, Swain R H A, 12th edn, Vol 1, p 345 et seq. Churchill Livingstone : Edinburgh
7. Fridovich I 1974 Superoxide radical and the bactericidal action of phagocytes. New England Journal of Medicine 290 : 624

8

Wound healing

The word *healing*, used in a pathological context, refers to the body's replacement of destroyed tissue by living tissue. It is therefore useful, at the outset, to enumerate the causes of tissue loss or destruction:

Traumatic excision, whether accidental or surgical.

Physical, chemical, and microbial agents. These all give rise to inflammation, and in sufficient amount lead to necrosis.

Ischaemia, which leads to infarction.

Hypersensitivity reactions to foreign proteins, or to products of organisms, are instances when the body's response to external agents can itself engender necrosis (see Arthus phenomenon, p. 185, caseation in tuberculosis, p. 216).

In insects, amphibians, and crustaceans the ability to replace lost parts has long been known, and is truly remarkable. Thus, if the lens of the eye of a salamander is removed a new lens develops from the adjacent iris; even the complex neural part of the retina, if destroyed, can be reformed from the outer pigmented layer of the retina. Other well-known examples of regeneration are the reformation of the amputated limbs of insects and newts, and of the claws of lobsters. The process whereby whole limbs are reformed is well developed in lower forms of life; it is complex, and resembles embryonic development or asexual reproduction. The process is termed *axial regeneration* by zoologists, but the term *reconstitution* is also used by pathologists. One would think that the ability to reform a lost limb or organ was so useful to survival that it would have been retained during evolution. Such has not been the case. The higher animals—including humans—do not have the ability to replace lost limbs following their amputation. Perhaps this is because sexual reproduction has been evolved and preserved at all costs as a means of improving and remoulding the species. 'If there were no regeneration there could be no life. If everything regenerated there would be no death. All organisms exist between these two extremes. Other things being equal, they tend towards the latter end of the spectrum, never quite achieving immortality because this would be incompatible with reproduction.'*

Axial regeneration[1]

The regeneration of the amputated arm of the newt has been extensively studied. The stump rapidly becomes covered by a layer of epidermal cells that slide in from

*Quoted from Goss R J 1969 Principles of Regeneration. Academic Press, New York.

the adjacent skin. The cells multiply to form an *apical cap*, and intimate contact of these cells with the stump, particularly its nerves, is an essential step in the regeneration process. After a brief inflammatory reaction the cells of the stump—fibroblasts, muscle cells, osteoblasts and other cell types—appear to revert from their differentiated form into a primitive cell type by a process termed *dedifferentiation.* Connective-tissue fibres—collagen, muscle, and bone—break down, and the cells of regeneration lie in an oedematous stroma that resembles the mesenchyme of the developing embryo. This mass of cells is termed the blastema. Its cells multiply rapidly in an avascular field in the first instance. Later there is vascularisation and differentiation: bone, muscle, tendon, nerves, and blood vessels are produced in a co-ordinated manner such that there is accurate replacement of the parts of the limb that were lost. No matter what the level of the original amputation, only the distal parts are replaced. Thus with a forearm amputation, a wrist and hand are formed but never an elbow. This rule of *distal transformation* has been summed up by the trite description of 'hands from elbows, but never elbows from hands'.

Wound healing in humans

In humans the cells adjacent to the area of damage fail to dedifferentiate, and no blastema comparable to that described above is formed. The healing process has two aspects:

Contraction, a mechanical reduction in the size of the defect occurring in the first few weeks (see below).

Replacement of lost tissue, which is brought about by migration of cells as well as division of adjacent cells to provide extra tissue to fill the gap. This can be accomplished in two ways:

Repair, the replacement of lost tissue by granulation tissue which matures to form scar tissue. This is inevitable when the surrounding specialized cells do not possess the capacity to proliferate, e.g. muscle and neurons.

Regeneration, the replacement of lost tissue by tissue similar in type. There is a proliferation of surrounding undamaged specialized cells. Regeneration is predominant when the cells comprising the tissue are capable of multiplication, and is well illustrated by the healing of a damaged liver.

It should be noted that the word repair is used in a rather arbitrary way by some surgeons and pathologists. Surgeons refer to the union of fractures or the closure of defects by various inert materials as examples of repair, but the latter is not even true healing, though it has an ameliorative effect. Some pathologists equate repair with healing and recovery and describe 'repair by resolution', 'repair by granulation tissue,' and 'repair by regeneration'. There is no doubt that such variation in the nomenclature is confusing, and in this book the terms resolution, regeneration, and repair are used strictly in accordance with the definitions given previously. The processes involved in healing may best be understood if each aspect is described in as clear a form as possible. The first of these is wound contraction.

Wound contraction[2]

Measurement. This is conveniently studied by excising a small, circular, full-thickness disc of skin from the back or flank of an animal. Figures 8.1 and 8.2 show the results of such an experiment. The size of the wound is measured at regular intervals, and it can be seen that after an initial period of 2 to 3 days there follows a period of rapid contraction which is largely completed by the 14th day. New tissue formation is not included, since the measurements are made from the original wound edges. The wound is reduced by approximately 80 per cent of its

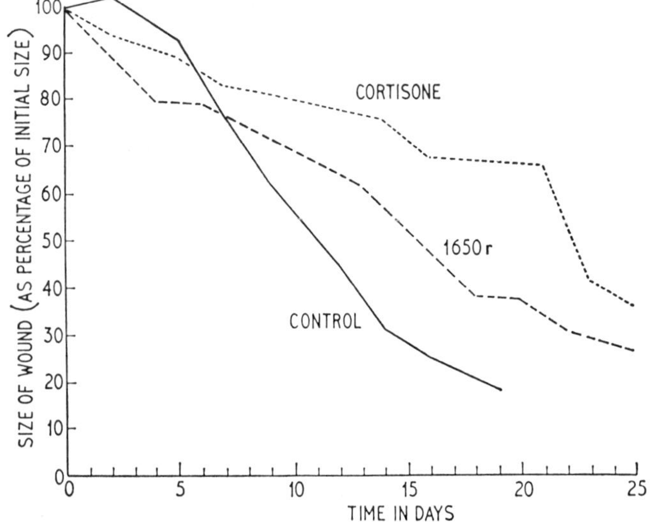

Fig. 8.1 Wound contraction in the rat. Daily administration of cortisone acetate causes considerable delay in the process. Irradiation with 1650 r immediately after inflicting the wounds has a similar delaying effect.

original size in the rat, but the actual extent of the contraction varies with the species of animal, and with the shape, size, and site of the wound. Contraction results in much faster healing, as less new tissue has to be formed. If contraction is prevented, healing is slow and a large ugly scar the result.

Contraction probably plays a similar role in the healing of wounds of the oral mucosa. In the non-keratinized mucosa scarring persists as on the skin, but in wounds of the keratinized mucosa of the gingiva, edentulous ridge, and the palate, only a small amount of scar tissue forms during healing and it soon becomes so inconspicuous that the actual site of the wound can no longer be found.

Cause of wound contraction. Contraction occurs in wounds at a time when granulation tissue is being actively formed, and it is generally agreed that it is in the granulation tissue at the edge of the wound (the '*picture-frame area*') that the mechanism for contraction lies. Present evidence suggests that the fibroblastic cells of granulation tissue can contract.[3] Indeed, their cytoplasm contains fibrillar components similar to that found in smooth muscle cells; hence they have been called *myofibroblasts*, and it is postulated that their contraction results in a remodelling of the granulation tissue such that the wound undergoes contraction.

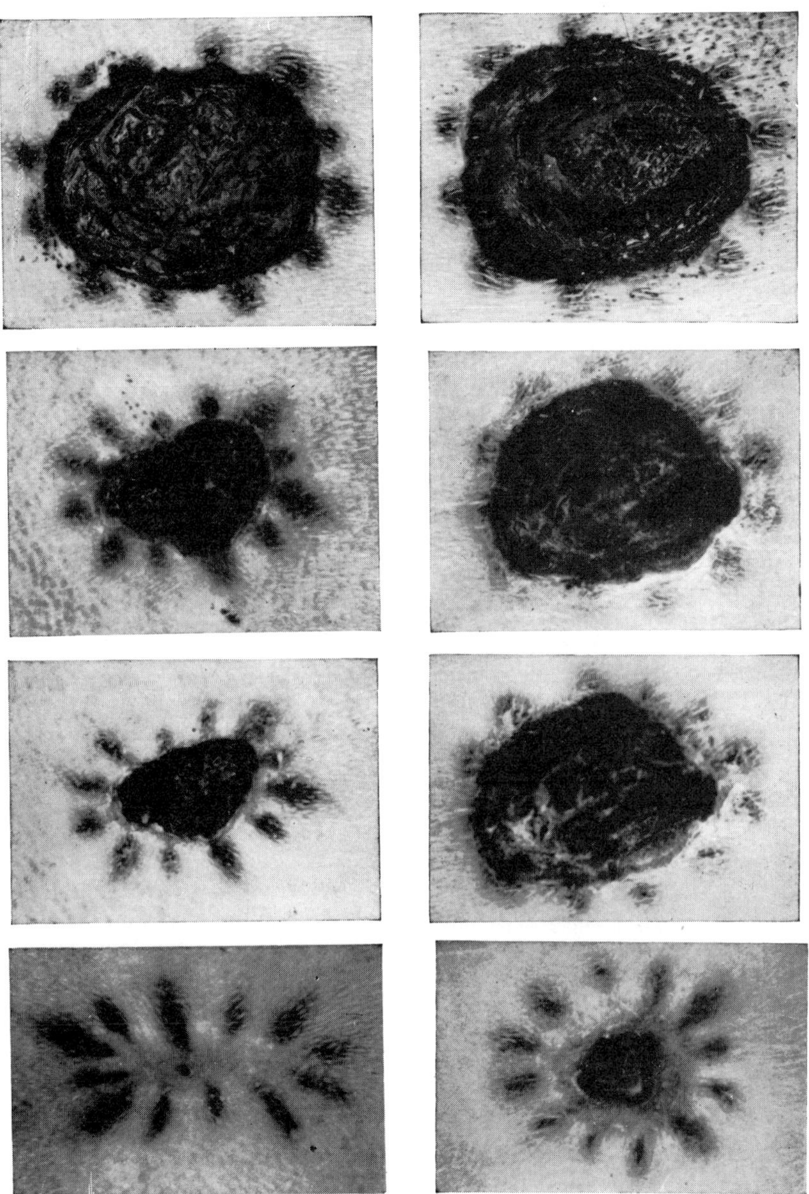

Fig. 8.2 Wound contraction in the rat and the effect of x-irradiation. The edges of the skin wounds have been tattooed with carbon so as to render them easily visible. Note how the delivery of 1650 r to the wound on the right has delayed the contraction process. (*From Blair G H, Slome D, Walter J B 1961 Review of experimental investigations on wound healing, British surgical practice: Surgical progress, Ross JP (ed). Butterworth, London.*)

Inhibition. Interference with the formation of granulation tissue, e.g. by *irradiating the wounded area* or the administration of *glucocorticoids,* causes considerable delay in wound contraction (Fig. 8.1). Interference with the formation of collagen, on the other hand, as in the vitamin-C-deficient animal, has no such effect.[4] The contraction of wounds may also be impaired following burns, and also if the raw area of the wound is skin-grafted.

Organization

Organization is one of the fundamental processes in pathology, and can be defined as *the ingrowth of fibroblasts and vascular endothelial cells into a blood clot or a fibrinous exudate to form granulation tissue.* In effect it results in the replacement of necrotic

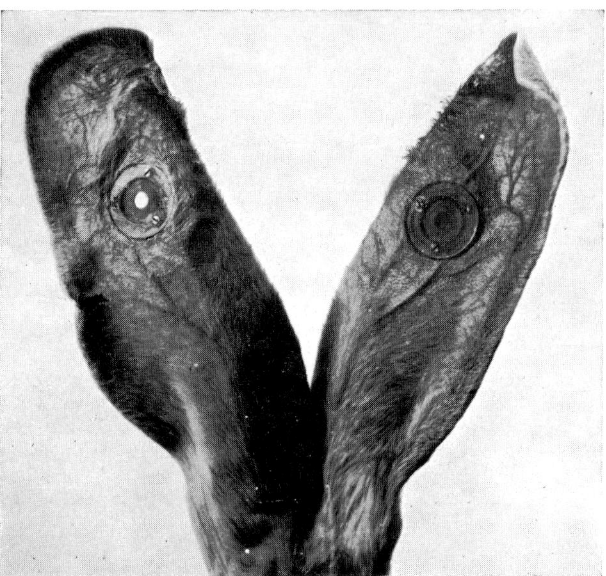

Fig. 8.3 Two rabbit ear-chambers in position. The one in the left ear shows the central area in which observations are made. In the chamber on the right the area of the central table is still filled with blood clot. (*From Blair G H, van den Brenk H A S, Walter J B, Slome D 1961 Wound healing. Pergamon Press, pp 46–53, in a symposium organized by Smith and Nephew Research Ltd.*)

tissue, fibrin, and blood clot by living granulation tissue. The four situations where organization is encountered are in an *inflammatory exudate* (this is especially important in chronic inflammation), a *haematoma* (especially if there is severe tissue damage as in wound healing), a *thrombus*, and an *infarct*.

The growth of granulation tissue can be studied experimentally using the rabbit ear-chamber technique[5] (Figs. 8.3, 8.4, 8.5). Four phases may be observed.

Haematoma formation. Blood clot soon occupies the table area of the chamber.

Traumatic inflammation. The damage caused by inserting the chamber sets in motion the phenomenon of acute inflammation in the surrounding tissue. An exudate containing fibrin and polymorphs therefore accumulates.

Demolition. The dead tissue cells liberate their autolytic enzymes, and other proteolytic enzymes come from disintegrating polymorphs. There is an associated mononuclear infiltration with macrophages. These are mostly derived from the blood monocytes, and their function is to ingest particulate matter, which they either digest or remove (p. 79).

Granulation-Tissue formation. Granulation tissue is formed by the proliferation and migration of surrounding connective-tissue elements. It is composed, in the first instance, of *capillary loops* and *fibroblasts* together with a variable number of inflammatory cells (Fig. 8.6). Initially this is a highly vascular tissue, but with the passage of time it develops into avascular scar tissue. The manner of its formation must be considered in more detail. Two stages may be recognized: there is first a stage of *vascularization*, and this is subsequently followed by *devascularization.*

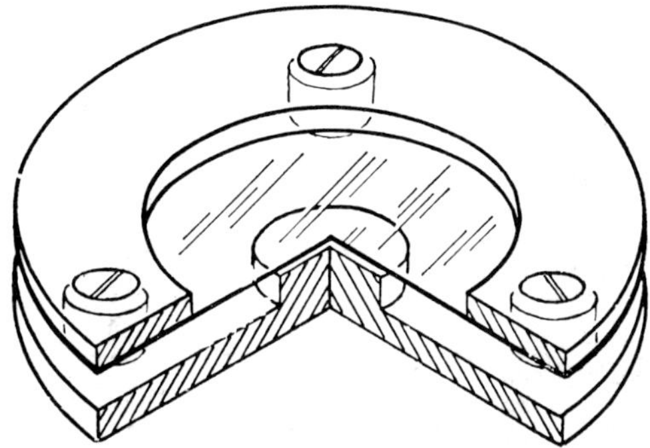

Fig. 8.4 Diagrammatic representation of one type of rabbit ear-chamber; a wedge has been cut out to show its construction. The chamber is composed of a Perspex base plate which has a raised central table and three peripherally arranged pillars. The cover-slip consists of a disc of mica supported at the edge by a ring of Perspex. The cover-slip is placed upon the three pillars, and held in position by screws which are inserted into threaded holes in the pillars. The height of the pillars is such that the gap between the top of the table and the mica is 50–100 μm. (Drawing by Mr S P Steward.)

Buds of endothelial cells grow out from the existing blood vessels at the wound margin, undergo canalization, and by joining with their neighbours form a series of vascular arcades. At first the newly-formed vessels all appear similar; the electron microscope shows gaps between the endothelial cells and a poorly-formed basement membrane. Protein escapes from these newly-formed vessels, and it is easy to imagine that the tissue fluid around them forms a very suitable medium for cellular growth. Very soon differentiation occurs. Some vessels acquire a muscular coat and become arterioles, while others form thin-walled venules. The remainder either disappear, or persist as part of the capillary bed.

At the same time as the vessels grow into the clot, the fibroblasts at the wound edge multiply and accompany the vascular invasion. Thus the clot is converted into a living vascular granulation tissue, and the process is known as *organization.* The fibroblasts (myofibroblasts, see p. 114) which accompany the capillary loops are large and plump, but gradually, as collagen fibrils form around them, the cells become elongated fibrocytes. Under light microscopy the fibrils are first detected as reticulin, but this gradually changes to mature collagen fibres. During this process of fibrogenesis the pH becomes alkaline. The fibroblasts are thought also to be responsible for the formation of the ground substance. Lymphatic vessels

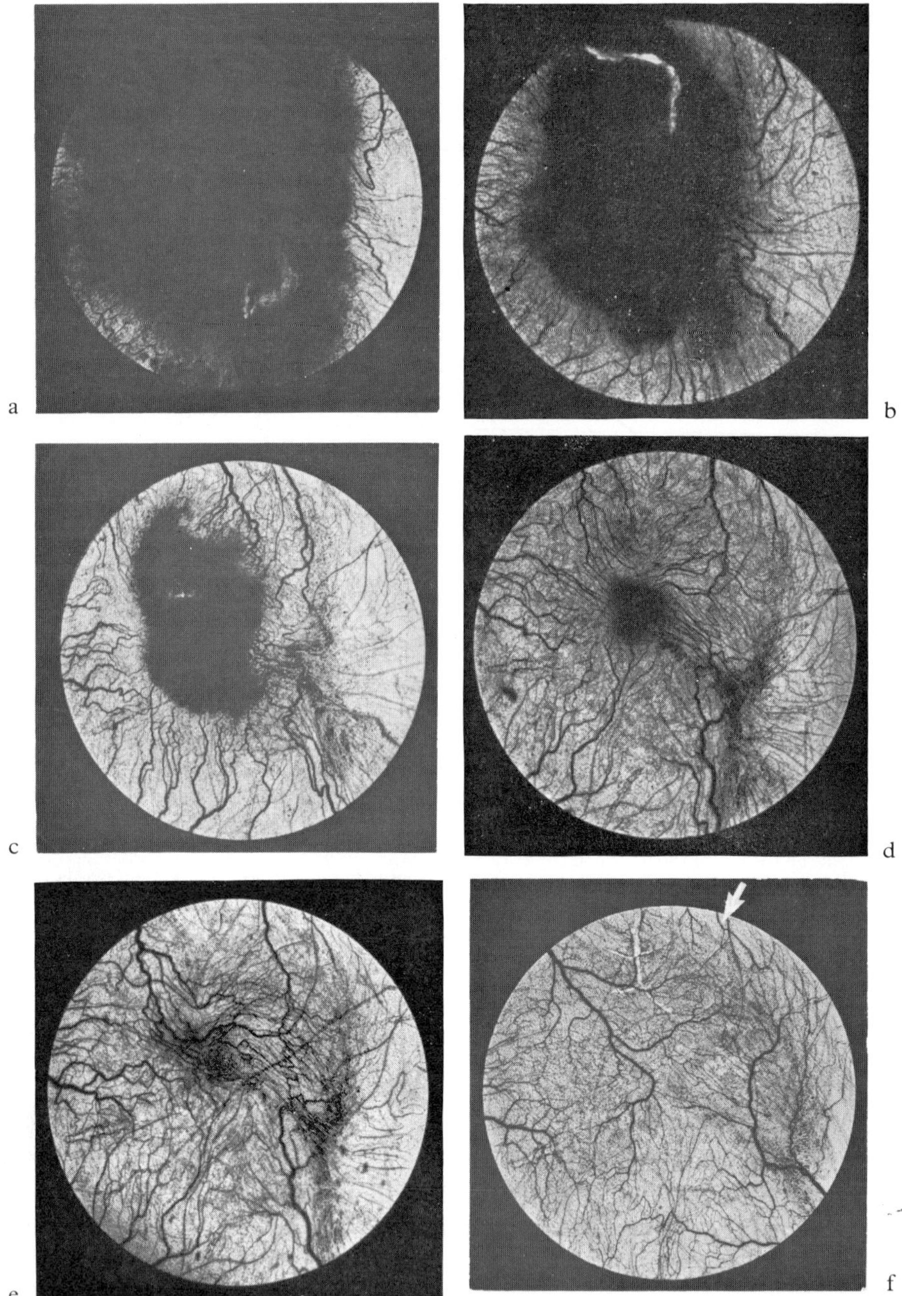

Fig. 8.5 Granulation tissue formation in the rabbit ear-chamber. Photographs taken at the following times after the insertion of the chamber: (a) 9 days, (b) 12 days, (c) 17 days, (d) 21 days, (e) 24 days, and (f) 44 days. At 9 days vessels are seen to be invading the dark clot in the centre, and by 24 days organization is complete. The large tortuous vessels are venules; the arterioles are more difficult to see at this magnification. The arrow in (f) indicates an arteriole which divides almost immediately. Note how by 44 days changes have occurred in the course of many blood vessels, although the original pattern of certain venules can still be recognized on the left-hand side of the picture. A lymphatic vessel is now visible at the top of the chamber. ×8.5.

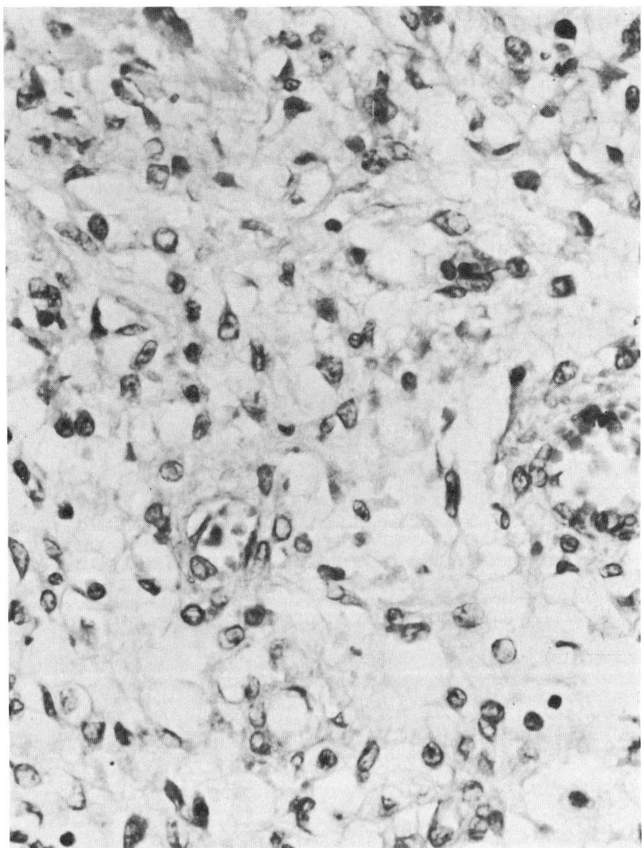

Fig. 8.6 Early granulation tissue. This is composed mostly of thin-walled capillaries. A few dilated vascular spaces are present, but they have not differentiated into arteries or veins. The intervening large, plump cells are fibroblasts. They have not yet started to lay down collagen fibres. × 160.

grow into the maturing granulation tissue in much the same manner as do the blood vessels, only later. The two sets of vessels do not anastomose. At the same time there is an ingrowth of nerve fibres to supply the arterioles, which are then capable of exhibiting contraction.

As maturation proceeds, so some vessels undergo atrophy and disappear. Others show thickening of their intimal coats and eventual obliteration of the lumen (*endarteritis obliterans*). This process of devascularization results in the formation of a pale avascular scar. Coincident with the devascularization there is often *cicatrization* of scar tissue with much local tissue distortion. This process must be clearly distinguished from contraction. *Cicatrization* (or *contracture*, as it is sometimes called) is a diminution in the size of a *scar* and is a late event; *contraction* is a diminution in the size of a *wound* and is an early event.

Although it is generally considered that collagen once formed remains for life, experimental evidence in animals suggests that it can be removed. The mechanism is not known, but that it does occur in the human is suggested by the way in which scars gradually become less obvious.

Tensile strength[2,6]

Another method of examining a wound is the estimation of its tensile strength. The strength of the wound is of great practical importance because it is the main safeguard against *wound disruption*, or *dehiscence*. Three stages may be recognized.

At first the strength of a skin wound is only that of the fibrin cementing the cut surfaces together. It is for this reason that skin wounds are held together by sutures, clips, or tapes. There then follows a period of increasing tensile strength which corresponds to the amount of collagen produced by the granulation tissue uniting the cut wound edges. Thus the increase in tensile strength parallels the increase of hydroxyproline in the wound area, since this is a reflection of the amount of collagen present (p. 37). Finally as the months go by the strength of a wound increases further.

The steady development of cross-linkages between collagen fibres (Ch. 2) is responsible for this steady increase in tensile strength. Experimental evidence suggests that collagen synthesis continues for many weeks. Since there is no increase in the total amount of collagen at this time, it is evident that there must also be collagen breakdown; presumably this is brought about by the action of collagenases. The balanced state of collagen synthesis and collagen degradation brings about a remodelling of the scar so that it reaches an optimum state. An imbalance could result in a weak scar (see scurvy and wound dehiscence) on the one hand, and keloid formation on the other.

Thus many factors influence the rate of increase of tensile strength. These are both local and general, and in the main are related to granulation-tissue and collagen formation.

HEALING OF SKIN WOUNDS[7,8]

Healing of a clean incised wound with edges in apposition[9]

This process is described as *healing by primary intention*, and is the desired result in all surgical incisions.

The following changes occur:

Initial haemorrhage results in the formation of fibrin-rich haematoma.

An acute inflammatory reaction occurs, and the fibrinous exudate helps to cement the cut margins of the wound together.

Epithelial changes. Within 24 hours of injury epithelial cells from the adjacent epidermis migrate into the wound and insinuate themselves between the inert dermis and the clot (Fig. 8.7 (B)). With well-approximated wounds by 24 hours a continuous layer of epidermal cells covers the surface. Overlying the area there is a crust or scab of dried clot. During the next 24 to 48 hours the epidermal cells invade the space where connective tissue will eventually develop; in this way a spur is formed (Fig. 8.7 (C)). The migrating cells of the epidermis do not divide. Mitotic activity occurs in the basal cells a short distance from the edge of the wound, and in the mouse this activity is maximal at 36 hours. Epidermal cells also migrate along suture tracks, and where the suture or the incision encounters a sweat gland or other skin appendage, epithelial cells are contributed from this source (Fig. 8.7 (C)). The stimulus for this epithelial growth and migration is not known. Experimentally it has been noted that cells in tissue culture continue to divide until they establish contact with similar cells, at which point mitosis stops. This has been called *contact inhibition* by Abercrombie; the mechanism is obscure.

A demolition phase follows the acute inflammatory reaction in the area of the wound.

Organization. By about the third day the wound area is filled with fibroblasts (myofibroblasts) and capillary buds growing in from the cut surfaces. This

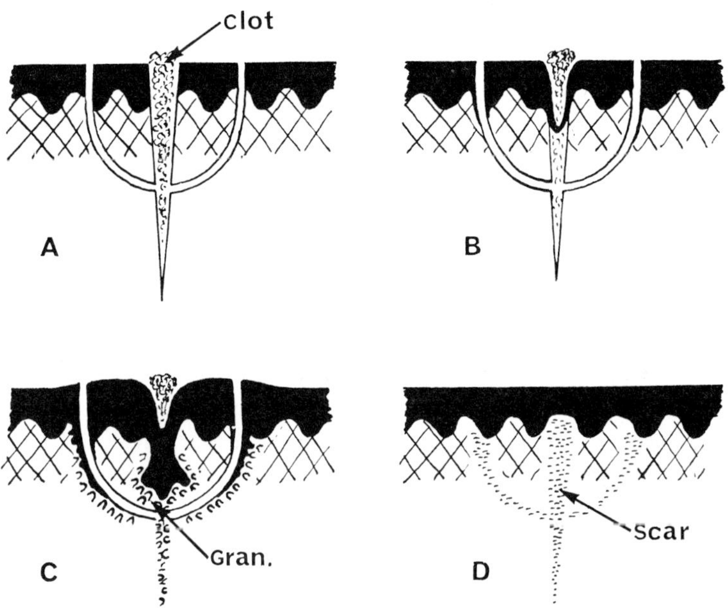

Fig. 8.7 Diagrammatic representation of the healing of an incised wound held together by a suture, the track of which alone is shown. The wound rapidly fills with clot (A) and shortly afterwards the epithelium migrates into the wound and down the suture tracks (B). Epithelial spurs are formed, and granulation-tissue (gran) formation proceeds (C). In D the suture has been removed, and scar tissue remains to mark the site of the incision and the suture tracks. The epithelial ingrowths have degenerated.

ingrowth occurs mainly from the subcutaneous tissues, with little or no contribution from the reticular layer of the dermis, which is inert. There may be some contribution from the papillary layer of the dermis. Collagen appears a day or two later. This granulation tissue appears to prevent excessive epithelial migration into the wound, and the epithelial cells which form the spurs and the lining of suture tracks degenerate and are replaced by granulation tissue. Only the surface epithelial cells persist, and these divide and differentiate so that a multilayered covering of epidermis is reformed. It first covers a vascular granulation tissue, but as devascularization proceeds the scar shrinks in size and changes in colour from red to white.

Epithelial cells are thus the first cells to be stimulated, and their presence excites a connective tissue response which in its turn inhibits the epithelial growth. The early role that epithelium plays in the process of wound healing has been stressed by Gillman, and explains the formation of an epidermoid cyst from epithelial remnants, and also the ugly punctate scars which appear if sutures are left in position for any length of time. Punctured wounds due to injections do not form such scars, because the wound is not held open and therefore no epithelial 'invasion' occurs. The use of adhesive tapes instead of sutures for closing wounds avoids these marks and produces a better cosmetic result.[10,11]

Healing of wounds with separated edges (*healing by secondary intention*)
Although stress is sometimes laid on the difference between healing by primary intention and secondary intention, the pathological changes in both are very similar. When there is extensive tissue loss, either by direct trauma, inflammatory necrosis, or simply failure to approximate the wound edges, a large defect is present which must be made good. The main bulk of tissue which performs this service is granulation tissue, and this type of healing is therefore sometimes known as *healing by granulation.* The term is, however, a poor one, since it wrongly implies that granulations are not formed in the simple incised wound. The differences between healing by primary and secondary intention are quantitative not qualitative.

In healing by secondary intention the wound edges are widely separated, so that healing has to progress from the base upwards as well as from the edges inwards. From the clinical point of view healing of a well-approximated incised wound (primary intention) is fast and leaves a small, neat scar. Healing by secondary intention is slow and results in a large, distorted scar. The difference lies in the type of wound and not in the type of healing.

The following account of the healing of a large uninfected wound is illustrated in Fig. 8.8

1. There is an initial inflammatory phase affecting the surrounding tissues. The wound is filled with coagulum, as described in simple incisions. This coagulum dries on its surface, and forms a scab in some wounds.

2. An important feature is *wound contraction*, which has already been fully described (see p. 114). Fig. 8.2 (p. 115) shows the changes in size of full-thickness skin loss.

3. As with incised wounds, the epidermis adjacent to the wound shows hyperplasia, and epithelial cells migrate into the wound. They form a thin tongue which grows between pre-existing viable connective tissue and the surface clot with necrotic material. The epithelial cells secrete a collagenase which probably aids their penetration between living and dead connective tissue.

4. Demolition follows acute inflammation, and the clot in the centre of the wound is invaded and replaced by granulation tissue. This grows from the subcutaneous tissues at the wound edge, and is important in causing wound contraction. Granulation tissue is also formed from the base of the wound, the amount from this source depending upon the nature and vascularity of the bed.

When the wound is viewed with a magnifying glass, the surface (under the scab) is deep red and granular, the capillary loops forming elevated mounds. It is very fragile, and the slightest trauma causes bleeding. It was this granularity which was responsible for the name 'granulation tissue'. The covering of the wound by granulation tissue serves an important protective role. If organisms are introduced into a recent wound, infection is likely to result, but not, however, if the wound is first allowed to granulate. Thus granulation tissue forms a temporary protective layer until the surface is covered by epithelium.

5. The migrating epidermis covers the granulation tissue, and in this way a mushroom-shaped scab is formed with a central attachment, which finally becomes nipped off (Fig. 8.8 (C)).

6. The regenerated epidermis becomes thicker, and sends short processes into the underlying tissue. These are transient structures and do not persist as rete ridges, for neither these nor the skin appendages are reformed in the human

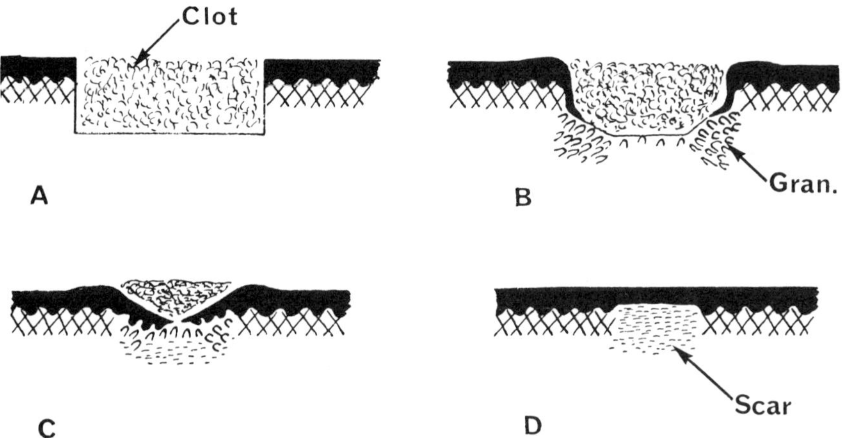

Fig. 8.8 Diagram to illustrate the healing of an excised wound. The wound is rapidly filled with clot (A). Epithelium soon migrates in from the margins to undermine the clot, which dries to form a crust. Granulation tissue (gran) grows into the wounded area, and is most profuse around the circumference where it is derived from the subcutaneous fat (B). Epithelial ingrowth continues and spurs are produced (C); these, however, do not persist, and the end-result (D) is a scar covered by epidermis which lacks rete ridges. During the healing process contraction has taken place so that the final scar is considerably smaller than the original wound.

subject. The epidermal incursions appear to stimulate the formation of granulation tissue, so that the scar gains thickness and is eventually level with the surface of the skin. The scar is at first pink, but the subsequent devascularization leaves it white.

It can be seen that with full thickness skin loss, part of the clot occupying the wound is organized but much of it is cast off. With partial thickness skin loss, as may occur following burns or at the donor site of a Thiersch graft, the area of the wound is covered by epithelium both from the wound edges and from the cut remains of hair follicles and sweat glands. Epithelialization is therefore very fast, and the granulation tissue which is formed is produced beneath the new epithelium.

Factors influencing repair

Although it would be desirable to analyse the factors which influence repair according to whether they affect granulation tissue formation, collagen production, contraction, etc., it must be admitted that in many instances we have insufficient information to adopt this policy. In practice, the factors which affect wound healing may be divided into two groups—those which act locally, and those whose influence is general or systemic. There are many factors which delay wound healing, but few are known which accelerate it. The following account consists therefore largely of the causes of delayed wound healing.

Local factors

Blood supply. Wounds in an ischaemic area, i.e. where there is a poor blood supply, heal slowly; for this reason injuries heal much more slowly in the pre-tibial region than in parts with a good blood supply, such as the face. The poor circulation in the skin of the leg in patients with varicose veins (with persistent oedema) or peripheral vascular disease causing ischaemia predisposes them to slow wound healing. Ischaemia secondary to pressure is an important factor in the causation and poor healing of *bedsores.* Any condition of chronic inflammation is liable to be accompanied by endarteritis obliterans and poor blood supply to the part; perhaps the best example of this is previous x-irradiation. Finally, the slow wound healing that sometimes is seen in old age may in part be related to a poor circulation.

Continued tissue breakdown and inflammation. Any condition causing continued tissue breakdown leads to persistent inflammation, and therefore delays completion of the healing process.

The most important examples are infection, the presence of a foreign body or irritant chemical, and excessive movement.

Infection. In an infected skin wound a scab does not form, and often the base is composed of dead tissue and inflammatory exudate forming a slough. Underlying this there is chronic inflammatory granulation tissue.

Foreign bodies and other irritants. The presence of a foreign body in a wound, even in the absence of infection, may delay healing. The over-enthusiastic use of irritating disinfectants may cause considerable delay in the healing of skin ulcers, and indeed, if hypersensitivity develops, may lead to extensive necrosis.

Movement. This delays healing by submitting the delicate granulation tissue to repeated trauma.

Poor apposition of the wound edges. This will obviously delay the healing of the wound. If the wound is adherent to a bony surface, this, by anchoring the wound edges, will tend to prevent contraction. This is well seen in wounds over the tibia, and also in chronic varicose ulcers.

Direction of the wound. Skin wounds made in a direction parallel to the lines of Langer heal faster than those made at right angles to them. *The lines of Langer*, first described in fact by Dupuytren in 1832, are due to the orientation of the collagen bundles in the dermis. The skin is less tensile in the direction of the lines than at right angles to them. In general they correspond to the direction of the crease lines, although the latter are in fact related also to the movements of the underlying muscles and joints. Skin incisions made across the crease lines tend to gape, and their healing is delayed. Therefore, when planning a surgical incision these should be taken into consideration. Wounds parallel to or in the crease lines are more satisfactory and the scars less visible.

Effects of previous wounding. Pre-existing wounds at a distance do not influence the healing of an additional skin wound. There is therefore no evidence of circulating wound hormone. Re-sutured wounds do, however, heal faster than do those sutured primarily, because the reparative process has already commenced. Severe trauma delays wound healing, presumably because of the adrenocortical response to the stress.

Exposure to ionizing radiation. Previous x-irradiation may reduce the vascularity of the part. Apart from this, x-rays inhibit wound contraction if given at the same time as the injury. The formation of granulation tissue is also delayed.

General factors affecting wound healing

Age. Wound healing is fast in the young, but is normal in old age unless there is some associated debilitating disease or ischaemia.

Nutrition. (*a*) *Protein deficiency.* Animals starved of protein show poor wound healing and deficient collagen formation. This abnormality may be corrected by administering proteins containing methionine or cystine, or by supplementing the diet with these amino acids only. Although cystine is not present in mature collagen, it is necessary for normal wound healing and collagen formation (see p. 39). Apart from an inadequate intake of protein the body may be deficient if there is excessive loss, as when there is a chronic discharging osteomyelitis or empyema.

(*b*) *Vitamin-C deficiency.* The observations of Lind on the effect of scurvy in sailors, and the finding that citrus fruit cured the condition is one of the classic descriptions in medicine. In spite of much research there are few who could not re-echo the words of Dr Grainger, who, writing to Lind concerning scurvy, noted that it was 'a subject of which I had read much but knew little'.[12]

Experimentally in guinea-pigs (scurvy does not occur in other rodents because they can synthetize vitamin C), wound contraction and epithelial regeneration proceed normally. Granulation tissue is produced, but is abnormal: the fibroblasts are arranged in an irregular manner and although they produce a little reticulin, normal collagen fibres are not formed. The wound is therefore very weak. Capillaries are unduly fragile and haemorrhages occur. In those who have teeth, swelling of and bleeding from the gingivae are characteristic. Vitamin C is necessary for the hydroxylation of proline prior to its incorporation into the collagen molecule (p. 38).

Although frank scurvy is uncommon, minor degrees of vitamin-C deficiency are not infrequent in patients who are on a marginal intake and who are in other ways stressed.

(*c*) *The role of zinc.*[13] The addition of zinc to the diet of rats has been shown to promote the healing of thermal burns and excised wounds. The mechanism is not known, but the fact that zinc is an important component of several enzymes may be related. The oral administration of zinc sulphate has been tried in humans, and a beneficial effect on wound healing claimed.

Glucocorticoids. In excessive amounts these inhibit the formation of granulation tissue and also delay wound contraction.

Temperature. It is the general experience that wounds of the exposed parts heal much more slowly in cold weather, and experiments on animals during hibernation have supported this observation.

Complications of wound healing

Wound dehiscence.[14,15] The bursting open of a wound is described as *dehiscence*, and it occurs when stress is applied before the wound has healed sufficiently. It is particularly serious in abdominal incisions, because it results in the exposure of the abdominal contents to the atmosphere outside. Increased intra-abdominal pressure combines with poor wound healing to precipitate this catastrophic event.

Cicatrization. This is a frequent complication of extensive burning of the skin, and may produce great deformity. Cicatrization involving hollow viscera, e.g. the intestine or the urethra, is an important cause of narrowing (*stenosis*) of the lumen.

Keloid formation.[16] Occasionally an excessive formation of collagenous tissue results in the appearance of a raised nodule of scar tissue called a keloid. The cause of this is unknown. Repeated trauma and irritation caused by foreign bodies, hair, keratin, etc., may play a part. Keloids are more common in the young, especially girls, in Black people, in tuberculous subjects, and during pregnancy. They are found most commonly in the region of the neck. They are especially frequent after burns.

Weak scars. If scar tissue is subjected to continuous strain, stretching may result. In elderly people the abdominal viscera may bulge through a weak scar to produce a local protrusion, or *incisional hernia.*

Implantation (or epidermoid) cysts. Epithelial cells which grow into the wounded area may persist, and their subsequent growth results in the formation of a small cyst. This should not be confused with a dermoid cyst.

Painful scars. Pain either local or referred may be experienced if a nerve is included in the scar tissue.

Pigmentary changes. Coloured particles introduced into the wound may persist and cause colouring or tattooing. Healed chronic ulcers sometimes have a russet colour due to staining with haemosiderin.

GENERAL READING

Blair G H, Slome D, Walter J B 1961 Review of experimental investigations on wound healing. In: Carling E R, Ross J P (eds) British Surgical Practice. Surgical Progress. Butterworth, London, pp 462–505

Douglas D M 1963 Wound Healing and Management: a monograph for surgeons. Livingstone, Edinburgh

Leading Article 1973 To heal the wound. Lancet 2: 84

Levenson S M, Stein J M, Grossblatt N 1966 (eds) Wound healing, proceedings of a workshop. Washington: National Academy of Sciences–National Research Council

McMinn R M H 1969 Tissue Repair 432 pp. Academic Press, New York

Peacock E E, van Winkle W 1970 Surgery and Biology of Wound Repair, 630 pp. Saunders, Philadelphia

Slome D 1961 (ed) Wound Healing. Pergamon, Oxford

REFERENCES

1. Rose S M 1970 Regeneration: key to understanding normal and abnormal growth and development. Appleton-Century-Crofts, New York. 264 pp
2. Walter J B 1976 Wound healing. Journal of Otolaryngology 5: 171
3. Gabbiani G, Hirschel B J, Ryan G B, Statko P R, Majno V G M 1972 Granulation tissue as a contractile organ. Journal of Experimental Medicine 135: 719

4. Grillo H C, Gross J 1959 Studies in wound healing: III. Contraction in vitamin C deficiency. Proceedings of the Society for Experimental Biology and Medicine 101: 268
5. Cliff W T 1963 Observations on healing tissue; a combined light and electron microscopic investigation. Philosophical Transactions of the Royal Society, Series B 246: 305
6. Forrester J D 1973 Mechanical, biochemical, and architectural features of surgical repair. Advances in Biological and Medical Physics 14: 1
7. Ordman L J, Gillman T 1966 Studies in the healing of cutaneous wounds. Archives of Surgery 93: 857, 883 and 911
8. Gillman T 1968 Healing of cutaneous wounds. Glaxo Volume 31: 5
9. Lindsay W K, Birch J R 1964 Thin skin healing. Canadian Journal of Surgery 7: 297
10. Rothnie N G, Taylor G W 1963 Sutureless skin suture. British Medical Journal 2: 1027
11. Murray P J B 1963 Closure of skin wounds with adhesive tape. British Medical Journal 2: 1030
12. Hunt A H 1941 The role of vitamin C in wound healing. British Journal of Surgery 28: 436
13. Leading Article 1975 Zinc in human medicine. Lancet 2: 351
14. Leading Article 1977 Burst abdomen—a preventable condition? British Medical Journal 1: 534
15. Leading Article 1977 Burst abdomen. Lancet 1: 28
16. King G D, Salzman F A 1970 Keloid scars. Surgical Clinics of North America 50: 595

9

Healing in specialized tissues

It is generally stated that the greater the degree of specialization of a tissue, the less well developed are its powers of regeneration. Certainly neurons are highly specialized and incapable of division, but degrees of specialization in cells are as difficult to define as they are amongst human beings. Is a liver cell more or less specialized than a simple unstriped muscle fibre? Liver cells show remarkable powers of proliferation, yet perform functions of which they alone are capable. Similarly, it is impossible to compare the degrees of specialization of the different types of epithelium, each of which has its own peculiar characteristics. It seems more likely that the power of regeneration is best developed in those organs and tissues which are most liable to injury, and the replacement of which has survival value for the individual and species.

Epithelial tissues

All covering epithelia show good regenerative power. This is hardly surprising since they are being continuously subjected to trauma, and their integrity depends upon their ability to replace the lost cells. Glandular epithelia, on the other hand, show erratic regenerative capacity.

Covering epithelia[1]

Squamous epithelium of skin. This shows good regeneration, although specialized structures like the rete ridges, hair follicles, sweat glands, and sebaceous glands are not replaced in man. The details of the epithelial changes in skin wounds, involving both movement and division of cells, have already been described (Ch. 8).

Oral epithelium. Complete regeneration occurs. The lamina propria and submucosa heal by repair, and scar tissue may remain in the lining mucosa but not in the masticatory mucosa.

Intestinal epithelium. Complete regeneration results in perfect replacement of lost epithelium, including, in the case of the small intestine, the crypts and villi. It is noteworthy that because there is normally a very high rate of mitotic activity in the epithelium of the small intestine, no further increase occurs at the wound margins. In passing, it should be noted that the remainder of the gut wall, including the muscularis mucosae, heals by scar tissue.

Stomach. Here epithelial regeneration is good. Acute ulceration of the mucosa of the stomach is a common event, but healing occurs rapidly and without any scarring, because the underlying specialized connective tissue and muscle are not destroyed. In chronic peptic ulcers epithelial regeneration is inhibited, the reason for which is not known. When healing does occur, the newly-formed epithelium may be of intestinal type, even showing well-marked villi.

Respiratory tract. Loss of epithelium, such as occurs in acute influenzal tracheobronchitis, is quickly followed by the division of basal cells leading to a reformation of ciliated pseudostratified columnar epithelium. Sometimes after repeated damage the new epithelium may change to simple columnar or squamous type (see metaplasia, p. 319).

Glandular epithelium

Liver.[2,3] The liver has remarkable powers of regeneration. In the rat resection of three-quarters of the organ results in such active division of the remaining cells that within two weeks the organ is restored to its original weight. The process could be regarded as a simple type of reconstitution, because it involves the co-ordinated growth of liver cells, blood vessels, bile ducts, etc.

In the human regeneration of liver cells is seen following any type of necrosis, provided the patient survives. The end-results of this regeneration vary so widely, depending upon the type of hepatic necrosis, that this important subject will be considered in Chapter 35.

Kidney. The renal tubular epithelium has considerable powers of regeneration; thus in acute tubular necrosis, in spite of extensive damage, complete return to normal may occur. This type of lesion is therefore most eligible for treatment with the artificial kidney (haemodialysis), since recovery is quite possible. When damage to the kidney results in destruction of a complete nephron, regeneration does not occur. Glomeruli once destroyed cannot be replaced.

Connective tissues

When conditions are favourable many of the specialized connective tissues show excellent regeneration. However, not infrequently adverse factors operate and these result in healing by repair.

Mesothelial lining of peritoneum and other serous cavities. Lost mesothelial cells are replaced from underlying connective tissue cells, which take on the appearance of flattened mesothelium. It has also been suggested that desquamated mesothelial cells can alight on the raw surface.

Synovium.[4] Synovial lining cells are also replaced from underlying connective tissue. The adjacent uninjured synovial cells are inert, and play no part in the process of healing.

Vascular endothelium.[5] In large arteries, e.g. the aorta, new endothelial cells arise by mitotic division of pre-existing ones, and slowly spread over the denuded area. It has been suggested that endothelial cells can also develop from deposited circulating mononuclear cells, but the evidence for this is not good.

Fat. Although fat cells may appear in fully mature granulation tissue, defects in fatty tissue are usually made good by fibrous tissue. The process of repair shows a characteristic feature during the demolition phase; the macrophages ingest large quantities of fat, becoming greatly swollen in the process. These *foam cells* form a prominent feature of traumatic fat necrosis (p. 64).

Cartilage. Regeneration in cartilage is generally poor. In the case of the hyaline cartilage of joint surfaces small defects are made good by regeneration. With larger injuries which involve damage to the underlying vascular bone, there is formed a haematoma which becomes vascularized and converted either into fibrous tissue or bone.

Tendon.[6] Regeneration in tendon is good, but the process is slow. It is said that the tendon ends should be accurately opposed and under some tension, otherwise union is by scar tissue.

Muscle.[7–10] It is generally taught that damaged muscle is not replaced, and that union is by scar tissue. In large destructive lesions of unstriped muscle a permanent scar remains to mark the site of the original injury, and this is well illustrated by the appearance of a healed chronic gastric ulcer. Although unstriped muscle cells appear incapable of division in postuterine life, the arterioles of granulation tissue acquire a muscular coat; the origin of these fibres is not known. There is also experimental evidence that smooth-muscle regeneration occurs when the taenia of the guinea-pig caecum is crushed.[7] Thus it would appear that smooth (unstriped) muscle has limited powers of regeneration.

In respect of striated muscle, when part of an individual muscle fibre is damaged, there may be limited regeneration with the production of new myocytes which later fuse to form a syncytial mass.[11] In a clean surgical wound of voluntary muscle, the sarcolemmal masses on either side of the incision may unite, so that the continuity of the muscle is restored, and in time no indication of the site of injury can be found. However, with extensive damage to muscle the architecture is destroyed, and healing is by scar tissue; this is seen following infarction.

Cardiac muscle shows no regenerative capacity, and once necrosis has occurred, as in infarction, a permanent scar remains. Under special circumstances cardiac muscle cells may form giant cells similar to those seen in voluntary muscle. It has been suggested that the Aschoff giant cell of acute rheumatic fever is of this nature (p. 512).

Bone marrow. Bone marrow provides an excellent example of tissue in which regeneration is complete.

Bone. The regeneration of bone as seen in the healing of a fracture is described in Chapter 37.

Nervous tissue. Adult nerve cells are unable to divide and therefore when a part of the brain or spinal cord is destroyed, new neurons are not produced.

Peripheral nervous system.[12,13] Following section of the axis cylinder the neuron shows changes described as *chromatolysis*. The cell swells and its Nissl granules disappear. These bodies are zones of endoplasmic reticulum studded plentifully with ribosomes, and their disappearance reflects dysfunction in the protein-synthetizing system of the nerve cell. The axis cylinder becomes irregular and varicose, and by 48 hours has broken up. The surrounding myelin shows splitting of the laminae, and later fragmentation. The Schwann cells enlarge, proliferate, and become filled with lipid droplets from the degenerated myelin. These changes were originally described as *Wallerian degeneration*. They affect the nerve fibre distal to the point of section and also, in myelinated fibres, a short area proximally up to the first node of Ranvier. The next stage is described as regeneration, but it should be remembered that it entails rather more than a mere replacement of the lost part of an individual cell. From the proximal portion of the cut axon numerous neurofibrils sprout out, and are seen to lie invaginated into the cytoplasm of the Schwann cells. They push their way distally through the Schwann cells at the rate of about 1 mm per day. Many of the fibrils lose their way and degenerate, but some reach an appropriate end-organ, and persist to form the definitive replacement axon. It is evident that accurate apposition of the cut ends of the nerve is of great importance in facilitating this process. The final process involves the reformation of the myelin sheath as the regenerating axon matures and increases in diameter.

The functional end-result of nerve damage depends on various factors: if the axons are damaged but the nerve trunk itself is not severed, an excellent result may be expected. When the nerve is severed, careful suturing and absence of infection are important. Functional recovery is more complete when a pure motor or sensory nerve is cut. Recovery from a lesion of a mixed nerve, like the median nerve of the forearm, is often poor.

Central nervous system.[14,15] Here oligodendroglia take the place of the Schwann cells in relation to nerve fibres. It is often stated that regeneration of central nerve fibres does not occur. The affected nerve cells show chromatolysis often followed by necrosis, and the destroyed tissue is replaced by proliferating neuroglia to form a dense glial scar. Nevertheless, there is considerable evidence that some regeneration is possible. In the clinical field it is noticeable that in patients with partial spinal-cord lesions, voluntary muscle strength seems to increase steadily for 9 to 12 months. This is generally attributed to improved utilization of residual undamaged pathways. In the lower animals regeneration of the long-tract axons in the spinal cord is a usual feature, and it is possible that some regeneration may occur in the higher animals, including the human being.

The mechanism of wound healing[16]

When one considers that in a healing wound there is cell and tissue production proceeding at a rate which exceeds that seen in the most malignant tumours, it is humiliating to admit how little we know of the mechanisms involved. We understand neither the signal which starts the process, nor the mechanisms which maintain and control it. Many workers have claimed that local wound hormones, or *trephones*, are responsible for stimulating the cell growth that is responsible for healing, but none has been isolated from animal tissue. In the plant world growth factors have, however, been found. Alternatively it has been postulated that removal of an inhibiting substance (*chalone*), normally present, is responsible for stimulating cell division.[17,18] Physical factors may play some part; for instance epithelial cells tend to maintain contact with each other and spread over surfaces. The migration of squamous epithelium in wound healing can be easily understood. However, the subsequent division of cells and the formation of a multicellular epidermis cannot be so explained. Although some general factors, such as food supply and hormones, affect wound healing, local factors far outweigh them in potency and probably in importance. In the control of cell division and maturation it is therefore local factors which are most likely to play the dominant role.

REFERENCES

1. McMinn, R M H 1960 The cellular anatomy of experimental wound healing. Annals of the Royal College of Surgeons of England 26: 245
2. Bucher, N L R 1967 Experimental aspects of hepatic regeneration. New England Journal of Medicine 277: 686 and 738
3. Verly, W G 1976 The control of liver growth. In Chalones, ed. Houck, J C, p. 401. North-Holland Publishing Company, Amsterdam
4. Levene, A 1957 The response to injury of rat synovial membrane. Journal of Pathology and Bacteriology 73: 87
5. Leading Article 1967 Endothelium and atherosclerosis. Lancet 2: 1239
6. Buck, R C 1953 Regeneration of tendon. Journal of Pathology and Bacteriology 66: 1
7. McGeachie, J K, 1971 Ultra-structural specificity in regenerating smooth muscle. Experimentia 27: 436
8. McGeachie, J K 1975 Smooth muscle regeneration, Monographs in Developmental Biology, Vol. 9, 90 pp. Karger, Basel
9. Gay, A J & Hunt T E 1954 Reuniting of skeletal muscle fibres after transection. Anatomical Record 120: 853
10. Carlson B M 1972 The Regeneration of Minced Muscles, Monographs in Developmental Biology, Vol. 4, 128 pp. Karger, Basel
11. Hay E D 1971 Skeletal-muscle regeneration. New England Journal of Medicine 284: 1033
12. Dyck P J, Thomas P K & Lambert E H (1975). Peripheral Neuropathy, Vol. 1, pp. 179–181 and 205–208. Saunders, Philadelphia
13. Walton J N (ed) 1974 Disorders of voluntary muscle, 3rd edn, see Wallerian Degeneration, pp. 239–244. Churchill Livingstone, Edinburgh
14. Windle W F (ed) 1955 Regeneration in the central nervous system. Thomas, Springfield
15. Leading article 1976 Any hope for the cut central axon? Lancet 1: 1224
16. Peacock E E 1973 Biologic frontiers in the control healing. American Journal of Surgery 126: 708.
17. Houck, J C (ed) 1976 Chalones, 510 pp. North-Holland Publishing Company, Amsterdam
18. Rytömaa T 1976 The chalone concept. International Review of Experimental Pathology, 16: 155

10

Chronic inflammation

Although the concept of chronic inflammation is in part a clinical one implying that the inflammatory process persists for a long period, pathologically it is best defined as *a process in which destruction and inflammation are proceeding at the same time as attempts at healing.*

The tissue response to injury has been divided into three phases: the initial vascular and exudative phenomena of *acute inflammation* are followed by a second phase of *demolition* which is accomplished by macrophage activity. The third and final phase is one of *healing*, by which lost tissue is replaced by the processes of *repair* and *regeneration.*

It is evident that complete healing can occur only when the acute inflammation and demolition phases are themselves completed. Since these are the consequences of the initial damage, it follows that healing results only when the cause of the inflammation is itself removed. If tissue damage continues, a disease process develops in which there is present a mixture of the phenomena of acute inflammation, demolition, repair, and regeneration. To such a lesion the term chronic inflammation is applied.

Causes of chronic inflammation

Any cause of tissue damage can, if it persists, lead to chronic inflammation. Three main groups can be recognized:

1. Infections. The body has a limited ability to destroy certain organisms, e.g. the tubercle bacillus and *Treponema pallidum.* Infection with these agents therefore commonly leads to chronic inflammation. Moreover, if local or general conditions impair the body's defences, an organism that usually produces a self-limiting acute inflammation may persist to cause a chronic one. Thus, *Staphylococcus aureus*, which can produce a boil that generally heals rapidly, can also produce chronic inflammation in some situations, such as in the bone marrow (see *chronic osteomyelitis*, p. 143). Any of the causes of delayed healing may so turn the scales against the host that there develops the 'frustrated healing' that chronic inflammation has so aptly been called.

2. Insoluble particulate irritants. Silica and asbestos are examples of irritant particles that the body cannot easily remove. Inhalation of such substances leads to persistent chronic inflammation of the lungs (see *pneumoconiosis*, Ch. 33).

3. Hypersensitivity. The development of hypersensitivity is an important factor in chronic infective diseases, of which tuberculosis is the prototype. Much of the chronic damage produced by persisting tubercle bacilli is mediated by damaging antigen-antibody interactions. There is also a group of diseases in which damaging antibodies are produced against the body's own tissues. This group of autoimmune diseases is typified by rheumatoid arthritis.

Classification of chronic inflammation

Chronic inflammation may be classified in several ways, none of which is ideal.

1. Clinical
2. Specific and non-specific
3. Histological
4. Granulomatous and non-granulomatous.

Clinical

Although chronic inflammation may follow in the wake of obvious acute inflammation, some irritants (e.g. tubercle bacillus) cause a mild or fleeting acute reaction which clinically may be completely missed. Nevertheless, they persist and lead to the development of a chronic disease. Clinically therefore two types of chronic inflammation may be described:

a. Secondary to acute inflammation
b. Starting *de novo.*

Specific and non-specific

Chronic inflammatory lesions have been subdivided in another way. Certain irritants cause a tissue reaction which is histologically characteristic. By examining such a lesion one can deduce its cause without either seeing or isolating the causative agent. Such a lesion is said to be *specific.* Tuberculosis, leprosy, and syphilis are included under this heading, and may be contrasted with the lesions of pyogenic organisms which are *non-specific.* Unfortunately, many lesions encountered in the specific diseases are not histologically characteristic, and therefore, strictly speaking, the term specific should not be used. Thus while the histological appearance of a gumma is fairly typical, the lesions of secondary syphilis are by no means diagnostic. The reaction is non-specific. Hence most authorities have dropped the term 'specific' in this connexion, but have retained 'non-specific' to describe any non-granulomatous reaction characterized by fibrosis and a small-round-cell infiltration.

Histological

The histological features of a chronic inflammatory lesion may be used in descriptive classification. Where polymorphs abound and abscess formation is present, the lesion may justly be called a *chronic suppurative inflammation.* Likewise when epithelioid cells are found grouped together in follicles resembling those found in tuberculosis, the term *tuberculoid* is frequently applied. Three variants occur:

a. Non-caseating tuberculoid reaction, as seen in sarcoidosis (Fig. 15.2)
b. Caseating tuberculoid reaction, as commonly seen in tuberculosis (Fig. 15.2)
c. Suppurative tuberculoid reaction, in which small abscesses filled with polymorphs are formed and are surrounded by a mantle of epithelioid cells. This is an uncommon reaction and is seen in coccidioidomycosis and lymphogranuloma venereum.

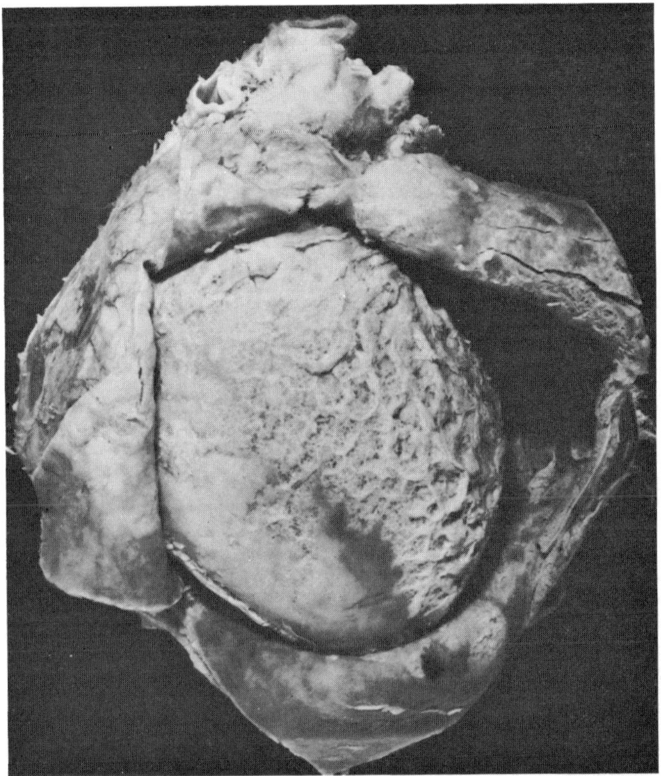

Fig. 10.1 Tuberculous pericarditis. The patient was a man aged 22 years, who had had pulmonary tuberculosis for 5 years. The specimen shows the opened pericardial sac, in which the heart is seen to be covered by a thick fibrinous exudate. Over the apex there is a layer of blood clot due to recent haemorrhage. The parietal pericardium is greatly thickened, and is also covered by fibrinous exudate and blood clot. (EC 12.1, *Reproduced by permission of the President and Council of the R.S.C. Eng.*)

Granulomatous and non-granulomatous

Some chronic inflammations are characterized by the formation of tumour-like masses composed of granulation tissue which is heavily infiltrated with inflammatory cells. These inflammations are sometimes called *granulomatous*, and such a reaction is frequently to be found in tuberculosis. By convention this disease and certain other chronic infections are often called the *specific infective granulomata*. It must be stressed that in fact not all lesions in these diseases are granulomatous, and that tumour-like masses can occur in other chronic inflammations not generally called granulomata, e.g. silicosis.

Granulomatous inflammation.[1] Some chronic inflammations are characterized by the formation of tumour-like masses, and the term granuloma has been applied to them. In some instances the mass is composed of inflammatory granulation tissue, and Virchow included this type of lesion amongst the granulomata. Most contemporary workers, however, use the term in a descriptive sense restricted to a microscopic appearance rather than related to the formation of a tumour-like mass. In this sense *a granuloma is defined as a chronic inflammatory reaction containing a predominance of cells of the macrophage series.* This includes both a diffuse infiltration of macrophages as well as the follicular type of lesion in which epithelioid cells are formed (tuberculoid reaction). Some pathologists restrict the term granuloma to a lesion characterized by the formation of epithelioid cells (and often giant cells also) arranged in follicular groups; in this case the terms granulomatous and tuberculoid are synonymous. Actinomycosis is often included in the group of granulomatous inflammations, even though the lesions are typically suppurative. It is evident that granulomatous inflammation is a term without a precise meaning, and it is wise not to use it without qualification.

Features of chronic inflammation

These are best considered under the headings of the three component reactions which together constitute chronic inflammation (Table 10.1).

Table 10.1 Components of chronic inflammation

Component	Tissue response
Acute inflammation	Polymorph infiltration Oedema Fibrin
Demolition	Macrophage formation Epithelioid-cell formation Giant-cell formation
Healing	
Repair	Granulation tissue Blood vessels Fibroblasts Collagen Neuroglia in CNS
Regeneration	Epithelial overgrowth Specialized connective-tissue overgrowth
Immune response	Lymphocytes Plasma cells Eosinophils

Acute inflammation

This is particularly well marked in chronic suppurative disease, for example osteomyelitis, empyema, and chronic brain abscess, to mention only a few examples. It is also typical of actinomycosis. Pus, rich in polymorphonuclear leucocytes, is very evident, and fibrin may not only be seen microscopically, but on occasions forms large masses easily visible to the naked eye (Fig. 10.1). Fluid exudation is also a feature of chronic suppurative disease, and if drained the continued protein loss may lead to hypoalbuminaemia (p. 432). Accumulations of protein-rich fluid are frequent in chronic inflammation of the serous sacs, e.g. tuberculous peritonitis.

Eosinophils are sometimes present in large numbers in the exudate in chronic inflammation. Whether this is a manifestation of hypersensitivity is not known.

Demolition[2–4]

This is accomplished by macrophages. These cells are derived from the emigrating monocytes of bone-marrow origin, and they constitute the bulk of granulomatous lesions. In some granulomata the monocytes are soon destroyed, but are replaced by new cells from the blood stream. This type constitutes the *high-turnover granulomata.* In other circumstances (*low-turnover granulomata*) the monocytes remain for many weeks in the tissues, and may undergo mitosis before entering a resting phase and subsequently developing into phagocytic cells. Some of these cells may morphologically resemble lymphocytes, and this has given rise to the concept, probably erroneous, that lymphocytes can develop into macrophages. In these low-turnover granulomata the proliferation of local histiocytes probably contributes to the macrophage population, and a constant recruitment for monocytes of bone-marrow origin is not required.

Chronic inflammatory lesions with a heavy macrophage infiltration are traditionally called 'proliferative'. It is now believed that macrophages arise both from exudation of blood monocytes and by the subsequent local proliferation. Nevertheless, an 'exudative' lesion is traditionally defined as one showing an exudate of plasma with fibrin and polymorphs.

Under certain circumstances macrophages become large and polygonal with pale, oval nuclei and abundant, eosinophilic cytoplasm. These cells are called *epithelioid cells*, from a resemblance in appearance to the epithelial cells of the epidermis. The epithelioid cells are not phagocytic, but avidly take up small particles by pinocytosis.

Precisely why macrophages differentiate into epithelioid cells is not clear, but they do so under a number of circumstances. Thus they do so when they have completely digested phagocytosed material, or have successfully extruded phagocytosed material by exocytosis. Epithelioid-cell formation is inhibited if phagocytosed material can neither be digested nor extruded. Thus the lepra cells in lepromatous leprosy and the foam cells found in xanthomata do not become epithelioid cells. In tuberculous granulomata, however, epithelioid cells are typical. Thus epithelioid cells appear to develop when the influx of macrophages exceeds the number required to ingest a non-digestible substance, or when the substance is digestible but not too toxic to the cells. It should be noted that when epithelioid-cell formation is marked, the cells tend to be grouped into follicles or tubercles. This contrasts with the more diffuse infiltration of phagocytic macrophages that do not differentiate into epithelioid cells.

When macrophages encounter insoluble material they frequently fuse together to form *giant cells.*[5] This occurs around exogenous foreign bodies like silk and talc, as well as around endogenous debris such as pieces of dead bone (sequestra), cholesterol crystals, and uric acid crystals. They are also formed in response to certain organisms such as the tubercle bacillus and many fungi. Three forms of these giant cells have been described.

Langhans giant cell. The nuclei are disposed around the periphery of the cell in the form of a horseshoe or a ring. These cells are particularly frequent in tuberculous lesions.

Foreign-body giant cell. In this type the nuclei are scattered haphazardly throughout the cytoplasm. In many lesions giant cells of both Langhans and foreign-body type are present, and the two should not be regarded as distinct types.

Touton giant cell. This type of giant cell is found in xanthomata (Figs. 10.2a and 10.2b). Its peripheral cytoplasm has a foamy appearance, and the nuclei surround a central area of clear eosinophilic cytoplasm.

Features of healing

Repair. Granulation tissue is prominent in many chronic inflammatory lesions. It contains:

1. Endothelial cells forming blood and lymphatic vessels
2. Fibroblasts forming collagen

The vascularity of the granulation tissue may give rise to haemorrhage. Thus bleeding occurs from the base of chronic peptic ulcers, the inflamed dilated bronchi in bronchiectasis, and in chronic gingivitis.

In chronic suppuration, the pus-filled cavity is lined by acutely inflamed granulation tissue which forms a pyogenic membrane.

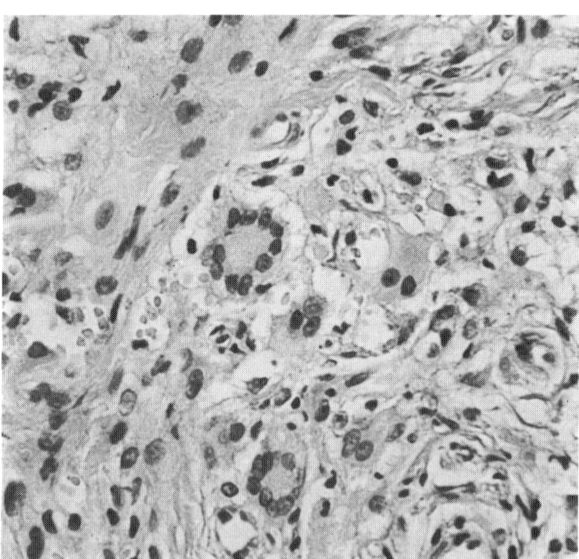

Fig. 10.2a Xanthoma showing Touton giant cell. The lesion consists of many foam cells some of which have fused to form giant cells. The cell in the centre is a typical Touton giant cell. The nuclei are arranged in a circular manner to form a wreath. The peripheral part of the cytoplasm is vacuolated due to its lipid content. The central part of the cytoplasm, enclosed by the nuclei, has a homogeneous, eosinophilic appearance. × 215.

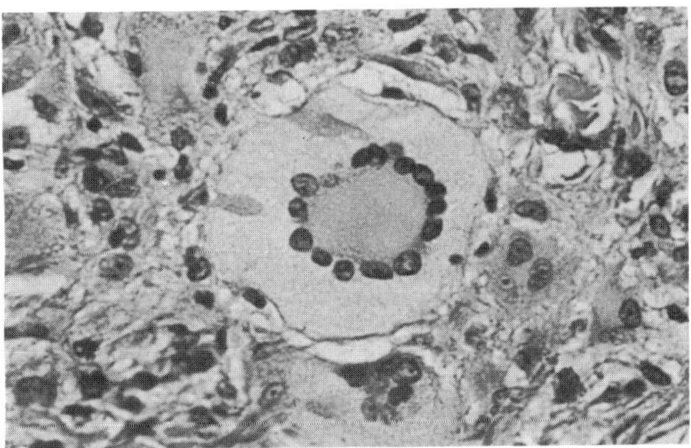

Fig. 10.2b Touton giant cell. This Touton giant cell differs from that shown in Figure 10.2a in that the peripheral cytoplasm is less vacuolated. The section is from a naevoxanthoendothelioma (juvenile xanthogranuloma). This curious lesion appears during the neonatal period as a rapidly-growing, red skin nodule which almost invariably involutes spontaneously. × 320.

Fibroblasts are prominent in most chronic inflammations. They lay down collagen, and the resulting scar formation is characteristic of many chronic inflammatory lesions. The proliferation of fibroblasts and their synthesis of collagen appears to be stimulated by a factor released from macrophages.[6] Fibrosis is especially well seen in fibroid tuberculosis, Crohn's disease, deep in the base of a chronic peptic ulcer, and in the wall of an abscess. If fibrin is the hallmark of acute inflammation, fibrosis can be considered the salient feature of chronic inflammation. As scarring proceeds, so the lumina of small arteries and arterioles are gradually obliterated by thickening of the tunica intima. This process is called *endarteritis obliterans* (Fig. 10.3). Ultimately a mass of dense avascular scar tissue is formed. Cicatrization may ensue and produce serious effects. For instance a chronic ulcer of the pylorus may lead to narrowing and obstruction of the lumen (pyloric stenosis).

Regeneration. When the tissue destroyed in chronic inflammation is of a type capable of division, regeneration rather than repair takes place. This is particularly obvious in surface epithelia. Indeed, regeneration may become so exuberant that the line of demarcation between it, hyperplasia, and neoplasia may be difficult to define. For this reason, cancer has frequently been ascribed to 'chronic irritation' (pp. 315 and 365).

The epithelial overgrowth at the edge of a chronic ulcer is sometimes quite remarkable, and may be misinterpreted by the unwary as cancer. The greatly divergent views expressed in the past on the frequency of malignant change in chronic peptic ulcer are largely due to the difficulties in interpreting the microscopic appearances at the edge of the ulcer.

The position is complicated by the fact that malignancy may indeed supervene on the exuberant regeneration of chronic inflammation. This is sometimes seen in chronic ulcerative colitis.

Evidence of an immune reaction

Although a few lymphocytes and plasma cells are found in uninflamed granulation

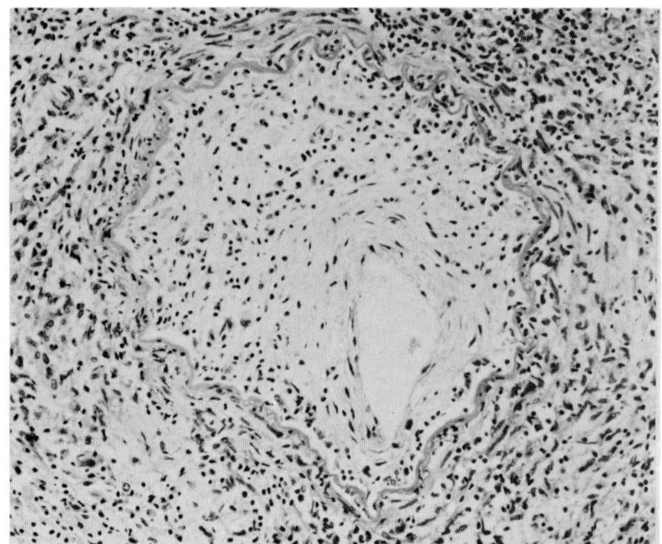

Fig. 10.3 Endarteritis obliterans. This is a section through a gumma. The periphery shows fibrous tissue heavily infiltrated by small round cells, but the central area is defined by the internal elastic lamina of a medium-sized artery. Inside this lamina there is a considerable proliferation of the more palely-staining tunica intima, which shows a moderate cellular infiltration. The lumen of the vessel is reduced to a small channel near the middle of the field. × 70.

tissue, many examples of chronic inflammation are characterized by a heavy infiltration by the cells (Fig. 10.4). Together these are called the cells of chronic inflammation, or *small round cells.* Frequently they assume a perivascular distribution, e.g. in syphilitic aortitis, and are presumably derived from the blood rather than from local lymphoid tissue or stem cells. Together with macrophages they are concerned with the processing of antigen and the local production of antibody.

There is little doubt that the plasma cells are engaged in the local production of immunoglobulin. They are derived from B lymphocytes, and are particularly prominent in the inflammatory lesions involving the skin adjacent to mucocutaneous junctions and in the mucous membranes themselves. Chronic gingivitis is characterized by a massive plasma-cell infiltration. Occasionally the plasma cells seem to contain one or more spherical, eosinophilic, PAS-positive, hyaline structures called Russell bodies (see Fig. 2.9, p. 16). When the cell dies these structures are released into the stroma. They are of no great significance, but should not be mistaken for fungi.

While some of the small round cells of chronic inflammation are B lymphocytes, others appear to be T cells and differentiate into sensitized T cells. As noted previously, some cells that appear to be of lymphocyte type are in fact resting monocytes and subsequently develop into macrophages. Because of the difficulty in distinguishing between these various types of lymphocytes the term 'small round cells' is convenient, for it distinguishes them from polymorphs and obvious macrophages.

Eosinophils are also involved in the immune response, but their role is complex (p. 79).

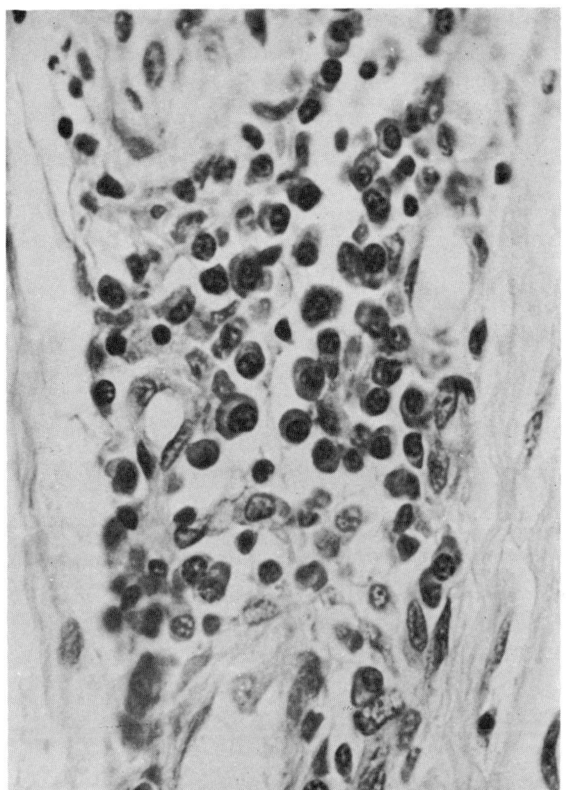

Fig. 10.4 Plasma cells. This is the section of a chronic inflammatory response in which plasma cells are predominating. The round and pear-shaped contour of the cells is well marked. Their nuclei are eccentric, and have a conspicuous cart-wheel disposition of clumped chromatin. The cytoplasm is comparatively darkly-staining due to its high content of RNA. The clear area adjacent to the nucleus is the Golgi complex. × 400.

General effects of chronic inflammation

The general effects of chronic inflammation depend upon the nature of the responsible agent and the extent of the lesion. In a localized foreign-body reaction there is no noteworthy response at all. On the other hand, in chronic infective disease like tuberculosis or actinomycosis there may be widespread changes in the RE system and in the blood stream. Remarkably little is known about the exact mechanisms involved.

Changes in the reticulo-endothelial system

Apart from the local accumulation of RE macrophages already described, the lymph nodes draining a chronic inflammatory lesion show hyperplasia. This may sometimes affect the sinus-lining cells ('sinus catarrh'), while at other times there is a marked increase in the number of germinal centres or small lymphocytes. These changes are related to the development of an immune response.

If organisms or their toxins gain access to the blood stream there may be a more generalized hyperplasia of the RE cells, producing enlargement of the spleen (splenomegaly) and lymph nodes (lymphadenopathy). Sometimes this is related to formation of antigen-antibody complexes in the blood stream, which are subsequently removed by the RE system. In other instances, e.g. leishmaniasis, there is a widespread parasitization of the RE cells.

The immune response

Antibody production is a prominent feature of most chronic inflammatory diseases. The antibodies may be immunoglobulins or of the cell-bound variety. The importance of hypersensitivity in chronic inflammation is described in Chapter 13.

The immune response may be reflected in definite morphological changes, and is an additional factor in the production of splenomegaly and generalized lymphadenopathy. Polyclonal gammopathy may occur, and finally the long-continued stress on the antibody-producing mechanism can lead to amyloid disease (p. 437).

Changes in the blood

The white cells frequently show changes which are related to the causative agent and to the extent of infection. These are considered later (p. 456). *Anaemia* is frequent, and is usually of the normochromic normocytic type. Repeated haemorrhages may lead to a hypochromic microcytic anaemia.

A rise in the erythrocyte sedimentation rate (ESR) occurs in many chronic inflammatory diseases, and is commonly used as an aid both to diagnosis and in assessing progress, e.g. in tuberculosis and rheumatoid arthritis (p. 436).

Other changes

Although 'toxaemia' is put forward as the explanation of many of the general symptoms, it cannot be regarded as anything more than a cloak for our ignorance. The following signs and symptoms are frequent and attributed to this state: tiredness, malaise, headaches, loss of appetite (anorexia), loss of weight, anaemia, loss of libido, and pyrexia.

Toxaemia is often assumed to be due to the liberation of endotoxins, but although such substances have been isolated from some organisms, e.g. *Esch. coli*, there are others, like the *Tr. pallidum*, in which no such endotoxins are known. Possibly toxic substances are formed when tissue is damaged either as a result of bacterial action or hypersensitivity. However, there is no direct evidence as to the nature of the endotoxins or the products of tissue damage which are responsible for the 'toxaemia' of infection.

Examples of chronic inflammation

The types of chronic inflammation can be graded as follows; those due to

1. Non-specific, pyogenic bacterial agents like *Staph. aureus* and *Esch. coli*
2. Inanimate foreign bodies
3. 'Specific' organisms, e.g. tubercle bacillus. This third group is so important that it is dealt with separately in Chapter 15

4. Ionizing radiation. This is described in Chapter 25
5. Hypersensitivity. This is discussed in Chapter 13. The collagen vascular diseases can be conveniently included in this group, though their aetiology is obscure.

The first group embraces a wide collection of conditions which are very commonly encountered in clinical practice. For the purpose of this discussion one important example has been selected.

Osteomyelitis

Acute osteomyelitis occurs most often in children at the metaphysis of one of the long bones of the lower limbs. This is the area which is most easily traumatized, and should this occur during the course of a *Staph. aureus* bacteraemia, the organisms become lodged in a haematoma and produce a metastatic lesion. A typical acute inflammatory reaction occurs, and owing to the rigidity of the bone the increased tension produced by the exudation causes compression of the blood vessels and subsequent ischaemia. Necrosis of marrow and bone therefore follows: pus is formed, and it tracks under the periosteum, thereby further imperilling the blood supply to the cortex. In this way quite extensive necrosis may occur, sometimes involving the whole shaft. This sequestrum acts as a foreign body; it cannot be easily removed, and it not only provides a focus for the growth of organisms but also prevents the adequate drainage of pus. Conditions are ideal for the development of chronic infection.

Pus ruptures through the periosteum into the muscular and subcutaneous compartments. Usually it is discharged on to the skin surface through sinuses.* The vascular periosteum attempts to reform the shaft of the bone by producing bone. This encases the sequestered shaft, and is called the *involucrum* (Fig. 10.5). The shaft is bathed in pus which escapes through holes, or *cloacae*, in the involucrum, and is then discharged to the surface. Osteoclasts slowly erode the sequestrum, detaching it at each end from living bone and slowly destroying it. This must be completed before healing can be accomplished. In practice this is seldom possible without elaborate surgical intervention. If nothing is done, the condition may lead to death as the result of pyaemia, 'toxaemia', or amyloid disease.

Chronic osteomyelitis is fortunately uncommon nowadays since the advent of antibiotic therapy, which is used in combination with early surgical drainage in the acute stage.

From a pathological point of view the disease illustrates many points. It shows how an acute infection can become chronic due to inadequate drainage of pus, as well as to the presence of a foreign body, in this case the sequestrum. Moreover, all the features of chronic inflammation are present. Acute inflammation is evident by the polymorphonuclear and fluid exudate, demolition by macrophages and osteoclastic activity, regeneration by bone formation, and repair by the surrounding scarring.

* A *sinus* is an abnormal channel, often lined by epithelium, which leads from the interior of the body to a free surface.

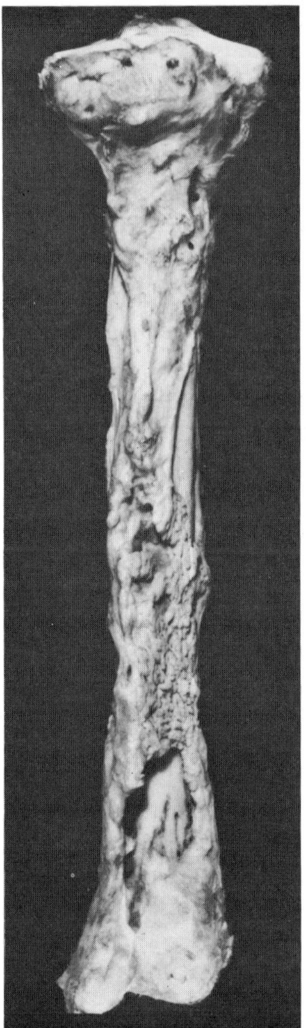

Fig. 10.5 Osteomyelitis of tibia. The extensive central sequestrum is largely encased in an exuberant involucrum formed from the detached periosteum. There is a cloaca at the base of the shaft, and through it the pitted sequestrum is clearly visible. (HS44.1. *Reproduced by permission of the President and Council of the Royal College of Surgeons of England.*)

Tissue response to insoluble inanimate foreign materials

The tissue response to these substances is very complex, but with the increasing use of metals and plastics in reconstructive surgery, it is a matter of considerable importance. In the root treatment of non-vital teeth a variety of compounds have been used. As they are in contact with vital tissues in the apical region, it is important that they should be non-irritant. Research on some of these compounds shows that, although most of them cause an inflammatory response when first inserted, this usually subsides within a few weeks.[7] It is probably true to state that all foreign materials are capable of producing an inflammatory response under certain circumstances. Nothing is truly inert. The factors which determine the severity of the inflammatory response are not completely understood, but the following are important:

The chemical nature of the material. The chemical stability and solubility are of great importance; thus stainless steel is more inert than ordinary steel.

Physical state of substance. Smooth, highly-polished surfaces provoke much less reaction than do rough, irregular surfaces. It is important to bear this in mind when inserting metal prostheses or pins. Finely divided or colloidal substances are particularly irritating. Nylon has been used in joint reconstruction, but the scratching and powdering which occur during use lead to a brisk foreign-body reaction.

Electro-chemical potentials. These are set up by the close proximity of dissimilar metals, and cause tissue damage. This is particularly important in orthopaedic and traumatic surgery. Plates and screws must all be of exactly the same composition, otherwise there is sufficient reaction to cause loosening of the screws. Even the metal scraped off the screwdriver may be enough to produce this effect.

The relatively insoluble foreign materials cannot be removed by the inflammatory reaction which they excite, and it follows that the lesions induced are typically chronic in character. Giant cells abound, and while most of these are of the foreign-body type, Langhans giant cells are also seen.

The extent of the reaction to foreign material depends on the nature of the material itself. A few important examples will be cited.

Examples of foreign-body reaction

Carbon. Tattooing consists of introducing carbon or cinnabar into the dermis. It excites a mild inflammatory response and is soon taken up by macrophages, in which it remains in the tissues indefinitely. The small amount of carbon which is deposited in the lungs of city-dwellers likewise causes little damage.

Metals. Vitallium and stainless steel cause little reaction when used in the form of polished plates, pins, arthroplasty cups, dental implants, etc. Tantalum, titanium, and zirconium are also used for their inertness. Other metals, e.g. iron, produce much more reaction, and in certain situations, e.g. the eye, can lead to serious damage.

Dental implants. There are four main types of dental implants: the subperiosteal implant, the needle (or pin), the screw, and the blade. These implants are inserted beneath the oral mucosa with a break in continuity, where a post projects through to support a crown, bridge, or denture. The implants are separated from the bone by a fibrous capsule sometimes referred to as a 'pseudoperiodontal ligament', although histologically it bears little resemblance to normal periodontal membrane.[8]

Many materials have been used—amongst these are cobalt chrome, alumina, and vitreous carbon. The implants excite a fibrous-tissue reaction, which is very little in the case of vitreous carbon.[9]

Suture material. Catgut excites a brisk acute inflammatory reaction which is soon followed by an infiltration of macrophages and giant cells. The strength of the plain catgut is reduced to half within two days, while for chromic catgut the

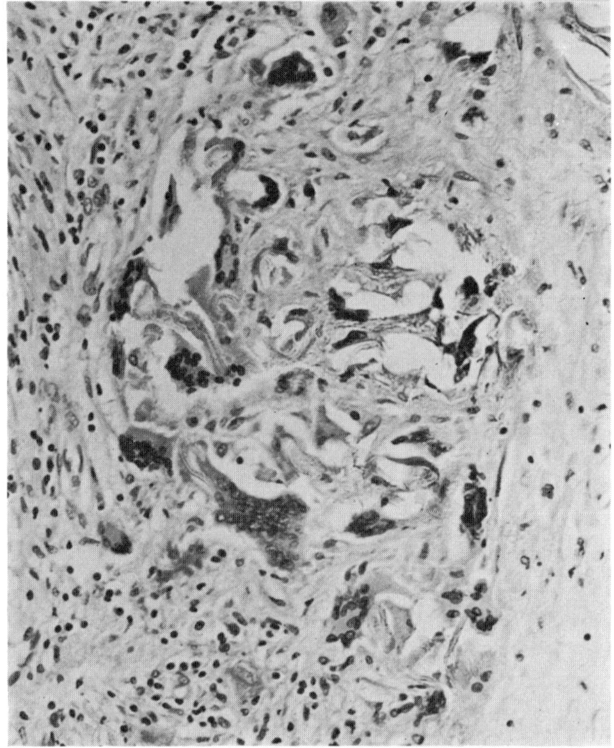

Fig. 10.6 Foreign-body reaction. This is a section through an old operation scar at the site of an unabsorbed nylon suture, which is not recognizable in the figure. There is a heavy accumulation of foreign-body giant cells, around which there are empty spaces. The whole is enclosed in dense fibrous tissue in which there is a moderate lymphocytic infiltration. × 100.

time is 10 days. Plain catgut is therefore unreliable, and should be discarded from general use. Fine chromic catgut should be used whenever absorbable material is indicated. The tissue reaction to nylon, linen, etc. does not readily remove the material, which therefore persists for a long period (Fig. 10.6).

Silica.[10] Small particles of silica are inhaled during the course of certain occupations like mining. An inflammatory response ensues in the interstitial tissues of the lungs, and this is later followed by dense nodular fibrosis. The precise manner by which silica causes such extensive destruction of lung is not known. The silica particles are phagocytosed by macrophages and being toxic destroy these cells. Lysosomal and other factors are released and these attract more macrophages to the area and also stimulate fibrogenesis (p. 139).

Many other dusts when inhaled into the lungs induce an inflammatory response which terminates in fibrosis. Such diseases are called the *pneumoconioses.* Silicosis and asbestosis are the most important.

REFERENCES

1. Adams D O 1976 The granulomatous inflammatory response. American Journal of Pathology 84:164

2. Ryan G M, Spector W G 1970 Macrophage turnover in inflamed connective tissue. Proceedings of the Royal Society B 175:269
3. Spector W G 1971 The cellular dynamics of granulomas. Proceedings of the Royal Society of Medicine, 64:941
4. Papadimitriou J M, Spector W G 1971 The origin, properties and fate of epithelioid cells. Journal of Pathology, 105:187
5. Carter R L, Roberts J D B 1971 Macrophages and multinucleate giant cells in nitrosoquinoline-induced granulomata in rats: an autoradiographic study. Journal of Pathology, 105:285
6. Allison A C, Clark I A, Davies P 1977 Cellular interactions in fibrogenesis. Annals of the Rheumatic Diseases, 36, Supplement p 8
7. Friend L A, Browne R M 1968 Tissue reactions to some root filling materials. British Dental Journal, 125:291
8. Biology and technology of oral prosthetic implants. 1974 Oral Sciences Reviews, 5
9. Hobkirk J A 1977 Tissue reactions to implanted vitreous carbon and high purity sintered alumina. Journal of Oral Rehabilitation, 4:355
10. Wagner J C 1977 Pulmonary fibrosis and mineral dusts. Annals of the Rheumatic Disease, 36, Supplement p 42

11

The immune response

Introduction

One of the characteristic features of the adult animal is its ability to distinguish between its own constituents ('self') and those of external, or foreign, origin ('non-self'). Foreign material excites a reaction which results in the elimination of the alien matter[1]. Since many of the foreign substances encountered are living organisms or their toxins, it follows that the reaction results in immunity to infection or limitation of its spread. For this reason the reaction is called the *immune response.* Presumably it has been evolved by animals during evolution as a means of self-preservation in a world teeming with micro-organisms.

The immune response is a reaction to foreign material and has two components. *Humoral immunity* is related to the formation of immunoglobulin antibodies. *Cell-mediated immunity* is attributed to sensitized lymphocytes (T cells) which are activated and either kill target cells directly (T killer cells) or secrete substances (lymphokines) which act locally. Both the humoral and the cell-mediated responses are involved in immunity to infection.

The immune response is intimately bound up with the function of lymphocytes and macrophages. This aspect will be examined in detail later in the chapter. It is important to realize, however, at the outset that there are believed to be several subpopulations of lymphocytes. Two major groups are concerned. Lymphocytes that are associated with the thymus developmentally are termed *T lymphocytes*, and are responsible for cell-mediated immunity. *B lymphocytes* are developmentally dependent on the bursa of Fabricius (or its equivalent in humans). They can be stimulated to produce immunoglobulins (humoral response), but often require T cell co-operation (*helper T cells*). Yet another group of lymphocytes (*suppressor T cells*) inhibits the immune response.

Under certain circumstances the elimination of foreign material is accompanied by a severe reaction—sometimes more severe than that caused by the material itself. The term *hypersensitivity* is therefore applied to such a reaction. It is evident that the 'immune response' is not concerned solely with immunity to infection, and for this reason it will be considered first in a general way rather than being linked with either immunity or hypersensitivity.

Properties of antigens

Any agent which is regarded as non-self is called an *antigen* and is capable of causing an immune response. This is often manifested by the development of specific globulins in the plasma called antibodies. These will be considered in detail later in this chapter, but it should be noted here that antibodies are highly specific, i.e. they react with the antigen which gave rise to them but to no other. Indeed, antigens may be defined in these terms. They are substances which react with specific antibody.

Antigens are high-molecular-weight substances, nearly always proteins, and are recognized as foreign by special features of their chemical structure—probably by particular configurations of their external shape. The areas of the molecular surface which are concerned are called *determinant sites*, or *epitopes*. It is possible to add new epitopes to a protein by the addition of quite simple chemical substances called *haptens*. The antigenic properties of the protein are altered by this procedure such that if it is introduced into a suitable animal, antibodies which are produced are specific for the hapten as well as for the carrier protein. Thus haptens are substances which are not antigenic in themselves, but which behave as antigens when combined with a suitable carrier protein. Indeed, one may regard the determinant sites on a protein antigen as haptenic groups so that all antigens are composed of a carrier protein plus haptens.

Haptens are of great importance in human pathology as a simple example will illustrate: iodine is not an antigen, but if applied to the skin of some individuals it acts as a hapten, and will combine with body proteins so that a new antigenic complex is formed. This stimulates the production of antibodies which are specific for iodine. The next occasion on which iodine is applied to the skin a damaging antigen-antibody reaction occurs and this produces a severe inflammatory response (*allergic contact dermatitis*).*

Between the two extremes of simple chemical hapten and true protein antigen there are many intermediate compounds, often polysaccharides and lipids, which are weakly antigenic when acting alone but powerfully so when acting as haptens combined with protein.

The humoral immune response

The humoral antibodies are mostly gamma globulins on electrophoresis, and by convention are called immunoglobulins (Ig).

When antigen is introduced into the body it is taken up by large phagocytic cells of the RE system. Following subcutaneous injection this occurs both locally and in the regional lymph nodes. With intravenous injection it is the sinus-lining cells of the bone marrow, spleen, and liver which are principally involved. This taking up by the RE cells appears to be the first step in the immune response. The next step is the *recognition* of the antigen as non-self, and this is usually performed by cells which do not themselves manufacture antibodies. The final step is the production of antibodies.

Factors influencing antibody production

A large number of factors affect the response of an animal to the introduction

* If it is proposed to use iodine as a preoperative skin disinfectant, a patch test should *always* be performed beforehand to eliminate the possibility of this reaction. This is done by applying iodine to a small patch of skin and reading the result 24 hours later.

of an antigen. The following account includes the important generalizations, but as with all generalizations, many exceptions will be found.

Genetic factors. The response to a particular antigen is probably determined by the animal's genetic constitution. Alleles at the Ir (immune response) locus are of great importance in the mouse, and this corresponds to the human HLA-DR region.

Previous contact with antigen. *Primary response.* When an antigen is introduced into an animal for the first time, there is an interval of about 10 days before antibody can be detected in the plasma (Fig. 11.1). There then follows a slow rise in titre which climbs to a maximum and then diminishes. This is the typical *primary response*, and it should be noted that the antibody titre reached is comparatively low, and that the first formed antibodies are IgM.

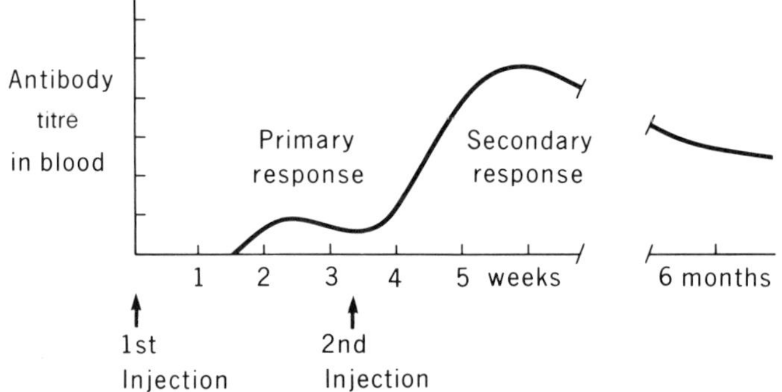

Fig. 11.1 Diagram showing the differences between a primary and a secondary response to an antigenic stimulus. (*Drawn by Margot Mackay, Department of Art as Applied to Medicine, University of Toronto.*)

Secondary response. When the same animal is injected with the same antigen on a second occasion, there is an immediate drop in circulating antibody due to its neutralization by the injected antigen. After 2 to 3 days there is a rapid rise in antibody titre which reaches a peak and again falls off, rapidly at first and later more slowly (Fig. 11.1). The final level of antibody is usually above the previous one. The secondary response is thus *quicker*, *of greater magnitude*, and *of longer duration.*

Furthermore, the type of antibody is generally IgG rather than IgM and has a greater affinity for antigen. That is to say the antibody combines more firmly with its appropriate antigen. This phenomenon has been termed *affinity maturation.* The explanation is probably that at the beginning of an immune response a large amount of free antigen is present and will bind to B cells with a wide range of receptor affinities. At a later stage in the response, the antigen is cleared more rapidly from the body and its concentration falls; hence B cells compete for the diminished supply of antigen and only those cells with highest affinity respond (see selective theory on p. 165).

It is evident that the first encounter with an antigen produces a change (termed *potential immunity*), such that future contact with the same antigen produces a big immune response.

The antibody titre already present. The presence of circulating immunoglobulin may depress or completely abolish the response to injected antigen. The implication of this should be remembered when artificial immunization is being attempted. Thus, the response to diphtheria toxoid is poor in infants, who have a high titre of transferred maternal antibody. The phenomenon can be used to advantage to prevent the sensitization of Rh-negative mothers who have recently given birth to Rh-positive children. If anti-Rh globulin is administered within 72 hours of delivery (or abortion), sensitization is inhibited.

Type of antigen. Antigens vary considerably in their ability to elicit antibody production. As a general rule those in particulate or insoluble form produce a better response than does soluble material. For this reason antigen precipitated with alum is used for diphtheria immunization (APT or alum precipitated toxoid). Freund's adjuvant is considered on p. 191.

Age of animal. This is a most important factor. The description of the immune response so far given applies only to the mature animal.

During early fetal life animals will accept foreign proteins without antibody production. In addition, they may be rendered incapable of reacting to the same antigen throughout adult life. This is called *specific immunological tolerance* and will be described in more detail later in this chapter.

Treatment designed to reduce antibody response. Several methods are available for suppressing the immune response. Some have been used in humans in attempts to prolong the life of homografts and treat diseases, such as systemic lupus erythematosus, in which tissue damage is thought to be caused by an immunological mechanism. All methods tend to be more effective in suppressing a primary response than a secondary one, and affect both the cell-mediated immune response as well as immunoglobulin antibody production.

Glucocorticoid administration. Continuous administration of prednisone is commonly used.

Administration of antimetabolite drugs, such as are used in the treatment of cancer, e.g. 6-mercaptopurine, cyclophosphamide, and azathioprine (Imuran).

Administration of antilymphocytic serum.[2,3] Antilymphocytic serum, prepared by the injection of lymphocytes from an animal of one species into one of another species, has been found to inhibit T-cell function. Its use in humans for inhibiting the graft reaction is under active study, but in a number of patients malignancy has followed its use.

Total body exposure to ionizing radiation.[4] This suppresses a primary response more than a secondary one. The dose necessary to suppress the immune response is dangerously close to the lethal dose and the method is seldom used in humans.

Depletion of small lymphocytes. Chronic drainage of these cells from the thoracic duct by establishing a fistula in the experimental animal causes depletion of lymphocytes and impairment of the immune response.

Anergy. See page 158.

Properties of the immunoglobulins[5]

Antibody activity in the plasma is due to a group of globulins which, on electrophoretic separation, form a broad band in the γ fraction together with some activity in the α and β regions. They are highly specific and react with their corresponding antigens in various ways, although this action may not always be demonstrable *in vitro*. The specificity of each antibody is thought to be determined by the precise amino-acid sequence of its polypeptide chains.

The *in-vitro* reactions between antigens and antibodies are considered later in this chapter, but it may be noted at this stage that in general the antibodies tend to neutralize their antigens and lead to their elimination. The antibody produced in an animal after the injection of an antigen is not a single distinct protein, for one antigenic compound may have several epitopes, and therefore antibodies of different specificities are produced. Furthermore, even the antibody possessing a single specificity is heterogeneous and consists of a group of proteins differing somewhat in molecular composition and size, and in electrophoretic mobility.

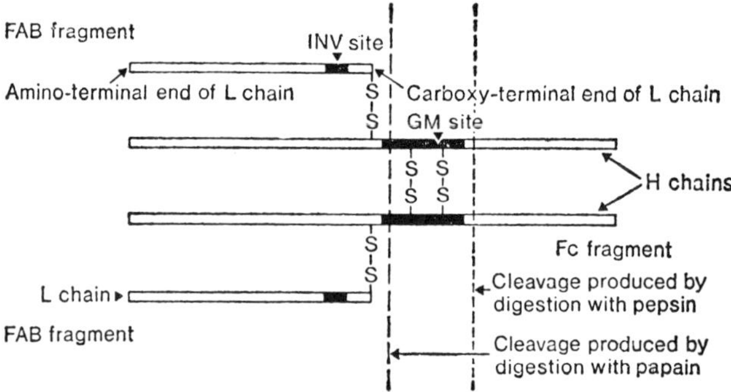

Fig. 11.2 Diagrammatic representation of the structure of IgG antibody. The molecule is composed of two light polypeptide chains and two heavy chains joined together by disulphide bonds. Digestion with the enzyme papain splits the molecule into three fragments, as indicated by the dotted lines. Two fragments are similar and have one antibody-combining site each (Fab fragments). The third fragment (Fc) can be crystallized, and has no antibody activity. The splitting action of pepsin is also indicated. The sites for the antigenic determinants governed by the *Inv* and *Gm* genes are shown.

Nomenclature and chemical structure. The plasma antibodies are now called *immunoglobulins*, with the designation Ig regardless of their electrophoretic mobility. Each molecule consists of four polypeptide chains—two light and two heavy chains held together by disulphide bonds. As explained in Fig. 11.2, the antibody-binding properties of the molecule reside in the Fab fragments, a fact which harmonizes well with the bivalent properties of most antibodies.

The amino-terminal ends of the light chains and the associated ends of the heavy chains are described as *variable*, because the amino-acids that constitute them vary both in type and in sequence in each molecule. In some areas the variable region displays much more variation than others. These are the *hypervariable* regions. Since antibody specificity is determined by amino-acid type and sequence, antibodies of different specificities can occur in any class of immunoglobulin. The carboxy-terminal ends of the light chains and the Fc fragments are more constant and are spoken of as the *invariable*, or *constant*, regions. These regions, particularly the Fc portion, convey the biological activities of complement fixation, skin fixation, placental transfer, and opsonic activity. The last is due to the binding of antibody-coated organisms to macrophages and granulocytes *via* the phagocytes' Fc receptor sites (p. 79).

The immunoglobulins are themselves antigenic when injected into other species, and immunoelectrophoretic studies have revealed that the light and heavy chains are not homogeneous. Human antibodies can be divided into *classes* depending upon specific antigenic determinants on the heavy chains. There are five types of heavy chains, which are named: γ, α, δ, ε, and μ. Each antibody molecule has a pair of identical heavy chains, and therefore five classes are recognized: IgG, IgA, IgD, IgE, and IgM respectively. Each class has been further subdivided into two *groups*: K for Korngold and L for Lipari, after the two workers who first recognized them. The difference lies in the light chains which are termed κ (kappa) and λ (lambda). Each molecule, whether IgG, IgA, IgM, IgD, or IgE, has either two κ or two λ chains, *but never one of each.* (See Fig. 11.3.)

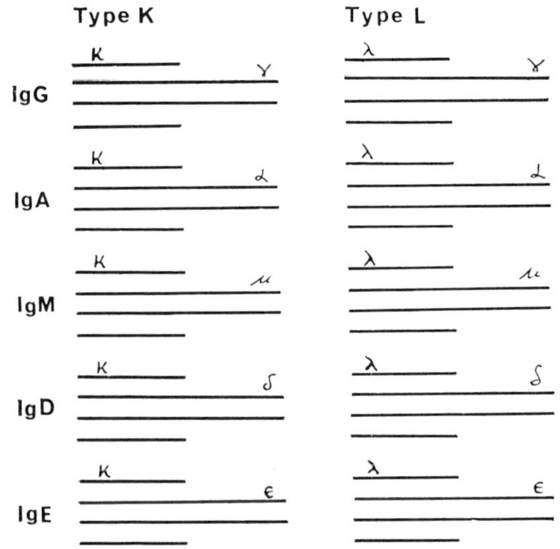

Fig. 11.3 Structure of the immunoglobulins. The classes resemble each other in that the molecules are composed of two identical light polypeptide chains and two identical heavy chains. The difference lies in their heavy chains. In any one class there are two types. In the K type there are two κ light chains, while in the L type there are two λ light chains. The molecular weight of the light chains is approximately 25 000 daltons, while that of the heavy chains is 50 000 daltons, thereby giving a total molecular weight of approximately 150 000 daltons.

Variants of the heavy chains have been found. Thus there are four of the γ chains, so that there are four subtypes of IgG—IgG1, IgG2, IgG3, and IgG4. Similarly, there are two subclasses each of IgA and IgD to add to the remarkable heterogeneity of the immunoglobulins.

IgG is the most abundant immunoglobulin present in the plasma. It is a 7S protein*, with a molecular weight of about 150 000 daltons and a structure as depicted in Figs. 11.2 and 11.3. It is the only immunoglobulin to cross the placenta.

IgA[6,7] is present in the plasma, but its highest concentration is found in

* The sedimentation constant is measured in Svedberg units, and is a measure of the rapidity with which macromolecules move when subjected to centrifugal force in an ultracentrifuge. The higher the constant the larger and heavier is the molecule. The 7S fraction of plasma contains the γ-globulins of MW 150 000 daltons, while the 19S fraction contains those of MW 10^6 daltons.

secretions of mucous membranes, and it is an important factor in preventing infection of mucous membranes. It is made locally in plasma cells and secreted as a dimer composed of two IgA molecules associated with a J chain and linked to a glycoprotein called secretory component. This *secretory*, or *transport*, *component* is manufactured by epithelial cells, and may serve to stabilize the IgA against proteolysis. IgA does not fix complement *via* the classical pathway, and its main function may be to react with antigens absorbed from the gut and other mucous membranes, and neutralize them without the damaging effects of complement activation.

IgD is of unknown function. It is possible that, as a component of the B-cell membrane, it may serve as an antigen receptor site.

IgE is a 7S fraction which is responsible for human anaphylaxis (p. 182) as well as for other type -1 hypersensitivity states such as asthma and hay-fever.

IgM is a 19S globulin with a molecular weight of 900 000 daltons—hence it is also called a *macroglobulin.* It consists of five 7S monomers associated with a J chain to form a pentamer. Because of its size, IgM is largely restricted to the intravascular compartment. In an immune response it is often the first immunoglobulin to be produced; this is later augmented by IgG.

Antigen-antibody union

There is only one way in which antibodies may be recognized and measured, and that is by their specific union with antigen.

When antibody is mixed with antigen a *primary union* occurs. Frequently there is no visible change but if the physicochemical conditions, e.g. pH, temperature, electrolyte concentration, etc., are appropriate, the primary union is followed by a variety of *secondary phenomena*, which can be seen or detected. They are therefore of great practical importance and are used to identify and measure antibodies. *Agglutination, precipitation*, and *complement fixation* are the most important.

Agglutination. When a particulate antigen, e.g. a bacterial suspension, is added to its antibody, the particles may adhere to each other to produce large visible clumps. This clumping is called *agglutination*, and the antibody is called an *agglutinin.* The detection of agglutinins in the serum of patients is frequently of value in the diagnosis of infectious disease. The highest dilution of serum which produces agglutination is called its *titre*, and a rising value is particularly significant. Occasionally the highest titres of antibody fail to agglutinate the antigen; this is called the *prozone phenomenon* (Fig. 11.4).

When the organism used is of the *Salmonella* group, the test is known as the *Widal reaction.*

It should be noted that agglutination tests may be used to *identify unknown organisms*, provided a supply of known antisera is available.

Agglutinins to red cells (*haemagglutinins*) are of great importance in haematology, and both the 'complete' and 'incomplete' types are described on p. 453.

Precipitation. Precipitation is the formation of an insoluble product when two soluble substances are mixed together. If a soluble antigen (e.g. a protein, a toxin, or an extract of an organism) is added to its specific antibody, a precipitate may form. The antibody is called a *precipitin*, and probably acts by virtue of the divalent antibody molecules joining up the antigen molecules to form a lattice.

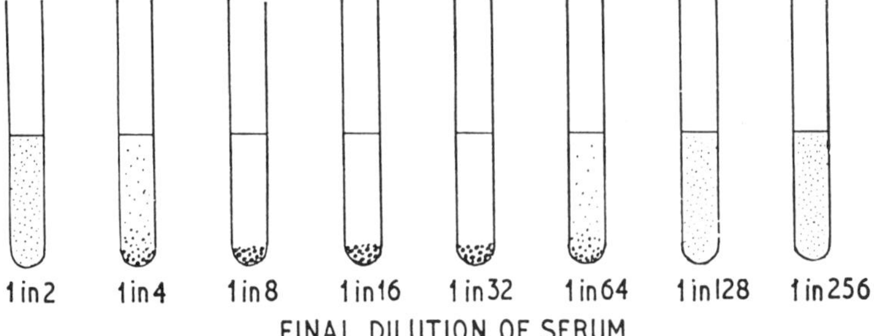

Fig. 11.4 Agglutination test. The titre of the antibody is 1 in 64. The failure of the first tube (1 in 2 dilution) to show agglutination is known as the prozone phenomenon, and is not uncommonly seen in *Brucella* agglutination tests.

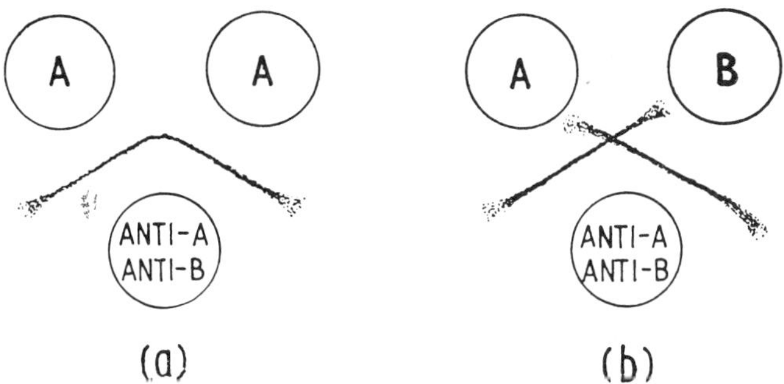

Fig. 11.5 Ouchterlony plates showing precipitin reactions. In (a) the precipitin lines join together, as they are both due to the same A-anti-A reaction. In (b) the lines cross, as they are formed by different antigen-antibody reactions.

Precipitins may be demonstrated simply by mixing the reagents in a test-tube, but a more sensitive method is to perform the reaction in an agar gel (Ouchterlony). Two cups are cut in an agar plate; into one is placed the antigen and into the other the antibody. Each now diffuses towards the other, and where they meet in optimal proportions a white line of precipitation appears (Fig. 11.5). Precipitin reactions are used in streptococcal grouping (Lancefield), in the identification of human blood and semen, and in the diagnosis of syphilis (Kahn test).

As with agglutination reactions, the prozone phenomenon may occur. This is particularly relevant in the diagnosis of syphilis. If the standard test for syphilis is reported negative in a case in which there is a strong suspicion of syphilis, the titre of antibodies should be estimated.

Radioimmunoassay and other methods are described in the footnote on page 255.

Complement fixation. This type of antibody, also called an *amboceptor*, produces an effect on its antigen only in the presence of a component of the blood called complement. *Complement* has been defined as the heat-labile activity in plasma which, in the presence of haemolysin, is cytotoxic to red cells. The details of the activation of complement are described on page 171.

Amboceptors may unite with their corresponding antigens and activate complement to produce some visible effect—for instance *lysis*. Antibodies which lyse red cells (*haemolysins*) or bacteria (*bacteriolysins*) are both of the complement-fixing variety. Under some circumstances the complement activation produces no visible effect, but it can nevertheless be detected indirectly. The *Wassermann reaction*, employed to detect syphilitic antibodies, is a good example of this. The test is explained diagrammatically in Table 11.1, in which it is seen that serum, heated to 56°C for 30 mins., is mixed with a standard quantity of complement and syphilitic antigen.* The object of heating ('inactivating') the serum is to inactivate the unknown quantity of complement which is normally present, so that a known, measured amount can be added to the reaction. The serum-complement-antigen mixture is allowed to incubate for a standard length of time. If the syphilitic antibody is present in the patient's serum, the antigen combines with it, and at the same time 'fixes' the added complement. The detector system is then added. It is also of antigen-amboceptor type, and utilizes red cells with their corresponding haemolysin. If complement has not been used up in the first reaction it is available for the second system. Therefore haemolysis of the red cells denotes an absence of syphilitic antibody, and the Wassermann reaction is negative. On the other hand, the absence of haemolysis indicates a positive reaction. Similar complement fixation tests are employed in the diagnosis of many other infections—being particularly useful in virology.

Opsonins. Opsonins are substances which render organisms more readily susceptible to phagocytosis. Polymorphs are in general able to phagocytose virulent organisms only if the latter are first coated with a specific opsonin. (See below.) This type of opsonin, and also the non-specific type, are also considered in the sections on acute inflammation (p. 78) and immunity to infection (p. 178). Opsonization also aids the clearance of organisms from the blood by the reticuloendothelial system.

Cytotoxic antibodies. Antibodies can destroy cells in two ways.

Complement-dependent lysis. IgM and certain subclasses of IgG can activate complement by the classical pathway and cause lysis (see p. 172).

Antibody-dependent cell-mediated cytotoxicity.[8,9] B lymphocytes, null lymphocytes, monocytes, and polymorphonuclear leucocytes have Fc receptors on their cell surfaces by which they can attach to IgG-coated cells. In the case of monocytes and neutrophils this is an opsonic effect, and is a prelude to phagocytosis. With lymphocytes the attachment results in cell death by some ill-defined mechanism that depends on close cell-to-cell interaction. The phenomenon of antibody-dependent cell-mediated cytotoxicity is yet another example of the co-operation between humoral and cellular components in the immune response. It is one mechanism whereby cancer cells and allografts can be destroyed by an immune mechanism.

Neutralizing antibodies. If the antigen has a particular biological property, for instance if it is a toxin, the corresponding antibody neutralizes this activity. Thus antibodies to toxins are called *antitoxins.*

Virus neutralizing antibodies probably coat the virus particles and prevent their attachment to cells (see p. 253). Syphilitic antibody causes the immobilization of

* The antigen is in fact a cholesterolized extract of heart muscle. This has been found to work in practice, but the precise reason for this is not clear. Treponemal protein can be used to make the test more specific.

the organism, a fact utilized in the *Treponema pallidum* immobilization test (p. 227).

Table 11.1. Wassermann reaction

First reaction	Second or detector reaction (haemolytic system)
Patient's serum with ? antibody heated to 56°C for 30 mins. (to destroy any complement which is present). + Antigen (standard quantity). + Complement (carefully measured amount).	Red cells (sheep). + Haemolysin (serum of rabbit immunized against sheep red cells). This is inactivated commercially to remove its complement. ? Complement unused.

It must be stressed that the immunoglobulins have been named according to the nature of the test used to detect them. In many cases a single antibody can perform several functions depending upon the conditions under which it is tested. For instance, an antibody may be capable of neutralizing toxin, e.g. diphtheria toxin, in an *in-vivo* experiment. It is therefore rightly called an *antitoxin.* However, *in vitro* it will produce a precipitate with its antigen and therefore be labelled a *precipitin.* Similarly a single antibody may perform the functions of precipitin, agglutinin, and lysin.

The cell-mediated immune response

In addition to the formation of immunoglobulins, the introduction of an antigen can lead to the production of sensitized lymphocytes which react specifically with the administered antigen.[10] This is the cell-mediated immune response, and is particularly well marked if the stimulating antigen is combined with Freund's adjuvant (p. 191) or is a component of the living cell. The sensitized cells are T cells and react with antigen, undergo blast-cell transformation, and release a number of agents called *lymphokines* which have a variety of actions.[11–13] These are ill-defined chemically, and it is not known whether there are a few agents having many actions or separate substances each with a specific effect. They may be listed:

1. *Migration inhibition factor (MIF).* This acts on macrophages and prevents them migrating in a tissue culture system. (See Fig. 13.3.) It may be supposed that MIF is important as a mediator of the demolition phase of acute inflammation and in chronic inflammation.

2. *Macrophage arming factor.* This substance is transferred to the cell membrane of macrophages, and has the property of conferring upon the macrophage the ability to act specifically with antigen. When the antigen is a tumour cell, the cell is killed. It should be noted that although armed macrophages react with specific antigen to become activated, the activated macrophages can then kill other cells non-specifically. A *macrophage-activating lymphokine* has been described, and it makes the cells more phagocytic and better able to kill organisms. It is evident that MIF, activating factor, and arming factor are closely related and may well be

important mediators of the demolition phase of acute inflammation and in chronic inflammation.

3. *Transfer factor.*[14] This substance specifically transfers sensitization to previously uncommitted lymphocytes. It therefore recruits new cells to the site involved, e.g. the site of infection.

4. *Lymphotoxin.* This agent has a cytopathic effect on cells, such as a monolayer of fibroblasts in culture.

5. *Skin reactive factor.*

6. *Chemotactic factors.* Probably several types are produced, and these affect either neutrophils, monocytes, or eosinophils.

7. *Mitogenic factor.* This causes blast transformation and stimulates mitosis.

8. *Interferon.*

9. *Immunoglobulin.*

An important feature of the cell-mediated immune resonse is that while the sensitized lymphocytes are reactive to a specific antigen, the subsequent events produced by release of lymphokines are non-specific.

In addition, the sensitized lymphocytes can kill target cells by some type of direct cell-to-cell interaction without the intervention of lymphokine production.[15]

Anergy

A loss of the ability to express a cell-mediated immune response is called anergy. Thus a person previously sensitive to tuberculin or mumps antigen becomes negative. Anergy is not uncommon in terminal states due to many causes, e.g. infections and malignancy. In cancer it is associated with a bad prognosis.[16] It is also a well-known feature of sarcoidosis, lepromatous leprosy, and measles. The pathogenesis is not known, and indeed may not be the same in all instances. Destruction of normal lymphoid tissue may be postulated as the mechanism in extensive malignant disease, Hodgkin's disease, and widespread sarcoidosis. However, this cannot be the explanation in early sarcoidosis or measles.

The action of blocking antibodies or of suppressor T cells may be involved, but non-immunological agents may also play a part. Thus a factor has been found in the serum of patients with Hodgkin's disease that inhibits the patient's T cells.

Effect of the immune response in the living animal

Ig antibodies can produce important effects in the living animal. They may provide *immunity* to infection, or cause immediate-type *hypersensitivity.* Likewise the cell-mediated response leads to the formation of sensitized lymphocytes that result in immunity to infection or cause delayed-type hypersensitivity. These effects are considered in the chapters which follow.

The antibody forming tissues

Before describing the cellular features of the immune response it is essential to understand the structure and development of the lymphoid tissues of the body. Much of our information stems from observations on the thymus and the bursa, particularly on the effects of thymectomy and bursectomy. These topics will therefore be described first.

The thymus.[17] The first lymphoid tissue to develop in mammals is the thymus. It contains an epithelial element in the form of reticular cells and Hassall's corpuscles. In addition there are many thymocytes which morphologically resemble lymphocytes.

Effects of thymectomy. Thymectomy performed shortly after birth can produce dramatic effects in some species. Mice, for example, appear normal for 3 to 4 weeks, and then a wasting syndrome usually develops which closely resembles runt disease (see p. 193). This is probably the result of microbial infection, for it does not occur in germ-free animals. Significantly there is a deficiency of small lymphocytes in the white splenic pulp, the paracortical zones of lymph nodes, and in the circulating blood. The animals exhibit an impaired ability to develop delayed-type hypersensitivity, and are tolerant of allografts and sometimes even of xenografts. These are all defects in T-cell function. The production of immunoglobulin to some antigens is normal, but to the majority there is impaired immunoglobulin production. This, as we shall see later, is due to a deficiency of helper T cells.

The bursa of Fabricius. In birds the second lymphoid organ to develop is the *bursa of Fabricius.* This is situated near the cloaca, and, like the thymus, has an epithelial as well as a lymphoid element.

Effects of bursectomy. Removal of the bursa of Fabricius, especially if combined with non-lethal total body irradiation, results in an immunologically deficient state characterized by a failure to produce immunoglobulins when suitable challenged by an antigen. It is possible that in mammals the intestinal lymphoid tissue corresponds to the bursa, for its removal in rabbits produces a similar failure in immunoglobulin production. This has been regarded as the gut-associated central lymphoid tissue. In humans it is thought more likely that its equivalent is in the bone marrow itself.

Lymph nodes. Lymph comes into the lymph node through the peripheral sinus, traverses the cortex, enters the sinuses of the medulla, and finally leaves through the efferent duct. The sinuses are lined by plump, *littoral*, or *sinus-lining cells*, which have eosinophilic cytoplasm and are phagocytic. Reticular cells are present and appear to be concerned with the formation of reticulin, which constitutes the connective tissue framework of the node. In the outer part, or *cortex*, of the node there are densely packed lymphocytes which are focally aggregated into *follicles.* In the centre of each follicle there is often a well-defined *germinal centre of Flemming.* This contains large cells which are generally called lymphoblasts. They show a high turn-over rate and therefore mitoses are abundant. In addition, the centres contain large macrophages which usually contain nuclear debris in their clear, abundant cytoplasm. On microscopy the macrophages produce clear spaces which have been likened to the stars in a starry sky.

The *medulla* of the node shows prominent sinuses and medullary cords of cells between them. These cells are mainly small lymphocytes together with a variable number of plasma cells and granulocytes.

Around the cortical follicles with their germinal centres, and between them and the medulla, there is a third zone which is packed with lymphocytes. This is the *paracortical zone*, which is a T-lymphocyte domain.

Small lymphocytes from the blood normally enter the lymph node *via* the post-capillary sinuses in the paracortical zone and subsequently leave the node in the efferent lymph. The lymphocytes therefore re-enter the blood stream through the thoracic duct. It follows that if this duct is exteriorized and drained, the body is steadily depleted of lymphocytes (mainly T lymphocytes). (See Fig. 11.6.)

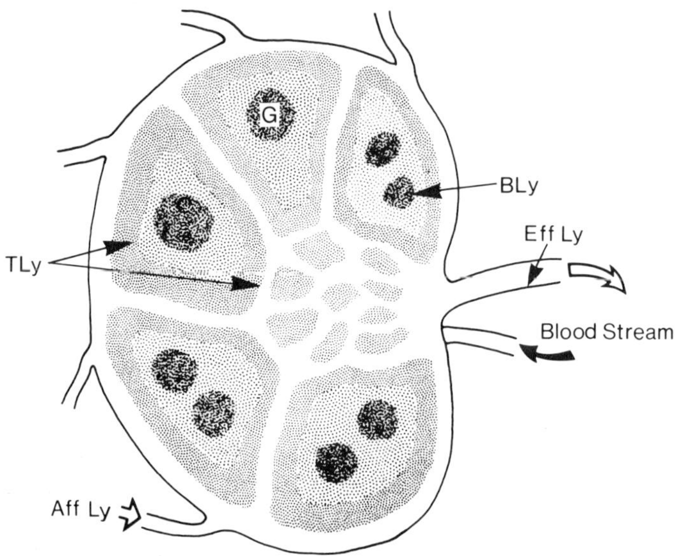

Fig. 11.6 Diagram of a lymph node. Lymph enters the node through several afferent lymphatic vessels (Aff Ly), and percolates through a meshwork formed by reticular cells and their reticulin fibres. In the medulla the fluid is collected into sinuses that are lined by phagocytic sinus-lining cells, which are members of the reticulo-endothelial system. The cortex contains collections of B lymphocytes (B Ly), some of which have one or more germinal centres (G). Surrounding these areas there is a mantle of T lymphocytes (T Ly); this is designated the *paracortical zone.* In the medulla there are groups, or cords, of B cells—both lymphocytes and cells that have differentiated into plasma cells. The B cells tend to remain in the node, and are therefore described as sessile. T cells, on the other hand, leave the node *via* the solitary efferent lymphatic vessel (Eff Ly), enter the blood stream *via* the thoracic duct, and finally return to a lymph node. They leave the blood stream by passing through the walls of the postcapillary venules in the paracortical zone. Lymph containing lymphocytes from tissues or other lymph nodes also enters the lymph node through the afferent lymphatics (Aff Ly). (*Drawn by Margot Mackay, Department of Art as Applied to Medicine, University of Toronto.*)

Spleen. In the spleen the blood passes through the central (malpighian) arterioles to enter the sinusoids which are, as in the lymph nodes, lined by phagocytic cells. In the red pulp there are reticular cells, lymphocytes, and plasma cells as well as occasional granulocytes and megakaryocytes. The lymphoid cuffs are situated around the malpighian arterioles, and the lymphocytes are thought to be derived from the blood as part of the re-circulation of cells as in the paracortical zones of the lymph nodes. Germinal centres may be prominent.

Development of the peripheral lymphoid tissues. It is evident that both the thymus and the bursa of Fabricius are essential for the proper development of the peripheral lymphoid tissues. It is believed that the primitive stem cells from the bone marrow that are destined for lymphoid differentiation (progenitor cells) migrate to the thymus and mature into T lymphocytes. The cells in the thymus (thymocytes) appear to be non-functional and do not take part in an immune response. They develop into functional T lymphocytes, probably under the influence of a thymic hormone (thymosin or thymopoietin). The mature T lymphocytes are released into the circulation and populate the thymus-dependent areas of the peripheral lymphoid tissue—the paracortical zone of lymph nodes, the white pulp of the spleen, and elsewhere (Fig. 11.7). They form about 70 per cent of the blood circulating lymphocytes.

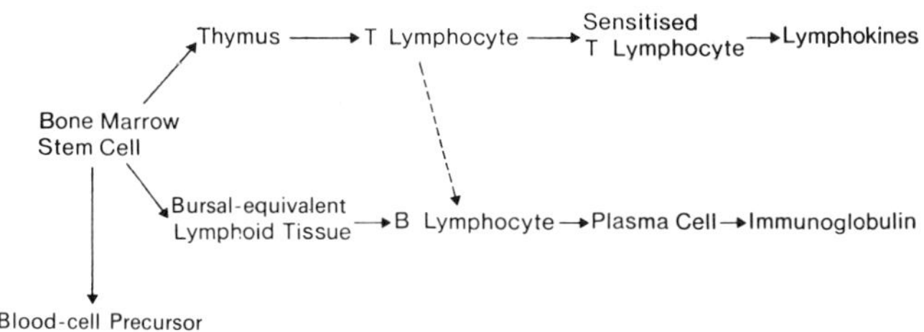

Fig. 11.7 Diagram showing the postulated development of the peripheral lymphoid tissue of the lymph nodes.

The primitive cells from the bone marrow which migrate to the bursa, or its postulated human equivalent, develop into B lymphocytes. These migrate to the B-dependent areas of the peripheral lymphoid tissue. These are the follicles (including the germinal centres of Flemming) and the medulla of lymph nodes, the lymph follicles of the gut, and the corresponding areas in the spleen. Thus, the thymus and the bursa are regarded as the *primary lymphoid tissues* which are responsible for the population of the *secondary lymphoid tissues.* T and B lymphocytes were the first types of lymphocytes to be recognized, but it is now believed that this simple division is an over-simplification, since subtypes of both B and T cells are known whilst others appear to be neither B nor T.

Properties of lymphocytes[18–23]

Properties of T lymphocytes. T lymphocytes have certain membrane markers by which they may be recognized. In the mouse the θ (theta) and the Ly antigens have been widely used in experimental studies; other surface antigens are determined by genes at the I region of the H–2 histocompatibility complex. This is the equivalent of the HLA-DR locus in the human (see p. 192). Anti-θ antibody in the presence of complement can be used to destroy T cells in experimental work. Human T cells have a sheep red-cell receptor. Hence, when human T cells and sheep red cells are mixed, the red cells form a rosette around the T cells (T-cell rosette or E rosettes). The ability to form these rosettes is a convenient method of identifying human T cells.

T cells can recognize antigen and respond to it by division and the subsequent formation of *memory T cells* and *sensitized (effector) T lymphocytes.* The nature of the antigen receptor on T lymphocytes is unknown, since antibody determinants cannot easily be detected on the cell membrane. Nevertheless, a special type of membrane-bound antibody has been postulated and called IgT.

Sensitized T cells can release lymphokines when they interact with specific antigen. This has been described on page 157. Furthermore, sensitized T cells can kill target cells to which they have been specifically sensitized by a direct cell-to-cell interaction. These cells are termed *killer T cells*, and form a subpopulation of T cells. If the target cells are labelled with ^{51}Cr, the release of radioactivity into the medium is a convenient method of estimating the cytocidal effect.

In addition to the antigen-sensitive T cells and the killer cells other subpopulations of T cells are known. *Helper T cells* are necessary for the humoral antibody response to most antigens (these are called T-cell-dependent antigens). Helper T cells are also needed for T cell activation in the cell-mediated immune response. Another subpopulation of T cells (*suppressor T cells*) can inhibit the immune response, either humoral or cellular or both.[24]

Properties of B lymphocytes. In contrast to T lymphocytes, B lymphocytes have well-defined immunoglobulin membrane markers. IgM determinants can be demonstrated by the use of fluorescein-labelled anti-Ig serum. As the B cells mature, so the IgM is often replaced by IgD determinants. This is the only known function for this antibody. The B cells also have receptors for complement components (C3 receptors), and the Fc component of immunoglobulin. The antibody determinants on B-cell membranes are the mechanism whereby B cells recognize specific antigen and respond to it by division and subsequent maturation into B memory cells and plasma cells. Plasma cells have a well-developed rough endoplasmic reticulum, and secrete immunoglobulin. It is believed that the specificity of this immunoglobulin is the same as that of the antibody on the B cell's membrane. *Thus an antigen reacts with and stimulates only those cells that are capable of forming antibody against it* (see selective theory).

B cells do not form rosettes with sheep red cells alone, but will do so if the red cells are first coated with anti-red-cell antibody (these are called EA rosettes). These rosettes are produced by attachment of the coated red cells to the C3 or Fc receptors on the B cell membrane.

Null cells. A small population of lymphocytes does not have the receptors associated with either B or T cells. Their role is not understood, but since they may have Fc receptors they can attach to antibody-coated cells and kill them. They are, therefore, also called *natural killer cells (NK cells)*.

Lymphocyte transformation

One of the most remarkable observations of recent times is that the small lymphocytes of the blood and lymph can be stimulated *in vitro* to become large cells with basophilic, pyroninophilic cytoplasm containing many free ribosomes, while their nuclei have nucleoli. These cells have been called *immunoblasts*, pyroninophilic cells, and blast cells. They exhibit DNA synthesis and mitotic activity, a feature which has led to them being intensively used in studies of human chromosomes. Blast cell change can conveniently be detected by the cells' uptake of tritiated thymidine.

Agents which lead to lymphocyte blast transformation and mitosis are termed *mitogens*, and include:

Lectins. These are proteins derived from plant tissue and have affinity for certain cell-surface carbohydrates. They include:

Phytohaemagglutinin, derived from red kidney beans; this substance was used originally to produce agglutination of red cells in experiments designed to facilitate the isolation of white cells from the blood.

Concanavalin A, derived from jack beans.

Pokeweed mitogen.

Antilymphocytic serum.

Bacterial lipopolysaccharide endotoxin.

Antigen-antibody complexes.

Other allogeneic lymphocytes.

Antigen, if added to lymphocytes from sensitized individuals.

If a sample of lymphocytes is exposed to a mitogen, the number of cells that undergo transformation varies; so also does the speed with which they respond. This is because some mitogens (phytohaemagglutinin and concanavalin A) stimulate T cells only, others (bacterial endotoxin) B cells only, while others (antilymphocytic serum and pokeweed mitogen) affect both types of cells. T-cell transformation occurs faster than does that of B cells. Hence, the number of cells that transform, and the speed with which they do so, is related to the number of B or T cells that is involved.

The precise role of the blast transformation phenomenon in the intact animal is not known, but various suggestions have been made.

Proliferating B cells can form the germinal centres of lymphoid tissue. Each centre may indeed be a clone derived from one cell. In other situations, e.g. the medulla of lymph nodes, the cells may differentiate into plasma cells. Others may revert to small lymphocytes and remain as memory cells.

Proliferating T cells can revert to small lymphocytes, and act as effector cells in a cell-mediated immune response; others remain as memory cells.

Functional steps in the immune response

The following steps may be postulated as occurring after the introduction of an antigen:

The recognition system. A mechanism must exist for recognizing an antigen as foreign. Furthermore, the system must have a *memory* so that the same antigen can be recognized again.

The processing system. Once having been recognized as an antigen, its determinants must be processed in such a way that specific antibody can be produced.

The production system. The final outcome of the immune response is the manufacture of antibody. This involves the synthesis of a range of specific proteins as well as the formation of immune lymphocytes. The production system must be *regulated* in some way, so that the immune response can be turned off when the antigenic stimulus is withdrawn.

The recognition system

A cell which is capable of recognizing antigen and of initiating an immune response, although not necessarily producing antibody itself, is termed an *immunologically competent cell.* There is considerable evidence that such a cell is morphologically a small lymphocyte and that both B and T types exist.

Precisely how the appropriate cells recognize the antigen is not known for certain. With B cells it is known that antibody determinants are present (either IgM or IgD), and it is probable that these act as receptors. In the case of T cells less is known about the possible receptors although again specific Ig has been postulated[23] (see p. 161).

The process of recognizing antigen is sometimes known as the *afferent limb* of the immune response. The actual production of immunoglobulins, or formation of effector T cells in cell-mediated immune responses, constitutes the *efferent limb.*

The processing system—number of cell types involved in the immune response

There is considerable evidence that both immunoglobulin production and the cell-mediated immune response involve the co-operative action of more than one type of cell.

Immunoglobulin production to many antigens is greatly enhanced by the activity of T cells. These helper T cells appear to release soluble substances (which may be included among the lymphokines) that, combined with the stimulus provided by the antigen, provide a signal for the B cells to produce specific antibody. Various soluble factors can provide this second signal; they may be either non-specific or else specific for the particular antigen. Antigens that do not require T-cell co-operation in order to provoke the formation of antibodies appear to act as B-cell mitogens. The relationship between B and T cells is very complex, for T cells can also act as suppressors to some immune responses. Thus, in some T-cell deficient animals there is an exaggerated immunoglobulin response to some antigens. The human counterpart of this situation is lepromatous leprosy, in which the abeyance of T cell function is combined with an excessive immunoglobulin response. Indeed, the polyclonal hypergammaglobulinaemia that results is responsible for one of the serious complications of leprosy: the combination of specific immunoglobulin with a lepra-bacillus antigen produces the immune complexes that cause a vasculitis (p. 225). The *erythema nodosum leprosum* that results and its pathogenesis parallel that of the Arthus reaction (p. 185).[25]

There is considerable evidence that *macrophages* are required for T-cell activation—not only in the activation of sensitized cells by antigen *in vivo* but also the non-specific stimulus provided by a mitogen *in vitro* (p. 162). It is probable that B-cell activation also requires macrophage co-operation, particularly those B-cell functions that require the aid of helper T cells.

Macrophages readily take up antigen, the bulk of which is metabolized. Some antigen, however, is retained and presented to the lymphocytes in such a form that it stimulates antibody production. This antigen probably remains on the cell membrane of the macrophage before presentation to the lymphocytes. Nevertheless, there is some evidence that antigen may enter the cell by endocytosis and be processed in some way. The transfer of antigen, or processed antigen, appears to be related to direct cell-to-cell contact, and lymphocytes can be observed to form clusters around macrophages. This process has also been interpreted as indicating that macrophages provide a nutritional role rather than indicating specific antigen presentation to the lymphocytes. Nevertheless, macrophages appear also to release a soluble *lymphocyte-activating factor* that can, under some circumstances, replace direct cell-to-cell contact. The situation is further complicated by the fact that macrophages can also act as suppressor cells; hence, both macrophages and T lymphocytes are involved in the complex regulation of the immune response.

Theories of immunoglobulin antibody production

Immunoglobulins are proteins, and it is reasonable to believe that their formation in the rough endoplasmic reticulum of plasma cells is largely determined by genetic information residing in the nucleus. The problem that has taxed immunologists is the mechanism whereby the body can be induced to produce new specific protein following external stimulation by an antigen. Two main theories have emerged.[26]

The instructive theory

It has been postulated that antigens play an instructive role, and that the extraordinary specifity of antibodies is related to the fact that antigens act as moulds, or templates, during antibody formation. The theory though superficially satisfying has many drawbacks. Antibodies being proteins are presumably produced under the influence of specific mRNA, and no mechanism is known whereby an exogenous protein could modify this process. Furthermore the theory assumes that antigen persists in the body throughout a period of antibody production—a period which is often measured in months or even years. There is little direct evidence that antigens can remain in the body for such long periods; indeed, the immune response is responsible for their rapid elimination.

The natural selection theory

This theory supposes that in the adult there are cells capable of mounting an immune response against any non-self antigen which the individual is likely to meet. The antigen selects these cells and stimulates them to grow and to produce antibody. The antigen thus determines the *quantity* of antibody produced, but not directly its *specificity*. This theory was formulated by Jerne, who envisaged the presence of innumerable cells each of which could make antibody of one specificity even in the absence of antigenic stimulus. Whether these innumerable types of cells are derived as a result of inherited genetic information, or whether they arise as a result of somatic mutation, perhaps in the thymus, is not known.

The theory has been extended by MacFarlane Burnet into the clonal selection theory; in one form or another this is the current concept of the immune response. According to the theory, antigen reacts with receptors at the surface of appropriate cells, and the reaction constitutes a signal for the cells to divide. In this way a clone* is developed. A further elaboration on the theory by Burnet and later Medawar supposes that during the early stages of embryonic development there

* A *clone* is a group of cells of like hereditary constitution which has been produced asexually from a single cell. The word is derived from the Greek klon, meaning a cutting used for propagation.

occur many somatic mutations in the immunologically competent cells. This results in the formation of a whole range of cells which between them are capable of mounting an immune response specific for any antigen which the body may subsequently meet. In the adult contact with antigen stimulates growth of these cells and in this way a clone develops; as it increases in size, so does antibody production increase.

It is obvious that if somatic mutation occurs so frequently that cells are produced which can form antibodies against all possible antigen, then inevitably some mutations will produce cells capable of forming antibodies against the host's own developing tissues. It must therefore be postulated that there exists some mechanism during *embryonic life* for the destruction, or inactivation, of these harmful, or *forbidden clones.* Any antigen present in the developing embryo is recognized as self, and at birth there are no cells present which make antibodies against it. According to this theory it is apparent that, if an antigen, normally foreign, is introduced into an embryo, it should be accepted as self, and the animal will exhibit *specific immunological tolerance*, that is to say, it will not make antibodies against this antigen. This in fact is what does happen.

Specific immunological tolerance

The administration of an antigen to an embryo results not in the formation of antibodies but in the acceptance of the foreign substance as 'self'. The phenomenon was first noticed when embryos were grafted with allogeneic cells, i.e. from an animal of the same species but of a different genetic constitution. So long as the grafted cells survived in the host the animals were tolerant of further grafts from the same donor, but not from those of any other donor. The tolerance was therefore *specific* and not due to a generalized depression of the immune response.[27]

Specific immunological tolerance to non-living antigens can also be induced, but it persists only for so long as the antigen remains. Repeated injections are therefore usually required.

Induction of tolerance. There are various ways in which tolerance may be induced.

1. Administration of antigen to a fetus or immature animal
2. Administration of massive doses of antigen to a mature animal
3. Administration of very small, often repeated, doses of antigen to young animals
4. Administration of antigen following extensive damage to the lymphoreticular system by ionizing radiations or cytotoxic drugs. Antibody formation is temporarily in abeyance, and regeneration of the immunologically competent cells occurs in the presence of antigen
5. Administration of antigen in an immunologically defective animal such as one subjected to neonatal thymectomy
6. Administration of certain antigens, e.g. picryl chloride by mouth.

Maintenance of tolerance. To maintain the state of tolerance the antigen must usually persist in the body, and this can be ensured either by injecting living cells as antigen or by the repeated injection of non-living antigens.

Explanation of tolerance. Many theories have been put forward to explain the remarkable features of immunological tolerance.

Production of tolerant cells. Under some circumstances antigen can act on immunologically competent cells to render them unresponsive. It has been suggested that if antigen acts directly on the cells they are rendered tolerant. If antigen is taken up by macrophages first, the immunologically competent cells are stimulated to initiate an immune response. This concept explains how *very large doses* of antigen can produce tolerance, for antigen can act directly on cells. Likewise *very small doses* of antigen may fail to initiate antibody production and yet can act on the immunologically competent cells to render them tolerant. Another possibility is that antigen-antibody complexes stimulate the immunologically competent cells to divide and lead to further antibody production. Tolerance is easier to produce if specific antibodies are absent and if the animal's capability of producing them is impaired, e.g. in fetal life and following x-irradiation and the administration of cytotoxic drugs.

Elimination of potentially reactive cells. It is possible that there is no such thing as a tolerant cell, but rather that the appropriate cell has been eliminated, as suggested by Burnet's theory. If this clonal deletion in fact takes place, one would not expect to find cells in a tolerant animal that were capable of binding the relevant antigen. In fact, such cells can be found. Refinement of the clonal deletion theory supposes that potentially reactive cells are rendered non-reactive by a process termed clonal abortion. The recognition of B and T lymphocytes has further complicated the issue. It is known that in immunological tolerance the tolerance may affect either the B or T cells—or both B and T cells. This may be illustrated with respect to tolerance to thyroglobulin. An animal does not normally make antibodies against this protein, and thyroglobulin normally circulates in the blood stream. The body is presumably tolerant to it. Yet injections of thyroglobulin combined with adjuvant lead to the production of antibodies. The explanation appears to be that, while T cells are tolerant, there are B cells which are capable of reacting if given a suitable signal—either derived from a T cell or by the use of adjuvant which could bypass the helper T-cell function.

Other explanations of tolerance have been put forward. It has been supposed that if antigen becomes attached to the cell receptors of a lymphocyte, it induces an immune response if there is limited cross-linking, but tolerance if there is extensive cross-linking with receptors so that the cell surface is virtually smothered by antigen. Various serum factors have been isolated which appear to be able to suppress an immune response; finally there is the question of suppressor T cells which, by overactivity, might produce tolerance. It is evident that there is no simple explanation of specific immunological tolerance, nor indeed is there evidence that there is only one mechanism involved. Tolerance is a state in which a particular immune mechanism is in abeyance, but whether this is due to a chemical repression or a physical elimination of the appropriate mechanism is undecided.

Conclusion

When an antigen gains access to the tissues of the body a complex series of events occur. The antigen is taken up by the phagocytic cells of the RE system, and this is followed by some permanent change in the population of antigen-sensitive cells. Usually the number of cells is increased—presumably by a specific selective process. Hence, when the antigen is encountered again more cells react, and either immunoglobulin or effector T cells are produced. These can result either in immunity or hypersensitivity—subjects which are described in greater detail in the chapters that follow. Sometimes the initial encounter with antigen results in a negative response to a second stimulus (i.e. tolerance). Whether this is due to production of suppressor or non-reactive type cells or to actual elimination of antigen-sensitive cells is not known, and may indeed vary under different circumstances. Nevertheless, the initial stimulus causes some change in response to a second encounter with antigen. Indeed an antigen may be directly defined in these terms: *it is a substance which when introduced into the body of a susceptible animal leads to an immune response which results in a specific change such that when the antigen is introduced on a subsequent occasion there is a response differing from that seen when the substance was first introduced.*

GENERAL READING

Gell P G H, Coombs R R A, Lachmann P J (eds) 1975 Clinical Aspects of Immunology, 3rd edn, 1754 pp. Blackwell, Oxford

Golub E S 1977 The Cellular Basis of the Immune Response, 278 pp. Sinauer Associates, Inc, Sunderland, Massachusetts.

Roitt I M 1975 Essential Immunology, 2nd edition, 260 pp. Blackwell, Oxford

Thaler M S, Klausner R D, Cohen H L 1977 Medical Immunology. 480 pp. Lippincott, Philadelphia

Turk J L 1978 Immunology in Clinical Medicine, 3rd edn. Heinemann, London

REFERENCES

1. Bellanti J A, Green R E 1971 Immunological reactivity: expression of efficiency in elimination of foreignness. Lancet 2:526
2. Leading Article 1975 Current status of antilymphocyte globulin. British Medical Journal 1:644
3. Leading Article 1976 A. L. G. and transplantation. Lancet 1:521
4. Taliaferro W H, Taliaferro L G, Jaroslow B N 1964 Radiation and Immune Mechanisms. Academic Press, New York
5. Cohen S, Milstein C 1967 Structure and biological properties of immunoglobulin. Advances in Immunology 7:1
6. Tomasi T B 1972 Secretory immunoglobulins. New England Journal of Medicine 287:500
7. Waldman R H 1971 Immune mechanisms on secretory surfaces. Postgraduate Medicine 50:78
8. Trinchieri G, de Marchi M 1975 Antibody-dependent cell-mediated cytotoxicity in humans. Journal of Immunology 115:256
9. Scornik J C 1974 Antibody-dependent cell-mediated cytotoxicity. Journal of Immunology 113:1519
10. David J R 1973 Lymphocyte mediators and cellular hypersensitivity. New England Journal of Medicine 288:143
11. Bellanti J A, Rocklin R E 1978 Cell mediated reactions. In: Immunology II, ed Bellanti J A. Saunders A, Philadelphia, Ch 9, p 225.
12. Leading Article 1973 Lymphokines. Lancet 1:1490
13. Leading Article 1978 Lymphokines: an increasing repertoire. British Medical Journal 1:62
14. Leading Article 1974 Transfer factor. British Medical Journal 2:397
15. Henney C S 1974 Killer T cells. New England Journal of Medicine 291:1357
16. Eilber F R, Morton D L 1970 Impaired immunologic reactivity and recurrence following cancer surgery. Cancer (Philadelphia) 25:362
17. Cantor H, Weissman I 1976 Development and function of subpopulations of thymocytes and T lymphocytes. Progress in Allergy 20:1

18. Craddock C G, Longmire R, McMillan R 1971 Lymphocytes and the immune response. New England Journal of Medicine 285:324, 378
19. Rowlands D T, Daniele R P 1975 Surface receptors in the immune response. New England Journal of Medicine 293:26
20. Parker C W 1976 Control of lymphocytic function. New England Journal of Medicine 295:1180
21. Seligmann M, Preud'homme J L, Kourilsky F M 1973 Membrane Receptors of Lymphocytes. North Holland Publishing Co, Amsterdam
22. Fu S M, Winchester R J, Kunkel H G 1974 Occurrence of surface IgM, IgD and free light chains on human lymphocytes. Journal of Experimental Medicine 139:451
23. Zuckerman S H, Douglas S D 1976 The lymphocyte plasma membrane: markers, receptors, and determinants. Pathobiology Annual 6:119.
24. Gershon R K, Cohen P, Hencin R, Liebhaber S A. 1972 Suppressor T cells. Journal of Immunology 108:586
25. Wemambu S N C, Turk J L 1969 Erythema nodosum leprosum: a clinical manifestation of the Arthus phenomenon. Lancet 2:933
26. Haurowitz F 1967 The evolution of selective and instructive theories of antibody formation. Cold Spring Harbor Symposia on Quantitative Biology 32:559
27. Leading Article 1975 Immunological tolerance. Lancet 1:555

12

Immunity to Infection

Immunity, or the ability to resist infection, is a property of all living creatures, and is highly complex. It has two components:

1. Immunity not dependent upon previous contact with the organism or its antigens
2. Immunity which is dependent upon previous contact with the organism or its products. This is acquired as a result of an immune response, and is either humoral or cell mediated.

IMMUNITY NOT DEPENDENT UPON PREVIOUS CONTACT WITH THE ORGANISM

All individuals possess an inherent ability to destroy invading micro-organisms, which is not dependent on the presence of antibodies or on the individual's previous contact with the organism or its antigens. The nature of this immunity is poorly understood but it may be considered under three headings.

1. *Cellular factors*
2. *Humoral factors*
3. *Genetic factors*—innate immunity.

Cellular factors

Organisms are phagocytosed by, and ultimately destroyed in, the polymorphs and macrophages.

Quantitative polymorph defects. If there is a decrease in the number of circulating polymorphs, liability to bacterial infection is increased. For this reason gingivitis and ulcerative pharyngitis are often a prominent feature of agranulocytosis or acute leukaemia. Inhibition of the acute inflammatory response reduces the numbers of phagocytes available locally. Glucocorticoid therapy has this effect, and predisposes to infection.

Qualitative polymorph defects.[1,2] The behaviour and functions of the polymorphs has been considered in Chapter 7. Abnormalities can be considered under the following headings:

1. Random movement

2. Chemotaxis
3. Adherence to bacteria
4. Phagocytosis
5. Intracellular bactericidal activity.

Each of these functions can be investigated, and many conditions with specific defects have been described.[3] One of the best known is *chronic granulomatous disease*. This disease affects males only, being inherited as an X-linked recessive trait. It is characterized by repeated infections, often staphylococcal, of the skin, lymph nodes, lungs, and other internal organs. The patient's polymorphs can phagocytose bacteria, but the characteristic 'respiratory burst' does not occur. The defect is in the hexose monophosphate shunt, but its precise nature is not known. In the absence of H_2O_2 production the H_2O_2–halide–myeloperoxidase mechanism is in abeyance, and, as noted previously, this plays a key role in bacterial killing.

Humoral factors

It has been known for a long time that blood and serum possess bactericidal power. For this reason blood is always well diluted with broth when it is cultured bacteriologically. The substances involved are not well understood, and in fact only two have been identified with any degree of certainty. *Natural oposonins* aid the phagocytosis of organisms of low-grade virulence (p. 78); *complement* has a more complex role.

Complement[4,5]

Complement was originally conceived by Bordet as a plasma component which aided, or complemented, the action of antibody. This notion stemmed from his observation that cholera vibrios cannot be lysed by antibody except in the presence of a heat-labile serum factor now called complement. It has since been discovered that complement consists of nine major components which are designated C1, C2, to C9. C1 in fact has three separate components which are held together in the presence of calcium ions. The activation of the early components of complement involves the formation of enzymes which cleave the next component by limited proteolysis. Cleavage products are suffixed by a lower case letter, e.g. C3a and C5a are cleavage products of C3 and C5. Components in an active state are symbolized by a bar over the component number, e.g. $C\overline{1q}$.

The component of complement that is most plentiful is C3 (previously often called β_1c), and indeed the activation of C3 by cleavage into C3a and C3b is a central feature of the complement pathway. Enzymes that act on C3 are termed C3 convertases, and can be generated in one of three ways:

1. *The classical pathway*, by the formation of the C3 convertase, $C\overline{42}$
2. *The alternate pathway*, by the formation of the alternate C3 convertase, $C\overline{3b}\overline{Bb}$
3. *Cobra venom factor*, with the formation of the C3 convertase, $CVF\overline{Bb}$.

Each of these will be examined in more detail.

The classical pathway of complement activation. The most intensively studied complement reaction is that of immune haemolysis initiated by the interaction of a site on the membrane of a red cell (the erythrocyte E) with a specific antibody A. The antigenic determinant may either be a natural constituent of the red-cell membrane, or an antigen or hapten artificially attached to it. In either event interaction with specific antibody results in the formation of a complex EA (Fig 12.1). It is now known that the first component of complement, C1, consists of three separate subcomponents. C1q is a molecule that resembles a six-flowered bouquet (see Fig 12.1), and it is thought that each 'flower' has an Fc combining site. Activation of C1q requires that at least two adjacent sites are bound to antibody. The C1q binding site on the antibody molecule resides in the

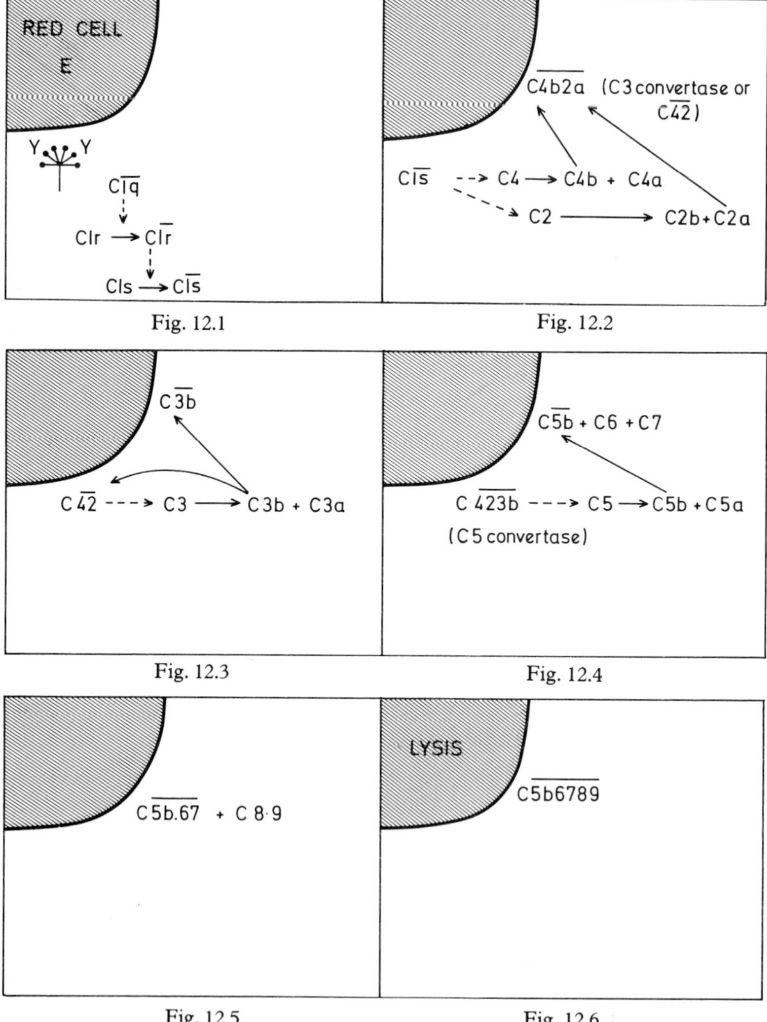

Fig. 12.1 Fig. 12.2 Fig. 12.3 Fig. 12.4 Fig. 12.5 Fig. 12.6

Figs. 12.1–12.6 The classical pathway of complement activation showing immune haemolysis of erythrocyte E with specific antibody A (depicted Y in Fig. 12.1).

Fc segment of the molecule, and it follows that at least two molecules of IgG must be attached to the C1q for the molecule to be activated. One molecule of IgM, on the other hand, with its five components, can directly activate C1q. The activated C$\overline{1q}$ activates the inactive C1r to the active enzyme C$\overline{1r}$, which in turn activates C1s to form a serine esterase C$\overline{1s}$ (Fig 12.1).

C$\overline{1s}$ acts on C4 and cleaves it into C4a and C4b. It also cleaves C2 into two fragments—C2a and C2b. C4b has a membrane-binding site, and attaches itself to the antigen against which the antibody has been directed but at a different site to the one occupied by the EAC1 complex. C2a binds to C4b, and the complex C$\overline{4b2a}$ (usually simplified to C$\overline{42}$) is a C3 convertase, being an enzyme capable of cleaving C3 (Fig. 12.2). The complex is unstable, and may revert to C4b by loss of the C2 component. However, under favourable conditions the active complex C$\overline{42}$ cleaves C3 into C3a and C3b. C3a (anaphylatoxin) is released into the fluid phase, whereas C3b randomly combines with membrane sites. When one of these sites is close to membrane bound C$\overline{42}$, C$\overline{423b}$ or C5 convertase is formed (Fig. 12.3). This enzyme converts C5 into C5b (Fig. 12.4). Together with C6 and C7 this forms a trimolecular complex C$\overline{5b67}$ which binds to a third site on the target cell membrane (Fig. 12.4). The trimolecular complex forms a binding site for C8, and this initiates cell lysis. Rapid lysis is effected by the final addition of C9 (Figs. 12.5 and 12.6). It will be seen that for complete lysis all terminal components of the complement cascade from C3 onwards must be activated. Also lysis of unsensitized cells can take place *via* non-specific absorption of C$\overline{5b67}$ on to cells. Although it might be imagined that innocent host cells might be damaged during an immune response, this danger is not great, since the complex is unstable and its ability to absorb on to cells rapidly declines.

The alternate pathway of complement activation. It is known that C3 and the terminal components of the complement pathway can be activated by a number of agents without the involvement of C1, C4, or C2. Zymosan (a polysaccharide derived from yeast), bacterial lipopolysaccharide endotoxin, and cobra snake venom are amongst the agents that can lead to generation of C3 convertase from the constituents of the blood other than C1, C4, or C2. Pillemer in 1954 was the first person to describe *properdin* as a plasma protein which in the presence of zymosan can generate a C3 convertase, and thereby activate C3 in the absence of an antibody. Additional factors (called factor A, factor B, and others) are required, as are magnesium ions but not calcium. Hence, Pillemer had demonstrated an alternative pathway which is probably identical with the alternate pathway mentioned above.

The initial steps in the activation of the alternate pathway are incompletely understood, and no clear account can be given at the present time. Under the influence of the initiating factor (e.g. zymosan), properdin is activated, and native C3 together with factor B and factor D can form a convertase which is capable of acting on C3 to generate C3b. Next there is an interaction of C3b with factors B and D to form a C3 convertase (C$\overline{3bBb}$), which will convert C3 to form more C3b and also activate C5. An important aspect of this mechanism is the positive feedback of C3b as shown in Fig. 12.7. It will be seen that one of the important actions of activated properdin is the stabilization of the labile C$\overline{3bBb}$.

The complement component C3 to C9 can be activated by the alternate pathway by a number of factors including aggregated IgA, IgE, and IgG4, immunoglobulins which previously were thought not to activate complement. The precise role of this pathway is yet to be determined, but abnormalities in it are known to affect immunity to infection, and its activation can explain how defects in the classical pathway may be circumvented. Thus C4-deficient guinea-pigs can exhibit the Arthus phenomenon. Furthermore, the positive C3b feedback cycle can act as an amplification mechanism regardless of whether the classical or alternate pathway is activated. One disease in which the alternate pathway appears to play a major role is paroxysmal nocturnal haemoglobinuria.

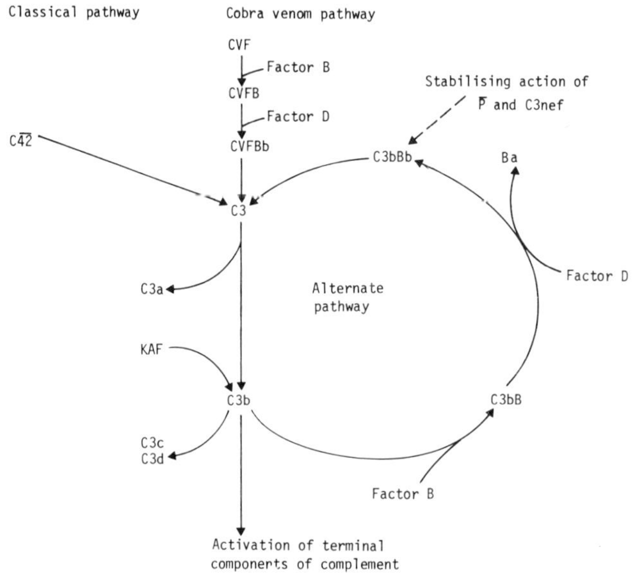

Fig.12.7 The alternate pathway to the activation of complement. The activation of properdin by zymosan, aggregated immunoglobulin, or bacterial endotoxin, in conjunction with factor B, factor D, and other factors is thought to cleave C3 to C3a and C3b. This step is poorly documented and is not shown in the diagram. C3b combines with factor B (also called C3 proactivator) in the presence of magnesium ions to form a loose complex C3bB. Factor D, which is a serine esterase, also called C3 proactivator convertase, cleaves factor B into Ba (which enters the fluid phase) and Bb which remains attached to C3b. The complex C3bBb is the C3 convertase of the alternate pathway, and can cleave C3 to form C3a and C3b. The latter can bind to cell membranes, cleave C5, and initiate the activation of the remaining components of the complement pathway. Note that C3 can be cleaved by two other factors: $C\overline{42}$ is the convertase of the classical pathway of activation. Cobra venom factor (CVF) is an analogue of C3b, and in conjunction with factor B and factor D forms the convertase CVFBb. Activated properdin ($\bar{P}$) and the C3 nephritic factor (C3nef stabilizes the labile C3bBb) help to give the feedback cycle of the alternative pathway another turn. Conglutinogen activator factor (KAF), by inactivating C3b to C3c and C3d, acts as a brake on the complement-activating mechanism.

Cobra venom activation of complement. It has been known since the beginning of this century that a factor in cobra venom (CVF) can activate complement without consumption of C1, C4, or C2. The factor is an analogue of C3b and combines with factor B. The complex is acted upon by factor D to form the stable active complex CVFBb. This mechanism is clearly not of any physiological importance.

Inhibitors of complement activation. *Temporal and spatial constraints.* Some of the activating factors in the complement cascade are unstable and readily disassociate. Furthermore, the spatial arrangement of the compounds is of importance. For example, C3b randomly combines with membranes sites, and only when in close proximity to membrane-bound C$\overline{42}$ is the C5 convertase formed.

C1 esterase inhibitor. This inhibitor forms a stable complex with C1s, and inhibits the enzymatic action of C1. Absence of the enzyme is associated with familial angio-oedema.

C3b inactivator, also called conglutinogen activating factor, or KAF. This enzyme degrades C3b, splitting it into C3c and C3d. The enzyme exposes a carbohydrate determinant in C3 that reacts with conglutinin, a protein normally present in the serum of cattle that is not an antibody but reacts specifically with C3.

Serum carboxypeptidase B. This enzyme inactivates both C3a and C5a.

Role of complement activation in disease. The activation of the entire complement sequence C1 to C9 is an important component in the defence mechanism because it leads to bacterial lysis. Bound C3 is recognized by receptors on polymorphs, macrophages, and lymphocytes, thereby allowing these cells to adhere to bacteria and attack them by phagoctyosis or some other cell-to-cell mechanism. C3a and C5a are anaphylatoxins which act on mast cells and cause histamine release. C$\overline{567}$ and C3a are also chemotactic factors. Thus complement activation modifies the inflammatory response in several ways.

Genetic factors

The immunity which is related to inherited constitution is known as *innate*, or *inborn, immunity*. It is manifest as *species, racial*, and *individual*.

Species immunity. This is the most absolute type of immunity known. Thus the spirochaete of syphilis infects the human with prodigious ease, and yet nearly all the other animals are immune. Likewise animals suffer from diseases to which humans exhibit immunity (e.g. distemper). It should be noted that saying an animal has innate immunity to an organism is an alternative way of saying the organism is avirulent to that animal.

Racial immunity. It is well established that different strains of an animal species may vary in their susceptibility to particular infections, e.g. tuberculosis in rabbits. Similar differences between human races probably exist, but are difficult to substantiate—Black people and the Irish are said to have a poor innate immunity to tuberculosis. Black races are more immune to malaria than are Northern Europeans. This is related to their possession of an abnormal type of haemoglobin (p. 46).

Individual immunity. Individuals differ considerably in the degree of immunity which they exhibit, but it is difficult to prove that this is innate and not acquired. Nevertheless, innate differences almost certainly exist.

These examples of innate immunity—species, racial, and individual—are dependent upon genetic make-up. In some instances the ability to mount an immune response is invoked, and sometimes the presence of a specific receptor for an organism or its toxin on a cell membrane is involved.

Recent work, mainly in thc mousc, has clarified the position to some extent. The ability to mount an immune response against a particular antigen (*immune responsiveness*) is inherited as an autosomal dominant trait. The responsible genes are the *immune response (Ir) genes*,[6] and are part of the major histocompatibility complex H-2.[7] The presence of an *Ir* gene determines an animal's ability to respond to a given antigen at all (responders and non-responders), the type of response (humoral or cell mediated), and the *level* of response (i.e. the amount of antibody produced, and whether it be IgM, IgG, etc.). The gene product has not been positively identified, but it appears to determine receptors on T cells primarily. The *Ir* gene has its human counterpart in the HLA-DR locus.

ACQUIRED IMMUNITY

Immunity dependent upon previous contact with the organism or its antigens

This type of immunity is dependent upon an immune response which may be either humoral or cell mediated. When the animal produces its own antibodies, the immunity is said to be *active*. When the antibodies are donated from another animal the immunity is described as *passive*.

Active immunity. This is produced as a result of the individual's own immune response.

Natural active immunity follows a natural infection with the organism. The subject may have been aware of the disease, or it may have been subclinical and have passed unnoticed. Subclinical attacks are very common with some infections, e.g. poliomyelitis and tuberculosis.

Artificial active immunity follows the injection of toxoids or vaccines.

Passive immunity. Preformed immunoglobulins may be passively transferred either naturally or artificially.

Natural passive immunity is seen in the newborn. The human fetus does not manufacture immunoglobulins unless infected *in utero* (see p. 166), and those which are normally present at birth are derived from the mother, having crossed the placenta. They are of the IgG variety, and confer some degree of immunity to infection on the baby for 3 to 6 months. Thus common viral diseases like measles and mumps are rare during this period.

Artificial passive immunity is deliberately induced by injecting immunoglobulin antibodies for prophylactic or therapeutic purposes. The antibodies may be obtained from the serum of an animal, usually the horse, or from another human. The protection afforded is short lived.

Adoptive immunity. This is the passive immunity acquired by transference of cells from an immunized individual. It has been demonstrated in the experimental animal, but not in the human because of the danger of producing a graft versus host (GVH) reaction (p. 193). The immunoglobulins are manufactured by the progeny of the transferred cells. This differs from the manner by which cells can transfer delayed hypersensitivity, in which it is the host cells that are changed (p. 189). The use of transfer factor in the human as a means of producing immunity is under investigation.

Mechanism of acquired immunity

The manner whereby acquired immunity protects the body against infection depends upon the type of organism concerned. With the toxic organisms (p. 101) the immunity is due to the action of *antitoxins*, while with the invasive group it is due to *antibacterial antibodies.*

Antitoxic immunity. Toxic organisms produce their effects by means of powerful, diffusible exotoxins which are highly antigenic. The antibodies (antitoxins) are capable of neutralizing the toxin, and act in the body by intercepting the toxin before it reaches susceptible tissues. Diphtheria provides a good example.

Immunity in diphtheria. Diphtheria bacilli alighting on a mucous membrane produce their effect, and indeed the disease, by elaborating an exotoxin. This acts on the local tissues, causing necrosis of epithelium and pseudomembrane formation, and is also absorbed by the blood stream and produces damage at distant sites, e.g. the heart, adrenals, and peripheral nerves. If the host has a high antitoxin level in the circulation, and therefore in the tissues and secretions, the toxin is rapidly neutralized, thereby depriving the organism of its main offensive weapon. It then becomes in effect avirulent, and is removed by the normal decontaminating mechanism of the part. A virulent organism attacking a host with a high antitoxin level is in the same position as an avirulent organism attacking a normal host.

Passive immunization consists of giving diphtheria antitoxin (prepared from the serum of an immunized horse), so that no further damage is produced by the toxin. The organism itself is not directly affected, but is soon destroyed by the host's defence mechanism. This treatment is effective only if given early in the course of the disease.

Active immunization. Since immunity to diphtheria is conferred by circulating antitoxin, active immunization is performed by inducing the subject to manufacture antitoxin. This is done by a series of *toxoid* injections. Toxoid consists of toxin treated with formaldehyde so that its toxicity is lost while its antigenicity is retained.

The other important toxic organisms, those causing tetanus and gas-gangrene, are described in Chapter 14. Immunity to them is also conferred by antitoxin, and closely resembles that seen in diphtheria.

Antibacterial humoral immunity. Invasive organisms contain a great number of antigens, and during the course of an infection many types of antibody appear in the plasma. Thus towards the end of the second week in typhoid fever antibodies appear which are specific for the surface and flagellar antigens of *Salmonella typhi.* They are easily detected as agglutinins (see Widal reaction, p. 154). Similarily, in syphilis precipitins and complement-fixing antibodies appear, and are detected by the Kahn and Wassermann tests respectively. The appearance of these antibodies is often of *diagnostic value*, especially if their titre continues to rise.

In infection with invasive organisms the antibodies which appear are *antibacterial*, in the sense that they are directed against bacterial components. They are detected as agglutinins, precipitins, complement fixers (amboceptors), antibacterial haemolysins, antihyaluronidase, etc. Which test is employed to detect them in clinical practice is arbitrary—it is often the one which is most convenient, or merely the one which was first discovered. The antibodies detected are not necessarily the ones which destroy the organism *in vitro* or *in vivo*. Therefore they do not necessarily provide immunity. A syphilitic patient with a strongly positive Wassermann test, far from being immune, is quite likely to be highly infectious.

Invasive organisms are destroyed in the body by two mechanisms: either they are digested by polymorphs or the phagocytic cells of the RE system, or they are lysed by the activation of complement. Antibacterial antibodies can provide immunity, and they do it by aiding one of these two mechanisms.

(*a*) They can act as *opsonins*. These neutralize the noxious surface antigens of certain virulent organisms, e.g. the capsular polysaccharide of pneumococci and the M protein of *Strept. pyogenes* (pp. 205 and 203), which repel or kill phagocytes at close quarters. An opsonized bacterium is easily phagocytosed. The importance of the Fc and C3 receptors on the cell membranes of polymorphs and monocytes has been described on page 79. Antibody-dependent cell-mediated cytotoxicity (p. 156) is another example of how immunoglobulins can aid in the destruction of bacteria, not only by phagocytes but also by lymphocytes.

(*b*) They can act as *amboceptors* (*bacteriolysins*) and activate complement. This bacteriolysis is seen in infections with *S. typhi*, *Vibrio cholerae*, and probably many other organisms. In many bacterial infections we have no satisfactory methods of detecting or estimating the titre of these protective antibodies. Hence *passive immunization*, produced by the administration of horse or human immunoglobulin, is not uniformly successful. The advent of chemotherapy as an alternative treatment has rendered serum therapy obsolete.

Active immunization can be induced by injecting a suspension of whole organisms called a *vaccine*. With some organisms a dead vaccine is used (e.g. TAB, which is a suspension of *S. typhi* and *S. paratyphi A and B*), but with others dead material is ineffective, and use is made of an attenuated (rendered avirulent) living vaccine (e.g. BCG in tuberculosis). Unfortunately, the factors which determine the virulence of invasive organisms are not clearly understood. Vaccines are prepared by a process of trial and error. Some are useful and others are not. Whooping-cough vaccine provides some protection, while staphylococcal vaccines do not. Moreover bacteria show considerable variation in their antigenic make-up, and a vaccine made with one strain will not protect against infection by another. Typhoid epidemics have occured in troops 'immunized' with TAB.

The local immunity produced by the presence of IgA in secretions is described on pages 96, 153, and 253.

Cell-mediated antibacterial immunity.[8] Infection with some invasive organisms leads to a cell-mediated immune response so that the lymphocytes and macrophages of the body are better able to destroy the organisms. This change is closely related to the development of *type*-IV *hypersensitivity* (p. 188).

Antiviral immunity. Circulating immunoglobulins play an important part in the destruction of viruses. By coating the virus, they prevent its attachment to the receptor site of the susceptible cell. Such a virus is soon destroyed by the humoral and cellular defences of the host. Other aspects of antiviral immunity, i.e. cell-mediated immunity and interferon, are considered in Chapter 16.

Summary of acquired immunity

Humoral factors

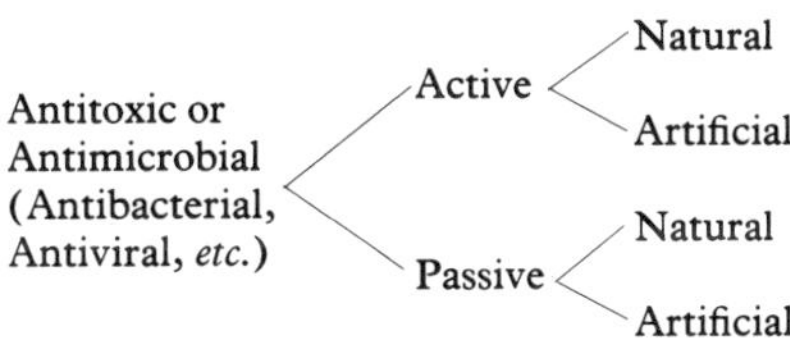

Cellular factors

Active cell-mediated immunity
Antibody-dependent cell-mediated immunity
Adoptive immunity

IMMUNOLOGICAL-DEFICIENCY DISEASES[9,10]

The primary group of immunological-deficiency diseases is uncommon, but its study has strengthened the view that the immune response has two separate components. In one group, typified by *congenital sex-linked agammaglobulinaemia*, there is a failure in development of the B lymphocytes and the subject is susceptible to repeated bacterial infections often resulting in early death. In another group there is thymic aplasia and a complete failure in T lymphocyte development. These individuals suffer from viral, fungal, and acid-fast bacterial infections. In the most severe type there is a complete failure of both T lymphocyte and B lymphocyte development, and life is limited to a year or two.

Acquired immunological deficiency is of much greater practical importance, and occurs in generalized lymphoma (particularly Hodgkin's disease), leukaemia, multiple myeloma, and occasionally in other types of malignant disease. It is also a feature of therapy with cytotoxic drugs and glucocorticoids. The cell-mediated immune response is depressed during certain infections, e.g. measles, German measles, and following measles vaccination. There is a similar anergy in lepromatous leprosy.

An interesting feature of the immunological-deficiency diseases, particularly the primary group, is the tendency for the subjects to develop malignant disease, particularly lymphoma. This lends some support to the concept that the immune reaction plays a role in eliminating malignant cells from the body.

REFERENCES

1. Bellanti J A, Dayton D H (edrs) 1975 The Phagocytic Cell in Host Resistance. Raven Press, New York
2. Leading Article 1976 Microbial killing by neutrophils. Lancet 1: 1393
3. Gallin J I, Wolff S M 1975 Leucocyte chemotaxis: physiological considerations and abnormalities. Clinics in Haematology 4: 567
4. Vogt W 1974 Activation, activities and pharmacologically active products of complement. Pharmacological Reviews 26: 125
5. Ruddy S, Gigli I, Austen K F 1972 The complement system of man. New England Journal of Medicine 287: 489, 545, 592 and 642
6. Green I 1974 Genetic control of immune responses. Immunogenetics 1: 4

7. Benacerraf B, Katz D H 1975 The histocompatibility-linked immune response genes. Advances in Cancer Research 21 : 121
8. Mackaness G B 1970 Cell-mediated immunity to infection. Hospital Practice 5 : 73
9. Hayward A R 1977 Immunodeficiency, Arnold, London, p 125
10. Hitzig W H 1976 Congenital immunodeficiency diseases, clinical appearance and treatment. Pathobiology Annual 6 : 163

13

Hypersensitivity, tissue grafts, and autoimmunity

HYPERSENSITIVITY

Hypersensitivity is a state in which, having experienced a primary response to an antigen, an animal reacts in an excessive way to a subsequent exposure to the same antigen. *Allergy* is sometimes used to denote a second response which is altered in quality rather than being simply excessive. It is very doubtful whether such a distinction is valid. Furthermore, both terms are used quite indiscriminately in the literature; in this book they will be used synonymously.

Two distinct types of hypersensitivity can be recognized. In one, the reaction to administration of antigen is immediate (within minutes), while in the other it is delayed for 24 to 48 hours. The distinction between these two types is of fundamental importance. The *immediate-type* hypersensitivities are related to the formation of sensitizing immunoglobulins. In *delayed-type* hypersensitivity the reaction is cell mediated.

It is now realized that immunoglobulins can cause hypersensitivity in various ways, and that in only one of these is the reaction immediate in the sense that this term is usually used. Indeed, injury due to immunoglobulins can be caused in three distinct ways, and these have been classified thus[1]:

Type I immediate-type hypersensitivity. This is commonly mediated by IgE, and is typified by acute anaphylaxis in the human subject.

Type II, or cytotoxic reaction. Antibodies, IgG or IgM, are directed against cellular or tissue antigens, e.g. as in haemolytic anaemia due to haemolysins.

Type III, due to antigen-antibody complexes. IgG is mainly involved.

In the *delayed-type hypersensitivities,* no such sensitizing antibodies can be demonstrated, and the hypersensitivity is cell-mediated. This type of hypersensitivity is classified as *type IV.*

TYPE I IMMEDIATE HYPERSENSITIVITY

The features of this type of hypersensitivity have been the subject of intensive study in animals. Anaphylaxis, which represents the most severe manifestation, will be described first as it illustrates the main features of this group.

Anaphylaxis[2]

Generalized anaphylaxis in the guinea-pig

If a guinea-pig is given an injection of a non-toxic protein, e.g. egg albumin, it shows no obvious discomfort. After about two weeks specific immunoglobulins appear in plasma. If a second injection of egg albumin is then given intravenously, antigen reacts with sensitizing antibody on the mast cells and the animal dies of generalized anaphylaxis (*anaphylactic shock*) within a few minutes. The following features should be noted:

1. Generalized anaphylaxis can be elicited by giving a single large *shocking dose* of antigen at a suitable interval after one or more sensitizing doses
2. The reaction is highly *specific* for the antigen
3. The shocking dose must be administered quickly, and the intravenous route is generally employed
4. The serum, or purified specific immunoglobulin, of a sensitized animal will passively sensitize a previously normal animal. The passive sensitization is not immediate but is made manifest after a time interval of several hours Thus the presence of specific immunoglobulin in the plasma alone does not confer sensitivity—present evidence suggests that the antibody must become fixed to cells
5. The cells which are sensitized (*target cells*) are mast cells; it is uncertain whether other cell types are also involved.

Cytotropic anaphylaxis. Anaphylaxis as described in the actively sensitized guinea-pig is called *cytotropic*, because it is the result of antigen reacting with antibody fixed to cells. The sensitizing antibody concerned migrates in the γ_1 band, and is of the 7S IgG type and has in the past been called a reagin. Other animals produce a similar type of sensitizing antibody, and in the human the most important belongs to the IgE class. A person sensitized by this type of antibody will exhibit erythema and a weal if a small quantity of antigen is injected into the skin (*cutaneous, or local, anaphylaxis*).

Mediators of cytotropic anaphylaxis.[3,4] The action of specific antigen on mast cells coated with specific IgE is to cause the release of the following agents: *histamine, 5HT, SRS-A, ECF-A, platelet activating factor,* and *prostaglandins.* These are described below. In addition, the platelets release vasoactive amines as part of the platelet release reaction.

Histamine. Histamine can be detected in the blood in acute systemic anaphylaxis, and is released if antigen is applied to sensitized tissue *in vitro.* Antihistamine drugs inhibit the production of acute anaphylactic shock.

5-*Hydroxytryptamine* (*serotonin*). This is present in the platelets of all species and in the mast cells of rats and mice. Its release may be important in anaphylaxis of these rodents.

Slow-reacting substance of anaphylaxis (*SRS-A*). If the lungs of a sensitized guinea-pig are perfused with a fluid containing antigen, histamine can be demonstrated in the fluid issuing at the beginning of the experiment. Alternatively, antigen can be added to lung chopped into small pieces. Later, another substance appears, which, when applied to isolated uterine muscle, causes a slow sustained contraction, unlike the more rapid 'kick' produced by histamine. This substance is a lipid of unknown composition, and might be responsible for the bronchospasm seen in the human subject. Histamine is not so important in this connexion; histamine-releasing compounds given to humans cause pruritus, oedema of the face, and hypotension, but not bronchospasm.

Eosinophil chemotactic factor of anaphylaxis (ECF-A). This is probably responsible for the local accumulation of eosinophils that is such a prominent feature of some local type-I hypersensitivity reactions in the human subject.

Platelet activating factor. This triggers the platelet release phenomenon and leads to the liberation of vasoactive amines from the platelets.

Prostaglandins. See p 86.

Kinins. There is evidence that kinin-forming enzymes are activated in anaphylactic shock.

Aggregate anaphylaxis. This type of anaphylaxis occurs in the actively sensitized rabbit, and is due to the formation of antigen-antibody aggregates in the circulation. The antigen-antibody complexes *activate complement*, and the chemotactic $C\overline{567}$ is released. Polymorphs join the aggregates and release their damaging lysosomal enzymes. The sensitizing 7S IgG antibody migrates in the γ_2 band on electrophoresis. In aggregate anaphylaxis there is *no cell fixation, histamine is not released,* and *antihistamine drugs do not protect.* Both *complement* and *polymorphs* are essential and the phenomenon falls into the type III, or immune-complex, group.

Cytotropic and aggregate anaphylaxis are best studied in pure form in animals passively sensitized with purified antibody of the appropriate type. Actively sensitized animals usually produce antibodies of both types, and anaphylactic shock in them is often a mixture of the two types. This accounts for the confusing past literature on this subject.

Although the manifestations of anaphylactic shock vary in different species, and even in the same species under separate conditions, two main effects are seen. These are:

1. *Spasm of smooth muscle*—either blood vessel or bronchial
2. *Damage to small blood vessels.*

When the reaction occurs in the human the manifestations are[5]:

1. *Bronchospasm*, with great difficulty in expiration. This sudden onset of wheezing dyspnoea is characteristic
2. *Generalized oedema*, often first detected as swelling of the eyelids, due to a generalized increase in vascular permeability. Sometimes *oedema of the larynx* adds to the respiratory difficulty
3. *Itching of the skin.* Erythema and urticaria are also common
4. *Pallor and low blood pressure. Death often follows.*

The sensitizing IgE has a great affinity for cells to which it becomes firmly attached. Very little need be present in the blood. Hence, unlike the situation in the guinea-pig, very small doses of antigen can cause acute anaphylactic shock. Although rare in the human subject, it is seen under several circumstances:

a. When horse γ-globulin is given to patients who are sensitized to horse protein, e.g. in passive immunization against diphtheria and tetanus, whether prophylactic or therapeutic
b. When a drug which is capable of acting as a hapten is injected into a patient who is sensitive to it. *Penicillin* is such a drug, and each year a number of people die of anaphylaxis from this therapy.
c. Following a bee sting in a highly sensitized person.

The danger of anaphylaxis should always be kept in mind by anyone administering animal serum or drugs by injection. At the first sign of anaphylaxis, 1.0 ml of a 1 in 1000 solution of adrenaline should be given by *intramuscular* injection and 0.5 ml repeated as necessary. Oedema of the larynx may necessitate an emergency tracheotomy.

Dust and food hypersensitivity

This group of hypersensitivity reactions occurs after the *ingestion* of certain foods and the *inhalation* of antigens contained in pollen and dust. The symptoms differ according to the route of absorption. The offending chemical may be a complete antigen or a hapten; the latter presumably combines with a carrier protein in tissue or plasma.

Types

Inhalation of antigens in pollen, horse dander, and dust usually produces watering of the eyes, symptoms referable to the respiratory tract, e.g. congestion of the nasal mucosa (*allergic rhinitis* or *hay-fever*), and *bronchial asthma* (p 539).

Ingestion of certain foods produces either *gastrointestinal symptoms* or *skin eruptions*. Shellfish, mushrooms, strawberries, and milk are among the numerous foods to which some people are allergic. Hypersensitivity to drugs is considered later.

Nature of lesions

The lesions are *exudative* in type and sometimes contain *eosinophils*. Histamine is almost certainly a mediator, and antihistamine drugs have an ameliorative effect.

Genetic influence: atopy

Patients with this type of hypersensitivity frequently give a family history of similar complaints. One may have hay-fever, another bronchial asthma, etc. It is the capacity to react to antigens in this peculiar way which is inherited, and the condition is called *atopy*. The subjects manufacture IgE, which has a marked capacity of adhering to cells and sensitizing them to the subsequent contact with antigen. These antibodies, although present in the plasma, cannot easily be detected by the conventional methods of precipitation, complement fixation, etc. They can, however, be demonstrated by *passive transfer*. Serum from a hypersensitive patient injected into the skin of a normal person renders that portion of skin sensitive to the antigen. This test is called the *Prausnitz-Küstner reaction*, after the two workers who demonstrated it in experiments on themselves.

Küstner was sensitive to cooked fish and transferred his hypersensitivity to Prausnitz.

Sensitive people can be detected by injecting a minute dose of the offending antigen into the skin. Erythema and a weal appear *within a few minutes.* It should be noted that if a large dose of antigen is given, especially if it is injected intravenously, the subject may exhibit anaphylactic shock. Unfortunately, the results of skin tests are not a reliable indication of a possible sensitization to anaphylaxis. The safest procedure, when administering foreign sera, is to give a small test dose subcutaneously and watch for any mild general reaction.

Atopic subjects are particularly liable to develop sensitization to anaphylactic shock. It therefore follows that before any injection is given to a patient, enquiry should be made into any personal or familial liability to hypersensitivity (infantile eczema, hay-fever, bronchial asthma, etc.).

Densensitization to immediate-type hypersensitivity

If it is desired to give an antigen (e.g. serum) to which an individual is sensitive, this may be done by giving small doses at frequent intervals. Although this procedure may avoid immediate serious complications, e.g. anaphylactic shock, and is loosely referred to as 'desensitization', it is doubtful whether it is ever justified. The injected antigen is rapidly eliminated, and is therefore of little therapeutic value. Furthermore, an acclerated type of serum sickness (p 186) may result and symptoms appear after a few days.

Another type of desensitization is sometimes attempted in patients with asthma, hay-fever, etc. Minute doses of antigen (e.g. pollen extracts) to which the subject is sensitive are injected at weekly intervals. The aim is to induce the formation of 'blocking antibodies' in excess. When the individual is next exposed to antigen, it combines with the circulating IgG blocking antibody, which therefore protects the IgE sensitized cells from the damaging effect of antigen. Unfortunately this procedure is not uniformly successful.

TYPE III HYPERSENSITIVITY REACTIONS

This type of hypersensitivity is dependent on the formation of damaging antigen-antibody complexes: hence, the alternative name *immune-complex disease.* The principles of this reaction are well shown by the experimental procedure described by Arthus.

Arthus phenomenon

Repeated weekly subcutaneous injections of an antigen, even into different areas, lead to progressively more severe local reactions; later injections produce haemorrhagic necrosis and ulceration. The reaction is due to the interaction of injected antigen with circulating sensitizing immunoglobulins.

Damaging antigen-antibody complexes are formed in the vessel wall, the complement system is activated, and this induces polymorphs to accumulate and release damaging lysosomal enzymes. The vessels become blocked, the wall is damaged, and haemorrhage and ischaemic necrosis follow (Fig. 13.1). The pathogenesis of the Arthus phenomenon bears some resemblance to that of aggregate anaphylaxis. However, in the Arthus reaction the antibody concerned is probably different, it must be present in much larger quantities, and finally the damaging antigen-antibody interaction is believed to take place in the vessel wall itself.

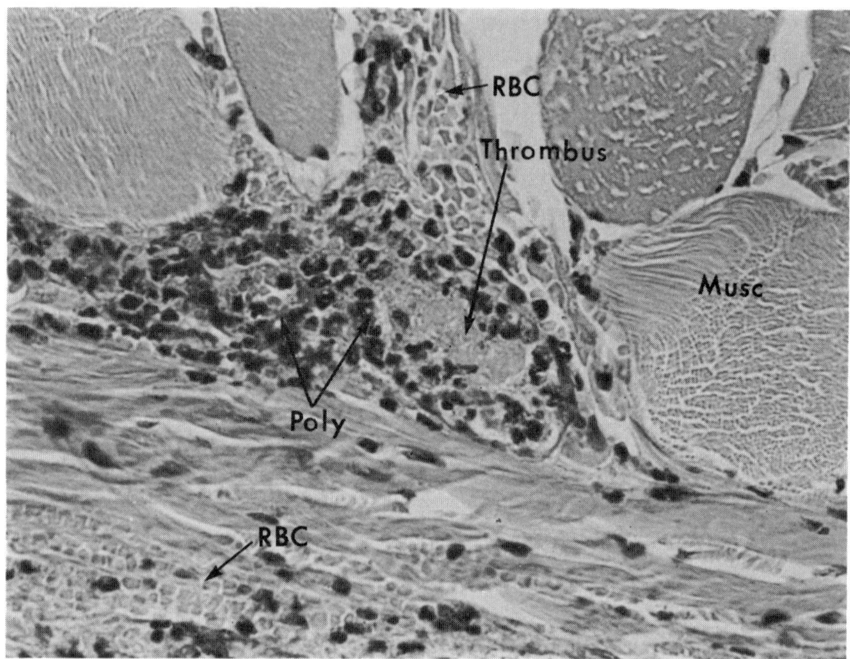

Fig. 13.1 The Arthus reaction. This section is taken from a rabbit, and it includes the subcutaneous tissues and the underlying muscle (Musc). The blood vessel in the centre is sectioned obliquely and shows occlusion of its lumen by thrombus. Its walls are heavily infiltrated by polymorphs (Poly), many of which are degenerating. Free red cells (RBC) in the tissues bear witness to the severity of the vascular damage. × 550.

Serum sickness

Serum sickness is a condition characterized by *fever, joint pains*, and *urticarial eruptions* that occurs 10 to 14 days after the administration of a *large dose* of foreign serum, e.g. horse γ-globulin. The pathogenesis is explained in Fig. 13.2. The injected antigen persists in the blood until the 10th day. At this time the immune response becomes evident by the disappearance of antigen from the blood (immune catabolism) and the appearance of immunoglobulins in the plasma. At first they form complexes with antigen, but as these are eliminated, free antibody appears in the plasma. The lesions of serum sickness are due to the damaging effect of immune complexes deposited at certain sites—skin, etc. Complement is activated, and polymorphs accumulate and release damaging lysosomal enzymes.

Microscopically the lesions of serum sickness are similar to those of the Arthus reaction, but are less severe. There is an acute vasculitis with polymorphs infiltrating the vessel walls. In addition, a glomerulonephritis is characteristic.

Chronic immune-complex disease.[6] If daily injections of antigen are given to an animal in doses such that antigen-antibody complexes with antigen excess are formed in the blood, a chronic glomerulonephritis develops. It is believed that some types of human glomerulonephritis have a similar pathogenesis, for example the renal lesions of systemic lupus erythematosus.[7]

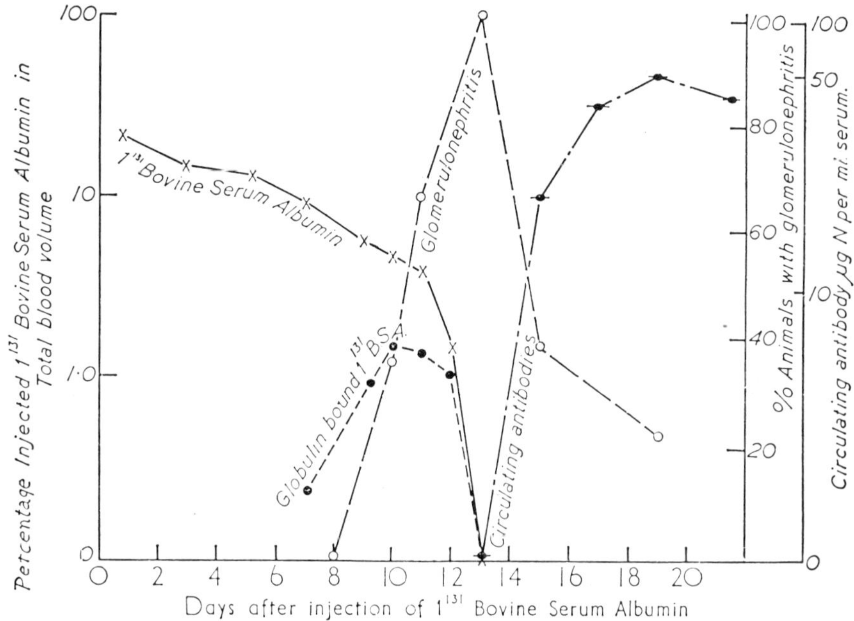

Fig. 13.2 Time relations between fall of circulating antigen, formation of antigen-antibody complexes, lesions of serum sickness (glomerulonephritis), and rise of circulating antibody in rabbits injected with large doses of ^{131}I-labelled bovine serum albumin. (*From Gladstone G P 1961. In: Florey H W General Pathology, 3rd edn, after Dixon J F et al 1959 in: Lawrence H S Cellular and humoral aspects of the hypersensitivity states. Harper and Row, New York, p 345*)

Drug hypersensitivity[8, 9]

Hypersensitivity to drugs is a common clinical event, and is due to the drug, or one of its degradation products, acting as a hapten and stimulating the formation of sensitizing antibodies. Virtually any drug can produce a reaction, but common offenders are penicillin, sulphonamides, aspirin, barbiturates, and quinine. Relatively few people given a drug manifest hypersensitivity, and the tendency to develop IgE-mediated effects is particularly marked in atopic individuals.

Types of drug reaction. The reaction may be *immediate* (type I reaction), and range from urticaria to severe, fatal anaphylactic shock. Sensitizing IgE antibodies are responsible. *Later drug reactions* begin several days after the administration of the drug, and have the features of immune–complex disease (type III reaction). Urticarial, papular, and petechial skin eruptions are common in addition to arthralgia and fever. The antibodies concerned are IgG or IgM. *Late drug effects* are thrombocytopenia, haemolytic anaemia, erythema multiforme, jaundice, and a syndrome resembling systemic lupus erythematosus. The pathogenesis of many reactions is unclear. In some instances, e.g. haemolytic anaemia, cytotoxic antibodies are present (type II reaction); they may be directed against the drug, as in pencillin-induced haemolytic anaemia, or against the red-cell surface antigens, an effect induced by α-methyldopa.

TYPE IV OR DELAYED-TYPE HYPERSENSITIVITY[10]

The simplest example of this type is bacterial hypersensitivity (bacterial allergy) as exemplified by the *Koch phenomenon.* It should be noted that the term bacterial allergy is somewhat inappropriate, because immediate-type hypersensitivity can also occur during bacterial infections. *Delayed-type hypersensitivity* is a more acceptable term, and it can occur in response to antigens of non-bacterial origin. *Cell-mediated hypersensitivity* is the most common currently used term, since it not only indicates that the antibodies concerned are cellular, but also distinguishes the reactions from certain immune-complex phenomena which take several hours to develop and are therefore difficult to distinguish, if the classification is based strictly on the time taken for the reaction to appear.

The Koch phenomenon

If tubercle bacilli are injected into a normal guinea-pig, there is an incubation period of 10 to 14 days followed by the appearance of a nodule at the site of injection. Ulceration follows and persists till the death of the animal. The bacilli spread to the local lymph nodes, finally reach the blood stream, and produce generalized miliary tuberculosis and death. The injection of more tubercle bacilli into an animal infected 4 to 6 weeks previously evokes a different type of response. A nodule appears in 1 to 2 days, ulcerates, and then heals. There is little tendency to spread to the local lymph nodes. This second type of response was described by Koch, and it should be noted that the reaction of a tuberculous animal to tubercle bacilli differs from that of a normal one in three important respects:

1. The incubation period is greatly shortened—this may be described as *hypersensitivity*
2. The lesion heals quickly
3. There is no spread. These are the features of *immunity.*

The heightened tissue response of the tuberculous animal can be demonstrated not only to the living tubercle bacillus, but also to extracts of the organism. Koch originally used 'old tuberculin', a crude extract of the bacilli, but more recently a Purified Protein Derivative (PPD) has been introduced.

The injection of a small quantity of PPD into a normal animal results in a negligible inflammatory response. In the tuberculous animal, however, there develops an indurated erythematous lesion which appears within 12 to 24 hours and reaches a peak by 48 to 72 hours. This is the *tuberculin*, or *Mantoux test*, and a positive result indicates the existence of hypersensitivity to tuberculoprotein. The injection of a larger quantity of PPD into a tuberculous animal leads to a generalized reaction with *fever* and in severe cases *shock* and *death.* This occurs with a dose of tuberculoprotein which would have no serious effect on a normal, unsensitized animal.

This type of hypersensitivity differs in many important respects from the type I reactions previously described:

1. The reaction is delayed—it takes at least 12 *hours* to develop as compared with a few *minutes*
2. Although there is some vasodilatation and oedema, the reaction is characterized by the accumulation of lymphocytes and macrophages rather than polymorphs
3. The reaction is not mediated by histamine, serotonin, kinins, or products of complement activation. The reaction is not blocked by antihistamine drugs, but is inhibited by glucocorticoids
4. It is not causally related to any known types of immunoglobulins, and cannot be transferred to another animal by serum transfusion
5. Delayed-type hypersensitivity can be transferred to a normal animal by the transfer of T lymphocytes. These cells are sensitized to antigen, and the delayed nature of the reaction is probably due to the time taken for them to accumulate at the site of antigen injection. The lymphokines (p 157) are the mediators for this reaction.

The state of passive hypersensitivity persists for as long as the injected cells live in the new host. In some way *the transplanted cells alter the host's own lymphocytes* so that these also take part in a delayed-type skin reaction which is subsequently elicited. In the *human subject,* delayed-type hypersensitivity can be transferred, not only by living cells, but also by extracts of white cells. Although described by Lawrence in 1955, the action of the *transfer factor,* which is one of the lymphokines, is not known but it is evidently very potent, for a single injection can render the recipient hypersensitive for many months.

***In-vitro* detection of cellular antibody.**[11] In spite of the potent effects exhibited by sensitized lymphocytes *in vivo*, the manner by which they produce tissue damage is poorly understood. As described on page 157, when T lymphocytes come into contact with specific antigen, a number of potent low-molecular-weight factors called lymphokines are liberated. Insofar as cell-mediated hypersensitivity is concerned, lymphotoxin is probably the most important, but other factors may recruit cells (migration-inhibition factor) and augment the inflammatory reaction (skin-reactive factor). The lymphokines can be demonstrated *in vitro*, and in practice two methods are commonly used to detect sensitized lymphocytes:

Migration inhibition effect. Lymphocytes and macrophages from the peritoneal cavity of a sensitized guinea-pig are placed in a capillary tube, and incubated in a suitable chamber containing culture fluid. Normally the cells migrate from the free ends of the tube to form tufts. These tufts do not appear if the cells from a guinea-pig showing delayed-type sensitivity are incubated in the presence of antigen (Fig. 13.3). If cells from a normal animal, mixed with about 10 per cent of cells from a sensitized one, are placed in a tube and cultured in the presence of antigen, *none* of the cells migrate. Hence a few sensitized cells can transfer information to cells *in vitro* just as they can *in vivo*. This is due to the action of transfer factor. It should be noted that lymphocytes from an animal sensitized towards immunoglobulin production and not delayed-type hypersensitivity do not show this phenomenon.

The effect of antigen on sensitized human cells can be assessed by using white blood cells from the buffy coat. If these are packed into capillary tubes, as described above, their migration is inhibited by the antigen to which the patient is sensitive.

Lymphocyte transformation. Lymphocytes from a sensitized animal, when incubated with the appropriate antigen, show transformation (p. 162). The number of cells transforming is not as great as with phytohaemagglutinin nor is it as rapid.

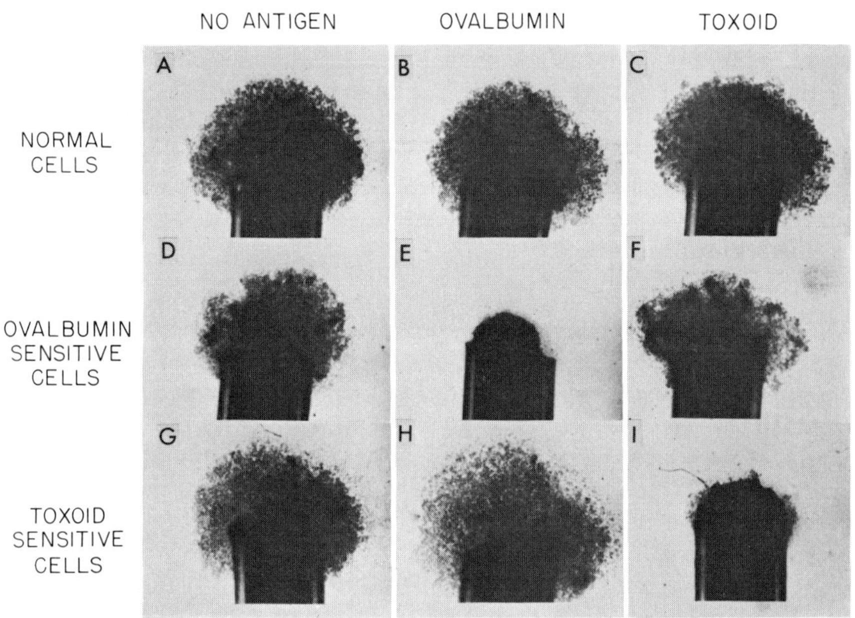

Fig. 13.3 Specific inhibition by antigen of the migration of cells from sensitized animals. The cells, mostly macrophages and lymphocytes from a peritoneal exudate, are placed in capillary tubes and incubated in a microchamber. Normally the macrophages migrate from the open end and produce a tufted appearance. The cells derived from animals with delayed-type hypersensitivity show no migration in the presence of the specific antigen. (*From David J R, Al-Askari S, Lawrence H S, Thomas L 1964 Journal of Immunology 93: 264*)

Examples of cell-mediated hypersensitivity

1. *Following infection.* A positive Mantoux reaction means past or present infection with the tubercle bacillus. Similar tests are available for other infections, e.g. leprosy, histoplasmosis, and coccidioidomycosis. Quite apart from their diagnostic value, delayed hypersensitivity reactions are probably responsible for many of the features of chronic infection. Much of the damage produced by the organisms is due to the host's own reaction.

2. *Allergic contact dermatitis.* This follows the application of a sensitizing chemical to the skin. The pathogenesis has been described previously (p. 149). The reaction is typically that of an acute dermatitis, and should not be confused with the erythematous, itchy, wealing type of skin reaction seen in immediate-type hypersensitivity.

3. *The graft reaction.* See below.

4. *Experimental.* It has also been described after certain experimental procedures in which antigen is injected with *Freund's adjuvant.* The latter consists of an oil-in-water emulsion mixed with tubercle bacilli. It is not known how this curious mixture can potentiate the sensitizing effect of an antigen.

Retest reaction.[12] If a positive tuberculin skin test is performed on a sensitive person, and the *same site* is retested with tuberculin at a later date, an accelerated reaction is observed. It appears at 2 hours and is maximal at 8 hours. The lesion is characterized by exudation of *fluid* and massive accumulation of *eosinophils.* Immediate-type hypersensitivity is not involved, but the mechanism concerned in the retest reaction is not known. Nevertheless, this phenomenon deserves further study, for many human diseases of an 'allergic' nature are also characterized by exudation and eosinophil infiltration, and some are curiously unresponsive to antihistamine drugs (e.g. bronchial asthma, allergic rhinitis, nasal polyps, etc.).

TISSUE GRAFTS[13,14]

In addition to its practical value in surgery, the transplantation of tissue has done much to extend our knowledge of the body's response to foreign tissues. To a considerable extent the fate of a graft depends upon its origin—the three types. autografts, homografts, and xenografts (heterografts), will therefore be described separately.

Autografts

An *autograft* is a graft of tissue made from one site to another site in the same individual. Provided the graft attains an adequate blood supply it usually lives and functions normally.

Autografts have found extensive use in plastic surgery. Whole-thickness flaps of skin may be used as pedicle grafts from one part of the body to another, or alternatively free grafts may be applied to raw surfaces, e.g. following burns.

In dentistry, teeth have been transplanted successfully from one part of the mouth to another.[15,16]

Homografts

A *homograft* is a transplant made from one individual to another of the same species. If the two individuals are *syngeneic* (*isogeneic*), i.e. of identical or nearly identical genetic structure, then the term *syngeneic,* or *isogeneic homograft* is used. Such a graft is accepted as 'self', does not provoke any immune response, and provided it attains an adequate blood supply persists indefinitely. In the human this situation occurs only with grafts exchanged between identical twins.

An *allogeneic homograft*, or *allograft* (often simply called a homograft), is a graft made between individuals of the same species but of different genetic constitutions.

As a general rule such a graft is always rejected due to the destruction of its cellular component by an immune response by the host. Three patterns of rejection are seen:

Hyperacute, due to the presence of preformed immunogobulin, as in the white graft reaction.

Acute, the most common reaction, and cell mediated.

Chronic, occurring after a year.

If, following the rejection of a allograft, another graft is applied to the same animal from the same donor, this second graft is rejected even more rapidly. This is known as the *second set phenomenon.*

The application of a second skin graft within a short time (about 12 days) of the rejection of the first results in the *white graft reaction*: the graft is not vascularized, but becomes pale, undergoes necrosis, and is cast off. The rejection is mediated by immunoglubulins, and a human counterpart is seen when a kidney graft undergoes hyperacute rejection due to a major ABO incompatibility or the pre-existence of antibodies to the graft.

If the second graft is applied after a longer interval, it shows early vascularization, but suddenly by the fourth or fifth day it becomes cyanosed and the surrounding skin shows marked erythema and oedema. The vessels thrombose and the graft undergoes necrosis. This is termed the *accelerated graft rejection phenomenon*, and is due to a cell-mediated immune response. This accelerated graft rejection can be transferred from one animal to another by the transfer of T lymphocytes. Graft immunity therefore resembles very closely the tuberculin-type of cell-mediated hypersensitivity.

Chronic rejection has been seen in human heart and kidney transplants. A year or more after apparent acceptance, the vessels of the graft become obstructed by intimal thickening and the organ suffers from progressive ischaemia. Humoral as well as cellular antibodies are involved in this type of rejection.

The vigour with which a graft is rejected is related to the type and amount of *transplantation antigens*[17] present in the graft but not represented in the host. Some tissues contain much antigen and these are rejected rapidly—thus in the human, skin transplants have met with little success. Renal grafts, on the other hand, are of great value. A start has been made in identifying the transplantation antigens in man, and it is now possible to match the host and graft more closely. The antigens are determined by genes which are part of a single complex called the HLA system.

The HLA (human leucocyte antigen) system.[18,19] The HLA system comprises a complex group of antigens which are present on the cell membranes of all cells other than erythrocytes. Their presence is determined by genes present at five closely associated major loci on chromosome number 6. These loci are designated HLA-A, HLA-B, HLA-C, HLA-D and HLA-DR. Every person receives two sets of alleles—one from each parent—and therefore the diploid cells contain a maximum of ten antigens for the whole HLA system. Since there are multiple alleles at each locus, the chances of two individuals having the same HLA type are very small indeed.

The human HLA system corresponds to the major histocompatibility system called H-2 in mice. In these rodents the system includes an area termed the Ia (immune associated) locus, and the antigens for which this codes are the major tissue antigens responsible for graft rejection. This region also controls the immune response (see p. 176). In humans it is thought that the HLA-DR locus corresponds to the Ia locus in mice. Since the genes that code for HLA antigens are closely associated with those that control the immune response, it is not surprising that particular tissue types are associated with certain diseases. Thus HLA-B27 is closely associated with ankylosing spondylitis.

Various attempts have been made to prolong the life of allografts (p. 151). In general these involve suppression of the immune response by ionizing radiation and the administration of cytotoxic drugs, but although the graft, e.g. a kidney, may live for several years, indefinite survival is very difficult to attain using present methods. Thus grafts whose function is dependent upon the continued survival of their cells (*homovital grafts*) are of limited value. This contrasts with a *static* graft, in which the cells die, but the matrix persists and performs an important function. The best example of this is a bone graft. The cells die, but the matrix remains and is gradually replaced by living host bone. Bone homografts are in fact as useful as autografts, because the osteocytes of the latter usually die through their failure to acquire an adequate blood supply in time. *Cornea* and *heart valves* are also used as homostatic grafts.

Homotransplantation of tissues in animals has provided much useful basic knowledge. The observation by Medawar that foreign cells injected into fetal or newborn mice were accepted as self and persisted indefinitely, led to the concept of *specific immunological tolerance,* since grafts from the same donor were accepted throughout the life of the treated animal. Furthermore, it was noted that if the injected foreign cells were immunologically competent (i.e. were small lymphocytes taken from adult animals), although they were recognized as 'self' and accepted, they themselves reacted against the host. The injected animals failed to thrive, and often died of a wasting disease called runt disease. This is an example of a *graft versus host (GVH) reaction.* It is occasionally seen when children suffering from an immunological deficiency disease are transfused with fresh blood containing living white cells, incompatible so far as the HLA antigens are concerned.[20,21]

Xenografts

An *xenograft,* or *heterograft,* is a transplant from one animal to another of a different species. Vital grafts are invariably rejected, but static grafts have found some use (e.g. pig heart valves).

AUTOIMMUNITY

Although it is evident that under normal conditions the body does not make antibodies against its own tissues, the mechanisms which prevent their formation may on occasion break down.

In theory antibodies could be made against the individual's own tissues (*autoantibodies*) under three circumstances:

1. **Alteration in antigenicity of tissue protein.** This may be due to:

Degenerative lesions. Following necrosis of tissue, e.g. the skin in burns, antibodies may be produced. It is evident that these antibodies are an effect of the disease and not its cause.

Attachment of hapten, e.g. allergic contact dermatitis (p. 190). A similar mechanism has been held to explain the aetiology of acute rheumatic fever. Streptococcal antigen might become attached to body proteins (e.g. of heart), and the antibodies produced against the altered proteins could cause damage. An alternative explanation is that the streptococci share a common antigen with the heart, so that antibodies to the organisms also react with the heart. Nevertheless, the most likely explanation of acute rheumatic fever is that it is an immune-complex disease involving streptococcal antigen in excess.

2. **Release of an antigen which has always been isolated.** It may be that some tissue products are anatomically isolated from the immunologically competent cells, and are therefore not recognized as 'self' when released into the blood stream following injury or disease. It has been postulated that thyroglobulin in the thyroid acini is one such substance, and that antibodies to it could damage the thyroid cells to produce Hashimoto's disease (p. 569). The evidence is not convincing.

3. **Altered reactivity of the immune mechanism.** In this case 'self' proteins would no longer be recognized. There is little doubt that this does sometimes occur. In chronic lymphatic leukaemia haemolysins are sometimes produced, and these may cause haemolytic anaemia. This is a good example of a condition caused by autoantibodies, and it indicates that the lymphoid tissue plays an important role in the immune response.

Experimental autoimmune disease. The injection into an animal of normal syngeneic or allogeneic tissue mixed with Freund's adjuvant may result in a disease of the respective organ, which is presumed to be due to autoantibody production. If thyroid is used, a condition resembling Hashimoto's disease is produced. If brain tissue is used, allergic encephalomyelitis results.

Types of antibody. It may be postulated that the autoantibodies will either be immunoglobulins or cell-bound. The immunoglobulins might be of any class and of one or two types:

1. *Organ-specific* immunoglobulins, whose specificity is directed against a determinant present in one organ, e.g. haemolysins and antithyroid antibodies.

2. *Non-organ-specific.* Antibodies directed against DNA, mitochondria, smooth muscle, and immunoglobulin determinants (rheumatoid factor) fall into this group.

Role of autoantibodies in disease processes

Antibodies may directly attack a tissue and cause damage. The immunoglobulins acquire destructive properties by activating complement, e.g. acute haemolytic anaemia due to a haemolysin. Sensitized T cells can also destroy cells, e.g. experimental allergic encephalomyelitis.

Autoantibodies can also combine with antigen and form damaging antigen–antibody complexes; sometimes complement is activated. The lesions of this immune-complex disease resemble serum sickness if acute, but if the process is chronic, the kidney is the organ most often affected[7] (see p. 569). Diseases in which the major lesions are caused by an immune mechanism may with justification be called autoimmune diseases. However, it must be stressed that the autoimmunity merely provides a mechanism in the pathogenesis of a disease. It does not provide the cause, which as noted below may be inherited or acquired.

Aetiology of immunologically mediated diseases

1. *Genetic factors.* There is a definite tendency for some autoimmune diseases, e.g. systemic lupus erythematosus and rheumatoid arthritis, to be familial. This is probably due to the fact that the immune response is itself regulated by genetic factors.

2. *Acquired factors.* Any extrinsic cause of disease can precipitate an autoimmune process. Certain drugs and sunlight can precipitate the onset of lupus erythematosus, and infections will on occasions produce autoimmune haemolytic anaemia (e.g. in mycoplasmal pneumonia). When the aetiology of a disease is clearly established, as in smallpox, the immunologically mediated manifestations of the disease, such as the skin eruption, are readily accepted as part of the whole condition. It is when the cause of a disease is not known, e.g. rheumatoid arthritis, that stress is laid on the autoimmune component of the illness. The label 'autoimmune disease' should not, however, delude one into thinking that one knows the cause of the disease—one has only described part of its pathogenesis.

Summary

From this brief account of the immune response and its relationship to hypersensitivity and immunity to infection, it is evident that the body's response to foreign material is very complex.

In response to antigenetic stimulation, the immune response may be humoral or cell mediated. Which occurs depends in part upon the nature of the initiating antigen and the method whereby it is presented to the body.

With *simple protein antigens*, or haptens which combine with body proteins, it is the immunoglobulin type of antibody which is produced. If the antigen is a bacterial toxin or component of a bacterium, the antibody can afford immunity to infection. Sometimes, the immunoglobulin antibodies are of such a type (IgE in the human) that they can sensitize the cells of the body to the action of antigen—this mediates hypersensitivity of the anaphylactic type. Sometimes antibodies form damaging complexes with antigen, and this leads to non-specific injury in various parts of the body; commonly the kidney and blood vessels are involved. This is immune-complex disease, or type III reaction. Occasionally antibodies are specific for a particular tissue, as when haemolysins are formed. This is the type II reaction.

When the body is invaded by *foreign living cells*, a cell-mediated immune response ensues. Sensitized lymphocytes when confronted with the appropriate antigen release a variety of lymphokines. These may attack the target cells directly or recruit macrophages and enhance the inflammatory response. The cell-mediated immune response can lead to the rejection of grafts and cause damage to the skin in acute allergic contact dermatitis. It can also mediate immunity to microbial infection, not only by directly affecting the organisms but also by exciting an inflammatory response and recruiting macrophages.

The role of the immune response appears clear enough when considering the action of immunoglobulins. Bacteria and their toxins are killed or neutralized. Hypersensitivity appears to be an unfortunate side-effect, but even this may have some beneficial effect in that it excites an acute inflammatory response.

The role of the cell-mediated immune response is less clear. Sensitized cells are thought to be important in the destruction of intracellular organisms and are therefore of survival value. The advantage of type IV hypersensitivity is, however, difficult to understand, since it seems to be a factor in prolonging the effect of some infections which thereby become chronic. Also the value of a response which eliminates foreign grafts is of no obvious evolutionary advantage. It has been suggested that the immune response, particularly the cell-mediated type, has evolved as a mechanism for eliminating invading organisms and also for the destruction of abnormal cells which have been produced in the body as a result of damage or genetic change. This scrutinizing action of the lymphocytes (*immunological surveillance*) has been suggested as an important homeostatic mechanism whereby neoplastic cells are recognized, destroyed and eliminated.[22] There is some increased incidence of lymphoma in individuals who are immunologically deficient, but no dramatic increase in the incidence of other malignant disease as would be expected if immunological surveillance by lymphocytes were a major defence mechanism against the development of cancer. Another suggested role of cellular immunity is that it has been evolved in mammals to prevent the invasion of the mother by fetal cells during gestation.

REFERENCES

1. Patterson R, Zeiss C R, Kelly J F 1976 Classification of hypersensitivity reactions. New England Journal of Medicine 295:277
2. Miescher P A, Mueller-Eberhard H J 1976 Textbook of Immunopathology, 2nd edn. Vols 1 and 2. Grune and Stratton, New York
3. Brocklehurst W E (1975) In *Clinical Aspects of Immunology,* ed Gell P G H, Coombs R R A, Lachmann P J, 3rd edn, p 821. Blackwell: Oxford
4. Orange R P, Austen K F, 1971 Chemical mediators of immediate hypersensitivity. Hospital Practice 6:79
5. Austen K F 1974 Systemic anaphylaxis in the human being. New England Journal of Medicine 291:661
6. Christian C L, 1969 Immune-complex disease. NewEngland Journal of Medicine 280:878
7. McClusky R T, Klassen J 1973 Immunologically mediated glomerular, tubular and interstitial renal disease. New England Journal of Medicine 288: 564
8. Dash C H, Jones H E H 1972 Mechanisms in Drug Allergy. Churchill Livingstone, Edinburgh
9. Coombs R R A, Hunter A, Jonas W E, Bennich H, Johansson S G O Panzanl R 1968 Detection of IgE (IgND) specific antibody (probably reagin) to castor-bean allergen by the red-cell-linked antigen-antiglobulin method. Lancet 1:1115
10. Turk J L 1975 Delayed Hypersensitivity, 2nd edn. North Holland, Amsterdam
11. Bloom B R 1971 In vitro methods in cell-mediated immunity in man. New England Journal of Medicine 284:1212
12. Arnason B G, Waksman B H 1963 The retest reaction in delayed sensitivity. Laboratory Investigation 12:737
13. Rapaport F T, Dausset J 1968 Human Transplantation, 278 pp. Grune and Stratton, New York
14. Russell P S, Winn H J 1970 Transplantation. New England Journal of Medicine 282:786, 848 and 896
15. Jonck L M 1966 An investigation into certain aspects of transplantation and reimplantation of teeth in man. British Journal of Oral Surgery 4:137
16. Shulman L B 1964 The transplantation antigenicity of tooth homografts. Oral Surgery, Oral Medicine and Oral Pathology 17:389
17. Berah M, Hors J, Dausset J 1968 Concentration of transplantation antigens in human organs. Lancet 2:106
18. Rosenberg L E, Kidd K K 1977 HLA and disease susceptibility: a primer. New England Journal of Medicine 297:1060
19. Various Authors 1978 The HLA system. British Medical Bulletin 34:213-316

20. Slavin R E, Santos G W 1973 The graft versus host reaction in man after bone marrow transplantation: pathology, pathogenesis, clinical features and implication. Clinical Immunology and Immunopathology 1:472
21. Elkins W L 1971 Cellular immunology and the pathogenesis of graft versus host reactions. Progress in Allergy 15:78
22. Leading Article 1972 Immunosuppression and malignancy. British Medical Journal 3:713

14

Some important bacterial infections

ACUTE PYOGENIC INFECTIONS

The organisms responsible for acute inflammation and the formation of pus account for some of the most important lesions seen clinically. Although most of the infections respond to antibiotic therapy, surgical drainage of abscesses is still often necessary. The most important members of this group of pyogenic bacteria are:

1. **Pyogenic cocci**, e.g. *Staphylococcus aureus, Streptococcus pyogenes*, pneumococcus, meningococcus, and gonococcus
2. **Gram-negative intestinal bacilli**, viz. *Escherichia coli*, *Proteus* species, and *Pseudomonas aeruginosa* (*Ps. pyocyanea*) and organisms of the genus *Bacteroides*.

Of these it is the staphylococcus, streptococcus, and Gram-negative bacilli which are of greatest surgical moment because of their capacity to produce infections in many different sites. Furthermore, they are of cardinal importance because they not only infect wounds and burns, but also act as secondary invaders in chronic ulcerative lesions from other causes, e.g. cancerous and tuberculous lesions of the skin and mucous membranes. By contrast the pneumococcus, meningococcus, and gonococcus tend to affect the lungs, meninges, and genital tract respectively.

The pathological effects of these bacteria are all essentially similar. There is an acute inflammatory response culminating in the accumulation of an exudate crowded with neutrophil polymorphs, which attempts to destroy the organisms. If the organisms are destroyed early in the inflammatory response there is resolution; otherwise the condition proceeds to tissue destruction and suppuration. The abscess so formed may burst spontaneously on to a free surface or else be drained surgically. If the pus is successfully drained, the destroyed tissue is replaced either by the regeneration of specialized tissue or by the formation of fibrous scar tissue. If pus becomes loculated and dead tissue remains, the circumstances are ripe for the development of chronic inflammation, as explained in Chapter 10. When the pyogenic lesion becomes chronic, there is an admixture of other cells to the polymorphs already present. Lymphocytes, plasma cells, macrophages, and eosinophils are all in evidence, as well as the proliferating connective-tissue and specialized cells of the part. Indeed, these organisms are responsible for the chronic non-specific bacterial inflammation that plays such an important role in everyday clinical practice. Sometimes if the body's resistance is very poor or if the organism is extremely virulent, there may be rapid local spread and generalized dissemination of organisms. In this case a fatal septicaemia or pyaemia may ensue.

Except in very localized infections there is a general body response reflected in a polymorphonuclear leucocytosis with an increased proportion of immature neutrophils in the blood. If the infection is spreading to any extent there is a variable constitutional reaction with fever and an elevation of the ESR (p. 436).

It is important to note the salient bacteriological features of these organisms because only by investigating their properties can a logical attempt be made to understand the diseases which they cause.

STAPHYLOCOCCI

Morphology. Staphylococci are Gram-positive, spherical organisms about 1μm in diameter, which tend to be arranged in grape-like clusters. They are non-motile, non-sporing, and non-capsulate.

Cultural characteristics. Staphylococci grow easily on most media. They are aerobic organisms, but can tolerate an anaerobic atmosphere quite well, i.e. they are facultative anaerobes. They grow best at 37°C. On blood agar, conspicuous, shiny, convex colonies appear within 24 hours, and these are pigmented. Most have a creamy white or dull yellow colour, but some species are golden, lemon yellow, and even red. Although pigmentation is no longer regarded as important, the organisms are still called *Staphylococcus albus*, when non-pathogenic (whatever the actual colour of the colony) and *Staphylococcus aureus* when pathogenic. *Staph. aureus* is sometimes called *Staph. pyogenes*, and *Staph. albus* is occasionally called *Staph. epidermidis*. Staphylococci are divided into these two groups according to their production of coagulase in the laboratory. The term non-pathogenic is not strictly true, for *Staph. albus* can produce infection (see p. 202).

Coagulase production. The important laboratory criterion of pathogenicity is the production of coagulase, an enzyme which coagulates plasma even in the absence of calcium. All pathogenic staphylococci produce coagulase, and are called *Staph. aureus.*

STAPHYLOCOCCUS AUREUS

Not all coagulase-producing staphylococci are equally virulent. Some produce mild skin lesions only, whereas others are responsible for epidemics of hospital infection of the most severe intensity. It is necessary to type the organisms in such an epidemic, so as to ascertain whether they are all of one strain or of many different strains (p. 92).

Typing. The basis of staphylococcal typing lies in the use of staphylococcal bacteriophage*, a virus which specifically lyses colonies of staphylococci. Any one

* Bacteriophage is often abbreviated to 'phage.'

bacteriophage can lyse only a few susceptible strains, thus each staphylococcus exhibits a distinct pattern of lysis: for example, a well-known epidemic strain of staphylococcus is lysed by phages 47, 53, 75, and 77, and is therefore typed 47/53/75/77. One of the most notorious epidemic strains is the phage type-80 staphylococcus. This was first recognized in Australia in 1953, and has since then wreaked havoc in many hospitals throughout the world.

Toxin production. The staphylococcus is an invasive organism, but the essential factors responsible for its virulence are not clearly defined. Nevertheless, some toxins are known, and these mainly have the characters of endotoxins. Some microbiologists, however, prefer to group these products under the heading of exotoxins. Be this as it may, there is no doubt that their action is considerably less potent than that of the enterotoxin, which is noted below. The most important of these is the *α-toxin,* which produces local tissue necrosis, and is lethal when injected intravenously. It is also haemolytic to red cells, and destroys white cells, i.e. it is a *haemolysin* and a *leucocidin.*

There is another staphylococcal toxin, the action of which is confined to white cells. It is called the *Panton-Valentine leucocidin.* Two other endotoxins are also described, and these have haemolytic and necrotizing actions.

In this list the three enzymes produced by staphylococci can be included:

Coagulase, which has already been described
Staphylokinase, which lyses fibrin by activating the plasmin system
Hyaluronidase.

Both staphylokinase and hyaluronidase are produced only by some strains and seldom in large amounts.

In addition some strains produce an exotoxin, called *enterotoxin*, which produces symptoms of food-poisoning when ingested. It is the only exotoxin produced by the staphylococcus, and unlike most exotoxins it is relatively thermostable.

Lesions produced by Staph. aureus. The typical staphylococcal lesion is a *circumscribed area of inflammation with suppuration.* Coagulase production has been suggested as an important factor in the localization of the infection by virtue of the copious fibrin formation that it induces. On the other hand, other authorities regard coagulase as a factor aiding spread of infection, because the deposition of fibrin acts as a protective covering for the organism and prevents its phagocytosis. It is evident that our ideas on the importance of coagulase in staphylococcal infection are still purely speculative. It seems likely that the local damage inflicted by the α-toxin leads to a considerable inflammatory reaction which in its turn successfully localizes and overcomes the infection.

Staphylococcal skin lesions are very frequent (Fig 14.1), and include boils, carbuncles, paronychia (inflammation of the nail-fold), impetigo, and its bullous variant in the newborn.

In *impetigo* the organisms invade the superficial layers of the skin and produce characteristic subcorneal bullae and pustules. This is common on the face and in children. The blisters soon rupture and become covered by a honey-coloured crust.

Folliculitis. Infection of the hair follicles is common, and the type of lesion produced depends on how deeply the organisms penetrate. Since pus is produced,

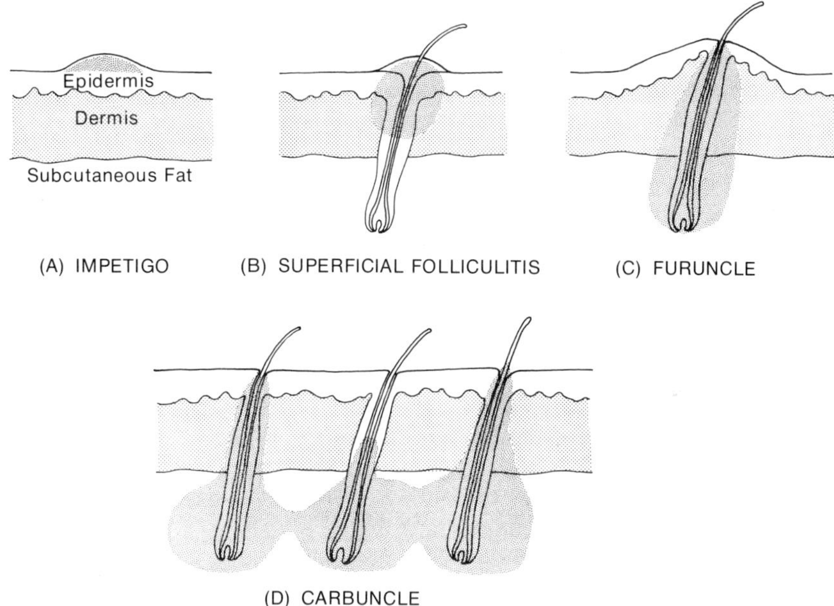

Fig. 14.1 Diagram illustrating some staphylococcal infections of the skin. (A) *Impetigo*. The infection is very superficial, and a pustule forms beneath the stratum corneum of the epidermis. (B) *Superficial folliculitis*. The suppurative inflammation involves the superficial part of a hair follicle. Clinically this appears as a small pustule; the condition is also called impetigo of Bockhart. (C) *Furuncle or Boil*. The infection involves an entire hair follicle, and in the inflammatory oedema produces a considerable swelling, which can be 1 cm or more in diameter. Nevertheless, a boil has one head only. (D) *Carbuncle*. The infection involves the subcutaneous tissues, and loculated pockets of pus are present. These pockets are formed between fibrous septa, which are not shown in the diagram. Note the multiple heads through which pus can be discharged. (*Drawing by Margot Mackay, Department of Art as Applied to Medicine, University of Toronto.*)

the term *pyoderma* is sometimes employed to include impetigo and folliculitis. In *superficial folliculitis* (*Bockhart's impetigo*) numerous small pustules are seen at the openings of adjacent hair follicles; the face and scalp are common sites. A somewhat deeper infection is seen in the beard area (*sycosis barbae*), and in addition to involvement of the hair follicle itself, there is much perifollicular inflammation. The lesions are very liable to become chronic.

A deeper more destructive infection of the hair follicle is the *boil*, or *furuncle*. Suppuration is the usual result, and pus is discharged from a single opening. A well-known regional type of boil is the *stye*, in which an eyelash is implicated. Boils are particularly common in the axillae and on the back of the neck, and they are often multiple in these sites due to the regional concentration of hair follicles and sebaceous glands. Nevertheless, each boil has its own 'head' through which it discharges its pus.

In a *carbuncle* the infection extends to the underlying fatty subcutaneous tissue and spreads laterally in this plane. The subcutaneous tissue is divided into compartments by fibrous septa which extend from the deep fascia to the dermis.

It therefore follows that when infection spreads a series of loculated abscesses is formed. The pus reaches the surface through hair follicles or sweat glands, and each abscess has its own 'head'. Thus a single carbuncle has multiple heads, each with one loculus. Extensive areas of skin become undermined, and they eventually slough off; a large granulating surface is produced as healing occurs.

Staphylococci are the commonest causal organisms in *infected wounds*, usually the result of cross infection in hospital.

*Bullous impetigo of the newborn** is the result of similar cross infection in maternity wards. Infected infants may transmit the staphylococci to their mothers during breast feeding. A *breast abscess* may be the result.

Two other important examples of cross infection are *bronchopneumonia* (p. 536) and *enterocolitis*.

Staphylococcal enterocolitis is an occasional cause of pseudomembranous colitis.

Staphylococci are the most important causal agents in *acute osteomyelitis* (p. 143).

Staphylococci may spread *via* the lymphatics to produce a *lymphadenitis* that may undergo suppuration. If the infection is not arrested, there will be massive blood-stream invasion to produce a fatal *septicaemia*. *Pyaemia* is not uncommon, and follows suppurative thrombophlebitis which may complicate any staphylococcal infection.

Staphylococcal food-poisoning is the only condition due entirely to the enterotoxin.

Occurrence. The reservoir of *Staph. aureus* is the anterior nares. About 40 per cent of healthy adults are nasal carriers and in a hospital population the figure may rise to over 70 per cent. From the nose they are transferred to the skin, particularly of the hands and perineum, where they multiply and spread. Staphylococci are also present in the faeces, though this is probably not an important source of infection except in patients with enterocolitis.

Staphylococcus albus

Staph. albus (coagulase negative) is a universal commensal of the skin and nose, and rarely produces infection. It occasionally leads to urinary-tract infections, especially in association with stones, and has recently gained prominence as a cause of opportunistic infection especially following surgery when foreign material is inserted. Thus it may cause endocarditis after open-heart surgery.

STREPTOCOCCI

Morphology. These too are Gram-positive, spherical organisms, slightly smaller than staphylococci. They tend to be arranged in chains which vary in length when they are cultured in fluid media. They are non-motile and non-sporing. Some strains possess very thin capsules called microcapsules.

Cultural characteristics. Streptococci grow less easily than staphylococci, but are also aerobes and facultative anaerobes. A few strains are obligatory anaerobes.

* The alternative name pemphigus neonatorum is best abandoned, since the staphylococcal disease of the newborn is not related to the pemphigus group of diseases (see Ch. 40).

They can be cultured on blood agar at 37°C, and within 24 hours, tiny, transparent, dewdrop colonies develop. Around these there may be a zone of haemolysis, and according to this the organisms are classified into three main groups:

α-haemolytic streptococci, which produce an ill-defined zone of partial haemolysis, which may be yellow or green in colour. These organisms are often reported as *Strept. viridans* or *Strept. salivarius*
β-haemolytic streptococci, which produce a sharply demarcated zone of complete haemolysis
Non-haemolytic streptococci. These are also called γ-type streptococci.

β-haemolytic streptococci are particularly important in producing serious pyogenic infections. Not all, however, are pathogenic to humans; some produce disease only in cattle and other animals. It is therefore important to distinguish between the different groups of β-haemolytic streptococci. This is done by Lancefield's method.

Lancefield grouping. β-haemolytic streptococci can be divided into 18 groups by a precipitation test, first described by Lancefield, according to the presence of a specific carbohydrate hapten, called the C antigen, in the wall of the organism. The great majority of human pathogens fall into Lancefield's group A, and a group-A organism is called *Strept. pyogenes*.

As described with staphylococci, *Strept. pyogenes* may also give rise to epidemics of infection, particularly in schools and barracks in association with acute glomerulonephritis. The necessity for typing the organisms may then arise.

Griffith typing. The technique used was first described by Griffith, who discovered that Group-A streptococci could be subdivided into over 50 different types depending on the presence of protein antigens on the surface of the organisms. These are called M and T antigens, and the M antigen is particularly important, because its presence is related to virulence. Typing is carried out by means of agglutination and precipitation tests using specific rabbit antisera. There seems to be little variation in the virulence of the different types, except that a few, especially type 12, are related to acute glomerulonephritis.

Toxin production. Like the staphylococcus, *Strept. pyogenes* is an invasive organism that produces powerful endotoxins and a single exotoxin. There are two haemolysins designated *streptolysin O* and *streptolysin S*. Streptolysin O is also cardiotoxic and leucocidic, whereas streptolysin S is a pure haemolysin. As the chemical nature of endotoxins is generally so poorly understood, it is reasonable to include the *M protein* among them. This is powerfully antigenic. It acts by interfering with phagocytosis, and the antibody formed against it is an opsonin (p. 178).

The organisms produce three enzymes:

Hyaluronidase
Streptokinase, which induces fibrinolysis by activating the plasmin system
Streptodornase, which lyses DNA. The name streptodornase is derived from the first letters of the syllables **deoxyribonuclease**.

The exotoxin referred to is the *erythrogenic toxin* responsible for the generalized punctate erythema characteristic of scarlet fever. It is produced by some strains only.

Lesions produced by Strept. pyogenes. The typical streptococcal lesion is a *spreading infection of the connective tissue called a cellulitis*. The poor localizing tendency has been associated with the hyaluronidase and streptokinase produced by most strains, often in large amounts. Abscesses occur much later than in staphylococcal infections, and the pus is watery and often blood-stained. It is probable that the streptodornase and streptokinase are responsible for this, because the viscosity of the pus is due to DNA and fibrin.

In recent years the virulence of *Strept. pyogenes* has declined so markedly that many of the classical streptococcal lesions which produced so much damage in years gone by are now rarely seen. By contrast staphylococcal lesions are commoner and more severe than ever.

Streptococci are occasional causes of *wound* and *burn infections*, and are also responsible for some cases of *impetigo*. *Erysipelas*, a spreading infection of the dermis, is a classical streptococcal lesion. It affects the face, and is seen as a raised, bright-red plaque with a sharply defined edge that steadily advances.

Streptococci are still important causes of *tonsillitis* and *pharyngitis* (streptococcal sore throat) and these may be complicated by infection of the middle ear (*otitis media*). Streptococci have a great tendency to invade the blood stream, with the development of *septicaemia*. This is quite a common complication of streptococcal infection of the uterus following labour (*puerperal sepsis*), which killed thousands of women before the introduction of aseptic techniques and chemotherapy.

If an infecting streptococcus produces the erythrogenic exotoxin, and the patient has no circulating antitoxin, the local lesion will be complicated by the effects of this toxin. A generalized punctate erythema appears, and the condition is called *scarlet fever*.

There is an indirect relationship between streptococcal infections on the one hand and *acute rheumatic fever* and *acute glomerulonephritis* on the other. Acute nephritis occurs about 10 days after an attack of streptococcal pharyngitis; after impetigo the period is often three weeks or longer. Acute rheumatic fever follows only on streptococcal pharyngitis, almost never on skin infections;[1] the current view is that both are manifestations of immune-complex reactions.

Occurrence of Strept. pyogenes. *Streptococcus pyogenes* is found in the throats of about 10 per cent of people, and in from 2 to 5 per cent it is also present in the anterior nares.

OTHER STREPTOCOCCI

Group-B streptococci (Strept. agalactiae). These organisms are not infrequently found in the female genital tract, and are recognized as a common cause of severe perinatal infection. The manifestations are those of respiratory distress with shock, septicaemia, and meningitis.[2]

Group-C streptococci and Group-G streptococci. These organisms may also cause puerperal infection and wound infection.

Alpha-haemolytic streptococci. *Strept. viridans* is not a single defined species, but is the collective name given to α-haemolytic streptococci. These organisms are invariable commensals of the mouth and throat, and a number of strains, e.g. *Strept. mitis*, *Strept. mutans*, and *Strept. sanguis*, have been incriminated in dental caries and periodontal disease. Of greater importance, however, is the association of *Strept. viridans* with subacute infective endocarditis, described on page 515.

Non-haemolytic streptococci. The non-haemolytic streptococcus is always present in the colon, hence its alternative names *Strept. faecalis* and *enterococcus*. If it leaves its normal habitat this organism can cause suppurative lesions of a type and distribution similar to *Escherichia coli.* It is a common cause of urinary-tract infection.

Anaerobic streptococcal infections. Anaerobic streptococci are normal inhabitants of the bowel, vagina, and mouth (particularly the gingival sulci). These were important causes of puerperal sepsis in the past, and occasionally are associated with *wound infection.* They may also be found in gangrenous lesions (p. 66).

THE PNEUMOCOCCUS

Diplococcus pneumoniae is closely related to the streptococci, and is sometimes called *Strept. pneumoniae*, but in fact it is better to regard it as a separate genus.

Morphology. The pneumococcus is an oval or lance-shaped coccus. The organisms are arranged in pairs with the long axes in line with each other. It is the same size as the streptococcus, and like it is Gram-positive, non-motile, and non-sporing. An important feature is the presence of a prominent capsule.

Cultural characteristics. It resembles the α-haemolytic streptococcus very closely, and both produce a diffuse greenish haemolysis of the surrounding blood agar.

Typing. Type-specificity depends on the polysaccharide hapten (the specific soluble substance, or SSS) present in the capsule of the organism, and it is this that determines its virulence. Over 70 different types of pneumococci have been recognized, but in practice pneumococcal typing is seldom carried out nowadays. Types 1, 2, and 3 are the most virulent, and are responsible for most cases of lobar pneumonia (p. 529). Types 5, 7, and 14 are also quite virulent, but the remainder appear to be commensals of the nose and throat, and cause little harm in healthy people.

Lesions produced. The most important pneumococcal lesion is *lobar pneumonia*, which is caused by one of the virulent strains, usually type 1, 2, or 3. Other types of pneumococci are sometimes implicated in bronchopneumonia (p. 533). Other primary pneumococcal conditions are *otitis media* and *suppurative sinusitis*, both of which may lead to *meningitis*.

THE GRAM-NEGATIVE INTESTINAL BACILLI

The members of this group, which are important causes of pyogenic infections, are *Escherichia coli*, *Proteus* species, and *Pseudomonas aeruginosa* (also called *Ps. pyocyanea*). Most of these organisms belong to the family *Enterobacteriaceae* which includes the numerous genera conveniently grouped together as the 'coliform organisms'. Of these the most important pyogenic member is the genus *Escherichia.*

Proteus is included, but *Pseudomonas* is excluded from it, because *Ps. aeruginosa* is only occasionally found as a commensal of the bowel, whereas the true *Enterobacteriaceae* are all native to the intestinal tract.

The group also includes the genus *Salmonella*, responsible for typhoid fever and food-poisoning, and the genus *Shigella*, responsible for bacillary dysentery. These two groups of organisms are not distinguished by suppuration, and are not described further.

Morphology. The *Enterobacteriaceae* are all Gram-negative rods 1 to 4 μm long. Most of them are vigorously motile, but there are some exceptions, e.g. *Klebsiella* species which are non-motile, and so also are the *Shigella* species.

Cultural characteristics. The organisms grow easily at 37°C, being aerobic and facultatively anaerobic. On blood agar, large greyish-white, irregular, shiny colonies are produced within 24 hours.

Colonies of some *Proteus* species tend to spread over the surface of the agar as a thin film submerging other bacterial colonies, a feature called 'swarming'.

Ps. aeruginosa produces a bluish-green pigmentation due to the formation of fluorescin and pyocyanin.

Biochemical reactions. The most important biochemical property of these organisms is their ability to ferment various sugars. This is used in their laboratory identification. Thus *Escherichia coli* ferments lactose, whereas *Proteus, Pseudomonas, Salmonella*, and *Shigella*, are unable to do so.

Occurrence. Unlike the pyogenic streptococci and staphylococci, these organisms may be regarded as normal inhabitants of the body, causing disease only when they leave their normal environment.

Esch. coli is always present in the bowel, and about a third of all human faeces harbour *Proteus*. *Ps. aeruginosa* is a more foreign type of organism, being found in only 3 to 16 per cent of faeces.

Pathogenicity. The pathogenic action of these organisms is believed to be due to an endotoxin, which as yet has been poorly defined. When they escape from the lumen of the bowel and invade the tissues, suppurative lesions ensue. Endotoxin is probably responsible for shock when large numbers of Gram-negative organisms enter the circulation (p. 408).

Lesions produced by the coliform organisms. *Esch. coli* and the other coliform organisms are always predominant in infective lesions derived from the bowel contents, e.g. *appendix abscess* and *generalized peritonitis following perforation of a hollow viscus*. It frequently infects *penetrating wounds of the abdomen*. It is furthermore the commonest agent in *urinary-tract infections*, reaching the kidney as part of a normal bacteraemia from the colon, or else being introduced into the bladder following maladroit catheterization.

Esch. coli is not infrequently present in sputum, and it may be an agent in producing *pneumonia*.

It should be noted that although *Esch. coli* is an inevitable and harmless inhabitant of the bowel, in recent years certain enteropathogenic strains have been isolated. These are of no special importance as causes of suppuration but they may produce epidemics of *infantile gastroenteritis*. The condition is most common in artificially-fed babies, and is probably spread by fomites and contaminated food.

Proteus organisms and *Ps. aeruginosa* have a similar range of pathogenicity, but as they are less frequently commensals of the bowel, they are much more frequently transmitted by cross-infection. Both are important causes of urinary-tract, respiratory, ear, and wound infections.

Salmonella typhi infection is described in Chapter 7. Intestinal infections due to *Salmonella* and *Shigella* organisms are considered in Chapter 34.

THE ANAEROBIC WOUND INFECTIONS

These infections are of great importance in clinical practice, not because they are common but because when they do occur they are serious. With the exception of infections with the anaerobic streptococci, bacteroides, and actinomyces, all are due to the clostridial group of anaerobic spore-bearers. The clostridial organisms are responsible for two extremely serious conditions, *gas-gangrene* and *tetanus*. Gas-gangrene is produced by the combined action of a number of clostridia, the most important of which are *Cl. welchii* (also called *Cl. perfringens*), *Cl. oedematiens*, and *Cl. septicum*, whereas tetanus is caused by a single organism, *Cl. tetani*. The rare, lethal form of food-poisoning, botulism, is produced by another clostridium, *Cl. botulinum*. This is not a wound infection but an intoxication which follows the ingestion of a heat-stable, potent exotoxin produced by the organism in poorly prepared food during its period of storage.

BACTERIOLOGY OF THE CLOSTRIDIAL ORGANISMS

Morphology. The clostridia are large, Gram-positive bacilli approximately 5 μm long. The most characteristic feature is the spore, which is produced whenever the organism finds itself in adverse conditions. It is usually central or subterminal, but in the case of *Cl. tetani* it is situated terminally, so that *Cl. tetani* is sometimes called the 'drum-stick bacillus'. These organisms are all motile and non-capsulate, with the exception of *Cl. welchii* which is non-motile and possesses a capsule.

Cultural characteristics. They all grow quite easily but most of them demand anaerobiosis, i.e. they are obligatory anaerobes. They are most conveniently cultured at 37°C on blood agar in the anaerobic atmosphere afforded by a McIntosh and Fildes jar. Robertson's meat broth, which consists of cooked meat suspended in infusion broth, is an alternative medium.

Biochemical reactions. Fermentation reactions are of considerable importance. Clostridia are divided into two categories, saccharolytic and proteolytic.

Saccharolytic clostridia ferment many sugars, e.g. lactose and glucose. They do not break down proteins, and they merely turn the meat in Robertson's medium a pink colour, due to the production of acid. The main pathogens of gas-gangrene, viz. *Cl. welchii*, *Cl. septicum*, and *Cl. oedematiens*, come into this category.

Proteolytic clostridia break down protein, and produce foul-smelling gases like hydrogen sulphide and ammonia. The meat in Robertson's medium becomes black due to the formation of iron sulphide. These organisms are also able to ferment sugars, but they are less active than the first group. The secondary putrefactive saprophytes of gas-gangrene, e.g. *Cl. sporogenes* and *Cl. histolyticum*, come into this category.

It is a fair generalization that the saccharolytic clostridia are the important pathogens in gas-gangrene and the proteolytic clostridia mostly saprophytes. However, the demarcation is not clear, since the proteolytic clostridia have some saccharolytic capacity, and, in addition, *Cl. histolyticum* is also pathogenic despite its predominantly proteolytic activity.

Toxin production. The clostridia are excellent examples of toxic organisms, the lesions they produce being due entirely to exotoxins. The infection is localized, but the systemic effects are far-reaching.

In the gas-gangrene group most work has been done on *Cl. welchii.* Five types have been described, type A being the human pathogen and causing gas-gangrene and food-poisoning. The important toxin of type A is called α-toxin. It is a lecithinase. In animals a local injection causes tissue necrosis, and larger doses are lethal. By virtue of its lecithinase activity it destroys the phospholipid components of red-cell envelopes, and is thus a powerful haemolysin.

The other toxins of *Cl. welchii* include a *hyaluronidase*, a *deoxyribonuclease*, and a *collagenase*. These enzymes play an important part in breaking down the intercellular ground substance and collagen fibres of tissues which are infected with *Cl. welchii*, and so aid the local spread of the organism.*

Cl. septicum and *Cl. oedematiens* produce powerful haemolytic and necrotizing exotoxins. *Cl. oedematiens* also yields small amounts of a lecithinase.

By contrast, *Cl. tetani* produces only two exotoxins. The important one is a neurotoxin called *tetanospasmin*, which is, of course, responsible for the convulsions of tetanus. Tetanospasmin has been separated in a pure crystalline form. It is an immensely potent poison, being second only to the exotoxin of *Cl. botulinum* in this respect. The other exotoxin is haemolytic, and is known as *tetanolysin.*

Occurrence. The spores of these organisms are widely dispersed in nature, and are especially plentiful in soil. The organisms are commensals of the human and animal intestine, and their spores are excreted in the faeces and returned to the soil in the form of manure. *Cl. welchii* is almost invariably present in the human bowel, but *Cl. tetani* occurs somewhat more sporadically. These spores must be expected in all environments, including the air and furniture of wards and even operating theatres.

By virtue of their ability to form spores in adverse circumstances, these organisms are resistant to heat and desiccation. Only well-devised sterilizing methods can destroy them.

Apart from the role played by *Cl. welchii* in gas-gangrene, certain specific strains are an important cause of *food-poisoning* when they contaminate meat in heavy culture. The symptoms, which may be quite severe and occasionally fatal, are dysenteric in type.

GAS-GANGRENE

Gas-gangrene may follow the contamination of a wound with the spores of the pathogenic clostridia. Considering the ubiquitous presence of these spores and the

* The description of proteolytic enzymes in saccharolytic organisms seems to be a contradiction in terms. But 'proteolytic' refers to the putrefaction of complex protein, and this is not done by the saccharolytic group.

rarity of gas-gangrene in civilian practice, it is evident that healthy incised wounds so contaminated do not develop infection. The essential factor necessary for spore germination is a reduced oxygen tension. This is present in irregularly contused or lacerated wounds containing much dead tissue, which has been devitalized as a result of compression or impaired blood supply. Foreign bodies like shrapnel or pieces of clothing will exert local pressure, and also favour pyogenic infection. Soil is particularly dangerous, in that the ionizable calcium salts in it lead to considerable tissue necrosis. Finally, any coincidental infection by aerobic pyogenic organisms serves to augment the anaerobiosis. The local injection of adrenaline has a similar effect by causing vasoconstriction.

It therefore follows that most gas gangrene is exogenous in origin, and is due to thc gross contamination of severely lacerated wounds. It is usually seen in battle casualties or in agricultural accidents. Occasionally gas-gangrene is endogenous, and occurs when a wound e.g. a high-thigh amputation stump, is contaminated with the patient's faeces.[3]

Spores of clostridia have been known to remain dormant in healed wounds, and to have germinated following surgical intervention. This is particularly important with regard to tetanus, and immunization is always advisable before surgery is performed on old war and agricultural wounds.

Pathogenesis and lesions. Gas-gangrene is never due to infection by a single type of clostridial organism; it is the result of a combined assault by numerous saccharolytic and proteolytic organisms working together. The true pathogens, *Cl. welchii*, *Cl. septicum*, and *Cl. oedematiens*, germinate, and the powerful exotoxins which they liberate produce local tissue necrosis. At this stage the proteolytic saprophytes, such as *Cl. sporogenes* and *Cl. histolyticum*, flourish on the dead material, and break it down into putrid products.

If the wound is merely superficial, it will discharge foul-smelling fluid in which there are bubbles of gas, but if it is extensive enough to implicate the underlying muscles, the florid anaerobic myositis typical of gas-gangrene develops.

1. There is a rapidly progressive necrosis of muscle fibres due to the necrotizing exotoxins of the saccharolytic clostridia.

2. The muscle carbohydrate is fermented by these organisms. Lactic acid and gas (mostly hydrogen and carbon dioxide) are formed. This is the origin of the 'gas' in gas-gangrene. At this stage it is odourless.

3. There is rapid spread of infection due to the destruction of local tissue barriers (e.g. endomysium and perimysium) by the hyaluronidase and collagenase present as components of the exotoxins. A whole muscle bundle may be affected with great rapidity. Indeed, gas-gangrene resembles an invasive infection in the extent of its local spread, but the organisms remain localized to one area. They show no tendency towards blood-stream invasion, except occasionally just at the time of death.

4. As the infection spreads, so the necrosis increases, due not only to the liberated exotoxins but also to the effect of ischaemia engendered by the pressure of the gas and exudate on the surrounding blood vessels. The area is tense, oedematous, and crepitant, and the muscle is odourless and brick-red in colour.

5. Following in the wake of the extensive necrosis there is progressive putrefaction, which is brought about by the proteolytic clostridia. These thrive on

and decompose the dead muscle, which becomes greenish-black in colour. Necrosis with superadded putrefaction is called gangrene (p. 65), and in this way these saprophytes complete the evolution of 'gas-gangrene'. It is at this stage that the characteristically foul odour appears.

6. During this local process there is a profound general toxaemia due to the presence of circulating exotoxins. It is manifested by shock and a rapidly-developing haemolytic anaemia, which is secondary to the effect of the lecithinase on the red-cell envelopes. It is this toxaemia which brings about the death of the patient.

The local pathological effects of gas-gangrene are those of acute inflammation with much muscle necrosis and spreading oedema. Polymorph infiltration is not conspicuous, at least not while the process is advancing. In the oedema fluid there are large numbers of organisms. The absence of polymorphis is strange; perhaps the powerful exotoxins exert a negative chemotactic influence.

Treatment. In the treatment of gas-gangrene it is usual to give a polyvalent antiserum against the exotoxin of the three main pathogens, as well as penicillin or tetracycline. For prophylaxis in cases of grossly contaminated wounds penicillin has replaced antiserum therapy. There is no doubt, however, that a complete wound toilet is the most important aspect of prevention.

The use of hyperbaric oxygen also has a place in treatment. The patient is placed in a special pressurized chamber in which oxygen is breathed at 2 to 3 atmospheres pressure absolute for periods of 1 to 2 hours. The treatment requires specialized knowledge as well as apparatus, and oxygen is potentially dangerous to the lungs when in high concentration.

TETANUS

The spores of *Cl. tetani* not infrequently contaminate wounds, but as with the gas-gangrene organisms a reduced oxygen tension is essential for germination. The conditions conducive to tetanus infection are therefore similar to those already described. Quite often the degree of trauma appears to be very mild, because an insignificant punctured wound, like the prick of a contaminated thorn, has quite commonly been the site of origin of a fatal tetanus infection.

Exogenous infection has also resulted in *surgical tetanus*, i.e. the introduction of spores into a wound during the course of a surgical operation. For such spores to germinate they must be presented with a nidus where conditions are relatively anaerobic. Foreign materials embedded in the tissues, e.g. contaminated catgut, talc, or cotton-wool, provide the necessary nidus, and these are the causes of surgical tetanus, which nowadays is fortunately very rare indeed owing to modern methods of sterilization.

Although tetanus is now uncommon in the Western world, the situation in the poorer countries is quite different; in them it is a leading cause of death among hospital admissions. Among the ways by which spores may be introduced into the tissues of the unprotected population are injecting quinine (for malaria), ear piercing, and applying soil (or even dung) to the umbilicus of the newborn.

Clinical features. The incubation period varies from a few days to several weeks, and the shorter it is, the worse is the prognosis. Tetanus developing from wounds of the upper extremities, neck, and face is said to be more frequently lethal than that arising after injuries to the lower parts of the body.

Tetanus is clinically a disease of the central nervous system. The local lesion may be so mild that only very careful search will reveal it, yet the exotoxin produced may be sufficient to cause death.

After peripheral absorption, the toxin reaches the central nervous system probably by passing along the motor trunks; it acts by interfering with the inhibitory impulses reaching the motor neurons. This accounts for the generalized increase in tone, and also explains *local tetanus*. This is the early tendency to spasms of those muscles controlled by the same spinal segment as that supplying the area infected. At first there is stiffness, but this is soon followed by increase in muscular tone and spasms. Spasm of the masseter muscles results in trismus (inability to open the mouth, or 'lockjaw').

Spasm of the facial muscles produces the characteristic *risus sardonicus*. Finally generalized tetanic convulsions occur. Death is due to asphyxia following involvement of the respiratory muscles.

Prophylaxis. Since tetanus may occur following quite trivial wounds, by far the best method of prophylaxis is active immunization. This is carried out by a course of three injections of tetanus toxoid, a formolized preparation of the exotoxin adsorbed on to aluminium hydroxide or phosphate. The second injection is given about 8 weeks after the first, and the third from 6 to 12 months after the second. This regime should be carried out on all infants, and is mandatory for people whose occupation carries a hazard of injury. Booster doses are recommended at 10-year intervals.[4]

In cases of deep wounds, particularly those with much ragged laceration of tissue or of a punctured type, prophylaxis is essential, and the procedure to be adopted depends on whether there has been previous active immunization or not.

If the patient has had a complete basic course of toxoid injections or a booster within the past 5 years, he is adequately immune, and nothing further should be done apart from local treatment of the wound. If the period since the last dose of toxoid exceeds 5 years, but is less than 10 years, a booster dose should be given. If, however, the period exceeds 10 years, immediate passive immunization must be performed, since any residual immunity may not be adequate to protect the patient even under the stimulus of a booster dose. If there is no history of active immunization, the need for passive immunization is even stronger. Nowadays in many countries passive immunization is carried out with *human tetanus immunoglobulin*, also called *tetanus immune globulin* (*human*), 250 units of which are given intramuscularly. This rarely causes untoward effects. Nevertheless, adrenaline should always be available.

In those areas where human immune globulin is still unavailable, the much less satisfactory and more dangerous *horse antitetanic serum* (*ATS*) must be used. There is such a great danger of anaphylactic reactions occurring that a small subcutaneous test dose must be given first. If symptoms such as a drop in blood pressure, tachycardia, or dyspnoea develop, adrenaline must be administered immediately. Treatment will in any case have to be abandoned, since the manifestations indicate that antibodies are already present in the patient's serum and these will neutralize any horse ATS that is given. If there are no adverse reactions, the remainder of the ATS can be given safely, but its immunizing effect is soon vitiated, since the foreign serum is cleared from the patient's blood much more rapidly than the homologous human serum. There is in addition the danger of serum sickness.

At the same time that the passive immunization is given, a dose of toxoid is also administered, but into a different limb. In the case of a patient who has never been immunized actively before, this constitutes the first of the three immunizing doses; in one who has allowed the respective immunity to lapse for more than 10 years, this is a booster dose. Since the toxoid is of the adsorbed type and is administered at a distance from the immunoglobulin, its action is not interfered with by the initially high level of passive immunity.

Gram-negative anaerobic intestinal bacilli

The Gram-negative intestinal organisms of the genus *Bacteroides* form the bulk of organisms in the faeces, and are present also as part of the normal flora of the mouth and vagina. They are non-spore-bearing, strict anaerobes. They cause wound infection, pelvic abscesses, otitis media, puerperal sepsis, and oral infections (p. 66), but in these instances their role is probably secondary to infection with more pathogenic organisms. Their presence should be suspected in any infection associated with a foul odour. The organisms may invade the blood stream and cause septicaemia and Gram-negative shock.

GENERAL REFERENCES

Cruickshank R, Duguid J P, Marmion B P & Swain R H A 1973 Medical Microbiology, 12th edn. Vol 1. Churchill Livingstone, Edinburgh. An excellent accoount of medical microbiology, with the accent on laboratory findings and the properties of bacteria and viruses

Wilson G S & Miles A A 1975 Topley and Wilson's Principles of Bacteriology Virology and Immunity, 6th edn. Vols 1 and 2. Arnold, London. An authoritative account of the whole subject

Youmans G P, Paterson P Y & Sommers H M 1975 The Biological and Clinical Basis of Infectious Diseases. Saunders, Philadelphia. An excellent account of medical microbiolgoy and infectious disease, with particular emphasis on the clinical features

REFERENCES

1. Wannamaker L W 1970 Differences between streptococcal infections of the throat and of the skin. New England Journal of Medicine, 282: 23 and 78
2. Leading Article 1977 Group-B streptococci in the newborn. Lancet 1: 520
3. Leading Article 1969 Postoperative gas gangrene. British Medical Journal 2: 328
4. Smith J W G, Laurence D R & Evans D G 1975 Prevention of tetanus in the wounded. British Medical Journal 3: 453

15

Tuberculosis, leprosy, syphilis, actinomycosis, and some fungal diseases

Introduction
Whereas the pyogenic infections produce an overt acute inflammatory reaction which may or may not terminate in resolution, there are a great number of other organisms which tend to set up the condition of chronic inflammation. In these there is usually great tissue destruction so that resolution is impossible and a chronic course invariable. During the progress of these infections acute exacerbations of an exudative type are not infrequent, and these are usually due to allergy. Tuberculosis, syphilis, actinomycosis, and the fungal, protozoal, and helminthic infections all come into this category.

There are no histological features common to all these lesions; in tuberculosis and histoplasmosis the macrophage is the prominent cell type, in actinomycosis there is a polymorph infiltration, while in syphilis there is a peculiarly non-specific infiltration of lymphocytes and plasma cells. The helminthic diseases are often associated with heavy eosinophil accumulations.

In the acute bacterial infections the causal organisms appear to produce damage by some direct action often by producing powerful toxins. From the many organisms responsible for chronic infection no satisfactory toxin has been isolated. The generally held view is that their destructive effect is the result of the development of cell-mediated hypersensitivity.

In the acute bacterial infections a long-lasting immunity often ensues, and this is usually due to the presence of immunoglobulins in the circulation. In chronic infections immunoglobulins may also be present, but though they may be valuable in the diagnosis of the disease, e.g. in the serological diagnosis of syphilis, they do not produce immunity against the disease. They will not passively transfer immunity when transfused into another person. There is evidence in some of these infections, notably tuberculosis, that a degree of immunity is acquired after an infection, but this is mediated by lymphocytes rather than being due to the development of specific immunoglobulins.

The body's general reaction to these infections depends on whether they are localized or generalized. In the latter case, there is fever, and severe constitutional disturbances are common. The ESR is considerably elevated and there is hypergammaglobulinaemia of the polyclonal type (p. 433).

TUBERCULOSIS

There are at least five distinct strains of *Mycobacterium tuberculosis*: the human, bovine, murine, avian, and piscine. The *human* and *bovine* strains are potential human pathogens, and the *murine* strain ('vole bacillus'), which is endemic in wild voles, has been used as an alternative to BCG (Bacille-Calmette-Guérin vaccine introduced in France in 1908) in active immunization against tuberculosis. The *avian* and *piscine* strains are pathogenic to birds and fish respectively, and have little human importance. The bovine organism is excreted in the milk of infected cows, and it used to be the cause of much intestinal and tonsillar infection in childhood. Nowadays bovine tuberculosis, acquired by *ingestion*, has almost completely disappeared from the list of human diseases in civilized countries owing to the eradication of tuberculous herds and the pasteurization of milk. It therefore follows that to all intents and purposes nearly all tuberculosis is caused by the human strain. The mode of infection is by the *inhalation* of organisms present in fresh droplets or the dust of dried sputum expectorated from an open case of pulmonary tuberculosis. Pulmonary tuberculosis is by far the most common type of disease encountered. *Inoculation* of the skin from *post-mortem* material is so uncommon as to be little more than a curiosity, and a primary tuberculous lesion of the oral mucosa is nowadays exceedingly rare.

Bacteriology. *Myco. tuberculosis* is a slender bacillus about 3 μm long, non-motile and non-sporing. Its most conspicuous feature is its waxy content which makes it impermeable to the usual stains. It slowly takes up heated stains, e.g. carbol fuchsin in the Ziehl-Neelsen method, and then resists decolorization even by strong acids and alcohols, i.e. it is *acid-fast* and *alcohol-fast*. It is Gram-positive, but Gram-staining is not performed because the methyl violet penetrates only with great difficulty. It grows very slowly and then only on complex artificial media. The Löwenstein-Jensen medium is one that is commonly used, and it takes several weeks at 37°C in an aerobic atmosphere for any growth to appear.

In recent years organisms have been isolated from human lesions which differ from the typical human or bovine strain in cultural characteristics, antibiotic resistance, or animal pathogenicity. These are the *atypical*, or *anonymous*, mycobacteria. Some organisms have been isolated from lung lesions, and of these there is one group which is closely related to the avian tubercle bacillus. Other mycobacteria cause chronic skin infections;[1] for instance *Myco. ulcerans* causes Buruli ulcer in Uganda, and *Myco. marinum* (*balnei*) leads to a skin infection that is acquired either in swimming pools or from tropical fish tanks.

Myco. tuberculosis is very resistant to drying, and it can survive in dust for several months. It is, however, very sensitive to the effect of ultraviolet radiation, and is rapidly killed in sunlight.

Pathogenesis of the tuberculous lesion. The following sequence of events occurs when tubercle bacilli are introduced into the tissues.

1. A transient acute inflammatory reaction with an infiltration of polymorphs. These cells are rapidly destroyed by the organisms
2. A progressive infiltration of macrophages derived from the monocytes of the blood

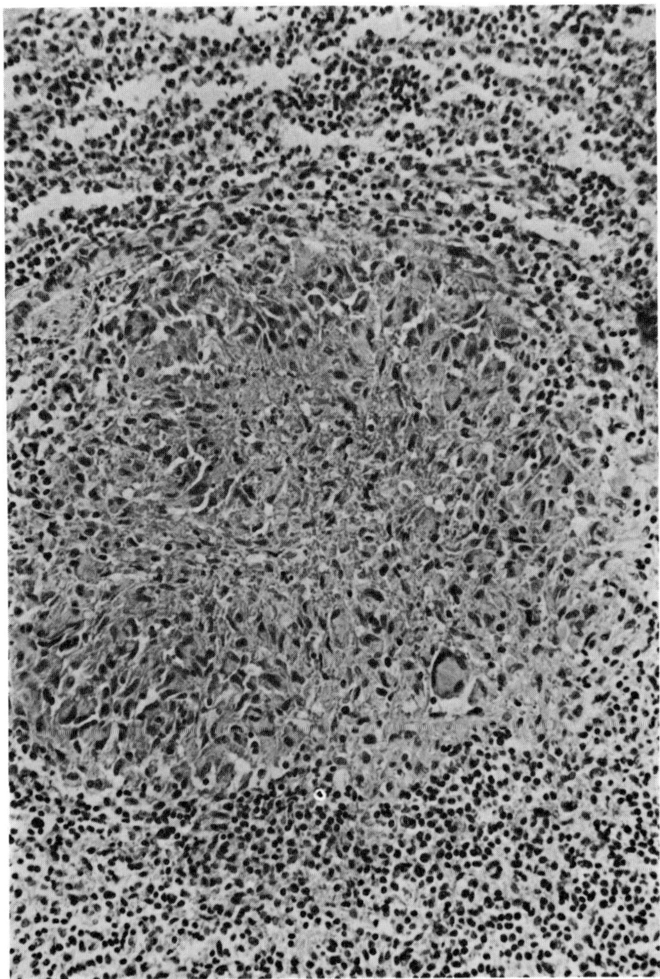

Fig. 15.1 A tubercle follicle. Note the central area of caseation surrounded by an ill-defined zone of epithelioid cells among which a Langhans giant cell is present. In the periphery there is a small round cell infiltration. × 120.

3. The macrophages phagocytose the bacilli. In a short time they change their character and become converted into epithelioid cells (p. 137)
4. Some macrophages, instead of becoming epithelioid cells, form giant cells which are usually of the Langhans type
5. Surrounding this mass of altered macrophages there is a diffuse zone of lymphocytes and fibroblasts
6. Within 10 to 14 days necrosis begins in the centre of this mass, which consists of altered macrophages and cells peculiar to the tissue of the part.

The *caseation* of tuberculosis is a very firm, cheesy type of coagulative necrosis, and it differs from other types of necrosis in that it has a very high content of lipid material, and shows little tendency towards autolysis. Histologically, caseation is

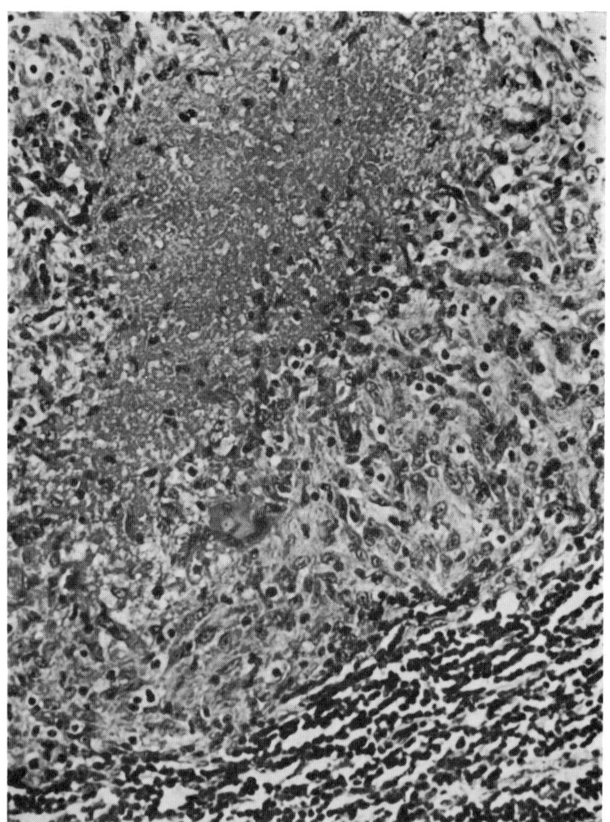

Fig. 15.2 A tubercle follicle. This is more advanced than the follicle in Fig. 15.1. There is a large area of caseation on the left-hand side, and it is surrounded by a dense zone of epithelioid cells in which a Langhans giant cell is present. At the right there is a small round cell infiltration. × 230.

associated with such great tissue disintegration that scarcely any structure is recognizable. Everything is merged into a brightly eosinophilic mass of amorphous debris.

Caseation is probably caused by the development of hypersensitivity to products of the bacilli, notably tuberculoprotein. It is not produced directly by toxins.

There is now produced the *tubercle follicle* (Figs. 15.1 and 15.2), which consists of a central mass of caseation surrounded by epithelioid and giant cells, which in turn are surrounded by a wide zone of small round cells. The appearance is characteristic of tuberculosis, though a similar picture is sometimes seen in the deep-seated fungal infections. For definite proof of a tuberculous origin organisms must be sought in the lesion.

Variations in the reaction to the tubercle bacillus. The common type of lesion described above is called *productive,* or *proliferative*, because its main components are cells rather than a fluid exudate. The acute caseous, and the chronic caseous, fibrocaseous, and fibroid types of tuberculosis are described in connexion with the lung (p. 219).

Another well-known type of lesion is the *exudative* form of tuberculosis. It is characterized by the outpouring of an inflammatory exudate rich in fibrin. There is a considerable infiltration of lymphocytes, and often many polymorphs are present, but epithelioid and giant cells are scanty. Exudative lesions are typical of tuberculosis of serous cavities. They are not necessarily more serious than productive ones.

The most serious type of lesion is *non-reactive tuberculosis*, in which there are extensive foci of caseation teeming with bacilli but showing virtually no cellular reaction around them. This type of disease is seen in patients with immunological deficiency and subjected to overwhelming infection: thus it may occur as a complication of leukaemia. The tuberculin test is usually negative in this type of tuberculosis.

The fate of the tuberculous lesion. The caseous focus may either cease to progress and heal by fibrosis, or it may soften and spread.

The hallmark of healing is fibrous tissue, and this is produced by the proliferating fibroblasts at the periphery of the lesion. In due course the area of caseation may be replaced by a solid fibrous nodule. Sometimes only a ring of fibrous tissue forms around the periphery, while the central mass of caseation undergoes slow *dystrophic calcification.* In this calcareous nodule organisms may still survive, and years later, when the resistance of the host breaks down, they may become active again.

The hallmark of activity is caseation and softening. If the lesion is spreading, bacilli are carried by macrophages into the surrounding lymphatics and tissue spaces. There they settle and set up satellite follicles, which by fusing with the primary enlarging lesion, produce a *conglomerate tubercle follicle.* Caseous material does not soften rapidly, due possibly to the presence of phosphatides that inhibit autolytic enzymes. Sometimes, however, *liquefaction* does occur, and this is attended by serious consequences.

There is no really satisfactory explanation for this softening. There is no doubt that it is associated with spread, and that the liquefied debris contains many bacilli, but it is not known whether this multiplication of organisms is the cause or the result of the softening. It has been suggested that the liquefaction is due to secondary infection, but this is untrue. Pyogenic infection may certainly complicate a tuberculous lesion, but liquefaction often occurs in the absence of such infection. The element of hypersensitivity is probably of considerable importance.

Once liquefaction has occurred, the debris contains large numbers of tubercle bacilli, and the whole is often called a *cold abscess.* Unlike a pyogenic abscess there are comparatively few cells present, and most of these are disintegrating. The term 'pus' is therefore inapplicable, as there are no pus cells. The term 'cold abscess' is equally inapplicable. In practice it is reserved exclusively for tuberculous lesions, even though in fact the suppurative lesions of actinomycosis may also be 'cold', as neither the heat, pain, nor redness seen in acute pyogenic infection is a marked feature of them. The liquefied debris ('pus') tracks towards a free surface and discharges there. In a lesion of the lung rupture soon occurs into a bronchus, and the disease spreads to other parts of the lung; much infectious material is also coughed up. A tuberculous abscess is lined by tuberculous granulation tissue. This consists of systems of tubercle follicles irregularly disposed in a mass of newly-formed fibrous tissue which is heavily infiltrated with lymphocytes and macrophages.

Whenever a tuberculous abscess opens to the exterior, the disease becomes more serious, firstly because of its *open*, infectious character, and secondly because the tubercle bacillus is an aerobic organism and proliferates much more profusely in an atmosphere of air. These features are well illustrated in the open, cavitating type of pulmonary tuberculosis.

Spread of tuberculosis in the body

The principles differ in no significant way from those of most other infections.

Local spread. The spread by macrophages has already been described.

Spread in serous cavities is seen in the diffuse pleurisy that may complicate lung lesions, the localized peritonitis found in cases of tuberculous salpingitis, and in tuberculous meningitis.

Spread along epithelial-lined surfaces is typified by the intrabronchial spread of tuberculosis that occurs when sputum is inhaled into adjacent lung segments. If the sputum is coughed up, it can produce *tuberculous laryngitis.* Tuberculous infection occasionally occurs on the tongue, lips, or gingivae. The ulcer so formed has an irregular outline with undermined edges. The most frequent lesion is an ulceration of the tongue, and the necrotizing tuberculous infection can spread to involve the pharynx, lips, and adjacent skin (*tuberculosis cutis orificialis*). The laryngeal and oral lesions are extremely painful, and fortunately are now rare.

If sputum is swallowed, the bacilli may infect the ileo-caecal area of the bowel and lead to tuberculous enteritis.

Lymphatic spread. This is a continuation of local spread. The result is a regional tuberculous lymphadenitis.

Blood spread. Organisms may reach the blood stream in one of two ways:

1. *As an extension of lymphatic involvement.* In an overwhelming infection the organisms enter the blood stream to produce *miliary tuberculosis.* The lungs, spleen, liver, kidney, and to a lesser extent other organs, are seeded with tubercle bacilli which produce numerous follicles about 1 mm in diameter. Clinically the patient is seriously ill and has a high fever. Sometimes only a few organisms enter the blood stream, and become lodged in various organs to produce metastatic lesions (see below).

2. *Direct involvement of a vein.* Blood spread also occurs when caseous hilar nodes directly implicate the adjacent pulmonary vein. If there is a discharge of large numbers of organisms into the blood stream, miliary tuberculosis occurs, but the lungs are often spared.

Tuberculous meningitis is almost invariably present in miliary tuberculosis, and is due either to involvement of the choroid plexus, or else to a small subcortical lesion (*Rich's focus*) rupturing into the subarachnoid space. Miliary tuberculosis is much more common in young children than in adults.

Metastatic lesions. In older children and adults it sometimes happens that only a few bacilli invade the systemic circulation. These may be destroyed by the RE system, or else become lodged in various sites to give rise to metastatic disease. Such a lesion may progress immediately to produce clinical effects, or else remain quiescent, only to undergo reactivation years later. This type of lesion is called *local metastatic tuberculosis*, and it accounts for most of the disease seen in surgical practice. Organs sometimes involved in this way are the *kidneys, adrenals, uterine tubes, epididymes*, and the *bones, joints*, and *tendon sheaths*.

Morphology of tuberculous infections

It has been recognized for a long time that the behaviour of tuberculous infection is quite different in children as compared to adults. At all ages the lung is the organ principally affected.

Childhood. In childhood the primary focus (*Ghon focus*) is a small wedge-shaped area situated at the periphery of the lung field. This subpleural focus may heal and produce no clinical illness, or else the infection spreads to the hilar lymph nodes, which become greatly enlarged and caseous. A conspicuous *primary complex* is the result. It either heals and calcifies, or else it spreads and the child dies of *miliary tuberculosis with meningitis*.

In days gone by the primary lesion was frequently in the pharynx, tonsil, gingiva, or palate. It appeared as a painless ulcer and was acquired by the ingestion of contaminated milk. Sometimes the primary lesion was in the oesophagus or small intestine and usually escaped clinical attention. In most cases the primary lesion was small and the major feature was the enormous enlargement of the regional lymph nodes—*mesenteric* or *cervical*. In all childhood lesions the feature in common is the small size of the primary focus and the tendency to extensive lymph-node involvement with the danger of spread to the blood stream and a fatal termination.

Adult life. In adult life the pulmonary focus is almost always apical or subapical (*Assmann focus*). The lesion either heals, or else it progresses, softens, and produces a cavity. Haemoptysis (the coughing up of blood), chronic cough, weight loss, low-grade fever, and a raised ESR are the main clinical features. Depending on the resistance of the patient there is a tendency for either fibrosis or extensive cavitation to occur. In severe cases great destruction of lung tissue eventually results (Fig. 15.3). A large cavity may be formed, and a vessel in its wall may be eroded, leading to severe haemoptysis. At any time caseous debris may be inhaled into other bronchi to produce tuberculous bronchopneumonia. This may occur on a small scale and result in extension of the disease, but if widespread it causes rapid caseation of a great area of lung tissue. The latter is associated with intense hypersensitivity, and the disease remains localized to the lungs. Lymph-node involvement is inconspicuous, and blood-spread dissemination is unusual. Death is the result of the local lung lesion which is called *acute caseous bronchopneumonia* ('galloping consumption'). There are severe constitutional symptoms due probably to the effects of hypersensitivity—these are described clinically as toxaemia, but no definite toxins have been isolated.

Chronic tuberculosis. Here the immunity of the host is adequate to cause some destruction of the bacilli, and healing by repair (fibrosis) occurs side by side with caseous destruction. Three types of chronic pulmonary tuberculosis are recognized: caseous, fibro-caseous, and fibroid, depending on the relative degrees of caseation and fibrosis. In longstanding fibroid tuberculosis the lung may be converted into a contracted mass of dense fibrous tissue, in which there may be little recognizable evidence of active tuberculous infection. Bronchiectasis is a

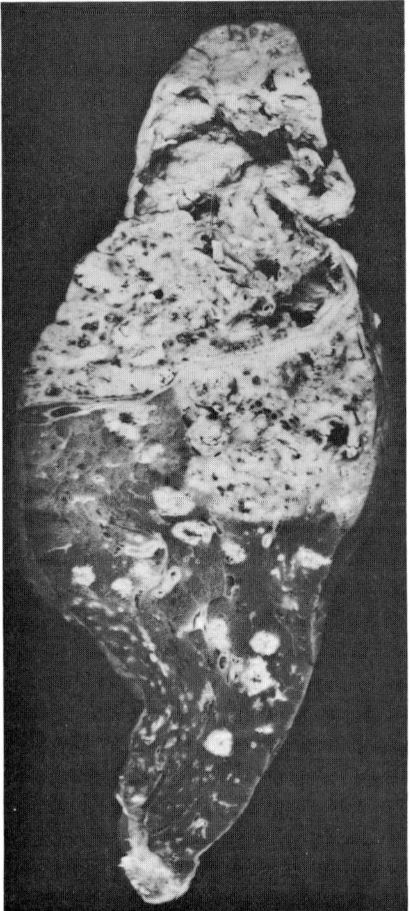

Fig. 15.3 Caseous tuberculosis of lung. The entire upper lobe and part of the apex of the lower lobe have been destroyed by caseous tuberculosis with extensive cavitation. Discrete areas of infection are present in the remainder of the lower lobe. (R37.1, *Reproduced by permission of the President and Council of the Royal College of Surgeons of England.*)

frequent complication of this type of disease, which is characterized clinically by dyspnoea, respiratory failure, and right-sided heart failure.

A similar type of pathogenesis occurs in other organs in the adult. Tuberculous enteritis, now a rare disease, is due to the swallowing of infected sputum in open pulmonary tuberculosis, and is characterized by a spreading ulceration of the wall of the ileum.

Another type of cutaneous tuberculosis, apart from tuberculosis cutis orificialis (p. 218), is *lupus vulgaris*. It nearly always involves the face with the ears and nose being commonly affected. The dermis shows a typical non-caseating tuberculoid reaction and the disease spreads by continuity. The course of lupus vulgaris is prolonged, and ultimately great tissue destruction and scarring result. Nevertheless, few organisms can be found in the lesions and the disease appears to be an infection in a person with considerable immunity. The source of the infection

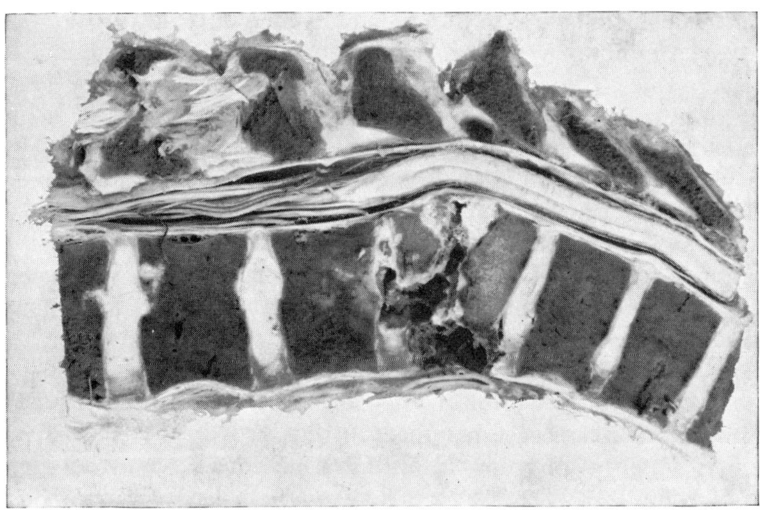

Fig. 15.4 Tuberculosis of spinal column (Pott's disease of the spine). There has been destruction of two adjacent vertebral bodies and the intervening intervertebral disc. The result has been collapse of the vertebrae, acute angulation of the spine, compression of the cord, and paraplegia. (S.49a.48, *Reproduced by permission of the President and Council of the Royal College of Surgeons of England.*)

may be from a previous pulmonary lesion, but often no other active tuberculosis can be detected.

Skeletal tuberculosis usually starts in the metaphyseal area of a bone, and it causes great local destruction. Unlike pyogenic osteomyelitis it destroys the epiphyseal cartilage with ease, and soon the neighbouring joint is affected. When softening occurs a 'cold abscess' is produced. Tuberculosis of the spine used to be quite common (Pott's disease), and was responsible for collapse of the affected vertebrae and great deformity (Fig. 15.4). Tuberculous 'pus' sometimes entered the psoas muscle sheath and tracked down, discharging on to the skin of the groin below the inguinal ligament.

The feature that all these adult lesions have in common is the tendency to extensive local destruction without much lymphatic involvement.

It is traditionally believed that the adult lesion is always secondary to a 'primary' lesion acquired during childhood, and that the difference in course of the two infections can be explained on the basis of allergy and immunity acquired during the 'primary' infection. Just as in the Koch phenomenon (p. 188), where the second dose of organisms remained localized and did not spread to the regional nodes, so it is that the 'secondary' adult lesion remains localized to the lungs and does not spread further afield.

It is becoming increasingly apparent that more and more young adults are Mantoux negative, a proof that they have not had tuberculosis in childhood, yet the incidence of the 'primary' Ghon type of lesion with massive hilar lymphadenopathy is not increasing in the adult population. It seems that even primary infections in adults start at the apex of the lung and do not produce much lymphatic involvement. Furthermore, there are very definite differences between the adult lesion and the Koch phenomenon. There is lymph-node involvement in the adult, though it is of microscopic extent only, and the lesion shows no particular tendency to heal as in the second infection of the tuberculous guinea-pig. The essential difference in behaviour between childhood and adult lesions appears to be due to tissue maturation; the older the patient the less is the tendency towards gross lymph-node involvement. The effect of a previous infection as an additional modifying factor cannot be excluded, but it is unjustifiable to label all adult lesions as secondary. The terms childhood and adult tuberculosis are much more accurate than 'primary' and 'secondary' tuberculosis.

The source of the organisms causing adult-type tuberculosis has been the centre of much discussion in the past. The pulmonary lesions were regarded as due either to *reactivation* of a quiescent primary lesion or to the development of a new lesion produced by a *reinfection* from some external source. In the past reinfection was probably of great importance, but nowadays it seems that adult-type lesions are themselves primary infections. In the case of other organs, e.g. kidney and bone, it is almost certain that tuberculosis is due to the reactivation of small lesions which were produced during a bacteraemic phase of a previous primary infection.

Factors determining the response of tissues to tuberculous infection

It is apparent that sometimes there is healing by fibrosis of a small tuberculous focus, and on other occasions there is caseation, liquefaction, and even a rapidly spreading fatal disease. The factors that determine the tissue response are:

1. The dose and virulence of the organism
2. The innate and acquired resistance of the body.

Innate immunity is of great importance in tuberculosis but is poorly understood (p. 175).

Age and Sex. During the first 5 years of life the body's resistance is poor and the mortality rate is high. From 5 to 15 years resistance is at its peak, but it breaks down during the early adult period of 15 to 30 years, particularly in women. After the age of 30 years resistance is quite high, but it breaks down again in old age, particularly in men.[2]

General health of the individual. *Malnourished people* in prison camps or slums have a poor resistance, and, of course, the overcrowding germane to such conditions predisposes to the rapid spread of disease throughout the community. Psychological stress and chronic debilitating diseases also lower the resistance. In this respect *diabetes mellitus* is particularly notorious in predisposing to a rapidly spreading type of infection. So also is administration of *glucocorticoids*. These drugs should be used with great caution in patients known to have, or to have had, tuberculosis.

Occupational factors. Those whose work carries the hazard of atmospheric pollution by particulate *silica*, e.g. tunnellers, miners, and quarrymen, arc liable to a spreading type of disease. *Asbestosis* is a less serious predisposing factor.

Acquired immunity and hypersensitivity. The effect of previous infection with tuberculosis was first described by Koch using guinea-pigs. Undoubtedly a primary infection with tubercle bacilli induces a state of immunity which is accompanied by delayed-type hypersensitivity to tuberculoprotein.

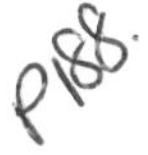

The really inscrutable feature of the Koch phenomenon is the immunity to the second infection. It is a very important consideration, because on it depends the advocacy of protective active immunization with BCG vaccine. It is clear that the immunity produced is in no way as effective as that seen in diphtheria or smallpox following an attack of the disease. It is certain that whatever type of immunity is produced, it is not due to specific immunoglobulins. The serum of a cured patient will not passively immunize another patient, as in diphtheria or measles. In fact, the serum of a tuberculous patient contains agglutinating, precipitating, and complement-fixing antibodies, but these have no protective action against the organism.

The acquired immunity in tuberculosis is cell mediated: the altered lymphocytes enable the macrophages to destroy the bacilli more effectively than they do in a primary infection. The macrophages of rabbits previously immunized with BCG, when grown in tissue culture, withstand parasitization by tubercle bacilli, whereas inactive macrophages from unimmunized animals have no such power. The precise nature of the cellular changes is unknown. In addition, the sensitized lymphocytes liberate lymphokines in the vicinity of the tubercle bacilli; these by inhibiting the random movement of the macrophages probably augment their local phagocytic activity. It is possible that the lymphokines have a directly lethal effect on the organisms as well.

The relationship between hypersensitivity and immunity has been much debated. Some authorities regard them as distinct and separable components, with hypersensitivity, by causing caseation and necrosis, being a harmful factor. On the other hand, it has been argued that the acute inflammation which hypersensitivity induces, does serve to bring many macrophages into contact with the bacilli very rapidly, and these cells are the essential agents in destroying the bacilli. Whatever may be the truth, it is generally acknowledged that so far as BCG vaccination is concerned, the benefits of immunity more than outweigh any possible harmful effects of hypersensitivity. BCG vaccination is usually offered to those whose profession brings them into contact with the disease and who are tuberculin negative.[3,4]

It should finally be noted that not only is the acquired immunity of partial degree, but also that it seems to have no effect in overcoming the primary infection. Even in Koch's phenomenon, though the second dose is overcome successfully, the animal still dies of its first infection. This indicates that an important mechanism of the immunity is the localization of the organism at a very early stage of the infection.

Treatment

Treatment with the chemotherapeutic agents streptomycin, para-aminosalicylic acid (PAS), isonicotinic acid hydrazide, ethambutol, and rifampicin has greatly improved the prognosis of tuberculosis. Nevertheless, the great improvements in social and economic conditions combined with facilities for early diagnosis have played the major role in the abolition of tuberculosis as an important cause of death in civilized countries.

SARCOIDOSIS[5,6]

Although of unknown aetiology it is convenient to consider sarcoidosis at this point, since its histological features closely resemble those of tuberculosis. The

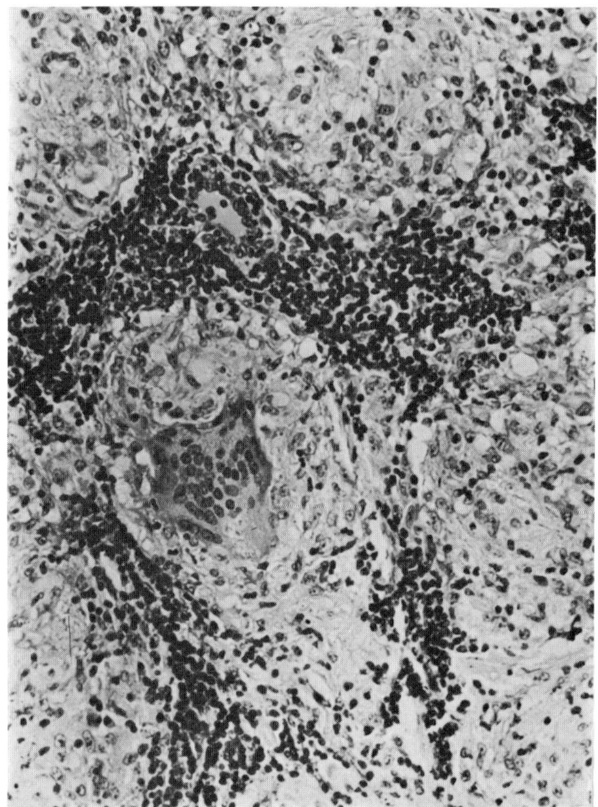

Fig. 15.5 Sarcoidosis. In this lymph node there are semi-confluent follicles of epithelioid cells without central caseation. A large giant cell is present, and is unusual in resembling that found in foreign-body reactions rather than a typical Langhans cell. × 230.

unit of sarcoidosis is a discrete follicle composed of plump epithelioid cells, in the midst of which a few giant cells may be found. The follicle is surrounded by a rim of lymphocytes and is therefore very like a tubercle follicle, but differs in that there is rarely any central caseation (Fig. 15.5).

Sarcoidosis is a generalized disease and affects the lungs (producing miliary lesions), the bones (especially those of the hands), the skin, eye, spleen, liver, lymph nodes, salivary glands, heart, and nervous system.

The lesions tend to heal with fibrosis, and in certain situations, e.g. the eye, brain, and lung, they can produce serious effects. The disease is not uncommon in Northern European countries.

LEPROSY

Introduction

Leprosy is caused by *Mycobacterium leprae*, which was one of the first bacteria to be incriminated as a cause of human disease and will probably be the last to be cultured in an artificial medium. Investigation of the disease, in particular the sensitivity of the organism to antibiotics, has been greatly hindered by our inability to grow the organism and the great difficulty encountered in infecting laboratory animals. So far, the organism has only been grown in the foot pads of mice and in the armadillo. In practice, pathological diagnosis depends on demonstrating the organism by Ziehl-Neelsen staining of smears or sections.

Although the disease is of great antiquity, it is uncertain whether the accounts in the Old Testament in fact describe leprosy. There seems little doubt that the disease was present in the Middle East before the birth of Christ, and during the Middle Ages it was common in Europe, having been introduced there by the returning Crusaders. The disease has now retreated from Europe and is endemic in the Far East, India, the Middle East, Africa, and Central and South America. The disease was probably introduced into the United States by the Negro slaves, and is still endemic in some southern states and Hawaii.

Mode of infection

The mode of infection is unknown, but the disease is probably spread by contaminated nasal secretions. The disease is generally acquired in childhood, and the first lesion is an insignificant scaly skin patch. This *indeterminate lesion* may heal spontaneously or progress to one of the two major forms of the disease.

Types of leprosy

Tuberculoid leprosy. This type of leprosy occurs in individuals with a high state of immunity. The skin lesions consist of one or several *well-demarcated* papules or plaques, which are associated with local nerves, causing the skin of the area to become anaesthetic. Microscopically the skin and involved nerves show a non-caseating tuberculoid reaction similar to that seen in early tuberculosis. Lepra bacilli are extremely sparse.

Lepromatous leprosy. In lepromatous leprosy the lesions consist of multiple macules, papules, and plaques, which are of *widespread distribution* and tend to be *symmetrical.* The lesions are *poorly delineated*, and often there is a diffuse infiltration of the skin. Microscopically the dermis is diffusely packed with macrophages, which are themselves stuffed with lepra bacilli. Since the lesions tend to occur in the cold parts of the body, the hands and face are particularly affected. The diffuse thickening of the skin of the face leads to a lion-like appearance (leonine facies). There is diffuse involvement of nerves, so that symmetrical peripheral neuritis is characteristic.

In lepromatous leprosy, the nasal mucosa is also infiltrated by bacteria-laden macrophages, and the destruction of the nasal bones leads to the characteristic appearance (Fig. 15.6). Because the nasal secretions contain a large number of bacilli, it is probable that this is the manner by which the disease is disseminated.

In lepromatous leprosy there is defective T-cell immunity, causing the lepromin reaction to be negative. As if to compensate for this, there is an overproduction of immunoglobulins, and the hyperimmunoglobulinaemia is associated with *acute reactional phases* that are a great hazard in leprosy. Exacerbation of the skin lesions, iridocyclitis, orchitis, nerve damage, fever, prostration, and death can occur during these acute phases, which may either develop spontaneously or be precipitated by ill-advised vigorous treatment. The

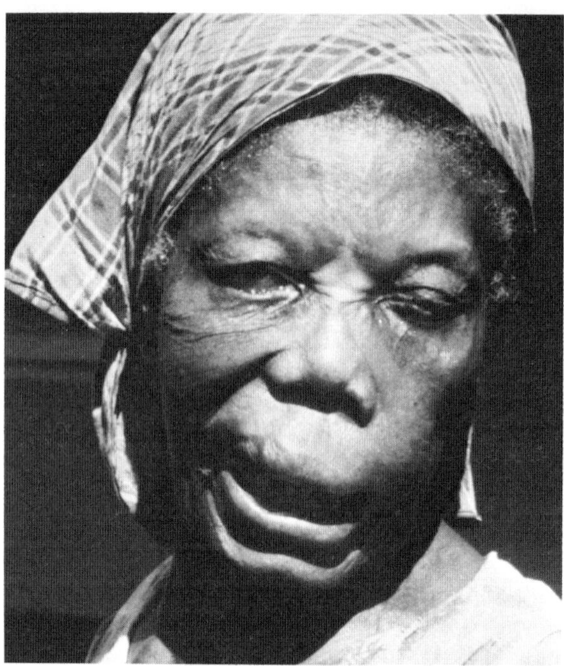

Fig. 15.6 Leprosy. This patient is a voluntary resident of a leper colony in the Caribbean. Years before this picture was taken she was found to be suffering from lepromatous leprosy, and has been taking a sulphone or other antileprous drug ever since. Her condition is not now infectious; indeed, she may be completely free of the lepra bacillus, although this is difficult to prove. Nevertheless, she exhibits some of the devastating effects of the disease. Inflammation of the nasal mucosa (rhinitis) accompanied by destruction of the nasal bones has resulted in collapse of the bridge of the nose. Repeated attacks of iritis have led to glaucoma and cataract so that the sight of both eyes has been gravely affected. The left eye is completely blind, but the right is able to detect movement and the difference between light and dark. Because the patient has a left-sided facial nerve paralysis, the muscles of the left side of the face do not move. This can be detected by the drooping of the left eyelid, and the failure of the left side of the mouth to move backwards when the patient smiles or talks.

damage is probably mediated by the deposition of immune complexes with antigen excess (see Ch. 13). The large number of bacilli present in the lesions provide the antigen for the formation of these complexes.

Leprosy provides a fascinating example of the effects that an immune response has on the pattern of an infection. In the tuberculoid type, T-cell immunity is well developed, few bacilli are present in the lesions, and the inflammatory response is characterized by a tuberculoid reaction with plentiful Langhans giant cells. The pattern of reaction is similar to that encountered in the common type of tuberculous infection. In lepromatous leprosy, on the other hand, T-cell function is in abeyance and vast numbers of bacilli are present in the lesions, which are characterized by a diffuse infiltration by macrophages ('lepra cells'). Occasionally an analogous situation is encountered in tuberculosis. In the terminal stages in miliary tuberculosis, the tuberculin test becomes negative, and the lesions teem with bacilli.

Borderline or dimorphous leprosy. Cases occur in which the clinical and pathological features are between the two polar types of tuberculoid and lepromatous leprosy. In these borderline cases, acute reactional states are particularly common, and the disease tends to terminate in one of the two major forms, often the lepromatous type.

Leprosy is a chronic disease that is now amenable to treatment with a number of chemotherapeutic drugs. The sulphones are the mainstay of these drugs, because they are not only effective but also readily available and cheap.

SYPHILIS[7]

Bacteriology and Serology. The causative organism *Treponema pallidum* is a delicate spiral filament, or spirochaete, about 10 μm long. It cannot be stained by the usual techniques, and is demonstrable in exudates by means of dark-ground illumination. In histological sections it is stained by special silver impregnation methods.

The organism has never been cultured artificially even in fertile eggs or tissue-culture systems, nor does animal inoculation play any part in the diagnosis of the disease. In fact, rabbits develop acute orchitis after the intratesticular inoculation of the organisms. This method is used to obtain a supply of spirochaetes for such procedures as the *Treponema pallidum* immobilization (TPI) test. An allied organism, the Reiter strain of spirochaete, can be cultured *in vitro*, and is used as a source of antigen in the Reiter protein complement fixation (RPCF) test.

During the course of infection a patient develops immunoglobulins of great importance. Two groups are recognized:

The Wassermann antibody. This antibody fixes complement in the presence of a phosphatide extract of heart muscle (cardiolipin). This antigen is used in the *standard tests for syphilis*, namely the *Wassermann complement-fixation test* and the *flocculation tests*, of which the *Kahn* and the *Venereal Disease Research Laboratory (VDRL) tests* are the most widely used. They are more sensitive than the complement fixation test but not more specific. Since the antigen can hardly be considered specific for the organism of syphilis, it is not surprising that a positive reaction is sometimes found in non-treponemal diseases, notably trypanosomiasis, leprosy, malaria, infectious mononucleosis, mycoplasmal pneumonia, and systemic lupus erythematosus. Pregnancy too, is occasionally associated with a false-positive reaction. The tests are positive in other treponemal diseases, e.g. yaws.

Treponemal antibody. The second group of antibodies which is formed reacts with treponemal protein. Some antibody activity is directed against protein common to several treponemes (group protein), whereas other antibodies are more specific. The following tests are employed.

Reiter protein complement-fixation (RPCF) test. This test is more specific than the standard test for syphilis and therefore gives fewer false positive results.

Treponema pallidum immobilization (TPI) test. When positive serum is incubated with a concentrated suspension of *Tr. pallidum* in the presence of complement, it leads to the immobilization of the spirochaetes as viewed under dark-ground illumination. The TPI test becomes positive a little later in the disease than do the standard tests, but it remains positive for the remainder of the patient's life with the exception of some cases in which the disease has been successfully treated early in its course. Being more specific, it is useful when there is a suspected false serology. Unfortunately the test is technically difficult to perform and needs a supply of pathogenic organisms.

Fluorescent treponemal antibody (FTA) test. Specific antibody adheres to *Treponema pallidum* and can be detected by applying fluorescein-labelled anti-human γ-globulin. Two antibodies are involved; one is group specific, reacting with *Tr. pallidum* and other treponemes, but the other is specific for *Tr. pallidum.* Both are formed in syphilis. The group specific antibody can be absorbed by Reiter treponemes, and the test (FTA-ABS) is as sensitive and specific as the TPI test. These two specific tests are performed only when the standard tests are equivocal, or when the results do not correlate with the clinical features of the case. No test is absolutely reliable, and none can distinguish between syphilis and yaws.*

Treponemal passive haemagglutination (TPHA) test. Formalised, tanned sheep red cells sensitized with material from disrupted *Tr. pallidum* are used as the antigen. The test is an alternative to the TPI and FTA-ABS tests.

Acquired syphilis

Apart from congenital syphilis, the infection is almost always acquired venereally, although on rare occasions it is transmitted by a blood transfusion, and a primary lesion can occur on the finger of an unfortunate dentist or physician who examines an infected patient. Nevertheless, considering how frequent it must be for the hands to come in contact with the treponema, the rarity of cutaneous chancres is curious. Evidentally the organism cannot easily infect the skin. Unlike the tubercle bacillus, *Tr. pallidum* is very rapidly destroyed both in water and by drying. Intimate direct contact is therefore necessary for infection to occur. The spirochaete is one of the most invasive organisms known. Once it penetrates the surface integument, it spreads along the lymphatics to the regional lymph nodes, and finally reaches the blood stream within a matter of hours. There is therefore systemic dissemination long before any local manifestation appears.

The disease is divisible into three stages with a latent period between each of them.

Primary syphilis. The typical lesion of primary syphilis is the *chancre*, which usually appears on the genital region 2 to 4 weeks after infection. It is an indurated nodule which breaks down to form an ulcer. It is characteristically painless, and is accompanied by a considerable *regional lymphadenitis* which is also painless. Extragenital chancres are not uncommon, e.g. around the anus in homosexuals, and on the lips, tip of tongue, tonsils, gingiva, or other part of the oral cavity.

The histological appearance is quite non-specific, consisting merely of a dense infiltration of lymphocytes, plasma cells, and a few macrophages in the dermis.

Even without treatment the chancre gradually heals, usually with little scarring.

* Yaws is a disease which has much in common with syphilis and is caused by *Treponema pertenue.* It is frequent in some tropical countries, and is not venereal in origin. The primary lesion is extra-genital, and this is followed by a secondary and tertiary stage. In the latter there are destructive skin and bone lesions, and these may affect the face and nose. Significant cardiovascular and central-nervous-system involvement is rare compared with syphilis. It is possible that *Tr. pallidum* developed as a variant of *Tr. pertenue* which became adapted to venereal transmission.

The fact that the spirochaetes become disseminated in the blood stream long before there is any local lesion suggests that hypersensitivity plays an important part in the process. The chancre is not comparable with a boil, for it is not a local inflammatory reaction tending to limit the infection. A possible explanation is that sensitizing antibodies are first formed in the cells at the site of entry and in the regional lymph nodes. During the incubation period the spirochaetes multiply in the RE system, and when liberated react with the sensitized tissue. This would explain the chancre and the lymphadenopathy quite well.

At a later stage the other tissues of the body become sensitized, and then the generalized lesions of secondary syphilis become manifest.

Diagnosis. The laboratory diagnosis depends on demonstrating spirochaetes in the exudate from the chancre by dark-ground illumination.

About 2 weeks after the appearance of the chancre, antibodies first appear in the blood. Blood serology should never be neglected in practice.

Secondary syphilis. Within 2 to 3 months after exposure the disease becomes clinically generalized. When syphilis was first introduced into Europe, this stage was severe enough to warrant the name, 'the great pox'. Nowadays it is much milder, and is characterized by the development of a skin eruption. This is widespread, symmetrical, usually not pruritic, and in addition to being present on the trunk is also seen on the face, palms, and soles. The lesions are generally erythematous papules, but may be of any type except vesicular or bullous. Other lesions are less common. In moist areas, e.g. the vulva, anal region, and axillae, plateau-like excrescences are formed (*condylomata*). In the buccal mucosa the flat lesions are called *mucous patches*, and shallow, serpiginous areas of ulceration also occur (*snail-track ulcers*). The muco-cutaneous lesions may be accompanied by constitutional symptoms which include low-grade fever, myalgia, moderate anaemia, iridocyclitis, and a generalized painless lymphadenopathy. Histologically the secondary lesions show a non-specific inflammatory infiltrate by lymphocytes, plasma cells, and macrophages. The secondary lesions resolve spontaneously and do not form scars. This is the phase of maximum infectivity; spirochaetes ooze out of the condylomata and mucous patches.

Diagnosis. The standard serological tests are always positive in overt secondary syphilis. If a negative result is reported in the face of strong clinical indications of syphilis, the *prozone phenomenon should be suspected* (p. 154), and the test repeated with suitable dilutions so that the titre of antibody can be measured. Organisms can be demonstrated in the exudates from mucous and cutaneous lesions.

The occurrence of the *Jarisch-Herxheimer reaction* is confirmatory evidence of a correct diagnosis of syphilis.[8] It consists of a transient episode of fever and malaise with an accentuation of the skin eruption within 12 hours of the commencement of treatment—generally an injection of penicillin. The reaction is presumed to be due to the massive release of bacterial antigens as the organisms are killed.

Tertiary syphilis. Local destructive lesions of a truly chronic inflammatory nature may appear 2 to 3 years after infection and continue to erupt sporadically for at least 20 years. Such lesions are rarely encountered nowadays: this is a tribute to the efficacy of penicillin, for syphilis is as common today as ever and indeed in some parts of the world is on the increase. The lesions of tertiary syphilis are

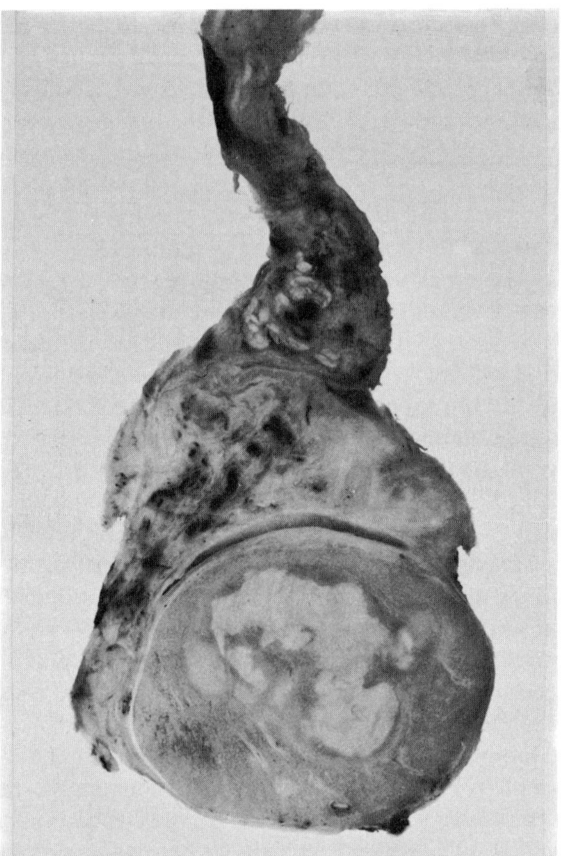

Fig. 15.7 Gumma of testis. The testis is replaced by an ill-defined area of gummatous necrosis, but the epididymis and spermatic cord are not affected. (EM6.1, *Reproduced by permission of the President and Council of the Royal College of Surgeons of England.*)

presumably due to marked hypersensitivity, since spirochaetes are few and the reaction to them is excessive. Two forms of lesions occur: *localized gummata* and *diffuse inflammatory lesions* characterized by parenchymatous destruction.

Localized gummata. The *gumma* is the classical lesion of tertiary syphilis. It is usually solitary, and consists of a large area of coagulative necrosis very similar in appearance to caseation, except that the tissue destruction is usually not quite so complete. Details of architecture can therefore still be faintly distinguished amid the debris. It is surrounded by an extensive zone of lymphocytes, plasma cells, and macrophages. Proliferating fibroblasts are plentiful, and much reparative fibrous tissue is laid down. Giant cells are much less numerous than in tuberculosis. The arteries in the vicinity show marked endarteritis obliterans.

Gummata are particularly liable to occur in the liver, testes (Fig. 15.7), subcutaneous tissues, and in bones, notably the tibia, ulna, clavicle, calvaria of skull, and the nasal and palatal bones. The destruction produced by gummata is exemplified by the perforated palate and the saddle-shaped nasal deformity seen in tertiary syphilis and characteristically in congenital syphilis.

Diffuse lesions. The really baneful effects of tertiary syphilis fall on the cardiovascular and nervous systems. In the former it is the thoracic aorta which usually suffers first. An infiltration of lymphocytes and plasma cells accumulates around the vasa vasorum of the tunica adventitia, and soon spreads inwards into the tunica media, where it destroys much of the elastic tissue which is essential for the integrity of the aorta.

The *syphilitic aortitis* that results weakens the wall so much that aneurysmal dilatation eventually ensues. Sometimes the disease spreads down to the aortic ring, which dilates and leads to aortic regurgitation. If the ostia of the coronary arteries are occluded at the same time, there is severe myocardial ischaemia as well.

Cerebral syphilis may be *meningo-vascular* or *parenchymatous*. In the former type there is focal meningitis and vascular occlusion due to endarteritis obliterans of the small vessels. Isolated cranial nerve palsies are quite common.

Parenchymatous neurosyphilis includes the two well-known conditions, general paralysis of the insane and tabes dorsalis. *General paralysis of the insane* is a chronic syphilitic meningoencephalitis in which the frontal lobes are particularly severely affected. This results in progressive dementia and often paralysis. *Tabes dorsalis* is a degenerative condition of the posterior columns of the spinal cord and the posterior roots of the spinal nerves. There is severe demyelination of the sensory tracts. This results in loss of sensation leading to trophic disturbances, and loss of postural sense, which produces the typical staggering gait.

The bones are sometimes affected by a diffuse type of syphilitic inflammation. There may be widespread periostitis, involving especially the tibia and the bones of the calvaria of the skull. The irregular thickening that is very apparent clinically is due to the laying down of new bone. This gives rise to the classical *sabre tibia*, and in the skull a rather typical worm-eaten appearance.

Diagnosis. The diagnosis of tertiary syphilis is primarily clinical, but it may often be substantiated by serological examination of the blood and cerebrospinal fluid. In most cases of overt syphilis this examination is strongly positive, and in neuro-syphilis the cerebrospinal fluid is generally more helpful than the blood.

Congenital syphilis

During the first 2 years of infection an untreated syphilitic mother is very liable to transmit the disease to her fetus, particularly after the fourth month of pregnancy, when the Langhans layer of the placenta becomes attenuated. Abortion may result, or else a severely affected infant may die soon after birth.

More frequently the child survives, and it may then exhibit early stigmata of infection like skin eruptions, snuffles, epiphysitis of the elbows, and wasting. Sometimes stigmata appear only in later childhood. The notched, peg-shaped Hutchinson's incisor teeth and mulberry molars (Moon's molars) due to syphilitic infection of the tooth germs during fetal life are well-known examples of this type of lesion, as are also interstitial keratitis (inflammation of the cornea), tibial periostitis (sabre tibia), and nerve deafness.

The histological appearances of these various lesions are all very similar, being combinations of the heavy cellular infiltration of secondary syphilis together with the gummatous destruction typical of the tertiary phase. In fact, congenital syphilis may be regarded as a combined secondary and tertiary syphilis occurring in a child whose primary lesion was placental.

ACTINOMYCOSIS[9,10]

Actinomycosis is characterized by chronic, loculated foci of suppuration occurring particularly in the region of the lower jaw. The human disease is caused by *Actinomyces israeli*, while a similar condition in cattle ('lump jaw') is caused by another organism, *Actinomyces bovis*.

Bacteriology. These organisms are Gram-positive filaments which have a tendency to branch. They grow in a colonial, bunched form particularly in animal tissues, where a densely felted mass of branching filaments matted together in an amorphous matrix is characteristic.

Although often called a mycelium, the term is not strictly correct since it is usually restricted to fungal growth. The filaments of *Actinomyces israeli* are much thinner than those of the fungi, and the organism is now classified as a bacterium of the family *Actinomycetaceae*, which also includes the genus *Nocardia*. In animal tissues the organisms grow in colonies consisting of a densely felted mass of filaments matted together in an amorphous matrix. Such a colony appears in the pus of actinomycotic lesions in the form of a small granule which is greyish-yellow in colour. This is called a *sulphur granule*. In artificial culture this colonial tendency is less pronounced, and the individual filaments remain more separate.

A colony formed in the tissues tends to be surrounded by a radial projecting fringe of club-shaped excrescences (*clubs*). These clubs are Gram-negative, and are not formed in artificial culture. It is believed that they are produced as the result of the deposition on to the colony of lipid material derived from the hosts's tissues. This radiating fringe around the colony gave rise to the alternative name *ray fungus* which has been loosely applied to *Actinomyces* organisms.

Diagnosis. The diagnosis of actinomycosis depends on finding sulphur granules in the copious pus that exudes from the abscess sinuses. The granules are crushed between two slides and stained, and also cultured anaerobically on blood agar.

Pathogenesis. *Actinomyces israeli* is a normal commensal of the mouth, and it is found especially in the tonsils and in carious teeth. Actinomycosis is an endogenous infection, and is not transmitted by contaminated pieces of straw and grass that have been sucked by cattle. It can follow a dental extraction, though considering the widespread distribution of the organism, the disease is surprisingly infrequent. It is not understood what local conditions must be fulfilled before the organism can invade the tissues and set up a progressive inflammatory reaction. It has been known to produce infection in a hand wound caused by hitting an assailant in the teeth ('punch actinomycosis').

The lesions. Actinomycosis commonly occurs in the *cervico-facial* region. Primary *ileo-caecal* infection is uncommon, and *pulmonary* lesions are rare.

The actinomycotic lesion starts as an acute suppurative inflammation, which then persists and progresses to intractable chronicity. As the organisms spread by direct continuity, large numbers of abscesses are produced. Some of these fuse together, but there is a tendency for individual foci of suppuration to remain discrete owing to the persistence of fibrous septa. This produces a characteristically loculated appearance, which is seen most typically in actinomycotic lesions of the liver (*honeycomb liver*).

Histologically the abscess cavities are crowded with pus cells which surround actinomycotic colonies (Fig. 15.8). The narrow septa between the abscesses are composed of fibrous tissue which is heavily infiltrated by polymorphs, lymphocytes, macrophages, and plasma cells. These fibrous septa are not merely the

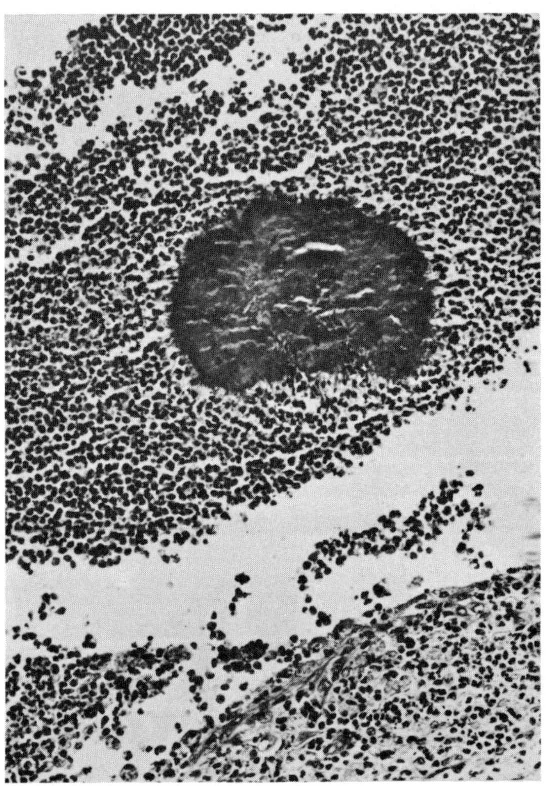

Fig. 15.8 Actinomycotic pus. This section shows a colony of actinomyces ('sulphur granule') in a dense mass of pus cells. × 150.

remains of destroyed parenchyma; they are produced by attempts at healing by repair, and the entire lesion is surrounded by a similar dense zone of fibrous tissue.

Spread of infection. The main mode of spread of the disease is by direct contact. Whereas other organisms move in the tissue spaces along preformed planes, the actinomyces extends slowly and inexorably onwards through the tissues. In cervico-facial actinomycosis there is direct spread to the adjacent muscles and bones. The mandible is the bone usually involved, but sometimes there is extension to the maxilla, and eventually the meninges and brain become infected. There is also progressive cutaneous involvement, and the abscesses discharge with the production of many sinuses. The appearance of a diffuse, indurated, painless area of suppuration in the area of the mandible discharging to the exterior through multiple sinuses is very characteristic of actinomycosis (Fig.15.9).

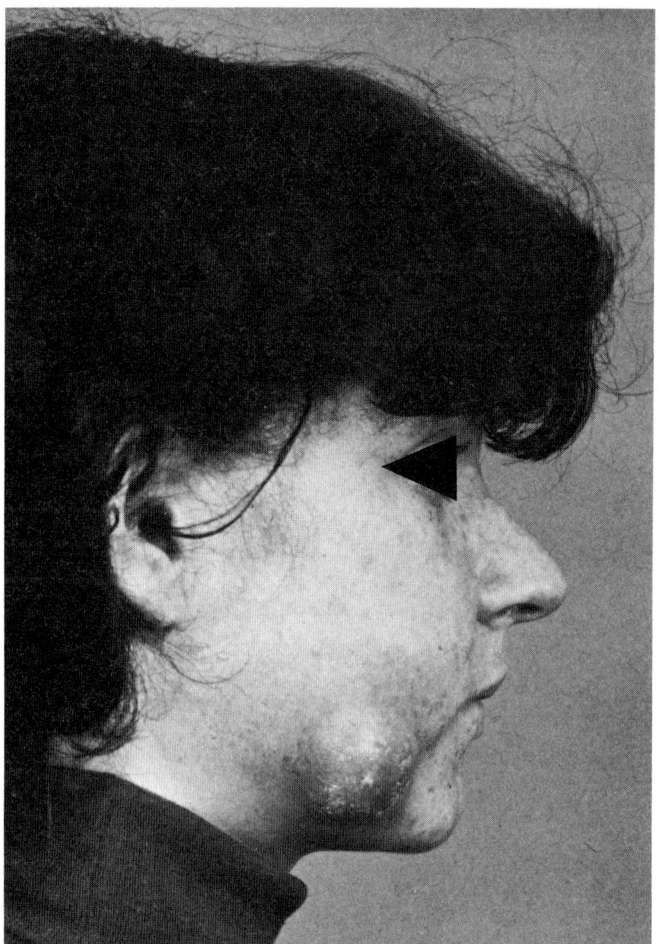

Fig. 15.9 Cervico-facial actinomycosis. There was a soft, fluctuant swelling over the lower part of the right side of the face, and the overlying skin was red and indurated. (Photograph by courtesy of Mr J W Frame.)

Similarly ileo-caecal actinomycosis spreads through the anterior abdominal wall with the development of discharging sinuses, and pulmonary actinomycosis erupts through the wall of the chest.

Lymphatic spread does not occur in actinomycosis; perhaps the filaments are too large to be accommodated in the lymphatic channels. Any regional lymphadenitis that may occur is attributable to secondary bacterial infection by staphylococci and coliform organisms.

Blood-borne spread, on the other hand, is important, and is typified by the spread of ileo-caecal disease by the portal vein to the liver, where the loculated actinomycotic abscesses of honeycomb liver are produced.

Treatment. Actinomyces organisms are very sensitive to the commonly-used antibiotics, and in practice penicillin and lincomycin are the most useful.

FUNGAL INFECTIONS

In the past fungi were regarded as plants without roots, stems, and leaves, incapable of photosynthesis because they lack chlorophyll. They are now regarded as neither plants nor animals, but are placed in a separate group. For practical purposes four varieties can be recognized:

Moulds, which grow as long filaments (*hyphae*), and which branch and interlace to form a meshwork, or *mycelium*
Yeasts, which grow by budding only
Yeast-like fungi, which grow partly as yeasts and partly as long filamentous forms called pseudohyphae
Dimorphic fungi, which can grow either as hyphae or as yeast depending on the cultural conditions.

The line of distinction between some higher bacteria (e.g. the *Actinomycetales* which includes the *Mycobacteriaceae*, *Actinomycetaceae*, and *Streptomycetaceae*) and true fungi is by no means clear-cut.

Superficial infections by fungi

A number of fungi are able to grow in the hair and the superficial layers of the epidermis, where they produce skin diseases typified by *ringworm*.

Ringworm, or tinea.
Ringworm is caused by a group of fungi which are termed *dermatophytes*, and have the property of digesting the keratin of skin or hair. The dermatophytes are moulds that grow as a mycelium and reproduce by the formation of various types of spores. Ringworm, which is due to invasion of keratin by one of the dermatophytes, can affect the scalp (causing *tinea capitis*, in which involvement of the hair shafts causes a bald patch), the body skin (causing *tinea corporis* with its variant *tinea cruris* affecting the inguinal region), the foot (causing athlete's foot, or *tinea pedis*), the hands (causing *tinea manuum*), and sometimes the nails (causing *tinea unguium*). Each type of ringworm has its own particular characteristics, but in general the lesions are erythematous, scaly, and sometimes vesicular, and tend to have a sharp, red, spreading border that gives the lesions a ring-like shape from which the disease acquired its name.

Diagnosis is easy: scrapings of nail or keratin can be examined by direct microscopy for hyphae; and from a culture one can readily identify the particular strain of mould responsible.

Candidiasis.[11]
Infection with Candida species is one of the most frequent fungal infections in the human subject. The organism most commonly involved is the yeast-like fungus *Candida albicans*. The common yeast form is seen in thrush, and is 1.5 to 5.0 μm in diameter and intensely Gram positive. It reproduces by budding, but sometimes the bud elongates to form a pseudohypha. This form can occur in cultures and is also characteristic of invasive candida infections, especially the lesions of systemic

candidiasis. The organism is a common commensal in the oral cavity, alimentary tract, and vagina. Infections occur when local or general conditions become suitable, but it must be accepted that the factors which govern the delicate balance between host and organism are poorly understood. The superficial infections of the mucous membranes appear as white patches called *thrush.* In the mouth this is very common in infants, especially premature ones, and may be accompanied by perianal lesions. Oral candidiasis can occur at any age during the course of any debilitating disease. It may also occur under dentures and orthodontic appliances, and can complicate other erosive disease, e.g. pemphigus vulgaris. Vaginal thrush is common during pregnancy, in those on the contraceptive pill, and in diabetes mellitus. Cutaneous candidiasis occurs around the corners of the mouth (*angular cheilosis*, or *perlèche*), in other moist intertriginous areas, and in the nail folds (*chronic paronychia*).

The important feature of candidiasis is that it is sometimes a serious opportunistic infection. With glucocorticoid therapy, in lymphomata, following the administration of cytotoxic drugs, and indeed in any disease in which cell-mediated immunity is impaired, oral lesions can extend down the alimentary or respiratory tracts to produce fatal results. The organism may invade the blood stream and lead to generalized systemic candidiasis in which lesions occur in many organs. Renal abscesses are usually prominent, but almost any organ may be affected and endocarditis is sometimes seen. Severe candidiasis is often a feature of the immunological deficiency diseases which affect the T lymphocytes.

Less extensive candida infections are seen in particular circumstances. Endocarditis can occur as a primary event, particularly in addicts who inject themselves intravenously with narcotics. Oral lesions can spread to produce extensive gastrointestinal infection following the prolonged administration of oral broad-spectrum antibiotics. Finally there are some types of primary immunological deficiency disease affecting the T lymphocytes in which there is *chronic widespread mucocutaneous candidiasis.*[12] These may be familial, and endocrine abnormalities, particularly hypoparathyroidism, may coexist. These conditions persist for many years and do not tend to terminate in generalized spread, nor is there usually a tendency for other infections to occur.

The tissue reaction to candida varies. In minor and superficial infections there is some tissue necrosis accompanied by a pyogenic response. Intra-epidermal pustules are seen in the cutaneous lesions. When the infection is overwhelming, as in generalized candidiasis, there is much necrosis and very little inflammatory reaction. Indeed, the lesions show massive accumulations of fungus and few host cells.

Deep-seated fungal infections

In certain parts of the world fungal infections are of considerable importance. In general the organisms are found in the soil, and infection is acquired by inhalation. A primary lesion occurs in the lung and in the majority of people healing follows. Occasionally, however, the organisms produce more severe damage and spread to involve other organs. These diseases therefore resemble tuberculosis in their pathogenesis. Furthermore, the tissue reaction to these organisms sometimes also closely resembles that seen in tuberculosis.

Cryptococcosis[13–15]

The causative organism *Cryptococcus neoformans* (previously called *Torula histolytica*) is a true yeast, and of world-wide distribution. The primary lung lesion is usually small and heals by fibrosis. Occasionally the organism becomes widely disseminated and in particular causes *meningitis*. This widespread dissemination is particularly common in patients with T-cell deficiency, e.g. Hodgkin's disease.

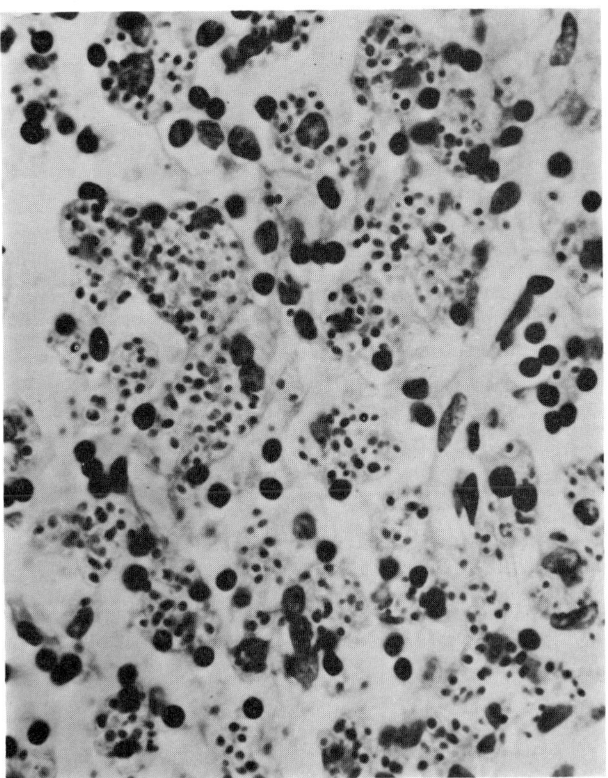

Fig. 15.10 Histoplasmosis. This section of spleen contains many macrophages crowded with *Histoplasma capsulatum* organisms. × 400.

Histoplasmosis[16, 17]

The causative organism *Histoplasma capsulatum* is a dimorphic fungus which has a world-wide distribution, and is endemic in the Mississippi Valley of the USA. The histoplasmin test, analagous to the tuberculin test, is positive in affected individuals.

The primary lung lesion resembles tuberculosis and usually heals with calcification. Occasionally cavitation occurs, and rarely there is blood-borne dissemination. This occurs most commonly in infants, and many of the internal organs are involved. Large numbers of organisms are then found parasitizing the RE cells (Fig. 15.10). Disseminated histoplasmosis may also occur in elderly debilitated subjects, usually men, and the infection is less widespread than in the infantile type. In some cases infection of the lips, mouth, nose, or larynx is the initial manifestation. In Africa, *Histoplasma duboisii* generally infects the skin.

Coccidioidomycosis[18,19]

This disease, caused by the dimorphic fungus *Coccidioides immitis*, is common in the desert regions of California and Arizona and also in the Chaco district of Argentina. Many of the inhabitants acquire a pulmonary infection, but this is either asymptomatic or accompanied by a self-limiting influenza-like illness called locally 'desert fever'. Occasionally the disease is progressive, and the destructive lung lesions closely resemble tuberculosis. Systemic spread to many organs may occur. Histologically the lesions show a suppurative tuberculoid reaction, the centre of each follicle being occupied by necrotic material containing many polymorphs.

North American blastomycosis

This is caused by infection with *Blastomyces dermatitidis*, a yeast with a thick double-contoured capsule. The primary lesion is usually pulmonary but may be cutaneous. It generally subsides spontaneously, but occasionally it progresses and widespread dissemination can then follow. Suppurative lesions occur in many sites, particularly the skin, bones, and lungs.

South American blastomycosis.

The causative yeast *Blastomyces braziliensis* multiplies by producing multiple peripheral buds so that the organism becomes surrounded by a 'row of beads'. The common primary site of infection is the nasopharynx, and ulcerative destructive lesions are produced. The lymph nodes are soon involved, and sometimes cervical lymphadenopathy is the presenting symptom. The disease tends to become disseminated and affect the lungs, skin, and other organs. It is commonly fatal unless treated.

Treatment of fungal infections

For generalized infections the antibiotic *amphotericin B* can be given systemically with a good effect. A less toxic drug *5-fluorocytosine*, is potent but unfortunately liable to induce drug-resistant strains.

For candidal infections these drugs can also be used. The imidazole derivatives *clotrimazole* and *miconazole* are also useful, and can be used both topically and systemically. The antibiotic *nystatin* is very effective for local treatment, but is not absorbed when taken by mouth and cannot be given parenterally.

GENERAL REFERENCES

See Chapter 14, page 212.

REFERENCES

1. Barker D J P 1974 Mycobacterial skin ulcers. British Journal of Dermatology 91 : 473
2. Leading Article 1969 Miliary tuberculosis in the elderly. British Medical Journal 2 : 265

3. Leading Article 1972 BCG vaccination. Lancet 2: 168
4. Leading Article 1975 BCG vaccination. British Medical Journal 4: 603
5. Scadding J G 1967 Sarcoidosis Eyre and Spottiswoode, London
6. Mitchell D N, Scadding J G, Heard B E, Hinson K F W 1977 Sarcoidosis: histopathological definition and clinical diagnosis. Journal of Clinical Pathology 30: 395
7. Sparling P F 1971 Diagnosis and treatment of syphilis. New England Journal of Medicine 284: 642
8. Leading Article 1977 The Jarisch-Herxheimer reaction. Lancet 1: 340
9. Cope V Z 1938 Actinomycosis, Oxford University Press, London
10. Bronner M, Bronner M, 1971 Actinomycosis, 2nd edn, pp 355, John Wright, Bristol
11. Winner H I, Hurley R 1964 Candida Albicans, Churchill, London
12. Leading article 1972 Candida infection, British Medical Journal 4: 505
13. Littman M L, Walter J E 1968 Cryptococcosis: current status. American Journal of Medicine 45: 922
14. Powell K, Christianson C 1973 Pulmonary cryptococcosis: clinical forms and treatment: a center for disease control cooperative mycosis study. American Review of Respiratory Diseases 108: 116
15. Symmers W StC 1960 In Recent Advances in Clinical Pathology, Series III, p 304. ed Dyke S C, Churchill, London
16. Schwarz J, Baum G L 1963 Histoplasmosis 1962. Archives of Internal Medicine, 111: 710
17. Cockshott W P, Lucas A O 1964. Histoplasmosis duboisii. Quarterly Journal of Medicine, 33: 223
18. Fiese M J 1958 Coccidioidomycosis. Thomas, Springfield, Illinois
19. Ajello L 1967 Coccidioidomycosis. University of Arizona Press, Tucson

16

Viral diseases

INTRODUCTION

It is useful at the outset, before considering the properties of viruses, first to define those of other small organisms with which they might be confused.

Bacteria

Bacteria are generally unicellular, but even the smallest is within the range of the light microscope (which resolves up to about 0.2 μm in diameter). They grow with variable ease on artificial cell-free media, though in this respect *Myco. leprae* and *Tr. pallidum* are exceptions, for as yet they have not been cultured artificially. The bacterial cell is complete, and contains DNA in its nuclear body and RNA in its cytoplasm.

Rickettsiae

Rickettsiae are unicellular organisms about 0.4 μm (400 nm) in size, and are visible under the light microscope. They resemble bacteria in reproducing by asexual binary fission, possessing both DNA and RNA, and having a *cell wall* containing muramic acid. They differ from bacteria in that they require living cells for growth, i.e. they are *obligatory intracellular parasites*. The rickettsiae produce the *typhus group of fevers* which have a world-wide distribution, and are transmitted by arthropods like lice, fleas, ticks, and mites, e.g. epidemic typhus is caused by *R. prowazeki* transmitted by lice. Another condition caused by a rickettsia is Q (query) fever, a febrile disease with chest symptoms. The causal organism *Coxiella burneti* is somewhat smaller than those of typhus.

Chlamydiae

These organisms have much in common with the rickettsiae but are smaller and more rudimentary. They are obligatory intracellular parasites and are cultivated in mice, yolk-sacs of fertile eggs, and in tissue-culture systems. Parasitized cells contain characteristic inclusion bodies, which are microcolonies of the organism. The *chlamydiae* are classified into subgroups A and B on the basis of the nature of the inclusion body.

Subgroup A chlamydiae, called *Chlamydia trachomatis*, cause five eye diseases—hyperendemic trachoma, inclusion conjunctivitis, TRIC ophthalmia neonatorum, TRIC punctate keratoconjunctivitis, and endemic trachoma—and two infections of the genito-urinary tract—lymphogranuloma venereum (LGV) and chlamydial urethritis and cervicitis in the male and female respectively. The word TRIC is derived from the first four letters of TRachoma and Inclusion and Conjunctivitis.

Chlamydia trachomatis consists of a number of different serotypes which are responsible for these various infections. Lymphogranuloma venereum is caused by one group of serotypes, hyperendemic trachoma by another group, and yet others cause the remaining ocular infections, often collectively called *paratrachoma*, and also chlamydial urethritis and cervicitis.

The most severe ocular disease of chlamydial origin is *hyperendemic trachoma*, which is responsible for blinding millions of people especially in Africa and Asia. It starts as a chronic conjunctivitis characterized by proliferation of the conjunctival epithelium and a heavy infiltration of the subepithelial tissues with lymphocytes and macrophages; ultimately discrete lymphoid follicles are formed so that granular elevations (follicles) are visible on the conjunctiva. The epithelium undergoes necrosis, and the subsequent ulceration and scarring cause the lids to become distorted by contractures. Furthermore, the inflammatory process involves the cornea and leads to ulceration. The deeper layers of the cornea are infiltrated by inflammatory cells, and there is progressive vascularization, thereby forming a *pannus*, which is subsequently replaced by scar tissue. Thus the cornea becomes opaque.

Inclusion conjunctivitis, *TRIC punctate keratoconjunctivitis*, and *endemic trachoma of sexual transmission*, the adult forms of paratrachoma, are chronic follicular conjunctival infections, usually of acute onset and commonest in young adults. The effects on the eye are similar to those of hyperendemic trachoma but are generally less severe. There is often an associated genital infection.

TRIC ophthalmia neonatorum is an acute mucopurulent conjunctivitis acquired during the infant's passage through the infected birth canal. It may become chronic and lead to pannus formation and scarring.

Lymphogranuloma venereum starts as a small papule or ulcer in the area of the external genitalia; this is followed in about 2 weeks by regional lymphadenitis, usually of a suppurative nature. During the healing stage there may be much scarring with lymphatic obstruction. This has serious effects in the female and can cause vaginal or rectal stenosis.

Transmission of chlamydia (subgroup A). Hyperendemic trachoma is transmitted directly from eye to eye. Paratrachoma is usually associated with a chlamydial urethritis and cervicitis; these are the commonest venereal diseases in the developed countries, and the infection is invariably transmitted sexually from genital tract to genital tract; occasionally infection is transmitted from the genital tract to the eye. Lymphogranuloma venereum is invariably venereal in transmission.

Subgroup B chlamdiae, called *Chlamydia psittaci*, cause *psittacosis* and *ornithosis* in the human subject, and similar diseases in birds, particularly those of the parrot family (psittacine birds) but also in other related species. The diseases are acquired by inhaling the infected aerosol or dust from birds which may have been handled as pets or killed for eating. Clinically the diseases may resemble influenza with rapid recovery, or else there may be progression to a severe pneumonia and death.

The regulations relating to the importation of psittacine birds have made psittacosis an uncommon disease, but occasional outbreaks still occur because native poultry and pigeons can harbour the organism.

Mycoplasmas

Mycoplasmas comprise a group of minute organisms of doubtful systematic position. They vary in size, but most are 200 to 250 nm. They possess no cell wall but only a limiting membrane. The result is *extreme fragility* and *pleomorphism*: granules, rings, coccoid forms, and fine filaments are all described. Because of their small size they pass through very fine filters, yet they resemble bacteria in being able to grow on artificial cell-free media.

The important human pathogen is *Mycoplasma pneumoniae*. At one time it was classified as a virus, and the disease it causes was erroneously called *virus pneumonia*. It responds well to tetracyclines. Mycoplasmas are also found in the mouth and genito-urinary tract, but it is doubtful whether they are pathogenic.

L-forms. These were first described by Klieneberger-Nobel working at the Lister Institute, London (L stands for Lister). When certain bacteria are faced with adverse circumstances, they swell up (and possibly fuse) into a large mass which then disintegrates into irregularly spherical granules which are plastic, refractile, and very fragile. They are minute, measuring 100 to 500 nm in diameter. They are penicillin-resistant irrespective of the general sensitivity of the strain from which they are derived. L-forms have been described in *Strept. viridans*, *Esch. coli*, and many other species. They pass easily through ordinary bacterial filters, and it is possible that they are present in bacteriologically 'sterile' filtrates. They bear a close resemblance to *Mycoplasma* organisms. An L-form returns to type when conditions are normal.

Viruses

Size is not a criterion in the definition of a virus because some of them are larger than the mycoplasmal organisms.

All viruses are obligatory intracellular parasites, but this is also a feature of the rickettsiae and a few bacteria.

The only feature which distinguishes viruses from all other organisms is that during the process of multiplication they enter a non-infective, or 'eclipse', phase (p. 246).

Viruses do not possess all the enzyme systems capable of synthetizing viral material; they are therefore dependent on the parasitized cell for survival and multiplication. Indeed, the essential difference between viruses and other organisms is that the synthetic processes that attend multiplication take place within the protoplasm of the infected cells in the case of viruses, but in the body of the organism itself in other infective agents.

GENERAL PROPERTIES OF VIRUSES

Size

Among the largest of the true viruses is the pox group responsible for smallpox, vaccinia, and similar diseases in other species of animals. These are about 250 nm in size, and a single virus particle when suitable stained is just visible under the light microscope. Viruses smaller than this cannot be seen by light microscopy, and therefore other methods of measurement are used.

Filterability. Their size can be assessed by their capacity to pass through specially graded filters. This is too inaccurate for precise measurements.

Sedimentation rate. A more modern method is ultracentrifugation using high-speed centrifuges. The larger the particle, the faster it falls.

Electron microscopy. The most accurate method at present available is electron microscopy, which has also imparted fundamental information about virus size,

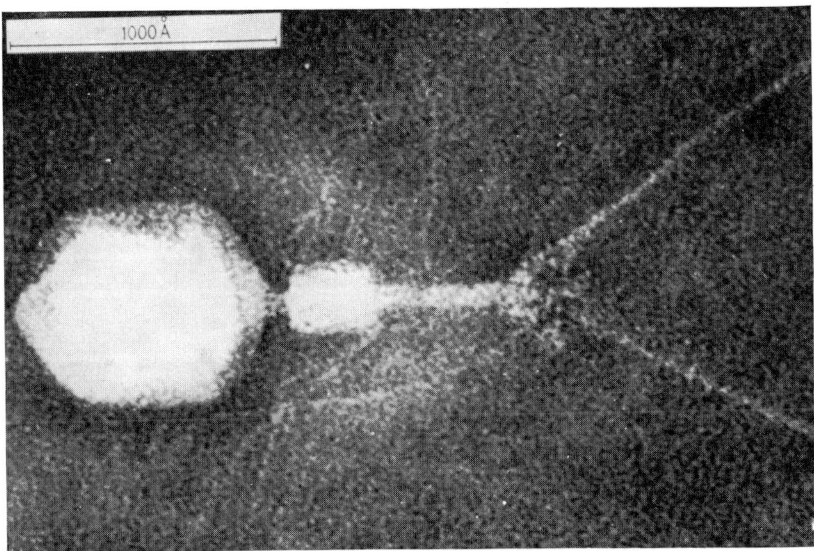

Fig. 16.1 The bacteriophage particle viewed under the electron microscope after negative staining. Note the following structures:
(*a*) The head, a bipyramidal prism. It contains the viral DNA.
(*b*) A central rigid core.
(*c*) A tail sheath which surrounds this central core. In the picture the sheath is contracted to the upper part of the core. It is attached to a hexagonal plate structure at the extreme end of the tail—it is unrecognizable in this picture.
(*d*) Tail fibres (six altogether) associated with the plate structure.
It is suggested that the plate and fibres are a means of attachment to the host. The components of bacteriophage have been compared to a micro-syringe system serving to inject the viral DNA into the host bacterium. × 300 000. (*From Brenner S et al 1959 Journal of Molecular Biology 1:281.*)

shape, and chemical configuration. Most viruses are less than 200 nm in size—varicella virus is 150 to 120 nm, and one of the smallest, that of foot-and-mouth disease, is only 20 nm.

Many viruses are spherical in shape, e.g. poliovirus, herpes-simplex virus, and adenovirus, some are filamentous, e.g. tobacco-mosaic virus and influenza virus, while bacteriophage has a characteristic tadpole shape (Fig. 16.1).

Chemical constituents

The basic composition of a virus particle, or *virion* (also called an *elementary body*), is a nucleic-acid core surrounded by a protein envelope called a *capsid*. In some viruses, e.g. herpesviruses and adenoviruses, the nucleic acid is DNA, whereas in others, e.g. the enteroviruses and myxoviruses, it is RNA. The heart of a virus is its nucleic-acid portion, for this controls the synthesis of new viral material when it infects a host cell.

The protein envelope is composed of sub-units built in a compact, regular manner around the nucleic-acid core. These protein sub-units are called *capsomeres*, and their arrangement is related to the shape of the virus. In spherical viruses they show a cubical or icosahedral symmetry, i.e. they are disposed around the core in the form of a regular icosahedron (a solid bounded by 20 plane surfaces each of which is an equilateral triangle). This is demonstrated in Figs. 16.2 and 16.3. Filamentous (or rod-shaped) viruses are surrounded by a helix of protein sub-units, i.e. they are arranged in a spiral around the central rod.

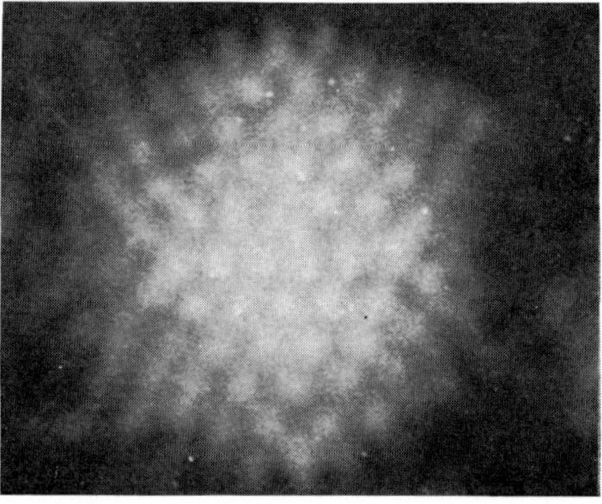

Fig. 16.2 A single particle (elementary body) of adenovirus embedded in electron-opaque phosphotungstate. The negatively-stained particle viewed under the electron microscope is seen to be composed of morphological units (capsomeres) of spherical shape packed in a symmetrical arrangement. It has been calculated that the total number of capsomeres around the central core of an adenovirus is 252. × 480 000. (*From Horne R W, Brenner S, Waterson A P, Wildy P 1959 Journal of Molecular Biology 1:84*).

The tadpole-shaped bacteriophage has a *binal* symmetry in its capsid, meaning that it is arranged differently around the head as compared with the tail (see Fig. 16.1).

Some viruses are also ensheathed in one or more outer membranes, or envelopes, composed predominantly of lipid, derived from the modified host cell or nuclear membrane prior to the release of the virus. Enveloped viruses, e.g. herpesviruses, myxoviruses, and togaviruses, are vulnerable to fat solvents such as ether and bile salts. The larger viruses, especially poxviruses, also contain carbohydrates, co-enzymes, and even some enzymes, e.g. lipase, catalase, and phosphatase, but none contains all the enzymes necessary for the metabolism of its own substance. It is for this reason that viruses are obligatory intracellular parasites.

Life-cycle and reproduction

The life-cycle of a virus is intracellular, and the details vary according to the virus, but the basic steps are similar for all viruses.

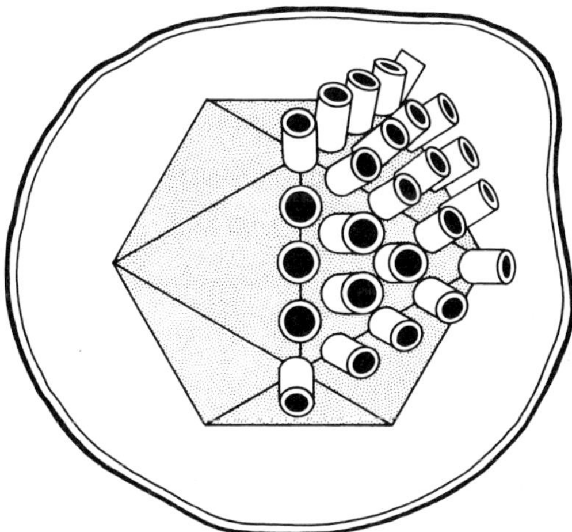

Fig. 16.3 Diagrammatic representation of a typical virus showing cubical symmetry. The core of the virus has the form of an icosahedron having 20 facets. It is covered by symmetrically arranged capsomeres, each consisting of a hollow tube. The covering of capsomeres constitutes the viral capsid. The virion (consisting of the genetic material and the capsid) has an outer membrane that is derived from the altered host plasma membrane or nuclear membrane. Not all such viruses possess an outer membrane. (*Drawing by Frederick Lammerich, Department of Art as Applied to Medicine, University of Toronto.*)

Attachment and penetration. The first stage is the attachment of the virus to a specific *cell receptor*, or *receptor site*, on the cell membrane. This *attachment phase* is followed by *penetration* of the virus into the cell.

Penetration. With bacteriophage the naked DNA is injected into the interior of the bacterium, while the protein coat, which acts as a microsyringe, remains exterior attached to the bacterial wall (Fig. 16.4). The mode of penetration of animal viruses is different, and both pinocytosis and phagocytosis are involved. With vaccinia virus in tissue cultures, the next step is removal of the protein coat and release of the nucleic acid.

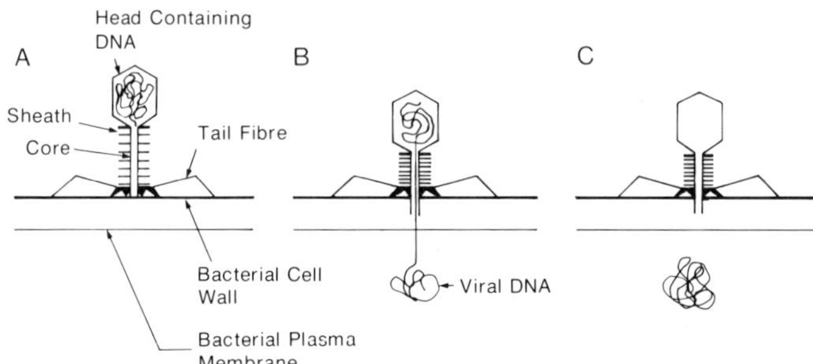

Fig. 16.4 Diagrammatic representation of the entry of bacteriophage into a bacterial cell. The bacteriophage consists of a head containing DNA, a rigid core surrounded by a sheath to which is attached a tail piece, and tail fibres. *A*. The first event in the entry of the phage is the attachment of the tail fibres to the receptors of the bacterial cell wall. *B*. Contraction of the sheath results in the injection of viral DNA into the bacterial cell substance. *C*. The protein component of the phage shown attached to the cell wall is subsequently lost, leaving the viral DNA within the substance of the bacterium. Here it can replicate and lead to lysis of the bacterial cell, or it can remain latent as prophage. (*Drawn by Sue Reynolds.*)

Eclipse phase. Once the nucleic acid has been released it becomes unidentifiable for a few hours. This is the all-important *eclipse phase* characteristic of viruses, and the nucleic acid is not infectious during this period.

It appears that the free nucleic acid is engaged in redirecting the cell's metabolism so that more viral nucleic acid and protein are produced. The eclipse phase takes from 1 to 30 hours. In DNA-containing viruses the DNA directs the formation of mRNA as well as virus-specific enzymes which take part in the formation of new virus material. With RNA-containing viruses the single-stranded RNA appears to act as mRNA. In some instances it directs the formation of DNA (p. 367). It is remarkable that a minute quantity of foreign nucleic acid can so dominate the cellular metabolism that, instead of forming normal cell substance, the cell is perverted into forming large amounts of the virus. This mode of reproduction (or replication) contrasts strongly with the binary fission of higher organisms.

Maturation and replication of the virus. In some viruses, e.g. the adenoviruses, the components are formed in the nucleus, in others e.g. the poxviruses, in the cytoplasm, and in yet others in both cytoplasm and nucleus. When the components are assembled into mature infective virus, they are soon recognisable as elementary bodies and escape from the cell either in a dramatic burst—as with poliovirus—or in a steady release from the cell surface—as with herpesviruses and orthomyxoviruses—or else very tardily after accumulating in the cell, as with adenoviruses.

Enveloped viruses receive an additional coat from a cell membrane. With herpesviruses the envelope is derived from the nuclear membrane; this membrane is not completely normal nuclear membrane, but one that has been modified by the presence of the virus and containing viral type antigens. The orthomyxoviruses incorporate modified cell membrane during the period of release, which takes about an hour. After release the virus enters other cells either by direct contact or after carriage by body fluids.

Some viruses produce globular intracellular masses which are easily visible under the light microscope. These are called *inclusion bodies* (Fig. 16.5). Some, like the intranuclear inclusions of herpesviruses, are formed as a result of cell degeneration. A few, like the inclusions of adenoviruses and reoviruses, are crystalline aggregates of virions. Most are composed of aggregations of developing virus particles bound together in a gelatinous matrix. Unlike *elementary bodies*, which are single mature virus particles, inclusion bodies are large (up to 20 μm in size). Some are acidophilic and others basophilic; some intracytoplasmic and others intranuclear. At one time they were of great moment in the diagnosis of viral disease; nowadays they are mostly of historical interest. Nevertheless, a few are worth noting:

(*a*) *Negri body*, an acidophilic body found in the cytoplasm of neurons in cases of rabies.

(*b*) *Guarnieri body*, an acidophilic body seen in the cytoplasm of epidermal cells in vaccinia and smallpox.

(*c*) The intranuclear bodies found in the epidermal cells in *zoster* and *herpes simplex*.

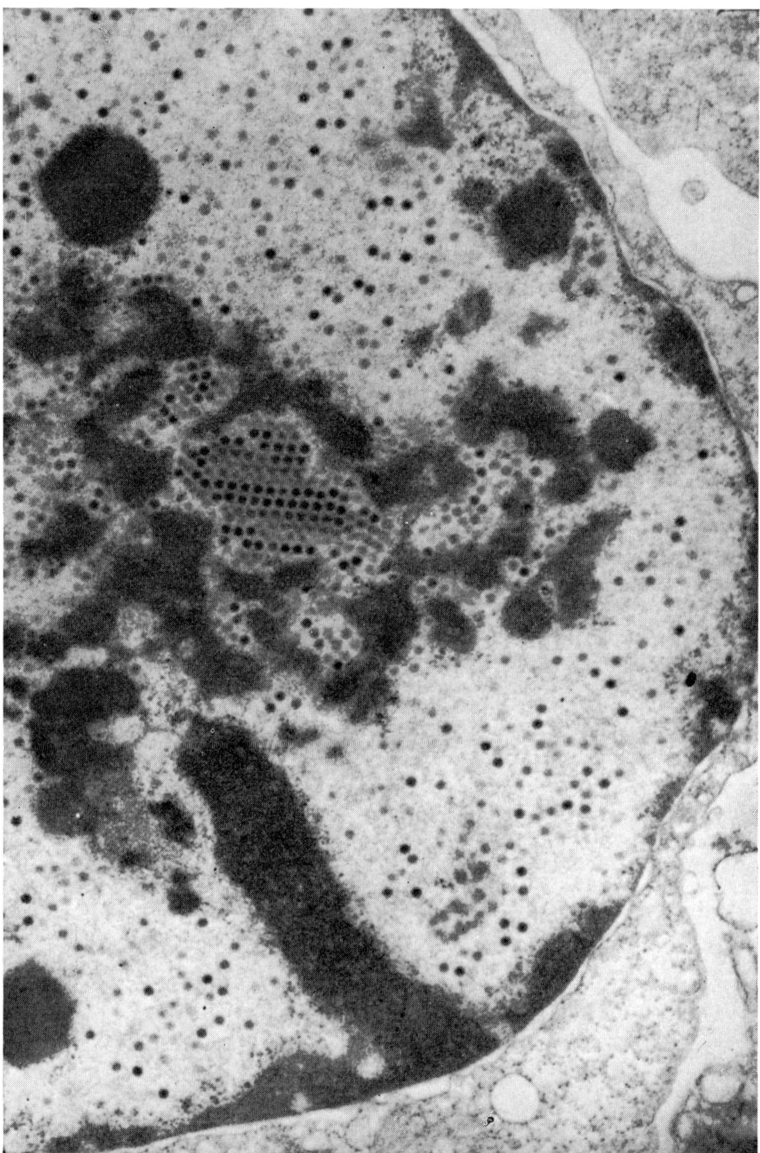

Fig. 16.5 Nuclear inclusion induced by adenovirus 12. The virus crystals in the centre are surrounded by very dense material with irregular contours. Many virus particles are dispersed in the nucleoplasm. ×24 000. (*From Bernhard W 1964 In: de Reuck A V S, Knight J (eds) Cellular injury, a Ciba Foundation Symposium. Churchill, London, p 215.*)

Reaction to environment

Unlike bacteria, most viruses are easily inactivated even at room temperature, and care must be taken to keep specimens frozen, if possible at −70°C. A few viruses are much more stable than this, however, and the viruses of poliomyelitis and vaccinia can survive at ordinary atmospheric temperatures for some weeks. The hepatitis viruses appear to be particularly resistant, but the most durable agent is that of scrapie, which withstands boiling for 3 hours.

Reaction to chemicals

Viruses are destroyed without difficulty by the chemical disinfectants used against bacteria; the scrapie virus is an exception, being able to survive in strong formalin solutions. One important property of viruses is their great resistance to a 50 per cent solution of glycerol, which kills non-sporing bacteria quite rapidly. Vaccinia virus is actually preserved in glycerol. No virus is susceptible to any antibiotic therapy in current use, but a few specific chemotherapeutic agents are now known.

Cultivation of viruses

Viruses multiply only in living cells, and at first the only systems that could be used were experimental animals and chick embryos. The discovery by Enders and his colleagues in 1949 that the virus of poliomyelitis could proliferate in tissue cultures of non-neuronal origin, e.g. human prepuce, heralded the modern era of virus research. Nowadays the vast majority of viruses are cultivated in tissue culture, a method which is cheap, simple, and efficacious.

1. *Animal inoculation* is reserved for those viruses which do not grow satisfactorily in tissue culture, e.g. some Coxsackie viruses.

2. *Chick embryo inoculation* is still used to culture some viruses. Characteristic lesions may be produced on the chorio-allantoic membrane by the poxviruses, and the amniotic sac is used for culturing influenza virus.

3. *Tissue culture* is the method of choice. The basis of this technique is that living cells are grown on the sides of test-tubes. Many viruses are able to multiply in these cells, in which they produce destructive changes. This is called a *cytopathic effect*, and is illustrated in Figs. 16.6 to 16.8. The changes are sometimes

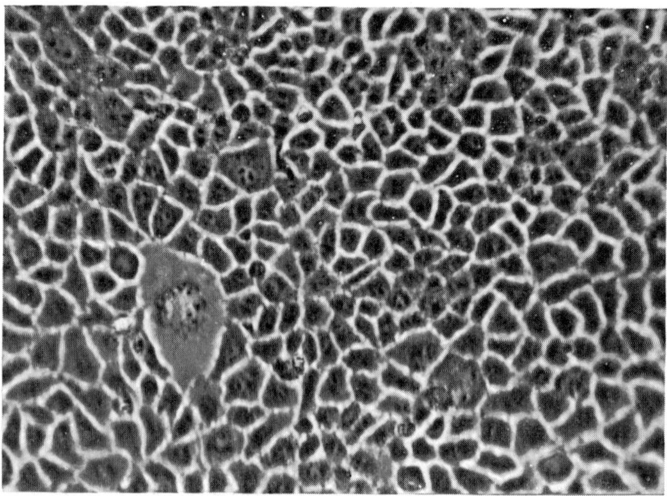

Fig. 16.6 Normal HeLa cells. Note the confluent sheet of plump polygonal cells with a conspicuous giant form. They are derived from a malignant epithelial cell line. (McCarthy phase contrast ×200.)

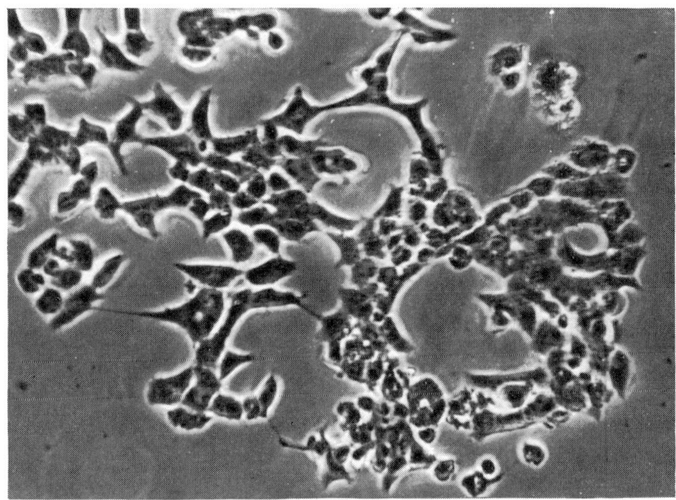

Fig. 16.7 HeLa cells infected with adenovirus. The sheet has been broken up, and the swollen, refractile cells form irregular masses. (McCarthy phase contrast × 200.)

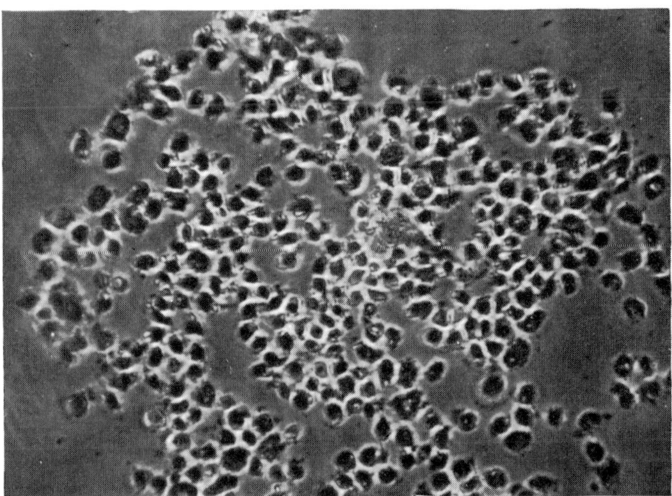

Fig. 16.8 HeLa cells infected with poliovirus. Note the severe disintegration of the cells. Poliovirus has a more destructive effect on cell cultures than does adenovirus. (McCarthy phase contrast × 200.)

characteristic of a specific virus, but in any case the virus can be identified by *neutralization tests* and *complement fixation* using specific rabbit antisera. If, for instance, a specific antiserum prevents a cytopathic effect in a cell system (or for that matter, if it prevents a lesion in an egg or a test animal), the virus is typed accordingly. The fluid in the tissue culture system provides the virus material. It also provides the source of antigen for performing complement fixation tests. The cell systems commonly employed in this way are monkey kidney cells, human amnion cells, and strains of cancer cells, e.g. the 'HeLa cell' derived from a carcinoma of the cervix of a woman named **He**len **La**ne.

Infectivity

Viruses produce disease even in minute quantities, and their degree of infectivity is so high that *epidemics are very common*, e.g. smallpox, influenza, and the common viral diseases of childhood.

Viral disease is by no means confined to vertebrates; there are insect infections like silkworm jaundice and sacbrood of bees, plant diseases like tobacco-mosaic disease, and also the very important group of bacterial infections due to bacteriophage.

Of the viruses pathogenic to the human subject many seem to attack one organ specifically, but the once fashionable concept of *tropism* is no longer valid. A 'neurotropic' virus like poliovirus multiplies in the cells of the small intestine, while the 'dermatotropic' virus of herpes simplex can produce encephalitis. There is as yet no entirely comprehensive classification of viruses, and therefore it is still very helpful to consider viral infections in terms of the organs or tissues that they usually infect:

Viruses attacking the skin: vaccinia, herpes simplex, and verruca vulgaris (the common wart).

Viruses attacking the central nervous system: enteroviruses, varicella-zoster, rabies, arthropod-borne viruses (arboviruses), mumps, and occasionally herpes simplex, measles, and vaccinia.

Viruses attacking the liver: hepatitis and yellow fever.

Viruses attacking the respiratory tract: influenza, adenoviruses, and the common cold viruses (rhinoviruses).

Viruses attacking the conjunctiva: herpes simplex and adenoviruses.

Viruses attacking the salivary glands and other secreting organs: mumps.

Generalized virus diseases often producing characteristic skin eruptions: smallpox, measles, rubella, chickenpox, dengue, and some enterovirus infections.

Tissue reactions to viruses

All considerations of the effects of viruses on the tissues of the body must start at a cellular level; viruses are intracellular parasites, and the damage they produce is directed primarily at the cell. This is followed secondarily by a local inflammatory reaction.

Cellular reaction. A cell infected with a virus may degenerate at once, or it may undergo proliferation which may or may not be followed by later necrosis, or it may show no change whatsoever.

This last effect is typical of what is called 'latent virus' infection. It is well known, for example, that many people harbour herpes simplex virus without showing any lesion. Similarly, many children are infected with certain types of adenoviruses early in life, and these remain in their tonsils and adenoids without producing conspicuous damage.

Whether a cell degenerates or proliferates depends on the type of cell involved and on the nature of the infecting virus. Labile cells, like those of surface epithelia, undergo continuous division throughout life, and so it is not surprising that some viral conditions of the skin have a proliferative tendency, e.g. verruca vulgaris.

Other cells described as permanent, e.g. neurons, cannot divide after birth, and viral infection of these is necessarily always destructive in tendency.

The skin is usually taken as a tissue in which the gamut of changes from immediate necrosis to indefinite proliferation is possible, as the following five infections demonstrate:

Foot-and-mouth disease causes a rapid swelling and necrosis of epidermal cells.

Vaccinia causes an early proliferation of the cells with necrosis following about 3 days later.

Fowl-pox causes a much more prolonged proliferation with necrosis supervening some weeks later.

Verruca vulgaris produces a massive proliferation which may last many months before involution occurs.

The *Shope papilloma of rabbits* is manifested by a neoplastic proliferation of cells, and malignancy may occur.

This is an instructive list, but many of the diseases mentioned are not relevant to the human being. Only in a few skin conditions, e.g. verruca vulgaris, is proliferation of cells a marked feature. There is no known example of human neoplasia directly attributable to viruses, a very important difference between human and animal viral disease. Nevertheless, some human tumours may be associated with viruses (see p. 368).

In most human viral diseases cellular destruction is the predominant lesion. The respiratory viruses destroy the surface epithelium, a tendency well marked in influenza, the viruses of hepatitis and yellow fever produce a characteristic necrosis of the liver, mumps produces destructive lesions of the acinar cells of the salivary glands and sometimes the pancreas, while the central nervous system may sustain permanent neuronal loss as a result of poliomyelitis and viral encephalitis.

Once the infection is overcome, there is rapid healing due to proliferation of neighbouring cells. The focal necrosis of virus A hepatitis heals so rapidly that needle biopsy of the liver performed after a few months may reveal no abnormality whatsoever. Neuronal destruction can be healed only by repair, i.e. gliosis, and hence permanent damage must sometimes be expected. It should be noted, however, that not every neuron infected with poliovirus is necessarily doomed. Many recover completely.

Inflammatory reaction. Secondary to the cellular damage there is a nondescript acute inflammatory reaction in the vicinity. This takes the form of vascular dilatation and an exudate containing lymphocytes and macrophages. Polymorphs are usually few in number. Most viral diseases are acute and of short duration, terminating in either rapid death or recovery. Exceptions to this are the tumour-producing viruses and perhaps certain neurotropic viruses.

Viral infections of epithelial surfaces are often complicated by secondary bacterial invasion: influenza is commonly followed by bacterial pneumonia.

It is noteworthy that viral infections, even the chronic ones, do not bring forth a predominantly macrophage response. Epithelioid-cell formation is never seen, nor indeed is any viral infection characterized by a granulomatous reaction.

The general body reaction to viral infection

Localization. Like other organisms, viruses first contaminate and infect a surface integument, either by inhalation (e.g. influenza), ingestion (e.g. poliomyelitis), or by the bite of an arthropod vector (e.g. yellow fever). Some viruses remain localized to their tissues of entry, e.g. verruca vulgaris virus and the rhinoviruses, while others become disseminated throughout the blood stream, and produce lesions in an organ remote from the sites of primary infection, e.g. poliomyelitis and yellow fever, or else lead to a generalized viral infection involving many organs, e.g. smallpox and measles. The systemic type of infection is associated with much more pronounced constitutional symptoms than the localized one, and a characteristic feature is the presence of high fever during the early viraemic phase. This is often followed by a remission, which is in turn succeeded by another spurt of pyrexia when the virus becomes clinically localized at its organ of destination. Localized diseases like the common cold and verruca vulgaris are accompanied by little, if any, constitutional upset.

Dissemination. The mode of dissemination of a virus in the body has been investigated with respect to mouse-pox. The virus enters the mouse's body through an abrasion in its skin, and multiplies there. Within 8 hours the virus reaches the local lymph nodes, and after further multiplication it invades the blood stream and is taken up by the RE cells of the liver and spleen. There it multiplies once more, and after 6 days it invades the blood stream in large amounts, and settles selectively in the epidermal cells of the skin. This phase of viraemia is accompanied by severe constitutional effects; still another 4 days elapse before a rash appears.

The initial 6 days of infection constitute the *incubation period*; the 4 days of severe illness, which may prove fatal in overwhelming infections, are the *prodromal period.* During this time virus material may still be cultured from the blood, but once the rash appears (10th day) there is a rapidly rising level of neutralizing antibody in the circulation. Human diseases like smallpox and measles have a somewhat similar pattern of dissemination, but the route of entry is through the respiratory tract.

Transplacental infection of the fetus is important in rubella infections and may lead to congenital abnormalities (p. 376). Other viral diseases transmitted across the placenta are herpes-simplex infection and Coxsackie-virus myocarditis.

Antibody response. Viral infections are accompanied by a high titre of immunoglobulins during the period of convalescence. The highest antibody response is encountered in those viruses which are widely disseminated in the circulation, and a life-long *immunity* may be expected after diseases like smallpox, measles, and mumps. Localized infections, like the common cold, also induce antibodies, but the degree of immunity is small, and recurrence is common. It must also be remembered that many viruses are of more than one type, e.g. there are 3 types of poliovirus and many types of human adenovirus. This is an additional reason for recurrent attacks of certain infections.

The element of *hypersensitivity* is also noteworthy in viral infections. The accelerated reaction following a second vaccination is a good example of allergy to vaccinia virus. The lesion appears within a day or two and resolves after about one week, whereas a primary vaccination reaction appears on the fourth or fifth day and reaches its zenith on about the tenth day. It takes about 3 weeks to heal and is occasionally complicated by systemic lesions. The close resemblance of this to the Koch phenomenon is obvious, except that here the element of immunity is much greater than in tuberculosis.

There is a strong allergic element in the skin eruption that occurs in the course of generalized infections like smallpox and measles. In such conditions there is an incubation period of about 2 weeks, and the skin is sensitized to viral products before the virus reaches it in full force. The analogy to the later intestinal ulceration of typhoid fever is very close.

Mechanism of the pathogenic effects of viruses

Viruses produce their harmful effects by virtue of the cell destruction they cause; no factors comparable with bacterial toxins have been demonstrated. It is believed that the cytotoxic effect of viruses is due to complex biochemical disturbances that accompany virus replication. In addition, there is also a delayed type of hypersensitivity.

The cause of death in viral disease is obvious when a vital organ is damaged directly, e.g. the liver in hepatitis. In the pox diseases the mode of death is less easily explained. Clinically there is a state of 'shock' reminiscent of the toxaemia of invasive bacterial infections, and it is suggested that this is due to virus invasion and damage of vascular endothelial cells.

Immunity to viral infections

The mechanism of immunity to viral infection is complex and has several components.

(a) **Immunoglobulins.** Immunoglobulins play an important part, especially in the disseminated infections. Viruses have a number of antigens, some associated with the nucleoprotein and others with the capsid and outer envelope. It is against these last two antigens that immunoglobulins act; by neutralizing them they prevent the virus attaching itself to a cell receptor. The extracellular complex is phagocytosed and destroyed. Intracellular virus is invulnerable to antibody. These plasma, virus-neutralizing immunoglobulins belong to the IgG class.

It is also to be noted that after recovery from an attack of poliomyelitis or following immunization with living attenuated virus administered orally, a subsequent dose of poliovirus does not flourish in the cells of the small bowel. This is due to the action of IgA antibodies produced locally in the intestine and present in the secretions. People who have been immunized with a killed suspension of poliovirus administered parenterally usually exhibit unhindered virus multiplication in the small bowel despite a considerable antibody response.

(b) **Cell-mediated immunity** plays an even more important role in viral infections than do the immunoglobulins. Thus in states of pure immunoglobulin deficiency (hypogammaglobulinaemia) there is usually an effective host response to systematic viral infections, whereas in states of T lymphocyte deficiency chronic, progressive, fatal viral infections, e.g. vaccinia, chickenpox, herpes simplex, and cytomegalic inclusion disease, are extremely common. The part the lymphocyte plays in viral infection is still obscure. It is known that a sensitised lymphocyte secretes interferon among the lymphokines; in addition, it is possible that the lymphocyte destroys the virus-infected cell directly, thereby killing intracellular virus.

(c) **Interferon.** The interferons are a family of antiviral proteins varying in molecular weight from 20 000 to 160 000 daltons which are produced by cells infected with a virus. This protein is non-toxic and non-antigenic to the host (and only feebly antigenic to other species), and has a remarkable effect in making the cells resistant to further viral infection. It 'interferes' with the proliferation of a second virus in the affected cell, and this effect has a very broad spectrum of activity. Inactivated virus is as effective in stimulating interferon production as is living virus. Interferon can be produced in many tissue culture systems, but its action is specific for the animal from which it was derived. There can be little doubt that it is important in checking the course of many viral infections. Whether it plays any part in the acquired cellular immunity of viral disease is uncertain. The administration of glucocorticoids inhibits the production and action of interferon; pyrexia, on the other hand, stimulates it. Interferon is thought to act by inhibiting the translation of viral mRNA. This it does not directly, but by inducing the formation of a second cellular protein called translation-inhibitory protein. Translation of host-cell mRNA is not interrupted; this explains why interferon is non-toxic.

Interferon is potentially an important therapeutic agent, but at the present time its use is experimental.

Chemotherapy of viral diseases

Viral multiplication is so intimately bound up with normal cell metabolism that the possibility of finding effective chemotherapeutic agents seemed remote even a few years ago. This gloomy forecast has, however, been proved to be ill founded, and a number of effective agents have been discovered.

Chemotherapeutic agents may act at any stage in the life-cycle of the virus from its initial attachment to the cell to the final stage of assembly of mature virus particles and their subsequent release. Some agents appear to act at different or several stages according to the particular viral infection.

Agents which have been found to be of some value include *5-iodo-2'-deoxyuridine* (*5-IDU*) in herpes infections and *adenine arabinoside* (*ARA-A*) in herpes-simplex and varicella-zoster infections. *Amantadine* is used in the prophylaxis of influenza A infection, and *marboran* has been of value in the prophylaxis of smallpox. Unfortunately many of these agents are toxic and unsuitable for systemic use in humans, but there is every indication that new, less toxic agents will be found.

The diagnosis of viral disease

In a few instances diagnostic *inclusion bodies* may be found (e.g. Negri bodies in rabies), or characteristic *elementary bodies* may be seen by light microscopy (e.g. Paschen bodies in the vesicles of vaccinia).

An important diagnostic procedure is the isolation of the virus from the patient's secretions using the living cell systems already described. The virus may then be typed by means of complement fixation and neutralization tests using specific rabbit antisera. Some viruses with a characteristic shape can be identified by electron microscopy. With negative contrast techniques virus may be detected within a few minutes of collecting the specimen, provided it is present at concentrations greater than about 10^6 per ml. For practical purposes this limits its use to examining specimens obtained from readily accessible sites which contain high concentrations of virus, e.g. poxviruses and herpesviruses from skin lesions and rotaviruses, adenoviruses, and hepatitis A virus from the faeces. The technique of immune-electron microscopy can distinguish between antigenically distinct but morphologically identical viruses; it consists of the detection of immune complexes after the specimen has been pre-incubated with a virus-specific antiserum.

Immunofluorescence techniques are also valuable in the rapid diagnosis of viral disease, and they are more sensitive than electron microscopy especially now that the quality of the reagents is satisfactory enough to minimize the amount of non-specific fluorescence. They are particularly useful in examining brain material for herpes-simplex virus and rabies virus and nasopharyngeal secretions for respiratory viruses.

Various *transport media* are available for conveying unfrozen specimens to the laboratory. The media consist of neutral balanced salt solutions containing a protein (eg. bovine serum albumin) and antibiotics. Viruses survive in transport medium for a number of hours or days according to the organism. In practice, a specimen should be sent to the laboratory as soon as possible and preferably the same day that it has been collected.

Antigen detection in diagnosis

The detection of viral antigen in blood or tissue fluids is a rapid and valuable aid to diagnosis in certain viral infections. It has found particular application in the investigation of patients and carriers of hepatitis B virus. The antigens are estimated by a variety of immunological techniques. Radio-immunoassay (RIA) is the most sensitive, commonly used method, but more recently the enzyme-linked immunosorbent assay (ELISA) and countercurrent immuno-electro-osmophoresis (CIEOP) have been introduced.*

Examination of convalescent serum. In convalescent patients there is invariably a rise in titre of antibodies against the agent. It is therefore important to obtain a sample of serum as early in the disease as possible (this furnishes a baseline against which to judge the subsequent rise), as well as a second specimen 10–14 days later. Antibodies may be estimated by a variety of tests including complement fixation, neutralization, RIA,* ELISA,* and indirect immunofluorescent techniques.

* Radioimmunoassay methods are used to estimate a wide range of substances, eg. viral antigens, antibodies, and hormones. Thus to estimate HBsAg, a quantity of antibody is attached to a suitable surface (the solid phase). This is allowed to react with patient's serum, and subsequently radioactive-labelled antibody is applied. By estimating the amount of radioactivity attached to the surface, the titre of antigen may be calculated. The enzyme-linked immunosorbent assay (ELISA) utilizes an enzyme as a marker instead of radioactive iodine. It is therefore a safer method for laboratory workers. In countercurrent immuno-electro-osmophoresis (CIEOP) the two reacting components are driven together under the influence of an electric field. This is less wasteful of reagents (and therefore a more sensitive method) than if the components simply diffused passively towards each other as in the original Ouchterlony precipitin method (p. 154).

In practice retrospective diagnosis made on serological grounds is the most important method of diagnosing viral disease.

SOME COMMON VIRAL INFECTIONS

Enteroviruses

The enteroviruses are a group of small, spherical, RNA-containing viruses found particularly in the cells of the intestine. They are members of a larger group called the *picornaviruses* (pico = small + RNA), to which the foot-and-mouth disease virus of cattle and the rhinoviruses that cause the common cold also belong. The enteroviruses are especially associated with neurological diseases. There are three subgroups:

The Coxsackie viruses, of which there are 30 types. They were first isolated in the town of Coxsackie in New York State in 1948, and are found quite frequently in the faeces of healthy children. They are responsible for a variety of clinical pictures including an upper respiratory, cold-like condition, and an illness which resembles paralytic poliomyelitis. They also cause *herpangina,* a febrile disease of children in which there are shallow greyish ulcers in the mouth and fauces, and *Bornholm disease,* in which there is agonizing chest pain.

The ECHO (Enteric, Cytopathic, Human, Orphan) viruses, of which there are at least 34 types. They are found quite commonly in children's faeces, and for a long time could not be associated with any disease—hence the name 'orphan'. It is now known that they produce a variety of febrile illnesses including some which mimic poliomyelitis and the common cold.

The polioviruses. Poliomyelitis is caused by the three types of poliovirus, of which type 1 produces the most severe disease. The disease is contracted by the ingestion of material which has been contaminated by virus-containing faeces. Faecal pollution of drinking water or swimming baths is a possible danger, as is also fly-borne contamination of food. Indirect contact with excretors, whose dirty hands contaminate fomites, is another source of infection.

Spread of virus in the body. It is believed that the virus proliferates first in the cells of the pharynx and the lower part of the small bowel. If it is not arrested at this stage, it enters the general circulation *via* the lymphatics, and it then multiplies in various extraneural sites like the spleen and kidneys. This marks the end of the incubation period, which usually lasts 7 to 14 days, but may extend up to 30 days. The next viraemic phase is ushered in by a febrile reaction, but even then the infection may be overcome. If the condition proceeds, the virus settles finally in the central nervous system which it reaches by the blood stream. It localizes itself specifically in the anterior horn cells and their medullary counterparts, and paralysis ensues.

A second mode of spread is directly up the peripheral nerve endings of the bowel and especially the pharynx. Opinions vary about the importance of this method of spread; it probably accounts for the bulbar type of disease that sometimes follows tonsillectomy and other operative procedures in the mouth.

It is evident that much has still to be learned about the pathogenesis of the disease. One thing is clear; many people are infected with poliovirus, and either show no illness at all or else have a mild febrile reaction. Only a small unlucky minority develop paralysis. Poliomyelitis is an excellant example of an infection that tends to be subclinical.

Factors aggravating the disease. The incubation period is shortened, and the liability to nervous-system involvement increased by the following factors: heavy exercise and fatigue, pregnancy, operative procedures, and active immunization with any antigen. When the disease follows immunization, it is called *provocation poliomyelitis*; it is believed that alum and other adjuvants in the vaccines and toxoids are the important factors. The mode of action is unknown, but it has been suggested that the focus of inflammation acts as a nidus for proliferation of the virus during the period of viraemia. It might then travel up the local nerve to the spinal cord. Active immunization procedures should be postponed during a poliomyelitis epidemic. So also should minor surgery, e.g. dental extraction.

Immunization. A consideration of poliomyelitis immunization is valuable as a general exercise in comparing the relative merits of dead suspensions to those of live attenuated viruses.

Active immunization. The first effective vaccine was devised by Salk, who used polioviruses grown in monkey kidney cells and subsequently inactivated by formolization. It is issued in trivalent form, containing types 1, 2, and 3, and requires at least three intramuscular inoculations, the second a month after the first, and the third about 6 months after the second. A high titre of circulating immunoglobulin should be produced, though often there is a disappointing response to type-1 virus, the most dangerous of the three. Immunity depends on the presence of IgG antibody. The resistance of the cells of the small bowel to subsequent infection by poliovirus is not altered.

Later Sabin produced a vaccine consisting of living attenuated strains of poliovirus which had undergone mutation after passage through mice. These attenuated viruses are given orally, and they closely simulate the natural disease except that spread does not occur to the nervous system. The immunity they produce depends not only on circulating immunoglobulin, but also on the presence of IgA in the small bowel, as has already been discussed. If a triple vaccine is given, a possible snag is that one virus might infect the cells first and interfere with the entry of the other two. In practice it is found that any interfering tendency is obviated by giving three doses of trivalent vaccine at monthly intervals. It must be stressed that the Sabin type vaccine leads to an infection of the intestine and a subsequent passage of virus in the faeces. It is almost inevitable therefore that the individual will infect other people, who in turn will become immunized. The possibility that the virus might mutate back to a virulent form has caused some concern, and indeed there is evidence that some cases of poliomyelitis in Britain are due to vaccine strains.

Despite this warning, there can be no doubt that the amount of poliomyelitis is very much less now than it was before the days of active immunization. Furthermore, virulent wild strains of poliovirus have been replaced by much less dangerous organisms derived from vaccine strains.

The oral vaccine has supplanted the inactivated one because it gives a better, long-lasting immunity and it acts more rapidly in a threatened epidemic. Despite its general safety it should not be given within 3 weeks of tonsillectomy or any immunization procedure.

The poxviruses

The poxviruses are a group of large DNA-containing viruses which produce vesicular and pustular skin lesions. Many animals have their own variety of pox disease, e.g. cow-pox, mouse-pox, etc. The human disease is smallpox.

Smallpox. The disease is acquired by the inhalation of infected particles from a patient directly or from fomites indirectly. The bedding is particularly dangerous, and numerous instances are on record where laundry workers have contracted the disease from contaminated bedclothes.

Spread in the body. It is believed that the primary lesions occur in the nasal mucosa and that this is followed by systemic spread to the RE system. After an incubation period of 10 to 14 days there occurs a phase of secondary viraemia during which the patient becomes ill. Some 4 days later the virus settles in the mucous membrane and skin giving rise to the characteristic rashes, the *enantham* and the *exanthem.*

Active immunization. The first really effective attempt at smallpox immunization was performed by Edward Jenner, who discovered that the natural pox infection of bovine animals, *cow-pox,* could produce a similar lesion in human beings, and protect them against smallpox infection.

Since then a third virus has emerged, *vaccinia virus.* Its origin is obscure, and although it may have arisen as a mutant of either cow-pox virus or smallpox virus, it now appears to be quite distinct from both.

In the human vaccinia virus applied to the skin with firm pressure by a needle (*vaccination*) produces a localized infection, and the subsequent immune response gives good, though temporary, protection against smallpox infection. Unfortunately vaccination is occasionally complicated by spread of the virus, either locally (*progressive vaccinia*), or to the rest of the skin (*generalized vaccinia*). A form of encephalitis with a 50 per cent mortality rate is another rare complication.

Though these complications are rare, it has become apparent that in many Western European countries the mortality due to them is greater than the indigenous smallpox mortality. It has therefore become the policy in Britain to dispense with the routine vaccination of infants and children, and reserve vaccination for those in immediate contact with a case of smallpox. Such vaccination of contacts within 3 days of exposure is usually effective. Of course, those whose occupation brings them into possible contact with the disease, e.g. doctors, nurses, and members of the armed forces, should be vaccinated regularly as long as they are at risk. Likewise, there are many countries, entry into which necessitates prior vaccination.

The most important contra-indication to vaccination is the presence of any widespread skin disease, especially atopic dermatitis. Vaccination should also be avoided in patients with any immunological deficiency syndrome especially of cell-mediated immunity, and also in those who are pregnant or who are being treated with glucocorticoids (unless there is an emergency).

There had been recent reports that no case of smallpox had occurred in the world for many months. Since no known carrier exists, smallpox may well be on

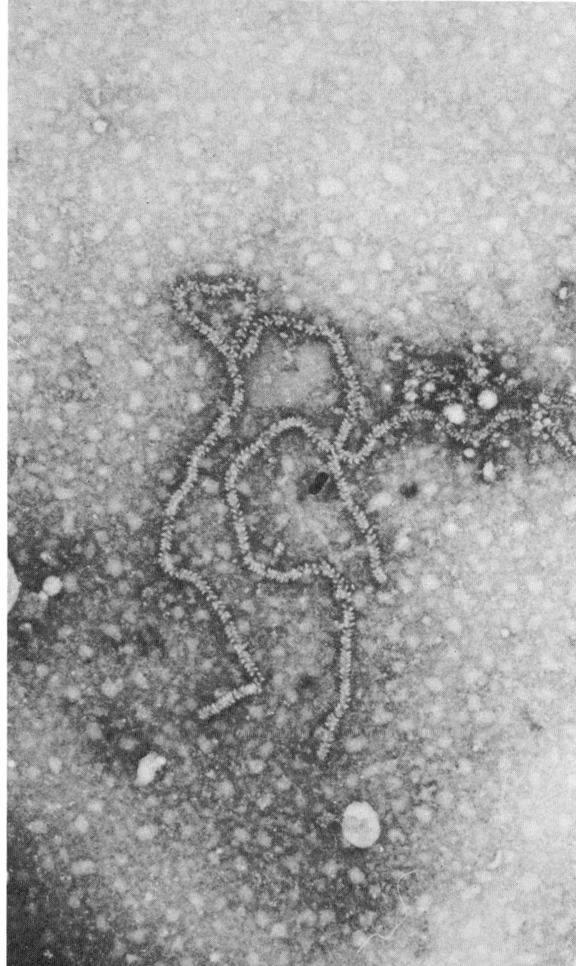

Fig. 16.9 A paramyxovirus. The covering membrane of the paramyxovirus has been ruptured; its RNA content has been released. The long thread of nuclear protein is surrounded by the capsomeres arranged in a helical fashion. × 117 450. (*Photograph by courtesy of Micheline Fauvel, Department of Medical Microbiology, Faculty of Medicine, University of Toronto.*)

the way to becoming extinct. In this event vaccination against the disease will be a thing of the past, and Jenner's true claim to fame will be the eradication of a disease rather than the development of a vaccine.*

Viruses affecting the respiratory tract

The number of viruses incriminated in respiratory infections is legion.

Orthomyxoviruses. The orthomyxoviruses are a group of medium-sized

* According to a WHO press release of 25 May 1978, the last confirmed case of smallpox was in Merka town, Somalia, with the onset of the skin eruption on 26 October 1977. If no new cases had occurred during the 2 years following that date, smallpox would have been regarded as extinct. Unfortunately there remains the hazard of reference laboratories that keep stocks of smallpox virus for research purposes. In September 1978 a woman died of the disease in Birmingham, England; it seems certain that she acquired the virus from the research laboratory which was located in the same building where she herself worked.

RNA-containing viruses. They are so named because they have a strong affinity for mucins. Thus, *in vitro* they can attach themselves to the mucroprotein receptors of red cells, and by forming bridges, cause the cells to agglutinate. The important human orthomyxoviruses are the *influenza viruses* of which there are three types. The *parainfluenza viruses* and the virus of *mumps* belong to a closely related group, the *paramyxoviruses,* which are slightly larger than the orthomyxoviruses (Fig. 16.9).

Adenoviruses. The adenoviruses are small DNA-containing viruses which have a proclivity for the mucosa of the upper respiratory tract and the conjunctiva.

Coronaviruses. These are a group of medium-sized, pleomorphic, RNA-containing viruses with a prominent envelope arranged into spikes, or peplomeres, which form a fringe of projections resembling petals. Their resemblance to a crown is the basis of the name coronavirus.

Many coronaviruses cause disease in animals, e.g. mouse hepatitis and avian infectious bronchitis. In the human being they are an important cause of upper-respiratory-tract infections of a cold-like type.

The common cold. The viruses that cause the common cold are called rhinoviruses. The rhinoviruses are of interest in requiring a temperature of 33°C instead of 37°C for successful culture. Their habitat in the nose is probably related to this temperature requirement. More thah 100 serotypes of this virus are known.

The arthropod-borne viruses

Arthropod-borne viruses cause yellow fever, dengue, sandfly fever, and a number of types of encephalitis of regional geographical distribution. Members of this group have been called *arboviruses,* but the group is in fact made up of several different families, e.g. *togaviruses* and *orbiviruses.* In addition to the diseases mentioned above, some arthropod-borne viruses cause *viral haemorrhagic fevers.* These are severe diseases which can also be caused by other viruses, e.g. the Marburg virus which was inadvertently imported from Germany in 1967.

Viral hepatitis

The two important diseases that come into this category are virus A hepatitis (previously called infective hepatitis) and virus B hepatitis (previously called serum hepatitis).

Virus A hepatitis occurs endemically in institutions like schools and military camps, and its main incidence is among children and young adults. The agent is excreted in the faeces, and infects other individuals after the ingestion of contaminated food. During the preicteric and early icteric phases of the illness it is present also in the blood. The disease is transmitted mainly by ingestion. No carrier state is known to exist.

Hepatitis A virus (HAV) is a small, 25 to 28 nm in size, RNA virus with cubical symmetry. It can be demonstrated in the faeces of patients for a few days after the onset of jaundice using electronmicroscopic techniques. It has not been grown in cell culture.

Virus B hepatitis is not usually acquired by the oral route, although it can be transmitted by ingesting contaminated blood. The virus is not usually present in the faeces, but it may be found in the blood for periods of over 5 years. It is transmitted not only by blood transfusion but also by the prick of a contaminated needle; the amount of blood or serum necessary to convey the infection need be as little as 0.01 ml. It is a major hazard among young drug-addicts, especially those who inject themselves intravenously ('mainliners'). People who handle blood, such as laboratory technicians, or work in haemodialysis units are also at risk.

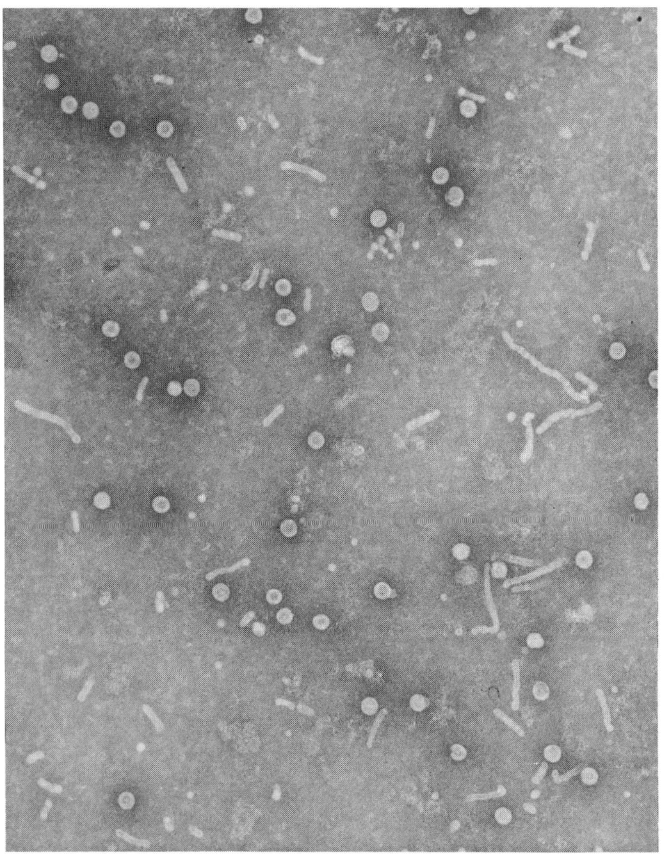

Fig. 16.10 Hepatitis B virus. This is a negative-stained preparation of hepatitis-B positive serum. Three types of particles can be seen: spherical particles 20 nm in diameter; elongated, tubular filaments up to 230 nm in length; and Dane particles, 42 nm in diameter, and having a double shell. × 119 700. (*Photograph by courtesy of Micheline Fauvel, Department of Medical Microbiology, Faculty of Medicine, University of Toronto.*)

Hepatitis B virus (HBV) is double shelled and 42 nm in size. It used to be called the *Dane particle.* It contains double-stranded DNA. It clearly belongs to a new family of viruses. It is found in the serum of patients and carriers, but it has not been grown in cell culture.

It possesses at least three separate antigens:

Hepatitis B surface antigen (*HBsAg,* which was first called *Australia antigen* because it was originally found in an Australian aborigine), which is found on the surface of the virus. It is also found on the 22 nm spherical particles and the long tubular forms, about 20 nm in diameter and of variable length, seen in the serum (Fig. 16.10). It displays antigenic heterogeneity: in addition to a common determinant 'a', all HBsAg particles possess two type-specific subdeterminants, either 'd' or 'y', and either 'w' or 'r'. Thus the four major serotypes are HBsAg /adr, ayr, adw, and ayw. Infection with one subtype may fail to confer immunity against a second infection with another subtype.

Hepatitis B core antigen (*HBcAg*), which is demonstrable only after disruption of the outer membrane of the virus. It is not found in the serum, but it may be found in the nuclei of the liver cells of monkeys and humans that have been infected with HBV.

The e antigen (*HBeAg*), which has three subtypes HBeAg/1, HBeAg/2, and HBeAg/3. There appears to be a close association between the presence of HBeAg in HBsAg-positive serum and the presence of complete HBV particles, so that HBeAg is a good marker of the potential infectivity of HBsAg-positive serum.

The diseases these two viruses produce are pathologically very similar: a widespread focal necrosis which usually recovers by complete regeneration. Nevertheless, there are distinct clinical differences. Virus A hepatitis has a much shorter incubation period than virus B hepatitis (15 to 40 days as compared with 60 to 160 days). Although the clinical features of the two conditions are very similar, the mortality rate is 0.1 per cent with virus A hepatitis and up to 10 per cent, or even higher, with virus B hepatitis. Both can kill with a fulminating infection that leads to massive necrosis, but as yet there is no evidence that HAV infection leads to chronic liver disease. On the other hand, about 10 per cent of cases of HBV infection progress to a chronic type of hepatitis, e.g. subacute or chronic active hepatitis, which may proceed to macronodular cirrhosis. Adults are more vulnerable than are children, and pregnant and older women are especially endangered. The most dangerous type of virus B infection is post-transfusion hepatitis, which has a mortality rate of from 10 to 20 per cent. This is attributable to the large dose of virus received and the poor state of health of the patient which necessitated transfusion. The over-all mortality rate is much less than this (about 1 per cent).

Prophylactic passive immunisation with γ-globulin is useful against HAV, but is of much less value in HBV infection because of the low antibody titre against HBV. Special high-titre HBV immunoglobulin is now available, and promises to be of value.

Virus B hepatitis is a good example of a condition in which antibodies can play a dangerous role in the progress of the disease. Immune-complex hypersensitivity effects, e.g. serum-sickness phenomena (urticaria and arthralgia) occur in 10 to 20 per cent of cases some days or weeks before the symptoms of liver disease occur. Occasionally there may be glomerulonephritis or polyarteritis nodosa.

Furthermore, immunologically deficient people, e.g. lepromatous lepers, those on immuosuppressants, and especially those with chronic renal failure, carry the antigen for long periods. Such people do not appear to suffer from liver damage, but they are potent transmitters of the agent. Many cases of hepatitis have occurred in doctors and nurses working in renal dialysis units, and a disturbingly high mortality rate has occurred in some centres.

In the general population the carrier rate varies from about 0.1 per cent in the

USA to over 10 per cent in some of the Pacific Islands. Perhaps primitive conditions, including tattooing, play a part in carrying infection around the community. Transmission by mosquito bite is another possibility, as these insects have been shown to harbour HBsAg, but it has not been shown that they transmit the disease. Spread by bed bugs is a possibility.

It has been shown that virus B hepatitis can spread naturally from person to person and that serum containing antigen is infectious when given by mouth. Thus the traditional teaching that virus B hepatitis be transmitted only by injection is not absolutely true; nevertheless, the great majority of infections are acquired parenterally. We know little about the excretion of the virus in the faeces and urine. The virus may also be present in the saliva, and be transmitted by kissing.

The presence of HBV in saliva presents a potential hazard to dentists. The following categories of patients have been suggested as presenting a particular hazard that requires special precautions for dental treatment.*

1. Patients with chronic renal failure who are receiving, or are likely to receive, regular dialysis treatment and patients who have had a renal or other organ transplant
2. Patients receiving long-term immunosuppressive therapy
3. Patients with haemophilia and others with haematological disorders who receive multiple transfusions of blood or blood products
4. Patients from institutions for the mentally handicapped. (Mentally handicapped patients living at home do not constitute a special risk)
5. Known drug addicts
6. Patients suffering from jaundice which is thought to be infective in nature and those who have suffered from such jaundice within the previous 6 months.
7. Patients who either live in, or have come from, areas where the carrier rate is high, e.g. Asia.

The detection of HBV antigens in the serum of blood donors has been a most important advance in blood-transfusion technique, and at last a means is available to protect recipients against this very unpleasant hazard. This is discussed in detail on page 255.

It should be noted finally that some episodes of acute viral hepatitis are not due to either HAV or HBV, nor even to such viruses as the Epstein-Barr virus or the cytomegalovirus, which occasionally produce a predominantly hepatic illness.

In the USA another as yet unidentified virus is the most common cause of hepatitis occurring after blood transfusion. Indeed, it is probable that there are a number of such viruses, but as yet there is no laboratory test to identify them. Provisionally this has been called non-A non-B hepatitis, and there are indications that the infection can be acquired by routes other than by transfusion and that non-A non-B viruses are responsible for some cases of chronic hepatitis.

* This recommendation is taken from a report by the Expert Group on Hepatitis in Dentistry published by Her Majesty's Stationery Office, London, 1979.

The herpesviruses

Varicella and zoster. Though the well-known clinical features of varicella (chickenpox) and zoster are poles apart, there is good evidence that they are both caused by the same virus.

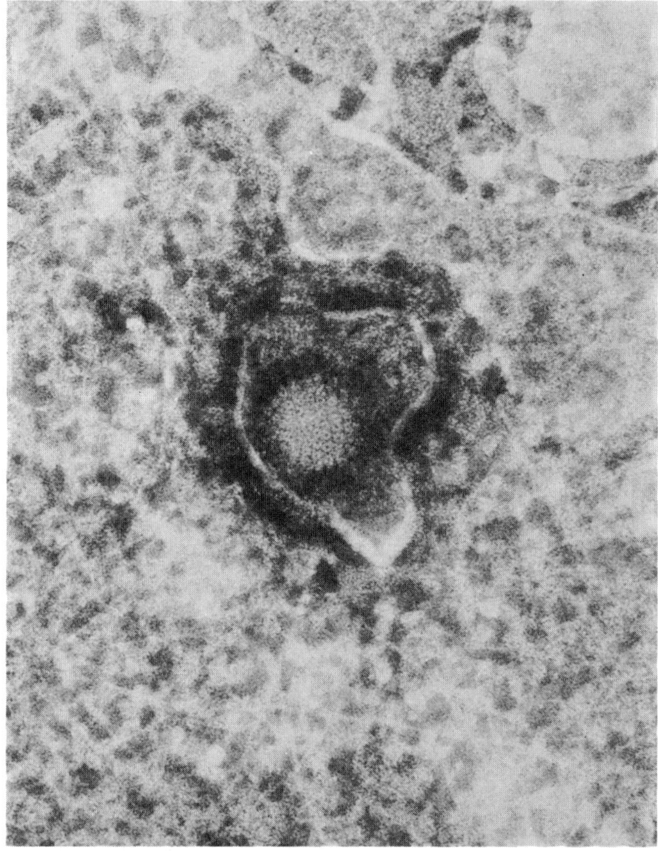

Fig. 16.11 Herpes simplex virus. The envelope, which is clearly delineated, is derived from the modified nuclear membrane of an infected cell. The hollow capsomeres of the virion are clearly visible. × 139 800. (*Photograph by courtesy of Micheline Fauvel, Department of Microbiology, Faculty of Medicine, University of Toronto.*)

Chickenpox has a pathogenesis similar to that of smallpox, and exhibits an enanthem involving the oral mucosa and an exanthem consisting of vesicles on the skin, which subsequently become pustular.

Zoster. Following an attack of chickenpox the virus may lie latent in the tissues, and in later life be reactivated by some physical or mental shock. It produces lesions specifically in the posterior root ganglia of the spinal, trigeminal, or facial nerves, and from there infection spreads down the nerve fibres to the skin. Pain followed by the development of a vesicular rash restricted to an area supplied by the nerve are characteristic. Children exposed to a patient with zoster often develop chickenpox.

Herpes simplex. The virus of herpes simplex is one of the most widely distributed viruses in human beings (Fig. 16.11). It is estimated that about 60 per cent of the population are affected. Of these only 10 per cent exhibit primary childhood lesions, such as *gingivostomatitis, keratoconjunctivitis,* and *vulvovaginitis.* Rarely the infection is more widespread.

Abrasions of the skin predispose to primary herpetic infection (*traumatic,* or *inoculation, herpes simplex*). A good example of this is the painful *herpetic whitlow,* which is seen in nursing attendants working in neurosurgical wards. These people acquire their infection while inserting endotracheal tubes into the mouths of unconscious patients. It is also seen in dentists.

Usually, however, the primary infection remains subclinical, and the virus remains latent in the cells of the host. This symbiosis tends to be disturbed by intercurrent infections, e.g. the common cold, pneumonia, and malaria, and even, in very susceptible victims, by menstruation, emotional strain, and exposure to sunlight. There then develop typical *herpetic blisters* (cold sores). These are most common on the *lips* near the mucocutaneous junction; the oral mucosa is rarely affected, and it should be noted that the common recurrent aphthous ulcers of the mouth are not due to herpes simplex. Occasionally the *conjunctiva* or *cornea* (dendritic ulcers) are affected. *Skin* lesions are common, and may be found on any part of the body. *Genital herpes* affects the vulva or penis and presents as recurrent blisters which rapidly break to form shallow, painful ulcers. A striking feature of recurrent herpes is that in any one patient the lesions usually affect the same site on each occasion. This suggests that the virus remains latent in either the skin or the supplying nerves. Babies born of mothers with active genital herpes may develop the dangerous *generalized herpes of the newborn.*

The precise localisation of the virus during the latent periods has been a matter for speculation. It cannot be identified in the skin between attacks, but it has been isolated from sensory nerve-root ganglia—trigeminal or sacral—examined at necropsy. It appears that the virus remains latent in nerve cells, but when conditions are favourable it is able to infect the skin and produce typical herpetic vesicles. The mechanism is therefore analogous to that encountered in zoster.

There are two antigenically distinct types of herpes simplex. *Herpesvirus hominis type 1* usually causes typical herpes febrilis of the face, mouth, pharynx, and cornea, and is also responsible for eczema herpeticum and herpes meningo-encephalitis. *Herpesvirus hominis type 2* usually causes herpes genitalis and vulvovaginitis, and also neonatal herpes. It should be noted that type-1 virus can cause genital infections, and likewise type-2 virus may be responsible for oral and skin lesions.

Epstein-Barr (EB) virus. This herpesvirus causes classical *infectious mononucleosis* (glandular fever) with a positive Paul-Bunnell test. It is also associated with Burkitt's tumour and nasopharyngeal carcinoma (see p. 368).

Rabies

Rabies is caused by a bullet-shaped virus belonging to the group of rhabdoviruses, which normally infect certain species of animals. The disease is rare in human beings, but it is of intense interest for two reasons. With one possible exception there has never been recorded a human case of rabies that survived. While many diseases are fatal, the mode of death in rabies is particularly unpleasant. An initial phase of excitement with spasms and convulsions is characteristic. Particularly common are painful contractions of the pharyngeal muscles initiated by attempts to swallow water. Hence the term *hydrophobia,* meaning that the patients fear water. The stage of excitement is followed by one of generalized paralysis, and death usually occurs within a few days of its onset. Treatment is entirely supportive; the only hope is that the diagnosis is wrong. The second reason for considering rabies important is that the infection is always a threat in North America and in continental Europe. Only in England is the disease virtually unknown and likely to remain so, owing to the strict quarantine regulations that are enforced.

Rabies is endemic in the fox population in Europe, whereas in North America it affects many species of animals, e.g. foxes, raccoons, and skunks. Following the bite of an infected animal the virus spreads to the nervous system *via* the nerve fibres. Rabies in dogs is invariably fatal within 10 days, and if a person is bitten by a dog, it is important to keep the dog under surveillance for this period. If the dog dies or is killed, examination of the brain for Negri bodies is an important investigation.

If the person is bitten by a rabid animal, or by an animal that escapes, the question of immunization is of paramount importance. It has been estimated that about 30 000 persons in the USA are given treatment each year for rabies immunization.

The original method of immunization against rabies was devised by Pasteur. He noted that rabbits infected with rabies developed a virus of fixed virulence. By taking the spinal cords of infected rabbits and drying them for varying periods, it seemed that the virus had lost its pathogenicity. Thus material derived from a rabbit spinal cord that had been dried for some time failed to produce rabies on injection into a human being. A series of 14 injections, each given at daily intervals, was administered—each one being from a rabbit cord preparation dried for a lesser period of time. Unfortunately, the injections are painful and produce ever-increasing local inflammatory reactions. The repeated injection of foreign spinal cord tissue can on occasion lead to an autoimmune encephalomyelitis. The problem with rabies prophylaxis is whether the risk of inducing a disabling encephalomyelitis outweighs the risk of developing rabies. Antiserum prepared in horses is now available, and vaccines prepared in duck eggs and tissue culture have been developed. The latter are used for immunizing animals, but whether they are sufficiently potent for human use, or indeed whether they are safe, has yet to be determined.

Papovaviruses*

The common wart is caused by an infection with a small DNA-containing virus (Fig. 16.12) which belongs to a group of organisms that also cause papillomata in animals, e.g. rabbits. The polyoma virus (p. 366) also belongs to this group as also does the SV-40 virus, a passenger virus quite commonly found in monkey kidney

* These viruses have also been called vacuolating agents since in cultures the infected cells show vacuolation. Similar vacuolated cells are also found in human warts. The name papova is derived from the first two letters of the words PApilloma, POlyoma and VAcuolating agent.

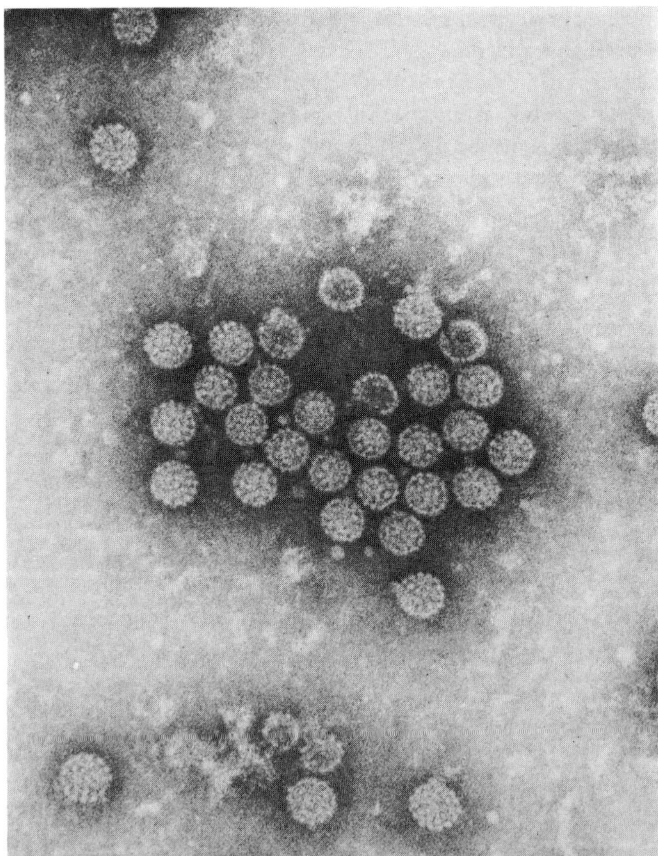

Fig. 16.12 A papovavirus (SV 40). This organism was found as a contaminant in a culture of African Green Monkey kidney cells. × 136 000. (*Photograph by courtesy of Micheline Fauvel, Department of Medical Microbiology, Faculty of Medicine, University of Toronto.*)

cells. Under some circumstances this virus is capable of inducing tumour formation in animals. It has not been proven to be harmful to humans.

Slow viruses

Scrapie is a lethal neurological disease of sheep which appears to be caused by an agent which is very resistant to heat and chemical disinfectants. The incubation period is several *years.* The nature of the agent is not clear, but there is interesting speculation as to whether any human counterpart exists to account for certain chronic diseases of the central nervous system.

Conclusion

The range of diseases caused by viruses is very large, and in many of them there are oral lesions; although these are often of little significance, some are useful in diagnosis. The enanthem often appears before the typical exanthem—Koplik's spots in measles are a good example of this. These resemble white grains of salt on a red background, and may be present on the buccal mucosa a day or two before the typical skin rash appears.

The increasing complexity of viral structure and reproduction which recent research has revealed is necessitating a reappraisal of the aetiology of many diseases. The phenomena of viral latency and the eclipse phase indicate that a failure to isolate a virus does not necessarily signify its absence. Similarly slow viruses, mycoplasmas, and the delicate and elusive L-forms of bacteria have not yet been sufficiently investigated for their role in disease to be assessed.

GENERAL READING

Cruickshank R, Duguid J P, Marmion B P, Swain R H A 1973 General Microbiology, 12th edn. Churchill Livingstone, Edinburgh. Chapters 50 to 52 give an account of rickettsiae, chlamydiae, and mycoplasmas. Chapters 12 to 14 give an account of the general properties of viruses. All of Part III is devoted to a detailed account of viral diseases.

Fenner F J, White D O 1976 Medical Virology, 2nd edn. 487 pp. Academic Press, London. This is a good working account of viral disease from a clinical as well as a microbiological point of view.

Wilson G S, Miles A A 1975 In: Topley and Wilson's Principles of Bacteriology, Virology and Immunity, 6th edn. Arnold, London, vol 1, p 1195–1247; vol 2, p 2343–2603. Vol 1 is devoted to the microbiological aspects and vol 2 to the clinical implications.

17

Some disorders of metabolism

GLUCOSE METABOLISM

The most important upset in glucose metabolism is diabetes mellitus. It is the great frequency of this disease, which affects about 3 per cent of the population, that has stimulated a vast amount of research into the metabolism of glucose, yet even today there are many aspects that are incompletely understood.

Glucose is used as a fuel by many of the body's cells, and is the only substance used by the brain under normal circumstances. Hence the maintenance of a blood-glucose level within narrow limits (3.0 to 5.0 mmol per litre, or 55 to 90 mg per dl in the fasting subject) is an important homeostatic mechanism. The blood level is mainly regulated by the balanced production of insulin, which lowers the blood-glucose level, and the activity of the liver, which can either store glucose as glycogen or produce glucose from glycogen (*glycogenolysis*) or non-carbohydrate sources (*gluconeogenesis*) (see Fig. 17.1).

Glucose homeostasis[1]

It is best to consider glucose homeostasis under the three headings:

1. Following glucose administration
2. In the postabsorptive state—following an overnight fast
3. During exercise.

Following glucose administration. Following the oral administration of glucose there is an increase in the amount of insulin released from the pancreas. This promotes the storage and utilization of glucose and prevents an undue rise in the blood-glucose level.

Following the absorption of glucose from the intestine, the rise in blood-glucose level stimulates the secretion of insulin from the pancreatic islets by a direct action. Insulin aids the entry of glucose into resting muscle and fat cells: these are the insulin-dependent tissues. Following the ingestion of 100 g of glucose, however, only about 15 per cent enters these tissues along insulin-dependent pathways. An additional 25 per cent escapes from the splanchnic bed and is utilized to meet the ongoing glucose needs of insulin-independent tissues, especially the brain. From 55 to 60 per cent is retained in the liver, for there is no barrier to the entry to glucose into liver cells, and this organ is well situated

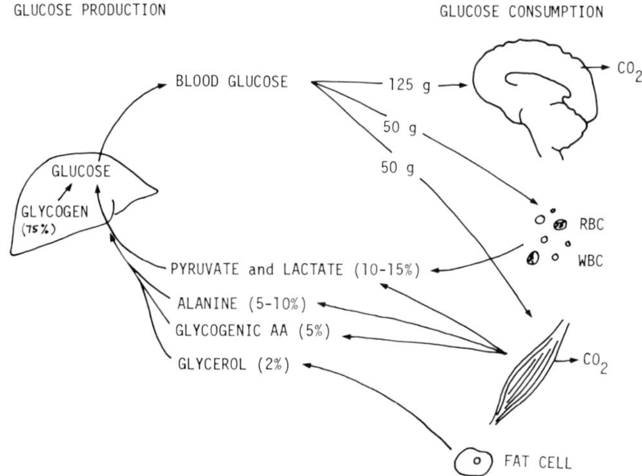

Fig. 17.1 Glucose balance in normal man in the postabsorptive, overnight-fasted state. Alanine forms the principal amino acid released from muscle, and is utilized by the liver to form glucose. The muscle can utilize glucose to form alanine, and this constitutes the glucose-alanine cycle analogous to the Cori cycle. In the latter, lactate and pyruvate formed from glucose in the muscle are released into the blood, taken up by the liver, and there converted into glucose. (*From Felig P 1975 The liver in glucose homeostasis in normal man and diabetes. In: Valance-Owen J (ed) Diabetes, University Park Press, Baltimore.*)

anatomically to intercept glucose from the portal vein and prevent it entering the systemic circulation. In the liver the glucose is utilized in the synthesis of glycogen and triglycerides.

It follows that in the normal person, even after a carbohydrate meal, the blood glucose does not rise above 9 mmol per litre (160 mg per dl); this forms the basis of the glucose tolerance test.*

In this test a fasting subject, previously on an adequate carbohydrate diet, is given 100 g of glucose by mouth. The blood glucose should not exceed 5 mmol per litre (90 mg per dl) at the start of the test nor 9 mmol per litre (160 mg per dl) an hour later; it should have returned to 5 mmol per litre after 2 hours. At a blood-glucose level of 10 mmol per litre (180 mg per dl) glycosuria may be expected.

In the postabsorptive state. If an individual fasts overnight, the liver and the insulin-dependent tissues (resting muscle and fat) show little glucose uptake. The insulin-independent tissues (brain, blood cells, and renal medulla) show a continued glucose uptake at a rate of 150 to 200 g per day; the blood-glucose level is maintained by the release of glucose from the liver (Fig. 17.1). The liver contains about 70 g of glycogen which provides an immediate source of glucose by glycogenolysis. The supply, however, lasts less than 1 day, and gluconeogenesis is stimulated; pyruvate, lactate, and alanine are used as the main raw materials for this. After 2 or 3 days gluconeogenesis is more important than glycogenolytic

* It should be noted that the normal levels of blood glucose cited in this chapter are somewhat lower than those found in older textbooks. This is because current biochemical methods measure the glucose content of blood specifically and not merely the content of reducing substances, of which glucose is the predominant component.

activity. Protein provides the ultimate source for this, a fact reflected in the brisk rate of nitrogen excretion that occurs early in starvation.

During exercise. In the resting state the major source of energy for muscular contraction is provided by the oxidation of fatty acids. During exercise the uptake of fatty acid is increased, but in addition there is a marked (up to 20-fold) increase in glucose uptake and oxidation. To compensate for this peripheral utilization, the liver releases glucose into the blood stream and the blood-glucose level shows little change. During short-term exercise the major source of this glucose is liver glycogen (glycogenolysis). During prolonged exercise gluconeogenesis plays an increasingly important role, because the liver's supply of glycogen is limited. The mechanisms involved in these changes are not well understood.

Secretion and actions of insulin

Insulin is synthetized in the beta cells of the islets of Langerhans as proinsulin, a polypeptide containing 81 to 86 amino-acid residues. The tail and head of this long polypeptide are joined by two disulphide bonds. By the action of peptidases the middle segment (termed the C peptide) is excised, leaving the two ends of the molecule to form the A and B chains of the insulin molecule; these remain united by the original disulphide bonds. The formation and excretion of C peptide has been used as a measure of the rate of insulin synthesis.

Insulin is formed in the rough endoplasmic reticulum; the product passes into the Golgi complex and is subsequently released as membrane-bound secretory granules. These mature to a crystalline form in the presence of zinc ions, and are finally released by a process of exocytosis. The actual movement and release of these granules is guided by microtubules and effected by the contractile proteins of the microfilaments. Calcium ions are required for this.

The major stimulus for both insulin synthesis and release is hypoglycaemia. Glucagon, gastrin, and other intestinal hormones also stimulate the islets of Langerhans, and the release of these hormones following oral administration of glucose plays a minor role in promoting insulin secretion.

The target cells of insulin are those of the adipose tissue and muscle, both of which have specific receptors: glucose transport into the cell is enhanced, and glycogen synthesis is increased. Insulin promotes the synthesis of protein from amino acids; it inhibits the breakdown of neutral fat (*lipolysis*).

Furthermore, insulin has two important effects on the liver: *glycogenolysis is inhibited* by small increments in insulin secretion; larger increments *inhibit gluconeogenesis.* The net effect of insulin is to lower the blood-glucose level; since the half-life of the hormone is from 3 to 4 minutes, the continuous and varying secretion of insulin is the main regulatory mechanism whereby the blood-glucose level is normally maintained within narrow limits.

Other hormones affecting glucose metabolism

Four other hormones have important effects on glucose metabolism:

Glucagon. This hormone is the secretion of the alpha cells of the islets of Langerhans. It is released whenever the blood-glucose level drops below 4 to 5 mmol per litre (80 mg per dl), and its main action is stimulating the liver to break down glycogen into glucose, which is then released into the blood. In the adipose tissue lipolysis is stimulated. It is evident that glucagon opposes the action of insulin.

Adrenaline. This raises the blood-glucose level by promoting glycogenolysis in the liver and muscles.

Pituitary growth hormone. This opposes the actions of insulin, thereby raising the blood-glucose level.

Adrenal glucocorticoids. These decrease glucose utilization in muscle and fat. Gluconeogenesis in the liver is stimulated, and the blood-glucose level rises.

DIABETES MELLITUS[2–5]

The discovery of insulin by Banting and Best appeared to provide both an explanation of the pathogenesis of diabetes mellitus and an effective treatment. Ironically, this outstanding discovery retarded further research into the true nature of the disease, so that even today its precise pathogenesis is not understood. It has become evident that insulin deficiency is only one factor in the disease. Many diabetic subjects need insulin in quantities far in excess of those required by a totally pancreatectomised individual. Some diabetics have a blood-insulin level that is normal or even above normal. Finally, insulin therapy can prolong the life of some diabetic subjects, but it fails to prevent premature death from the cardiovascular complications or the onset of blindness. The life expectancy of a diabetic patient is still below that of the normal individual.

Aetiology of diabetes mellitus

Diabetes mellitus may be regarded as a syndrome characterized by a relative or absolute deficiency of insulin. Three major types of the disease may be recognized.

1. Hereditary diabetes mellitus. This is by far the commonest type, but although the disease is clearly familial, the precise mode of inheritance is not decided. The current trend is to incriminate a dominant gene which renders the individual liable to develop diabetes, but is not itself the only cause. It is possible that about 25 per cent of the population possess this gene, but only 2 to 3 per cent actually develop the disease.

2. Diabetes mellitus associated with other endocrine disorders. Diabetes is encountered in Cushing's syndrome (and following glucocorticoid therapy), acromegaly, and phaeochromocytoma. Under these circumstances the disease is due to the overabundance of hormones that antagonise insulin. To this is probably added the hereditary factor, since ultimately the islet cells may become exhausted or unresponsive.

3. Diabetes associated with pancreatic disease. Diabetes is occasionally encountered as a complication of chronic pancreatitis, cystic fibrosis, and total pancreatectomy.

The islets of Langerhans

These show a variety of changes, but in about one-third of cases no abnormality can be detected. In early-onset diabetes a lymphocytic infiltrate ('insulinitis') may be present. If the patient had marked hyperglycaemia before death, the beta cells show vacuolation due to an accumulation of glycogen. Longstanding diabetics may show atrophy of the islets with replacement by amyloid or fibrous tissue. Thus the changes give no hint of the cause of diabetes mellitus. Exhaustion due to genetic error, destruction by autoantibodies, and a viral infection are amongst the suggested causes.

Clinical types of diabetes mellitus

The disease occurs in two main clinical forms:

Growth-onset diabetes. This form affects children and young adults, and appears to be due to an absolute failure of the pancreas to secrete insulin. Polyuria (due basically to the osmotic diuresis promoted by the glycosuria, polydipsia, and polyphagia are characteristic symptoms. The disease is severe, wasting is marked, and without treatment the patient dies in diabetic coma. Insulin is particularly valuable in saving the lives of these patients.

Maturity-onset diabetes. This form occurs typically in middle-aged and elderly subjects, and is usually associated with obesity. The amount of insulin in the blood may be normal or reduced, but it is not absent. The disease is generally mild, there is no great risk from ketosis, and treatment by diet alone is often successful particularly if this leads to weight loss. Since this type of diabetes can occur in younger patients also, the name is somewhat misleading.

Pathogenesis of diabetes mellitus

The fundamental error in the common types of diabetes is not understood. It appears that the pancreas is unresponsive to an increase in the blood-glucose level. Thus in the early diabetic, after the ingestion of glucose, there is no early burst of insulin production, and a transient *hyperglycaemia* develops. This is due to an impaired hepatic uptake of glucose and a consequent entry of an abnormal quantity into the systemic circulation. A later release of insulin may be so excessive that the patient next develops *hypoglycaemia.*

The hyperglycaemia of diabetes leads to an increased peripheral utilization of glucose, an effect particularly evident in the mild, maturity-onset disease. There is enough insulin present to prevent lipolysis, so that fat continues to accumulate and the patient becomes obese. Nevertheless, there is considerable doubt about the relationship between obesity and diabetes. On the one hand, it may be that obesity provides a stress that promotes the development of the disease in those individuals who are genetically predisposed. On the other hand, it is possible that obesity is an effect of the disease during the early stages of its development, as described above.

In the severe diabetic the virtual absence of insulin leads to augmented lipolysis in the adipose tissues, so that free fatty acid is released and transported to the liver. The glycerol component contributes to the formation of glucose, while the remainder is used in the production of ketone bodies. Ketosis and diabetic coma are, therefore, common.

In the severe diabetic there is hyperglycaemia even in the fasting state; peripheral utilization by the insulin-independent tissues continues unabated, and the accumulation of glucose in the blood is due to overproduction by the liver. This continues despite the hyperglycaemia. The raw materials for this gluconeogenesis are amino acids (particularly alanine) released from the peripheral tissues, especially the muscles. The continuous production of glucose and its subsequent loss in the urine lead to loss of weight. Thus the growth-onset diabetic becomes wasted unless treated.

Although diabetes mellitus is usually associated with diminished insulin production, some patients (particularly the obese, maturity-onset type) have a normal or raised blood insulin level. The presence of insulin antagonists may be the explanation of this.

Diagnosis of diabetes mellitus

Four stages of the disease are recognized:

Prediabetes. This subject has the inherited tendency to develop the disease, but has neither symptoms nor detectable biochemical abnormality. Diagnosis is impossible until after the subject has developed diabetes.

Chemical diabetes. Symptoms are absent, and the fasting blood-sugar level is normal. The glucose tolerance test is, however, abnormal. A random blood-glucose determination is of little value in diagnosis at this stage. To avoid the tedious 3-hour glucose tolerance test, one may take a single blood sample 2 hours after a carbohydrate meal as a screening test.

Latent or stress diabetes. The patient is asymptomatic and has a normal glucose tolerance test. The test becomes abnormal if glucocorticoids are given to provide an additional stress.

Overt or clinical diabetes. Symptoms are present, the fasting blood glucose is raised, and glycosuria is present.

Complications of diabetes mellitus

Diabetic ketosis and coma. This is most common in the growth-onset type of the disease, and may be precipitated by the patient's failure to administer his insulin. Vomiting and abdominal pain may be severe enough to simulate an abdominal emergency.

Hyperosmolar non-ketogenic coma. This condition is generally encountered in patients with maturity-onset diabetes, and may be precipitated by an acute illness, such as an infection or a myocardial infarct. The plasma glucose level is very high and may exceed 55 mmol per litre (1000 mg per dl). The osmotic diuresis that this engenders leads to hypovolaemic shock. The effect of the dehydration is most marked on the central nervous system—coma is characteristic, and fits occur in about one-third of cases.

Cardiovascular disease. These is good evidence that diabetics are more prone than normal people of the same age group to develop atheroma, peripheral vascular disease, gangrene of the toes and feet, and ischaemic heart disease. This tendency does not seem to be related to the severity of the diabetes nor to the efficiency of the treatment; indeed, treatment with tolbutamide and phenformin may actually increase the mortality from cardiovascular disease.

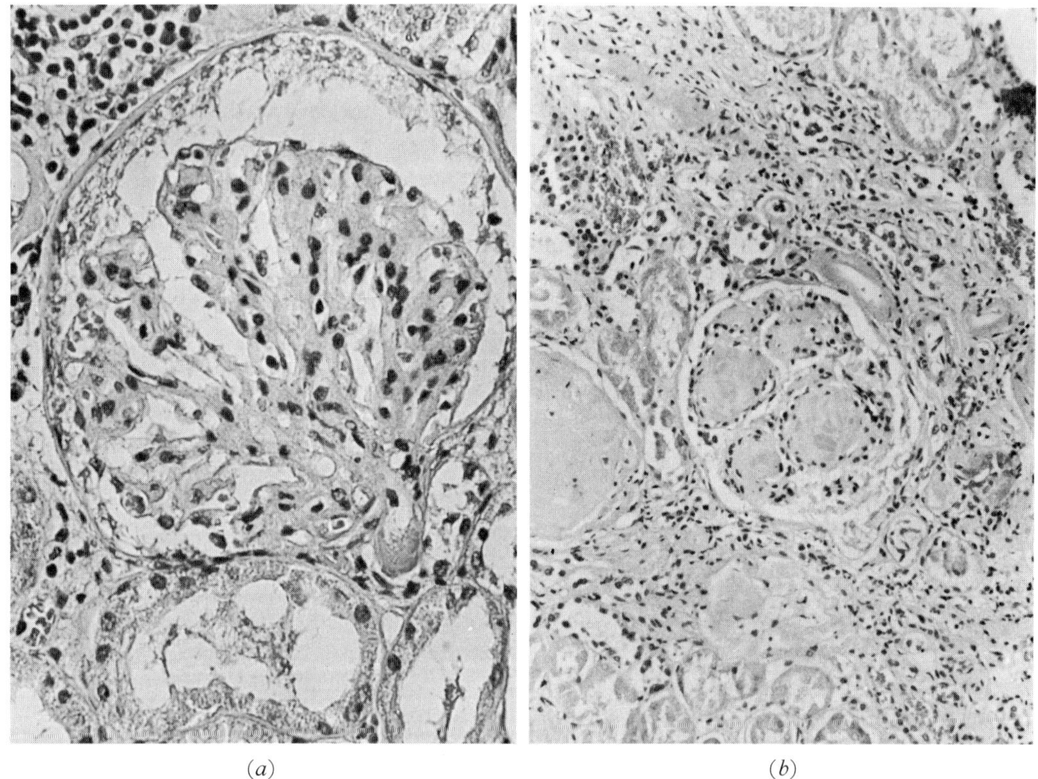

(a) (b)

Fig. 17.2 Diabetic nephropathy. (*a*) Diffuse glomerulosclerosis. There is considerable mesangial proliferation and thickening. Note the hyalinized afferent arteriole entering the glomerular tuft. × 250.

(*b*) Nodular glomerulosclerosis. There are focal accumulations of hyaline material disposed especially in the peripheries of the glomerulus. × 100.

Diabetic microangiopathy. A thickening of the basement membrane of capillaries has been described in the skin, muscles, kidney, retina, and other parts of the body.

Diabetic nephropathy. The common *diffuse glomerulosclerosis* involves thickening of the basement membrane of the glomerular vessels together with mesangial proliferation and an increase in the amount of basement-membrane-like material in the mesangium (Fig. 17.2 (a)).

The most characteristic change is, however, *nodular glomerulosclerosis,* described by Kimmelstiel and Wilson. In this there are focal depositions of basement-membrane-like material in the peripheral parts of the glomeruli, thereby forming nodules of varying size (Fig. 17.2 (b)). These nodules stain strongly by the PAS method.

Urinary-tract infection is common in diabetic subjects, especially women, and papillary necrosis may occur; clinically this is characterised by haematuria and the rapid onset of renal failure.

Glomerulosclerosis itself leads to proteinuria which may be of sufficient intensity to produce the nephrotic syndrome. In the terminal stages nitrogen retention and renal failure occur.

Changes in the eye. The retinal microangiopathy causes ischaemic changes, microaneurysm formation, and bleeding (diabetic retinopathy). *Cataract formation* is another important complication of diabetes; it is little wonder that the disease is one of the leading causes of blindness in the world.

Neuropathy. Ischaemic damage to peripheral nerves leads to a variety of effects, e.g. pain, loss of sensation, and paralysis.

Liability to infection. Diabetic patients are susceptible to bacterial infections, especially of the skin, lungs, and urinary tract. The mechanism is incompletely understood, but abnormal polymorph function (chemotaxis and bactericidal action) may be of importance. Vaginal candidiasis is a troublesome complication in diabetic women.

PURINE METABOLISM[6,7]

GOUT

Gout is a disease of great antiquity. It is characterised by hyperuricaemia, recurrent attacks of a characteristic acute arthritis, and the development of tophi. Deposite of urates in the cartilages of joints lead to chronic arthritis. The clinical features of gout were well recognised by Hippocrates, and the classical condition was described by Thomas Sydenham, who was himself a sufferer. The disease is commoner in times of plenty than during wars and famines; it is a malady of the affluent rather than the poor. Among its famous victims were Martin Luther, Isaac Newton, Samuel Johnson, and the Pitts. Gout responds well to colchicine, a drug still in current use and introduced into North America by Benjamin Franklin, yet another famous person afflicted by the disease.

Gout is now regarded as a symptom complex of multiple aetiology. In some cases, labelled *primary gout,* there is often a strong hereditary factor. In others, labelled *secondary gout,* there is an obvious associated disease that is the primary cause. In both types there is an upset of purine metabolism, either overproduction of uric acid or a failure in its excretion by the kidneys.

Degradation of purines. The degradation of nucleic acids by nucleases results in the formation of the free purine and pyrimidine bases. Adenine and guanine are converted to hypoxanthine, which is acted upon by xanthine oxidase to form xanthine. In the human this is converted into uric acid and excreted.

The drug allopurinol acts as a xanthine-oxidase inhibitor, therefore reducing the amount of uric acid that is formed; it is of value in preventing hyperuricaemia and its effects in patients in renal failure and in those being treated with cytotoxic drugs.

Under normal circumstances up to 5 g of free purine are formed daily, but only 0.5 g are excreted; the remainder is salvaged and recycled. An important element in this salvage of purines is the enzyme hypoxanthine-guanine phosphoribosyltransferase.

Pathogenesis of primary gout

Overproduction of uric acid. This is a feature of many patients with primary gout, but in most of these the precise biochemical error is not known. In a few families there is a low level of the enzyme hypoxanthine-guanine phosphoribosyltransferase, and purines are excreted as uric acid rather than being recycled. These patients exhibit neurological signs as well as gouty arthritis and renal stones.

Renal handling of uric acid. Uric acid passes freely into the glomerular filtrate, and most of it is reabsorbed by the tubules; 80 per cent of the uric acid excreted in the urine is derived from tubular secretion. A reduction in the normal secretion of urate per nephron has been demonstrated in some patients with gout, and is prominent in those in whom there is no evidence of uric-acid overproduction.

It is evident that many defects in the metabolism of purines can result in the clinical state of gout. There may be an overproduction of purines, with or without impaired renal excretion of uric acid. A familial tendency is well established in primary gout, but the exact mode of inheritance is not known in most instances. The situation is comparable to that encountered in diabetes mellitus; it is probable that the tendency to develop gout is inherited but that other factors are of importance in actually precipitating the onset of the disease. The development of obesity and overindulgence in alcohol are important factors in this regard.

Clinical features of gout

Gout may be divided into three phases:

1. *Asymptomatic hyperuricaemia.*

2. *Acute gouty arthritis.* This generally affects the first metatarsophalangeal joint; occasionally it is bilateral. There is a sudden onset of severe pain with fever and rigors. The pain becomes intolerable, but without treatment it slowly subsides over a period of days or even weeks. Further acute attacks may occur affecting either the same or other joints. Over 50 per cent of untreated cases develop permanent joint damage and tophi (deposits of urates).

The attacks appear to be caused by the precipitation of crystals of monosodium urate in the joint cavity. Phagocytosis by polymorphs leads to release of damaging lysosomal enzymes; acute inflammation, rigors, and fever follow as a consequence of this.

3. *Chronic gouty arthritis.* The progressive deposition of monosodium urate in the articular cartilage leads to the degeneration of the cartilage, pannus formation, and eventual fibrous or bony ankylosis. Similar deposits of urate in the adjacent bone, synovium, and soft tissues complete the picture of chronic gouty arthritis. As the chronic changes advance, so renal insufficiency develops and acute attacks occur less frequently and are more mild. No joint is exempt, but the legs are affected more often than the arms; distal joints are affected more frequently than the proximal ones. Tophi also occur in the cartilages of the ears, and in bursae (especially the olecranon and prepatellar), tendons, and soft tissues generally. There may be much deformity (Fig. 17.3).

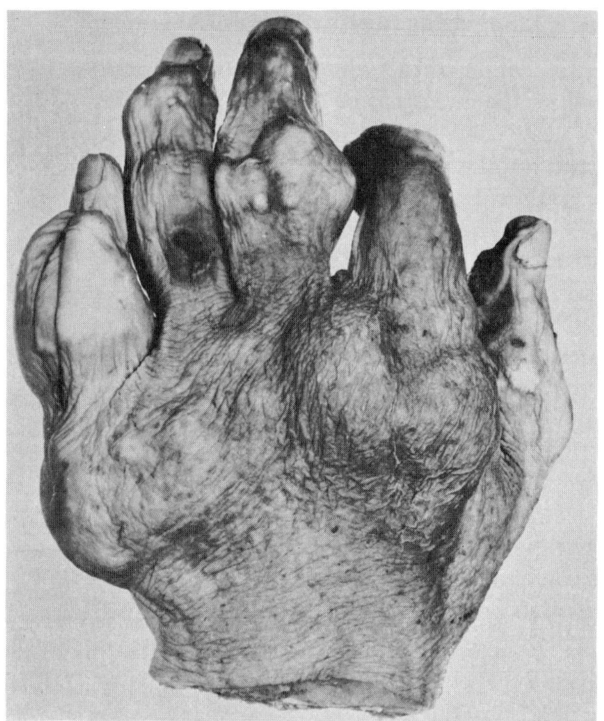

Fig. 17.3. Gout. This left hand shows the effects of severe, chronic gout. There are irregular swellings on the dorsum corresponding with the position of the metacarpo-phalangeal joints. Similar swellings are present over the interphalangeal joints, where opaque, chalky deposits are visible through the atrophic skin. (S88.1, *Reproduced by permission of the President and Council of the R.C.S. Eng.*)

Microscopically a tophus consists of sheaves of urate crystals and a surrounding granulomatous reaction with numerous foreign-body giant cells (Fig. 17.4).

Renal lesions of gout

Between 20 and 40 per cent of patients with gout develop uric-acid stones; in about 20 per cent the urolithiasis is the first indication of the disease. Apart from the changes secondary to urolithiasis (obstruction and infection), the kidneys often show a glomerulosclerosis which is probably secondary to ischaemia. Hypertension is present in about one-third of the patients.

Secondary gout

Hyperuricaemia and secondary gout can occur under two circumstances:

1. *Overproduction of uric acid due to increased cellular turnover,* as in the leukaemias especially after treatment with cytotoxic drugs. Chronic haemolytic anaemia (e.g. sickle-cell anaemia) and psoriasis are other examples of conditions in which there is an increased cellular turnover.

2. *Impaired renal excretion.* This is encountered as a complication of the

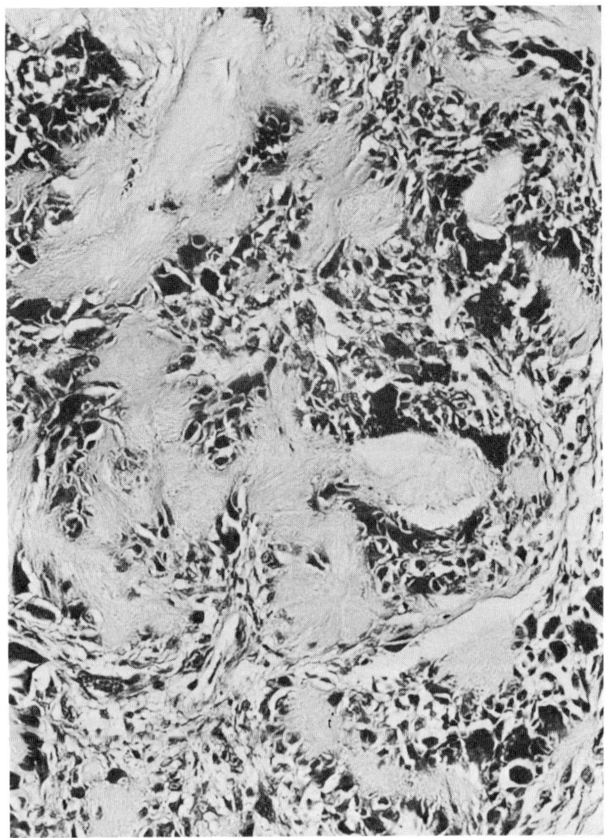

Fig. 17.4. Gout tophus. There are deposits of crystalline sodium urate surrounded by exuberant foreign-body giant-cell systems. × 100.

administration of certain drugs, chiefly the thiazide diuretics, and of renal damage. Lead poisoning in particular causes chronic renal damage that may be complicated by gout.

REFERENCES

1. Levine R, Haft D E 1970 Carbohydrate homeostasis, New England Journal of Medicine, 283: 175 and 237
2. Vallance-Owen J (ed) 1975 Diabetes, 208 pp. University Park Press, Baltimore
3. Leading Article 1975 Heritability of diabetes, British Medical Journal, 4: 127
4. Zonana J, Rimoin D L 1976 Inheritance of diabetes mellitus, New England Journal of Medicine, 295: 603
5. Irvine W J 1977 Classification of idiopathic diabetes, Lancet, 1: 638
6. Wyngaarden J B, Kelley W N 1972 In: The Metabolic Basis of Inherited Disease, eds Stanbury J B, Wyngaarden J B, Fredrickson D S, 3rd edn., pp 889–968. McGraw-Hill, New York
7. Leading Article 1973 Mechanism of gouty inflammation, British Medical Journal, 4: 125

18

Disorders of nutrition

With the world population expanding at an estimated rate of 70 million each year, it is likely that starvation and malnutrition will become increasingly common. The effects of total starvation will first be described.

STARVATION[1–3]

Metabolic changes during starvation

The body's stores of glucose and glycogen are sufficient for only 1 day's metabolic needs. The protein supply and the triacylglycerols (triglycerides) of adipose tissue provide enough energy for an additional 3 months in the average individual. For a fat person there are enough energy reserves for about 1 year's survival. After an overnight fast (the post-absorptive state) the insulin-dependent tissues (e.g. resting muscle and fat) cease to take up glucose. Insulin-independent tissues (e.g. brain), on the other hand, continue to utilize glucose at a rate of 150 g per day. The liver releases glucose at a similar rate in order to maintain a normal blood-glucose level.

Immediate changes in starvation. The brain normally uses only glucose as fuel; after the first day of starvation the blood-glucose level is maintained by the new glucose formation in the liver, in which amino acids, particularly alanine, are used as fuel. The amino acids are provided by the breakdown of protein. Because the nitrogen component is excreted as urea, the body is in negative nitrogen balance.

The triacylglycerols of adipose tissue are broken down to glycerol and fatty acids. Fatty acids are converted into ketone bodies in the liver, and these are used directly by most organs of the body instead of glucose.

Later changes in starvation. After the first week of starvation the breakdown of protein declines rapidly, and gluconeogenesis continues at a reduced rate. A change occurs in the brain's metabolism such that it is able to utilise ketone bodies, particularly beta-hydroxybutyrate, instead of glucose. Starvation can now continue until all the stores of body fat are utilized. When the supply of fat has been exhausted, only protein remains. The muscle masses decline and death soon follows.

During starvation the body conserves energy by reducing energy output. The starved individual is apathetic, lacking interest in life. Hypothermia is a danger in cold climates. This picture of starvation differs from that of the patient with anorexia nervosa, who is usually restless (see Ch 39).

The oedema of starvation affects the dependent parts and is due to the laxity of the subcutaneous tissues as well as to hypoalbuminaemia.

The wasted appearance of the starving person is all too familiar. The lax, dry skin and wasted muscles are matched by wasting of the internal organs. In particular, with advanced starvation the intestine becomes increasingly thin; hence, when treating a starving patient one must give frequent small feeds if the person's life is to be saved.

Protein-calorie malnutrition in childhood. Protein-calorie malnutrition is regarded as a spectrum of disease with marasmus at one end and kwashiorkor at the other end.

Nutritional marasmus. Marasmus is the name given to starvation in infants. It is due to deficiency of both protein and calories, and is encountered in infants under 1 year of age. It is a common condition in the developing countries of the world, and is usually due to cessation of breast feeding when the mother again becomes pregnant. The child exhibits the wasted appearance of starvation and in addition shows lack of growth. In those who survive, dwarfism is a frequent complication. As with starvation in adults, the marasmic child is very susceptible to infection; tuberculosis and dysentery often complete the lethal process initiated by starvation.

Kwashiorkor. This is a syndrome observed in children between the ages of 1 and 3 years. Its name is derived from a local African word denoting illness in a child displaced from the breast by a subsequent pregnancy.

Kwashiorkor is due to a low protein intake in the presence of an adequate carbohydrate supply. It is characterized by a fatty liver and marked oedema of the subcutaneous tissues. The inadequate protein supply leads to defective pigment formation: the hair becomes pale and even red in Black African children, and the skin often depigmented and shows hyperkeratosis and flaking.

THE VITAMINS

Definition and classification

Vitamins are organic substances that the body cannot manufacture and that are necessary for normal metabolism; only 10 such substances are known in the human being. If these substances are present in insufficient quantity, disease results. The 10 vitamins essential for good health are listed below in Table 18.1.

Table 18.1. The essential vitamins

Fat-soluble	Water-soluble
Vitamin A	Vitamin C
Vitamin D	Vitamin B complex:
Vitamin K	Thiamine
	Riboflavin
	Niacin
	Pyridoxine
	Cobalamin (B_{12})
	Folate

CAUSES AND EFFECTS OF INDIVIDUAL VITAMIN DEFICIENCIES AND EXCESSES

Vitamin A (retinol)

Vitamin A is one of the fat-soluble vitamins. In herbivorous animals the carotenoid pigments, such as the carotenes of plants and vegetables, are converted into vitamin A in the intestine, absorbed, and subsequently stored in the liver. Human beings acquire their supply of vitamin A either from the carotenoids in vegetable matter (e.g. carrots, beetroot, and green vegetables in general) or as the vitamin itself from animal or dairy produce. The concurrent absorption of fat and the presence of bile salts in the intestine favour vitamin-A absorption.

Causes of vitamin A deficiency. This is usually due to a deficient diet. This nutritional problem usually occurs in Indonesia, parts of Asia, India, the Middle East, and Latin America; it is almost unknown in North America and Europe. Vitamin-A deficiency does, however, occur as a complication of the malabsorption syndrome.

Effects of vitamin A deficiency. *The eye.* Vitamin A forms an essential component of rhodopsin, a pigment in the rods of the retina. By absorbing light, rhodopsin initiates an electrical impulse that is transmitted to the brain and is interpreted as light. The first sign of vitamin-A deficiency, therefore, is *night blindness.* Apart from this one known biochemical action of vitamin A, its other functions remain a mystery in spite of much research. It is known that vitamin A regulates the structure of certain epithelial cells. In vitamin A deficiency the epithelia of the genito-urinary tract, the trachea, the nose, and the conjunctiva all tend to undergo squamous metaplasia. The most important effect is in the eye. The conjunctival epithelium loses its mucus-secreting goblet cells and becomes keratinized, thereby taking on the characteristics of epidermis. The lacrimal ducts show hyperkeratosis, so that the eye becomes dry and subject to cracking and infection. The condition is called *xerophthalmia.* In due course the cornea becomes cloudy; with infection it can soften (*keratomalacia*), so that the globe may become perforated. The lens is then extruded, and blindness results. Indeed, vitamin-A deficiency is a leading cause of blindness in the world.

The skin. The skin shows dryness and follicular plugging, but whether these changes are specific for vitamin-A deficiency is not clear.

Other effects. The replacement of respiratory-type epithelium (with its goblet cells and cilia) by keratinized squamous epithelium is a factor in the production of respiratory infections. Nevertheless, in the presence of a normal amount of vitamin A there is no evidence that an excessive intake can prevent respiratory infections. The time-honoured practice of giving children large quantities of vitamin A (in cod-liver oil) in order to prevent colds and respiratory infections appears to be quite ill-founded. Indeed, such a practice can cause toxic effects (see below).

In spite of the dramatic changes seen in epithelium in vitamin-A deficiency, the biochemical nature of the defect is unkown. If a small piece of skin is grown in organ culture and subjected to vitamin-A deficiency, it soon shows hyperkeratosis. If an excess quantity of vitamin A is now added to the medium, the epithelium changes to a goblet-cell, mucus-secreting type. There is no evidence, however, that excess vitamin A in the human can convert normal keratinized epidermis into mucus-secreting epithelium.

Toxicity of vitamin A. Very large doses of vitamin A are toxic and can cause an increase in intracranial pressure with headache, blurring of vision, vomiting, and drowsiness. This effect has been described by Arctic explorers when they ate polar-bear liver, which is a very rich source of vitamin A. Chronic poisoning can cause loss of hair, bone pains, calcification of ligaments and tendons, hyperpigmentation of the skin, liver damage, and psychiatric symptoms.

Vitamin D

Vitamin D is present in all fat-containing animal products, but its richest source is cod-liver oil. Vitamin D is also formed in the skin by the action of ultraviolet light on 7-dehydrocholesterol. The actions of vitamin D and the effects of hypo- and hypervitaminosis D are described in Chapter 19.

Vitamin E

Vitamin E includes a group of fat-soluble substances that act as antioxidants. In humans vitamin E deficiency has been described in premature infants and in patients with cystic fibrosis with severe steatorrhoea.

Vitamin E has been regarded as a panacea by some enthusiasts, but unfortunately it cannot delay the effects of senility nor decrease the incidence of coronary-artery disease.

Vitamin C (ascorbic acid)

Human beings share with other primates, the guinea-pig, and certain birds the inability to synthetize vitamin C. The main dietary sources of this vitamin are citrus fruit, currants, berries, green vegetables, and potatoes. Vitamin C is necessary for the synthesis of collagen, and the main effect of vitamin C deficiency is *scurvy*. This is characterized by a bleeding tendency, the cause of which is probably poor anchorage of the smaller blood vessels in a thin, watery intercellular substance devoid of adequate collagen fibres. The site of bleeding varies according to the age of the patient. As noted in Chapter 8, *wound healing* is greatly impaired.

Adult scurvy. Bleeding often first takes place into the skin, being first detected around the hair follicles, which also show follicular hyperkeratosis. Cutaneous ecchymoses may follow minor trauma. There is also bleeding into muscles and along fascial planes, particularly at points of mechanical stress. A very characteristic finding is gingival haemorrhage, which occurs only in those who have teeth: the gingivae become spongy, swollen, and ultimately ulcerated. There may be severe bleeding with later superimposed infection.

Anaemia is common in scurvy and is due to the effects of haemorrhage as well as to concomitant multiple nutritional deficiencies.

In the past scurvy plagued sailors on long sea voyages, since the disease first becomes manifest about 2 months after commencing a deficient diet. For example, Vasco da Gama is reported to have lost 100 men of his 160-man crew on his journey around the Cape of Good Hope in 1497. James Lind (1716–1794), a British naval surgeon, introduced oranges, lemons, and limes into his sailors' diet in 1747, thereby preventing the lethal effects of scurvy and earning the name 'limey' for his countrymen.

Scurvy in infants and children. Milk and milk products are often a poor source of vitamin C, especially if the milk has been stored or processed. Consequently scurvy can develop in infants at about the age of 8 months.

In infantile scurvy the outstanding feature is subperiosteal haemorrhages, which are very painful; these are rare in adults. On the other hand, although bleeding can occur elsewhere, gingival lesions are not seen in infants unless the teeth have erupted.

Osseous lesions are also seen in infantile and early childhood scurvy, since there is an impaired formation of osteoid. An x-ray of a scorbutic bone shows generalized rarefaction due to osteoporosis, which is particularly well marked at the metaphyseal ends of the shaft. By contrast, the zones of provisional calcification are very dense; in the long bones this density appears as a transverse line at the junction between the epiphysis and the end of the shaft. There is heavy calcification of the cartilage with foci of fragmented spicules of calcified cartilage forming during the period of retarded longitudinal growth. The epiphysis may be fractured at the line of junction and undergo displacement and dislocation. Microscopically there is little evidence of bone formation either beneath the periosteum or at the margins of the calcified spicules of cartilage in the metaphyseal zone. Instead there is an accumulation of cells of fibroblast type embedded in a loose-textured, oedematous ground substance. These cells are in fact osteoblasts, and they start to lay down osteoid as soon as ascorbic acid is administered. The subperiosteal haemorrhages follow the disruption of the collagenous attachments (Sharpey's fibres) from the cortex of the bone. There is also an impairment in the formation of dentine, and the teeth may be loosened from the alveolar bone.

Vitamin B complex

Thiamine

Thiamine is a coenzyme necessary for several steps in carbohydrate metabolism. In the absence of this vitamin, lactic acid and pyruvic acid accumulate in the blood instead of entering the Krebs cycle. The vitamin is widely distributed in foodstuffs. Thiamine deficiency was once prevalent in the Far East, where polished (highly milled) rice formed the staple diet (the process of milling removes most of the thiamine from the rice). Thiamine deficiency is now much less common in the world generally, but is still encountered in the Far East, particularly in persons of all ages living in isolated communities, in infants, and in pregnant women. In North America it is sometimes encountered in chronic alcoholics.

Effects of thiamine deficiency. The early symptoms of thiamine deficiency, which is called beriberi, are vague: weakness, ankle oedema, and paraesthesiae and numbness of the legs. At any time one of the two major forms may develop.

Wet beriberi. In this form the accumulation of lactic acid and other vasodilator chemical agents causes so much vasodilatation that high-output heart failure develops. The outstanding feature is extensive oedema with an accumulation of fluid in the serous sacs. Sudden death from heart failure is not uncommon.

Dry beriberi. The outstanding feature of this form is peripheral neuropathy. Numbness and anaesthesia are the result of sensory-nerve damage, whereas weakness and muscle wasting are the effects of motor-nerve involvement. The patient eventually becomes bedridden.

Riboflavin[4]

Riboflavin is a constituent of many foods, and is a component of several enzymes that play a vital role in metabolism. Yet the lesions associated with riboflavin deficiency are ill-defined. A sore mouth is an an early symptom: the angles of the mouth become macerated and later develop cracks (angular stomatitis or perlèche), the lips become sore, dry, and cracked (cheilosis), and the tongue becomes smooth and sore (glossitis). A scaly dermatitis, resembling seborrhoeic dermatitis, develops later, and affects the face and the scrotum or vulva.

Niacin (nicotinic acid)

As with thiamine and riboflavin, niacin is widely distributed in plant and animal food and is also a component of important enzymes. A deficiency of niacin causes pellagra, a disease so named because of the rough skin (from the Italian pelle agra, or 'rough skin') that is present. Pellagra is a disease of poor peasants who subsist chiefly on maize (American corn). Although this cereal contains niacin, the vitamin is in a bound form.

Pellagra was once common in Spain and Italy. It became widespread in the USA in the early years of the present century, but has been largely eliminated by improved economic conditions. Nevertheless, it is still sometimes encountered in chronic alcoholics.

The symptoms of pellagra are most easily remembered as the *three Ds.*

Dermatitis. Erythema, superficially resembling a sunburn, develops on the sun-exposed areas. This may progress to blistering and a chronic type of dermatitis.

Diarrhoea. This is one of the principal gastrointestinal symptoms. A smooth, sore tongue of 'raw-beef' appearance is another common finding.

Dementia. Mental changes are common; they may take the form of acute delirium, or a more chronic manic-depressive state followed by progressive dementia. There may also be neurological accompaniments, such as peripheral neuritis, ataxia, and visual and auditory disturbances.

Death (the fourth D) was a common end-result of pellagra before the advent of vitamin therapy.

The modern view is that pellagra results from a diet that is poor in protein and reduced in nicotinic acid, riboflavin, and haematopoietic factors; toxic or antivitamin substances may also be involved.

Pyridoxine (vitamin B_6)

Pyridoxine is also a component of important coenzymes. Dietary deficiencies are unusual, but pyridoxine deficiency has been reported as a complication of drug therapy, particularly isoniazid (for tuberculosis). It has also been reported as a complication of the oral contraceptive. The effects of pyridoxine deficiency are vague; dermatitis, cheilosis, angular stomatitis, and glossitis have all been noted.

It is evident from this short account that thiamine, riboflavin, niacin, and pyridoxine are widely distributed in food and that deficiencies are due to an unbalanced or inadequate diet. Such dietary deficiencies are generally the effect of poverty, ignorance, or alcoholism. It follows therefore that multiple deficiencies are often present in the same patient, and it is proper practice to prescribe a mixture of these members of the vitamin B complex.

Cobalamin (vitamin B_{12}) and folate

These vitamins are necessary for red-cell maturation. Their absence leads to a megaloblastic anaemia (Ch 30).

THE MALABSORPTION SYNDROME

The small intestine has two main functions, (1) the intraluminal digestion of food, mainly by the action of pancreatic enzymes aided by the bile salts, and (2) the absorption of nutrients, which is often aided by enzymes in the brush border of the absorptive cells that complete the process of digestion. An abnormality of the function of the small intestine may lead to a failure in digestion or absorption. This failure may involve a single substance or it may be of a more general nature, involving the absorption of many components of the diet, in which case the effects are far-reaching, if severe, constituting the malabsorption syndrome. It is useful first to consider the normal mechanisms involved in the digestion and absorption of nutrients.

Carbohydrates. Starch, which constitutes a major component of the diet, is hydrolysed by salivary and pancreatic amylase to oligosaccharides and then to disaccharides, mostly maltose. The oligosaccharides together with maltose and other disaccharides, such as sucrose and lactose, are hydrolysed by specific disaccharidases, e.g. maltase, β-galactosidase (lactase), and sucrase, that are an integral part of the intestinal luminal surface. These enzymes are situated in the brush border of the intestinal cell, being probably a component of the glycocalyx. Monosaccharides (glucose, galactose, and fructose) are the end-result of carbohydrate digestion, and are absorbed by two specific and separate mechanisms: glucose and galactose are actively absorbed by a common mechanism, while fructose utilizes a separate mechanism. The hydrolysis of disaccharides is a rapid process, absorption being the rate-limiting factor; lactose provides the only exception to this rule, since it is only slowly hydrolysed. This relative lack of lactase activity in the human intestine is the explanation of the lactose intolerance so frequently encountered clinically. The absorbed monosaccharides are passed into the portal blood stream and thence to the liver.

Proteins. After the partial hydrolysis of protein by the pepsin of the gastric secretion, the pancreatic trypsin, chymotrypsin, and carboxypeptidases continue the process of digestion; polypeptides, dipeptides, and finally amino acids are produced. Dipeptidases and tripeptidases associated with the mucosal cells complete the process of hydrolysis, and the dipeptides and amino acids so produced are absorbed by an active transport mechanism. Some amino acids share a common mechanism, and it is therefore understandable that in certain genetic defects there is an impaired absorption of a specific group of amino acids, for example cystine, arginine, ornithine, and lysine in *cystinuria* (p. 9).

Fat. Bile salts play an important part in fat absorption, since they have an emulsifying, detergent effect which aids the action of pancreatic lipase. The bile salts also aid fat absorption by forming micelles with fatty acids and monglycerides. About 25 per cent of ingested lipid is hydrolysed to glycerol and fatty acid, while the remaining 75 per cent remains at the monoglyceride stage. Fatty acids and monoglycerides are absorbed into the intestinal cells, after which they follow one of two pathways depending upon the chain length of the fatty-acid component. Fatty acids (and their associated monoglycerides) of long chain length (C16 to C18 fatty acids) are esterified to triglyceride and very low-density lipids. These, in combination with apoproteins (p. 435), form chylomicrons and very low-density lipoproteins, which enter the lacteals. In contrast to this, fatty acids of medium chain length (C8 to C10 fatty acids) are not esterified, and pass directly to the portal circulation where they are bound to albumin. On reaching the liver, the medium-chain fatty acids are mostly metabolised to CO_2 acetate, or ketones. Any medium-chain fatty acids not metabolised thus are converted into long-chain fatty acids and then esterified to triglyceride. It follows that a patient with impaired fat absorption due to lymphatic blockage will fare better on a diet containing medium-chain fatty acids than on one containing the long-chain fatty acids.

Even in the absence of pancreatic enzymes a considerable portion (60 to 80 per cent) of ingested fat is absorbed by mechanisms that are not clearly understood. The faecal fat is partly of endogenous origin, being derived from desquamated epithelial cells, and partly the residue of undigested food. The composition of the fat is modified by bacterial action in the colon. An increase in the amount of fat in the faeces is a common finding in the malabsorption syndrome, and is called steatorrhoea.

Disorders of intestinal absorption

A failure in the absorption of nutrients may be due to a derangement of either digestion or absorption. Three classes of disorder may be recognized:

1. The defect may be specific for a particular food component; this is usually associated with an enzyme defect, e.g. lactose intolerance.

2. There may be a lack of major digestive fluid, e.g. the gastric juice following total gastrectomy, the pancreatic juice in pancreatic disease, or the bile in bile-duct obstruction.

The gastric juice is not essential for digestion, apart from the secretion of intrinsic factor and its vital part in the absorption of vitamin B_{12}. Nevertheless, even a partial gastric resection leads to a degree of general malabsorption, because after gastrectomy there is a much more hurried passage of food in the intestine, and digestion is rendered less complete. Hence considerable loss of weight and an iron-deficiency anaemia are not uncommon.

3. There may be a gross abnormality of the small intestine itself such that many processes are affected..

In the last two groups there is a defective absorption of many food components, that of fat being particularly severely affected. The clinical state is that of the *malabsorption syndrome.*

Specific defects of absorption

Carbohydrate maldigestion and malabsortption. The effects of a failure to digest and absorb carbohydrate are mainly attributable to the osmotic pressure exerted by the unabsorbed oligosaccharides or monosaccharides. Soon after ingesting the offending carbohydrate the patient feels bloated and the abdomen becomes distended. Furthermore, bacteria convert the carbohydrate to fatty acids, which appear to irritate the intestine; abdominal colic and diarrhoea may result.

Idiopathic lactase deficiency in adults. This is a common condition, its prevalence showing a racial incidence, being commonest in Oriental groups. The individual experiences no trouble during infancy or childhood, but only later exhibits intolerance to milk, which is eliminated from the diet in order to avoid symptoms.

Protein malabsorption. There are a number of inherited diseases in which there is a defective absorption of specific amino acids or groups of amino acids. Cystinuria has already been noted.

General malabsorption syndrome

If the functions of small intestine are markedly impaired a state of severe undernutrition results. The digestion and absorption of protein, carbohydrate, and fat are variably affected, and in addition there may be defective absorption of vitamins and minerals.

Causes of the malabsorption syndrome.[5] These may be either extrinsic or intrinsic.

Extrinsic causes of malabsorption may be gastric, pancreatic, or biliary, and are related to impaired digestion of food products or intestinal hurry.

Intrinsic causes are due primarily to defective intestinal function, and are related both to impaired absorption and disturbed enzyme action in the mucosal cells themselves. These will now be considered.

1. Intrinsic disease of intestine itself. A good example of such a condition that leads to severe malabsorption is the *sprue syndrome.* It is typified by atrophy of the intestinal villi, the cause of which is not known (Fig. 18.1.). Two types of sprue syndrome are recognised:

a. *Tropical sprue,* which is seen extensively in the Far East. It is not related to gluten sensitivity, but it often responds to oral antibiotics.

b. *Gluten-induced enteropathy,* which in children is called *coeliac disease* and in adults *non-tropical sprue.* The intestinal lesions and symptoms can be relieved by a diet that is low in gluten, a protein contained in flour. There is a marked familial incidence, the condition probably being inherited as an autosomal dominant trait with incomplete penetrance. Whether the gluten damages the small intestine by a directly toxic action or indirectly by an immunological reaction is not known.

Malabsorption may also follow other diseases of the small intestine, for example lymphoma, congenital lymphangiectasia, amyloidosis, and ischaemia. The intestinal hurry associated with diabetes mellitus and the Zollinger-Ellison syndrome are other causes.

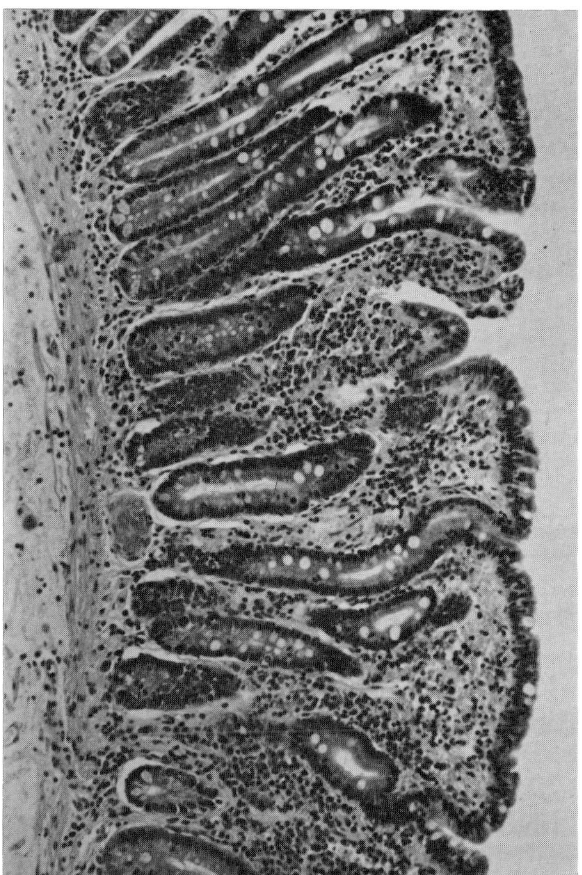

Fig. 18.1 Gluten-induced enteropathy (coeliac disease, or non-tropical sprue). This section from a jejunal biopsy shows the typical flat surface and absence of villi. The lamina propria is heavily infiltrated by lymphocytes and plasma cells. × 200.

2. The blind loop syndrome, also called the *stagnant bowel syndrome*, may complicate any condition in which blind loops of bowel are found either as a result of disease (e.g. Crohn's disease) or surgical procedures.

It is generally accepted that the mechanism of malabsorption in this syndrome is an upset in the intestinal bacterial flora. Normally the small bowel is virtually sterile (p 96). But blind loops, abnormalities in peristalsis, and gastro-colic fistulae all allow bacterial proliferation to occur.

3. Surgical resection of the small intestine. This, if extensive, leads to a serious reduction of the absorptive area. Such a resection may be necessitated by abdominal gunshot wounds, recurrent Crohn's disease, or massive intestinal infarction.

Effects of malabsorption

The effects of malabsorption may vary from subclinical disturbances to fatal malnutrition, depending on the portion of small bowel affected and the extent of the disease. The lack of absorption of essential nutrients may produce some effects similar to those of starvation, such as weight loss and generalised body atrophy.

Fat absorption is usually severely affected. If much fat—some of it undigested—is passed in the faeces, these will be pale and bulky.

Carbohydrate absorption is often affected, and the excess carbohydrate in the bowel is fermented by resident bacteria. The resulting gas renders the stool frothy and offensive.

Protein absorption is affected in intestinal and pancreatic steatorrhoea. If the hypoproteinaemia is severe enough to produce generalized oedema, an additional protein-losing gastroenteropathy should be suspected (p. 432).

Vitamin absorption. The vitamin-B complex may be inadequately absorbed, producing effects already described. Vitamin-C absorption is rarely impaired. The fat-soluble vitamins tend to be more severely affected, the lack of vitamins A and K producing characteristic effects. The malabsorption of vitamin D is aggravated by a concomitant binding of calcium to fatty acids in the bowel. Important effects of this dual interference with calcium absorption are a negative calcium balance, mild hypocalcaemia, a tendency to tetany, and in more prolonged cases osteomalacia. There may also be osteoporosis due to protein deficiency. Malabsorption of folic acid and vitamin B_{12} produces a megaloblastic type of anaemia.

Mineral absorption. An impaired absorption of iron is common, and this leads to hypochromic, microcytic anaemia. Other minerals that may be poorly absorbed are sodium, potassium, magnesium, and chloride (as well as calcium previously noted). Malabsorption may therefore be accompanied by symptoms of dehydration and muscular weakness.

It is evident that the effects of intestinal malabsorption are diverse, producing widespread disorder in many of the body's organs. This emphasises the importance of the small intestine in the economy of the whole body.

Cystic fibrosis

An important cause of pancreatogenic malabsorption is *cystic fibrosis*, also called *fibrocystic disease of the pancreas* and *mucoviscidosis*. It is inherited as an autosomal recessive trait, and is often referred to as the commonest hereditary disease of White populations; by contrast it is very rare in Blacks and almost unknown in Orientals. It is remarkable for the considerable variety of its presentations.

The *pancreas* is frequently involved: the gland secretes a thick mucus that obstructs the ducts, which dilate, and the gland undergoes atrophy. The disease sometimes develops *in utero*, when the absence of pancreatic enzymes leads to such viscosity of the intestinal contents (meconium) that intestinal obstruction (*meconum ileus*) and even perforation may ensue. More commonly the child later develops a chronic malabsorption syndrome which is often accompanied by constipation.

Pulmonary involvement is also common. The thick mucus blocking the bronchi is a powerful predisposing factor to infection and subsequent bronchopneumonia, which may become chronic and be complicated by lung abscesses. Indeed, chronic lung disease is a feature of most cases of cystic fibrosis that survive for several years.

Occasionally the *liver* is affected and cirrhosis later develops. There may also be *salivary-gland* involvement. A remarkable feature of the disease is the high content of sodium chloride in the *sweat*; this is due to an increased secretion by the eccrine sweat glands. This forms the basis of a useful diagnostic test for cystic fibrosis. Treatment is mainly palliative. The malabsorption syndrome is combated by giving pancreatic extract with each meal. The diet should be high in calories and protein with a moderate content of fat and supplements of the fat-soluble vitamins. Physiotherapy helps to relieve the bronchial obstruction due to the accumulated viscid secretions, and antibiotics will prevent lung infections. In young children the penicillin group is best. Tetracycline is acceptable in those over 8 years of age, but in younger children its effects on the developing dentition lead to a disfiguring greyish-brown discoloration of the teeth. In these patients general anaesthesia should be avoided where possible because of the tendency to chest infections.

REFERENCES

1. Lehninger A L 1975 Biochemistry, 2nd edn. Worth Publishers, New York. See Chapter 13 pp 335–360 for a description of the vitamins and pp 840–845 for a description of starvation
2. Cahill G F 1970 Starvation in man, New England Journal of Medicine, 282: 668
3. Truswell A S, Wright F J 1974 In Davidson's principles and practice of medicine, ed Macleod J, 11th edn. pp 111–172 Nutritional factors in disease, Churchill Livingstone, Edinburgh
4. Rivlin R S 1970 Riboflavine metabolism, New England Journal of Medicine, 283: 463
5. Morson B C, Dawson I M P 1972 Gastrointestinal Pathology, pp 299–335, Blackwell, Oxford

19

Calcium metabolism and heterotopic calcification

Introduction

In addition to providing rigidity to the bones, calcium ions play an important role in many physiological functions. The permeability of cell membranes is affected by the calcium-ion concentration of the extracellular fluids: elevation of the calcium concentration reduces permeability. The calcium ion is important in regulating the electrical properties of membranes; thus, hypocalcaemia increases excitability (see tetany). Calcium plays an essential role in muscle contraction. It is involved in the release of preformed hormones from the endocrine glands, as well as playing a part in the formation of the cyclic AMP that is generated in target cells when acted upon by the relevant non-steriod hormones. Finally, it will be recalled that calcium is important in many steps of blood clotting as well as in the activation of complement.

The total body content of calcium is about 1 kg. The average North-American diet involves an intake of 600 to 1000 mg, and a rather similar quantity (about 600 mg) enters the gastrointestinal tract in the various digestive secretions. In all, about 800 mg of calcium is absorbed per day, and this involves a net gain of about 200 mg. This is approximately equal to the urinary loss, so that the individual is in calcium balance. Calcium is absorbed in the duodenum by an active transport mechanism, but the greatest amount is absorbed in the remainder of the small intestine. Its absorption is reduced in vitamin-D deficiency, uraemia, and in the malabsorption syndrome. The presence of phytic acid and an excess of unabsorbed fatty acids inhibit absorption.

Role of bone

Since bone constitutes the main repository for calcium, it is not surprising that it plays a vital part in calcium metabolism and that upsets in calcium balance can cause severe bone disease.

The osteoid tissue of bone is manufactured by osteoblasts, and after a 5 to 10-day period of extracellular maturation this osteoid undergoes mineralization with the deposition of calcium salts in the form of hydroxyapatite. Bone salts are deposited first in the region of the gap between tropocollagen molecules; their composition is not fixed, since ions other than calcium and phosphate are involved in their formation, e.g. magnesium, sodium, potassium, and fluoride. Initial mineralization of bone is a rapid process, about 70 per cent of the total salts being deposited within a few hours. The remaining 30 per cent are deposited slowly over a period of several weeks. The mechanism of normal mineralization of osteoid is not well understood. If the calcium-phosphate ion product of extracellular fluids is reduced, osteoid calcification does not take place normally and large amounts of osteoid remain unmineralized. This is the defect found in rickets and osteomalacia. As bone matures, so the osteoblasts become trapped within it and form osteocytes. These cells are not inactive, and are in communication with each other by means of delicate processes that lie in the canaliculi. The osteocytes are bathed in a fluid which is in equilibrium with the bone, but is separated from the general extracellular tissue fluids. The osteocytes play an important, though ill-defined, role in bone homeostasis: thus if they die the bone crumbles and is removed. There is considerable evidence that osteocytes are able to demineralize the bone adjacent to them and also remove its osteoid matrix. This process is called *osteolysis*, and is probably of great importance in the hour-to-hour regulation of the plasma calcium level. Having mobilized calcium by the process of osteolysis, the same cell can subsequently lay down more bone. It is generally agreed that the multinucleate osteoclast is capable of mobilising calcium from bone by removing both the salts and the protein matrix. This destructive osteoclastic activity is probably of great importance in the general remodelling of bone that is continually taking place.

It is evident that the processes of osteolysis and osteoclastic resorption both involve the simultaneous removal of bone salts and bone matrix. The bone salts presumably enter the fluid surrounding the osteocytes and osteoclasts, but are not immediately able to diffuse into the plasma. Nevertheless, diffusion between this pericellular fluid and that of the extravascular extracellular space ultimately occurs, and the interchange of salts between bone and plasma is of vital importance in the regulation of plasma calcium levels. The mechanism involved is not well understood, but is governed by three factors: parathyroid hormone, vitamin D, and calcitonin. The actions of these substances is considered after a review of the normal plasma calcium levels.

Plasma calcium

The normal plasma calcium is remarkably constant in health and is about 2.4 mmol per litre (9.5 mg per dl). It exists in three forms:

1. *Ionized calcium.* This component is diffusible and constitutes about 1.1 mmol per litre (4.5 mg per dl). It is the most important fraction, and it is maintained at a constant level by the regulatory mechanisms to be described.

2. *Non-ionized, diffusible calcium.* This is the smallest fraction (0.25 mmol per litre, or 1 mg per dl), and is present for the most part as citrate.

3. *Protein-bound calcium.* This component (1 mmol per litre, or 4 mg per dl) is bound mostly to albumin and is therefore non-diffusible.

It is the total plasma calcium that is usually measured in clinical practice, and in the absence of a marked alteration of plasma proteins, it is a good guide to the level of the ionized fraction. The normal concentration lies between 2.3 and 2.6 mmol per litre (9.2 and 10.4 mg per dl).

CALCIUM BALANCE

In spite of a varying diet, the amount of calcium absorbed from the intestine, the amount excreted in the urine, and the amount deposited or withdrawn from bone are so regulated that the level of plasma ionized calcium remains constant. The actions of parathyroid hormone, vitamin D, and calcitonin are vitally concerned in this homeostatic mechanism.

Parathyroid hormone

There is a continuous secretion of hormone from parathyroid glands, but the rate of secretion is influenced by the plasma ionized calcium level: a fall in calcium level stimulates parathyroid secretion, and a rise in clacium level inhibits it. The parathyroid hormone is a polypeptide containing 84 amino-acid residues; it acts on its target organs by activating cyclic AMP. Its major targets are bone, kidney, and intestine.

The effects of parathyroid hormone on bone. Parathyroid hormone promotes the resorption of bone by osteoclasts as well as promoting osteolysis by osteocytes. Thus the bone minerals are mobilized, and osteoid is removed. Osteoclasts appear to be directly stimulated so that their number increases (see hyperparathyroidism).

The initial action parathyroid hormone on osteoblasts is to inhibit their action, but there is evidence that it can later stimulate them to produce bone. Hence the action of parathyroid hormone on bone is somewhat complex, although the over-all picture is that of resorption.

Effects of parathyroid hormone on kidney. A characteristic effect of the hormone is to increase phosphate excretion. The result of this is that the plasma phosphate decreases in spite of the continued release of phosphate from the bone. The hormone, on the other hand, increases calcium reabsorption from the kidney, and this, together with the calcium released from the skeleton, results in a rise of plasma calcium. The increased level of ionized calcium leads to an increased glomerular load of calcium; the result is an increased quantity of calcium passed in the urine (*hypercalciuria*). Thus hyperparathyroidism is characterized by hypercalcaemia and an over-all calcium loss from the body. Another important action of parathyroid hormone on the kidney is to increase the rate of synthesis of 1,25-dihydroxycholecalciferol which is a vitamin D (see later).

Effects of parathyroid hormone on intestine. The hormone tends to increase the absorption of calcium from the intestine and augment the activity of vitamin D.

Parathyroid hormone thus appears to be the major factor regulating the level of plasma ionized calcium. By its action it mobilizes calcium from the bone and retards the excretion by the kidney. The regulation of parathyroid hormone secretion is determined by the plasma ionic calcium level by a simple feed-back mechanism.

Vitamin D[1–3]

The two important forms of vitamin D are irradiated ergosterol (ergocalciferol), which is present in a diet containing artificially fortified foods and is also called vitamin D_2, and the natural vitamin D produced in the skin by ultraviolet radiation of 7-dehydrocholesterol, and called cholecalciferol or vitamin D_3. The originally described vitamin D_1 has been found to be a mixture.

Both vitamins D_2 and D_3 are first hydroxylated in the liver to 25-hydroxy compounds called 25-hydroxycholecalciferol, 25-HCC, or 25-OHD_3 in the case of vitamin D_3. The 25-HCC is further hydroxylated to 1,25-dihydroxycholecalciferol, also called 1,25-DHCC or 1,25-$(OH)_2D_3$ in the kidney. This is believed to be the final active metabolite. This final hydroxylation is promoted by low plasma levels of calcium or phosphate and by parathyroid hormone, prolactin, and possibly growth hormone.[4] A similar second hydroxylation occurs in respect of vitamin D_2.

The main action of vitamin D is to aid the absorption of calcium from the gut. There are several suggestions as to how this is mediated. It may be that the vitamin stimulates an active transport mechanism or that it promotes the formation of a calcium-binding protein in the intestinal wall. There is considerable confusion regarding the action of vitamin D on bone. In physiological concentrations vitamin D probably has no direct effect, but in pharmacological doses it exhibits a parathyroid-hormone-like action on bone.

Although parathyroid hormone and vitamin D both play important roles in maintaining calcium homeostasis, the action of vitamin D is the more vital. Patients with hypoparathyroidism can be maintained on vitamin-D therapy and additional calcium. On the other hand, the absence of vitamin D leads to severe skeletal disease, and no substitute for the vitamin will prevent it.

Calcitonin

This hormone is a polypeptide containing 32 amino-acid residues and has the effect of lowering the plasma calcium level. It is secreted by the C cells of the thyroid gland, but the precise role of this hormone in calcium homeostasis is not known. Although tumours of C cells occur (medullary carcinoma of the thyroid) no upset in calcium metabloism has been described in the patients.

DISORDERS OF CALCIUM METABOLISM

Disorders of calcium metabolism form a complex group of topics, and will be described under five headings: vitamin D deficiency, hypoparathyroidism, hyperparathyroidism, hypocalcaemia, and hypercalcaemia. Some interrelationships between these conditions are depicted in Figure 19.1.

VITAMIN-D DEFICIENCY

The body obtains vitamin D from the food and by synthesis in the skin under the influence of ultraviolet light. An inadequate diet (particularly in those countries where there is not much sunlight) and the malabsorption syndrome will therefore lead to its deficiency.

A deficiency of vitamin D results in an impaired absorption of calcium from the intestine and consequent hypocalcaemia. There is a diminution, or even a complete cessation, of calcification of cartilage and osteoid.

Rickets

In the growing child calcification of the epiphyseal cartilage does not occur at the growing ends of the long bones. The cartilage therefore does not die and instead continues to grow, so that the epiphyses undergo enlargement at the bone ends with greatly delayed ossification.

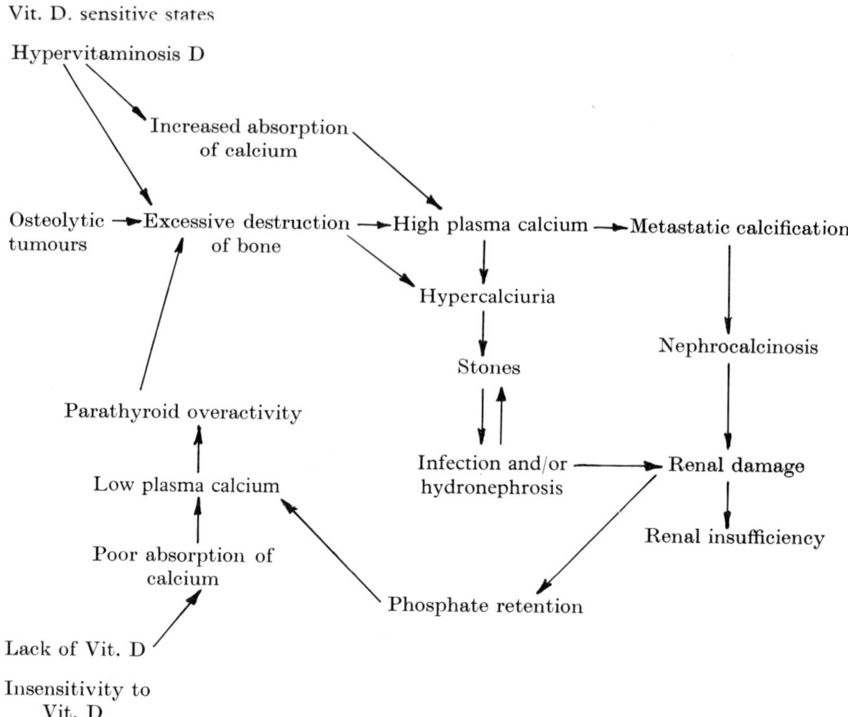

Fig. 19.1 Diagrammatic representation of the important effects of disturbed calcium metabolism. The effects of parathyroid hormone and dietary calcium intake on vitamin D are not shown (see pp. 294 and 295).

Similarly, the costo-chondral junctions are enlarged, producing the clinical deformity called the 'rachitic rosary'. Growth of bone length is impaired, and the child is dwarfed. Even the osteoid which is formed is poorly calcified, and the weakened bones are liable to deformities and fractures: knock-knees, kyphosis (forward curvature of the spine), and other deformities are common.

In infants there is a thickening of the frontal and parietal eminentia, and flattening and thinning of the occipital region (craniotabes), and there may be delayed eruption of the teeth. Fortunately, this florid picture of rickets is rare in civilized countries.

Vitamin-D resistant rickets. There are a number of hereditary conditions in which rickets occurs in spite of an adequate vitamin-D intake. Usually this is associated with an abnormal excretion of amino acids in the urine, excessive excretion of phosphate in the urine, and hypophosphataemia.

Osteomalacia

The counterpart of rickets in the adult is osteomalacia. It is more common in women, because pregnancy imposes an additional drain on the supplies of calcium.

In the normal adult bone is continually being remodelled; it is removed by osteoclasts and replaced by osteoblasts laying down osteoid which promptly calcifies. If this calcification fails, the bones consist largely of osteoid and the result is osteomalacia: there is an abundance of osteoid but poor calcification, in contradistinction to osteoporosis, where the matrix is normally calcified but reduced in quantity.

All bones are affected, but it is the weight-bearing regions where the most severe effects are seen. Severe pelvic distortion may cause complications in subsequent pregnancies, and collapse of the vertebrae gives rise to pain due to compression of the spinal nerves in the intervertebral foramina.

HYPOPARATHYROIDISM

The most common cause of hypoparathyroidism is damage to the glands or their blood supply sustained during thyroid surgery.

Hypoparathyroidism is characterized by hypocalcaemia which causes tetany and convulsions and the other effects noted on page 299. Hyperphosphataemia is also present. These changes are also found in pseudohypoparathyroidism, a rare condition in which the parathyroids are normal but there is end-organ unresponsiveness to parathyroid hormone.

HYPERPARATHYROIDISM

Excessive secretion of the parathyroid glands may occur as a primary or a secondary condition.

Primary hyperparathyroidism

The first account of this disease was published in 1743 by a Welshman, Sylvanus Bevan. It is generally due to an idiopathic hyperplasia of the parathyroid glands, but sometimes a simple adenoma is responsible; rarely the tumour is malignant.

Primary hyperparathyroidism can present in a variety of ways. The best known is classical *osteitis fibrosa cystica, or von Recklinghausen's disease of bone*, in which intense osteoclastic resorption leads to destructive cystic changes involving many bones. Bone pain is a prominent symptom, pathological fractures are common, and sometimes tumour-like masses of osteoclasts are formed.

These *brown tumours*, as they are called, closely resemble giant-cell tumours of bone (p. 596), and are seen typically at sites which normally contain haematopoietic tissue: the skull, jaw, ribs, and spine. The brown coloration is due to the content of haemosiderin.

Occasionally the first indication of the condition is a cyst-like lesion of the jaw. The radiographic description is of a 'ground-glass' appearance of the affected bone. There is resorption of bone, and although the lamina dura may be lost, the teeth are not usually affected. The diagnosis may be confirmed by finding the characteristic biochemical changes described below.

More commonly the resorption of hyperparathyriodism is generalized, and the bone disorder is less conspicuous and presents as generalized osteoporosis. In these cases the hypercalcaemia causes the characteristic effects (p. 299). Death is due to renal failure. If the plasma calcium reaches very high levels (above 5 mmol per litre, or 20 mg per dl). there may be a *hypercalcaemic crisis.* There is shock, haemoconcentration, anuria, and death preceded by confusion and coma.

Another well-known presentation of hyperparathyroidism is recurrent renal-calculus formation. These cases are usually of long standing, bone lesions may be absent, and the systemic effects of hypercalcaemia are often mild.

The biochemical changes of hyperparathyroidism are a raised level of plasma calcium (it may rise to 5.5 mmol per litre, or 22 mg per dl), a lowered level of plasma phosphate, and an increased urinary output of calcium. The plasma alkaline phosphatase is usually considerably raised. Metastatic calcification in the usual sites is common, and is aggravated when renal failure develops. Often this renal failure is caused by metastatic calcification in the kidneys, so that a vicious circle is set up.

Secondary hyperparathyroidism

Hyperplasia of the parathyroids occurs in many types of osteomalacia and rickets. It is the hypocalcaemia that stimulates the glands into activity. In some cases the parathyroid hormone secretion is sufficiently marked to initiate osteoclastic activity in the bones, and therefore in addition to the changes or rickets or osteomalacia there develop those of osteitis fibrosa cystica. This type of response occurs only occasionally, and renal disease is the usual antecedent.

Renal osteodystrophy (renal rickets). Chronic renal disease, especially in young people, is sometimes attended by skeletal lesions which comprise a mixture of calcification defects—osteomalacia (or rickets according to age) and osteitis fibrosa cystica. Metastatic calcification affecting principally the kidneys, arteries, and subcutaneous tissues sometimes occurs.

Tertiary hyperparathyroidism. It is now recognized that some cases of longstanding parathyroid hyperplasia secondary to malabsorption or chronic renal failure may undergo adenomatous change. Hypercalcaemia then develops.

Ectopic parathyroid-hormone syndrome. A number of patients with malignant disease have hypercalcaemia without evidence of metastatic bone disease. This syndrome is due to the elaboration by the tumour of a substance resembling parathyroid hormone. Squamous-cell carcinoma of the lung and carcinoma of the kidney are the usual culprits.

HYPOCALCAEMIA

Causes. The following are important causes of hypocalcaemia.

In association with hypoalbuminaemia. Since the ionized, diffusible calcium level is normal, tetany does not occur.

Hypoparathyroidism. This is described on page 297.

Renal failure. Phosphate retention leads to hyperphosphataemia and a reciprocal lowering of the plasma calcium. Another important factor is deficient formation of 1,25-hydroxyvitamin D with a consequent impairment in the intestinal absorption of calcium.

Vitamin-D deficiency.

Widespread osteoplastic metastases. These may utilize so much calcium that hypocalcaemia results. The usual primary source of the tumour is the prostate.

Infantile hypocalcaemia. Neonatal tetany is well recognized and is due to functional immaturity of the parathyroid glands during the first 2 days of life.

Acute pancreatitis. Hypocalcaemia in this condition can be attributed partly to the deposition of calcium salts in the foci of fat necrosis (dystrophic calcification), and partly to the release of glucagon from the damaged pancreas.

Effects of hypocalcaemia. 1. Tetany and epileptiform convulsions. There may also be mental disturbances, especially states of depression and anxiety.

In milder hypocalcaemia, where there are no clinical symptoms, there are two simple manoeuvres which may elicit latent tetany: (a) *Trousseau's sign*, which is a spasm of the interossei and of the adductor and opponens muscles of the thumb following the inflation of a sphygmomanometer cuff on the upper arm to above the systolic blood pressure for up to 3 minutes, and (b) *Chvostek's sign*, which is a twitching of the muscles of that side of the face when the branches of the facial nerve in the parotid gland at the angle of the jaw are tapped. If Trousseau's sign takes more than 2 minutes to elicit, it is of doubtful significance. Chvostek's sign has been found in from 2 to 20 per cent of normal people.

The actual manifestations of tetany usually commence with paraesthesiae of the hands and feet, and these are followed by classical carpopedal spasms. In severe cases there may also be spasms of the diaphragm, abdominal muscles, and back. Spasm of the glottis in children leads to the alarming manifestation of *laryngismus stridulus.*

2. Abdominal pain of obscure origin. It may be due to smooth-muscle spasm.

3. Electrocardiographic changes: a prolonged QT interval principally in the ST segment.

4. A predisposition to eczema in chronic cases. There is also an increased incidence of *Candida albicans* infections of the skin.

5. Cataract, a well-known complication of chronic hypocalcaemia. The cause is uncertain.

HYPERCALCAEMIA

Causes. An increase in the level of plasma calcium occurs in the following conditions:

Primary hyperparathyroidism. This important condition is described on page 297.

Hypervitaminosis D. Excessive administration of vitamin D leads to hypercalcaemia and generalized metastatic calcification. The parathyroid-hormone-like activity of vitamin D potentiates this action.

Vitamin-D-sensitive states. The hypercalcaemia sometimes encountered in sarcoidosis is probably due to increased sensitivity to vitamin D.

Destructive bone lesions. Extensive destruction of the skeleton by osteolytic metastases of carcinoma, multiple myeloma, or Hodgkin's disease may lead to the release of excessive amounts of calcium.

Miscellaneous causes. Prolonged immobilization, compulsive milk drinking, and hyperthyroidism are occasionally associated with hypercalcaemia. In the rare *congenital hypophosphatasia* hypercalcaemia and hypercalciuria are associated with low alkaline phosphatase level in the plasma and a clinical picture that resembles rickets.

Effects of hypercalcaemia 1. Fatigue, lethargy, and muscle asthenia.

2. Anorexia, nausea, and vomiting. Constipation is prominent, possibly due to the muscular hypotonia.
3. Pruritus, an unexplained symptom.
4. Psychotic manifestations.
5. Symptoms of progressive renal dysfunction starting with polyuria due to an unresponsiveness of the distal and collecting tubles to antidiuretic hormone. There is an accompanying thirst, which may also be due to the high plasma calcium directly stimulating the hypothalamus. This is followed by disturbances in pH regulation and glomerular function, which terminate rapidly in renal failure. Indeed, the renal effects of hypercalcaemia are the most lethal aspect of the condition.
6. Electrocardiographic changes: a shortened QT interval and depressed T waves. These are seldom of diagnostic value.
7. Metastatic calcification.
8. Peptic ulceration. This is particularly common in primary hyperparathyroidism, but can occur in other types of hypercalcaemia also. The excess plasma calcium releases gastrin.
9. Pancreatitis, both acute and chronic. This again is seen most often in association with primary hyperparathyroidism, but can occur in other types of hypercalcaemia also. The mechanism is unknown (as indeed is that of pancreatitis generally); suggested factors include stones forming in the pancreatic ducts and the ionised calcium favouring the conversion of trypsinogen to trypsin in the pancreatic ducts.

HETEROTOPIC CALCIFICATION

It is convenient to conclude this account of calcium metabolism with a description of *heterotopic calcification.* This is defined as the deposition of calcium salts in tissues other than osteoid or enamel. Because calcium salts are radiopaque, their deposition is conspicuous on x-ray examination, and heterotopic calcification has therefore come to assume an importance in diagnostic radiology which far outweighs its pathological significance.

Microscopically calcium salts appear as granular deposits which stain a very deep blue colour with haematoxylin. Two quite distinct types of heterotopic calcification are recognized. *Dystrophic calcification* is the deposition of calcium salts in dead or degenerate tissue. The plasma levels of calcium and phosphate are normal and abnormal local conditions are the cause of the calcification. In *metastatic calcification* there is an upset in calcium metabolism and the calcification takes place in certain normal tissues.

DYSTROPHIC CALCIFICATION

The cause of dystrophic calcification can be considered under two headings: (1) calcification in dead tissue, and (2) calcification in degenerate tissue. Though the distinction between the two may be somewhat arbitrary, this forms a convenient division.

Calcification in dead tissue. Calcification is frequent in caseous tissue and remains as a permanent memorial to a previous tuberculous lesion, e.g. in the lung or hilar lymph nodes. Dead parasites (e.g. *Trichinella spiralis*), areas of fat necrosis (in pancreatitis), artheromatous material, and thrombi provide other examples of dead tissue that may calcify.

Calcification in degenerate tissue. Calcification is not uncommon in the fibrous tissue of scars or a chronic inflammatory lesion, e.g. in chronic tonsillitis or a treated lesion of bacterial endocarditis. Degenerate areas of tumour may calcify, and this forms the basis of *mammography*, in which radiographs of the female breast are examined as a means of detecting a carcinoma that cannot be felt.

METASTATIC CALCIFICATION

Metastatic calcification is caused by a disordered metabolism of calcium and phosphate, and although in the common type (following hyperparathyroidism) the calcium salts are truly metastatic, being derived from bone, there are other conditions in which the excess calcium is absorbed from the gut. Nevertheless, it is convenient in practice to use the term 'metastatic calcification' to cover both these varieties, and it will be used in this context in the account that follows.

Generalized metastatic calcification is usually due to hypercalcaemia, but occasionally, as in renal osteodystrophy, a high plasma phosphate appears to be the precipitating factor. The bone salts are deposited in certain sites of election.

Kidney. This is the most frequent and important site. Deposition occurs especially around the tubules, where severe damage is produced. The condition is called *nephrocalcinosis*, and it may lead to renal failure (see Ch. 36). In addition, calculi often form in the pelvis and ureter, where they may predispose to infection and cause further renal damage. *Renal failure is therefore a prominent feature of generalized metastatic calcification whatever may be the primary cause.*

Lung, stomach, blood-vessel walls, and the cornea are other sites frequently affected. Slit-lamp examination of the eye is indeed of use in diagnosing the condition during life.

Causes of metastatic calcification. The following causes of metastatic calcification can be recognized:

Hyperparathyroidism. Primary hyperparathyroidism is due to parathyroid hyperplasia, adenoma, or rarely carcinoma. *Secondary hyperparthyroidism* is generally caused by renal failure.

Excessive absorption of calcium from the bowel. Hypervitaminosis D and vitamin-D sensitive states, e.g. in sarcoidosis.

Destructive bone lesions. Widespread osteolytic metastatic carcinoma in bone and multiple myeloma are both sometimes complicated by metastatic calcification.

GENERAL REFERENCES

Fourman P, Royer P 1968 Calcium Metabolism and the Bone, 2nd edn. Blackwell, Oxford, pp 656
Nordin B E C 1973 Metabolic Bone and Stone Disease. Churchill Livingstone, Edinburgh
Paterson C R 1974 Metabolic Disorders of Bone, Blackwell, Oxford, pp 373
Vaughan J M 1975 The Physiology of Bone, 2nd edn. Clarendon Press, Oxford, pp 306

REFERENCES

1. Raisz L G 1972 A confusion of vitamin D's. New England Journal of Medicine 287:926
2. Kodicek E 1974 The story of vitamin D from vitamin to hormone. Lancet, 1:325
3. Leading Article 1974 Cholecalciferol metabolism. Lancet 1:492
4. Leading Article 1977 Vitamin D and the pituitary. Lancet 1:840

20

The collagen vascular diseases

The term collagen disease was coined by Klemperer in 1942 to describe a group of disorders in which the primary lesion appeared to be damage to collagen. *Lupus erythematosus*, *dermatomyositis*, *progressive systemic sclerosis*, and *polyarteritis* are now included in this group, and each will be described in this chapter. *Acute rheumatic fever* and *rheumatoid arthritis* can also be included, but they are described elsewhere.

The evidence for these diseases being primary disorders of collagen is by no means convincing, but because they all possess certain features in common it is convenient to group them together. Since blood vessel involvement is as constant a feature as collagen damage the term *collagen vascular disease* is currently used.

LUPUS ERYTHEMATOSUS

Lupus erythematosus may occur as a localized skin disease or it may be a multisystem disease. The two types will be described separately, and the interrelationship between them discussed later.

Chronic discoid lupus erythematosus (DLE)

This type of lupus erythematosus has been recognized for many years by dermatologists as a skin condition that occurs particularly on the face and other exposed areas of the body and is worsened by exposure to sunlight. The lesions consist of well-defined erythematous scaly papules and plaques. The epidermis shows atrophy, and as the lesions heal there is scarring with disturbance of pigmentation. Telangiectasia is often present and the appearances are described as poikilodermatous. When the scalp is involved, there is loss of hair (alopecia). Indeed, lupus erythematosus is an important cause of alopecia with scarring; the lesions are very similar to those produced by lichen planus and scleroderma of the scalp. The oral mucosa is affected in about 15 per cent of cases of chronic discoid lupus erythematosus; the lesions are erythematous and hyperkeratotic, so that a type of leukoplakia is produced.

Systemic lupus erythematosus (SLE)

In systemic lupus erythematosus there are widespread lesions affecting many organs. The disease varies considerably in severity. The onset may be acute with fever, elevated ESR, lymphadenopathy, splenomegaly, malaise, and joint pains.

On the other hand, the onset may be insidious with the development of a skin rash later to be followed by evidence of other organ involvement.

The skin may show lesions identical to those of chronic discoid lupus erythematosus, but in the acute phase of the disease it merely shows erythema and oedema of the sun-exposed areas. Typically, this affects the nose and both cheeks, thereby giving the classic 'butterfly rash'. Lesions in the oral mucosa may occur, and tend to be haemorrhagic or ulcerative. Other important features of systemic lupus are arthritis, pericarditis, pleurisy, endocarditis and glomerulonephritis (Fig. 20.1). A nephrotic syndrome can occur, but progressive renal damage

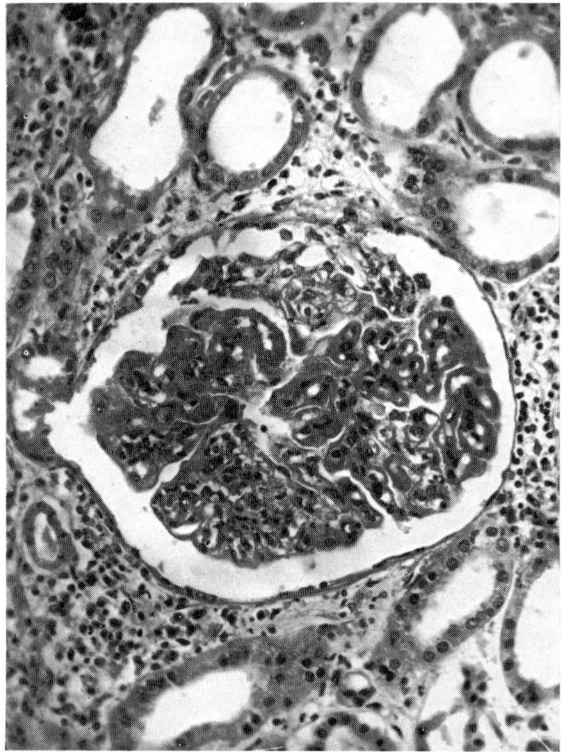

Fig. 20.1 Systemic lupus erythematosus. This glomerulus shows the typical 'wire-loop' lesion. The thickened capillary wall stains brightly with eosin, because there is subendothelial deposition of immune complexes. Not all the basement membrane is affected. This accounts for the patchy appearance of the lesion in the glomerulus. × 240. (*From Heptinstall R H 1960 Diseases of the kidney. In: Harrison C V* 11 : (*ed*) *Recent advances in pathology 7th edn, Fig. 4.11. Churchill, London, p 103.*)

commonly develops and the patient dies in renal failure. When the brain is involved in SLE there can be severe psychiatric disturbances, and indeed these may be the presenting symptoms. Raynaud's phenomenon is common in SLE.

A prominent feature of SLE is the presence of many autoantibodies in the serum. Acute haemolytic anaemia can occur, and the Coombs test is sometimes positive. The serological tests for syphilis may also be positive. The rheumatoid factor is present in about 30 per cent of cases.

The important antibodies, from a diagnostic point of view, are those that react specifically with nuclear antigenic components. Antinucleoprotein and anti-DNA antibodies can be demonstrated in most cases of the active disease. The antibodies may be detected by immunofluorescence: the patient's serum is applied to a section or smear of tissue, and the antinuclear antibody that adheres to the nuclei is detected by subsequently applying fluorescein-labelled anti-IgG and examining the tissue by ultraviolet microscopy. Many patterns have been described but four are commonly recognized.

1. *Homogeneous pattern.* The entire nucleus is seen to fluoresce evenly. This pattern is associated with an antibody against nucleoprotein—the same antibody that is responsible for the LE test (see below).

2. *Peripheral or rim pattern.* This pattern is associated with antibodies to DNA and nucleoprotein. Renal involvement is more common with this pattern.

3. *Nucleolar pattern.*

4. *Speckled pattern.* This pattern is characteristic of the mixed connective-tissue disease.*

A less sensitive method of detecting antinuclear antibodies is to search for the *LE cell phenomenon.* This was the first specific laboratory test described in the diagnosis of SLE. When normal human leucocytes are incubated for about 2 hours with the serum of a patient with SLE, some neutrophils are found to contain a homogeneous basophilic mass of nuclear material. Such neutrophils are called LE cells. The mass is derived from a necrotic leucocyte nucleus that has been acted upon by the antinuclear antibody. Its subsequent phagocytosis by a polymorph produces the LE cell.

The skin changes in lupus erythematosus are similar in both types of the disease. There is hyperkeratosis, epidermal atrophy and hydropic degeneration of the cells in the basal layer. The dermis shows oedema and a periappendageal lymphocytic infiltrate (Fig. 20.2).

The cause and pathogenesis of SLE are not understood. A disease very similar to it, and encountered in Aleutian minks, is caused by a viral infection. Virus-like particles can be found in the lesions of human SLE, but they have not been cultured and their nature remains undetermined. There seems little doubt that SLE is a disease in which many autoantibodies are formed, particularly against nucleic acid, but whether the antigen is the patient's own nucleic acid or whether it is foreign—possibly viral—nucleic acid is not known. It is probable that the disease occurs in persons who are genetically susceptible, since there is an increased incidence of autoantibodies and autoimmune diseases in relatives of patients with SLE. It may well be that in these susceptible individuals various factors can trigger the formation of autoantibodies, and that the immune-complexes that are formed damage the blood vessels of the skin, kidney, and other organs to produce the syndrome of systemic lupus.

The precipitating factor may be a viral infection, the administration of a drug, or exposure to sunlight.

The cutaneous lesions of chronic discoid lupus erythematosus cannot be distinguished from those found in some cases of SLE. Occasionally patients with DLE progress to SLE but this is a rare event. Both diseases are commoner in the

* The term mixed connective-tissue disease has been applied to a syndrome having features of SLE, progressive systemic sclerosis, and dermatomyositis. The condition has a good prognosis, since renal complications are uncommon and the response to prednisone is good.

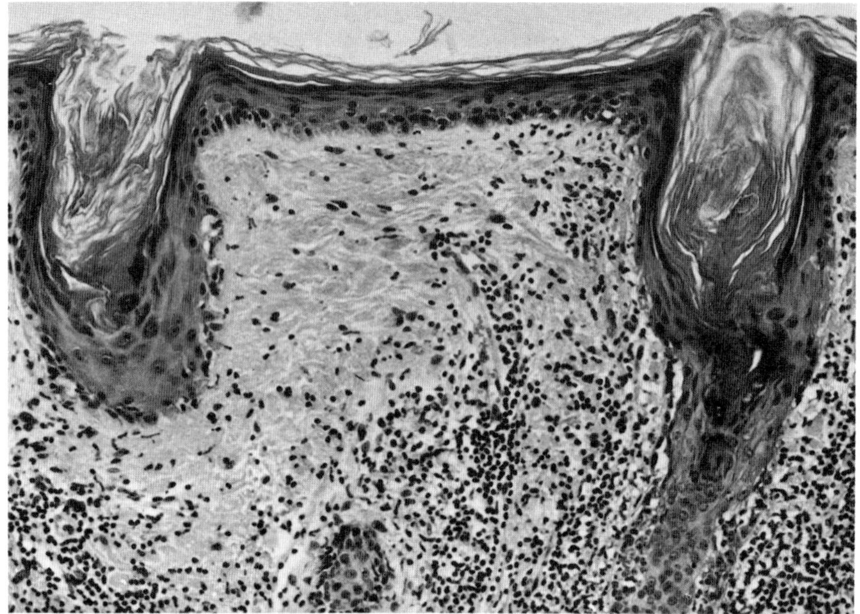

Fig. 20.2 Chronic discoid lupus erythematosus. The epidermis shows atrophy which, in this slide, is particularly marked around the orifices of the hair follicles. There is hyperkeratosis, and the hair follicles are atrophic and their mouths filled with keratinous plugs. The basal layer of the epidermis is poorly seen, and in some areas there is a vacuolated appearance due to hydropic degeneration of the basal cells. In the dermis there is a patchy lymphocytic inflammatory infiltrate which has a tendency to be arranged around hair follicles. In the follicle on the right, the inflammatory infiltrate is closely applied to the epithelial cells so that the junction between the two is poorly seen. × 120.

female, a tendency more marked with SLE. Thus the two diseases appear to be distinct entities, and their inter-relationship remains to be clarified.

DERMATOMYOSITIS

The combination of muscle inflammation (myositis) causing progressive weakness of the proximal limb muscles and a variety of skin rashes constitutes this extraordinary disease. The occurrence of oedema and a purplish-red heliotrope erythema, particularly around the eyes, is characteristic. Skin and muscle biopsies help to establish the diagnosis. The disease may run a fulminating, fatal course, or it may be indolent and chronic. In patients over the age of 40 years dermatomyositis is often associated with a malignant tumour of some internal organ. Hence, a thorough search for carcinoma should be undertaken. The common sites (e.g., lung, gastrointestinal tract, and kidney) should be investigated if no specific signs or symptoms indicate the location of the tumour.

SCLERODERMA

Like lupus erythematosus, scleroderma can occur in two forms. The purely cutaneous disease is called *morphoea*, whilst the generalized form is termed *progressive systemic sclerosis*.

Morphoea

The dermis becomes thickened, fibrous, and bound down in this form of the disease. One or more plaques of affected skin are present, and they usually have a faintly purple or mauve colour, particularly at their edges. Rarely the lesions are widespread. Sometimes they are linear, and the underlying muscle and even bone may be affected. This is particularly well marked in the *fronto-parietal type* (*en coup de sabre* from the resemblance to a sabre cut). This lesion starts with fibrosis of the

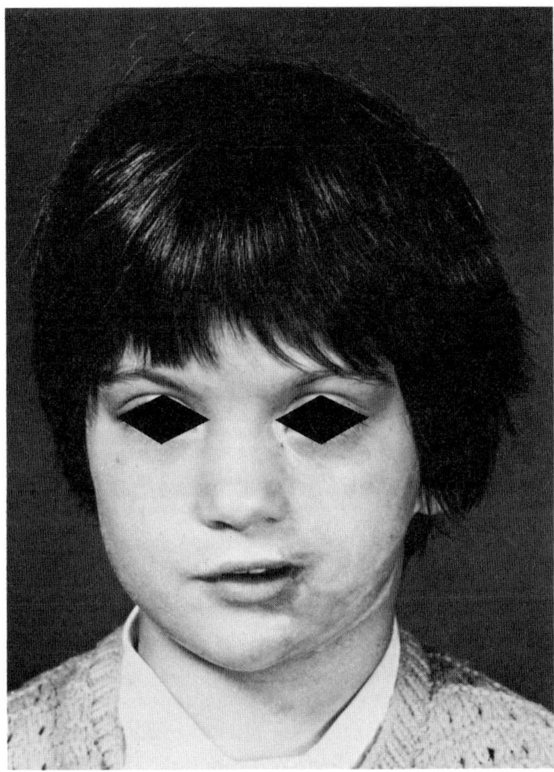

Fig. 20.3. Morphoea affecting the left side of the face of a child aged 7 years. The resulting facial hemiatrophy has led to shrunken appearance of the tissues. (Photograph by courtesy of Professor T. D. Foster.)

affected skin of the face. A linear, depressed groove appears on the fronto-parietal region, extending into the scalp and producing an area of alopecia. The underlying soft tissue and bone atrophy can extend to involve the facial bones, including the alveolar bone. Facial hemiatrophy and alterations in the teeth are the end-result (Figs. 20.3 and 20.4).

Progressive systemic sclerosis (systemic scleroderma)

In the systemic variety there is widespread, bilateral involvement of the skin, the face and hands often being first affected. The earliest feature is usually Raynaud's phenomenon. Next the skin becomes smooth, shiny, firm to the touch, and bound down to underlying structures. When this affects the face, an immobile, mask-like appearance with pinching of the nose is characteristic. The hands are at first

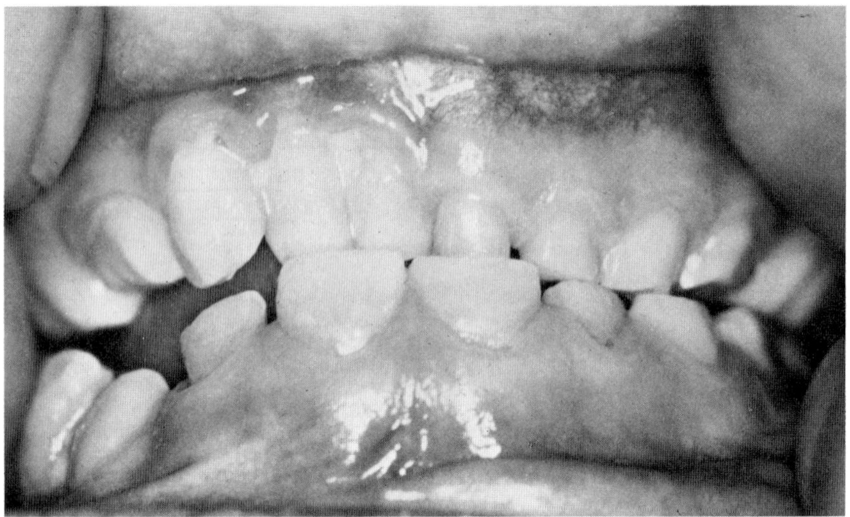

Fig. 20.4. Morphoea affecting the left side of the face of a child aged 7 years. This picture comes from the same case as Fig. 20.3, and shows the changes in the mouth. There is loss of alveolar bone, and the gingiva has receded from the lower incisors. (Photograph by courtesy of Professor T. D. Foster.)

swollen, but later, as fibrosis occurs and movement becomes limited, there may be atrophy of soft tissues, particularly of the pulps of the fingers and the terminal phalanges. The appearance is then described as *sclerodactyly*. Ulceration of the finger tips and dystrophic calcification of the pulps (*calcinosis cutis*) is a well-recognized event. Telangiectatic vessels are commonly seen on the face, and morphologically resemble those of hereditary haemorrhagic telangiectasia (p. 382). The combination of calcinosis, Raynaud's phenomenon, sclerodactyly, and telangiectasia has been separated as a distinct variant called the *CRST syndrome.*

In progressive systemic sclerosis there is always involvement of internal organs. Characteristically there is fibrosis of the oesophagus, and oesophageal reflux may lead to a foul taste in the mouth. Radiographic motility studies are diagnostic even before the patient experiences dysphagia. Other parts of the intestinal tract may also be involved. A characteristic oral radiographic finding is widening of the periodontal membrane. Fibrosis can occur in the lungs, heart, and elsewhere, but the most serious effect is in the kidneys. Although vascular involvement is unusual in scleroderma it is a predominant feature in the kidneys, where medium-sized vessels become obstructed and small arterioles in the glomeruli show fibrinoid necrosis. The changes are identical with those seen in malignant hypertension, and the progressive vascular obstruction leads to renal failure.

POLYARTERITIS NODOSA

Classical polyarteritis nodosa

This type of polyarteritis, first described in the last century, usually affects middle-aged males, and is characterized by an arteritis involving medium-sized muscular arteries of organs. The inflamed arterial walls become necrotic and infiltrated with both inflammatory cells and fibrin, which gives the appearance of *fibrinoid necrosis*. The weakened vessel walls bulge, and the aneurysms so formed are responsible for the designation 'nodosa'. The lumen of the affected vessels becomes obstructed by thrombus, and the disease is characterized by ischaemia and infarction affecting many organs, particularly nerves, spleen and kidney. Renal failure, often with hypertension, is a common end-result of this fatal disease.

Variants of polyarteritis nodosa

The classic polyarteritis nodosa described above is relatively uncommon, but many variants have been described recently. Often, when the vessels affected are small, the term *microscopic polyarteritis* has been applied to these lesions. In some of them, the precipitating cause appears to be an infection, whereas in others hypersensitivity to a drug has been implicated. In none of them is the pathogenesis at all clear; an immune-complex type of vasculitis has been postulated, however. Some of the recognized syndromes are as follows:

Lethal midline granuloma. This disease usually affects young males. It commences with bleeding from the nose and is characterized by a vasculitis with much necrosis affecting the nose and nasopharynx. This terrible disease produces extensive necrosis and gangrene affecting the nose and nasopharynx. Without treatment death is invariable and results from local infection, massive bleeding, or bronchopneumonia.

Progressive allergic granulomatosis. This variant usually commences with asthmatic attacks and pneumonia. Infarcted areas of lung excite a granulomatous reaction that closely resembles tuberculosis histologically.

Wegener's granulomatosis. This disease is defined as a microscopic polyarteritis affecting kidneys, lungs, and upper respiratory tract. In the last site, the lesions may resemble those described in lethal midline granuloma. Death is usually due to renal failure.

It is not clear whether these variants of polyarteritis represent a single disease or are completely separate entities sharing one morphological component—namely, a necrotizing vasculitis. However, necrotizing vasculitis can occur in other conditions. Thus it is a prominent component of septicaemia, malignant hypertension, and the Arthus reaction; it is also encountered in rheumatoid arthritis, lupus erythematosus, and progressive systemic sclerosis.

SUMMARY

The validity of grouping these diseases under the heading of collagen vascular disease is dubious. Mixed cases occur with patients who exhibit features of several diseases. Thus some have lesions of scleroderma with vasculitis, or lupus erythematosus with rheumatoid arthritis. The occurrence of such cases suggests that there is a common mechanism, but it does not prove a common cause. The presence of autoantibodies is another feature that these diseases have in common, being the most striking in lupus erythematosus and the least evident in polyarteritis. Until the origin and pathogenesis of these diseases are discovered, it is convenient to refer to the group collectively as the 'collagen vascular diseases', since they share many features. Thus, they all produce widespread lesions affecting many organs, and often they exhibit a marked constitutional effect such as fever, raised erythrocyte sedimentation rate (ESR), and hypergammaglobulinaemia. This tendency is least marked in progressive systemic sclerosis. All the diseases respond to glucocorticoid therapy as well as to other immunosuppressants such as azathioprine. Presumably, these act by suppressing autoantibody formation, thereby inhibiting the formation of new lesions. Once again progressive systemic sclerosis is the odd man out and is least responsive to therapy.

GENERAL REFERENCES

Leading article 1972 Wegener's granulomatosis. Lancet 2: 519

Minkin W, Rabhan N 1977 Mixed connective tissue disease. Archives of Dermatology 112: 1535

Peltier A P Estes D 1972 In Pathobiology Annual, vol. 2, ed. by Ioachim H L, p 77–109 (antinuclear antibodies)

Talbott J H 1974 Collagen-Vascular Diseases 285 pp. Grune and Stratton, New York

21

Disorders of growth

Most organs of the body possess a considerable reserve of tissue, which can be brought into play whenever additional work is demanded of them. At rest the inactive cells are maintained by an intermittent blood flow through their supplying capillaries. This mechanism results in an economical use of the circulation and explains why noxious substances spread by the blood stream may nevertheless produce patchy effects. When more work has to be performed, the shut-down vessels dilate and the organ shows active hyperaemia. This is well illustrated by the tremendous increase in blood flow through the salivary glands which occurs during periods of active secretion.

Growth potentiality of cells

In addition to this reserve mechanism, organs or tissues subjected to prolonged excessive strain respond by increasing their bulk. This may be done by either increasing the size of each constituent cell, or increasing the total cell number; which of these events occurs depends upon the growth potentiality of the cells involved. Three classes of cells are described.[1]

Labile cells. These cells, also called continuous replicators, undergo division throughout life to replace those lost through differentiation and subsequent desquamation.

The cells of lymph nodes, bone marrow, and most of the covering or protective epithelia (skin, endometrium, alimentary, respiratory, and urinary mucosa) come into this category.

Stable cells. These cells, also called discontinuous replicators, rarely divide in adult life, but never lose their ability to proliferate if suitably stimulated. This group includes most of the secretory epithelial structures (liver, kidney, pancreas, and endocrine glands).

Permanent cells. These non-replicating cells, typified by neurons, are incapable of multiplication. For practical purposes muscle cells fall into this group.

The factors which control the growth and differentiation of cells are largely unknown. Nevertheless, abnormalities in these two functions are frequent, and form an important aspect of many disease processes. They may be considered under three headings:

1. *Quantitative abnormalities of cellular growth*

2. *Abnormalities of cellular differentiation*
3. *Neoplasia,* a topic so important that it is considered separately in the succeeding chapters.

QUANTITATIVE ABNORMALITIES OF CELLULAR GROWTH

EXCESSIVE GROWTH

Tissues composed of labile or stable cells respond to an increased demand for work primarily by multiplication. Permanent cells either show no morphological change (neurons), or else only an increase in size (muscle). Even stable and labile cells usually show some increase in size. An increase in the cell number is called *hyperplasia,* and an increase in individual cell size is *hypertrophy.* Both are usually related to a tangible stimulus, which is often a basically physiological one acting to excess. The most important stimulus is an *increased demand for function.* As will be seen, this may take the form of increased muscular work in response to an abnormal load, an increased production of the blood cells in response to hypoxia or infection, a thickening of protective epithelium in response to external trauma, or an increased secretion of a gland in response to some external need.

Hyperplasia

Definition. Hyperplasia is the increase in size of an organ or tissue due to an increase in the number of its specialized constituent cells. Enlargements due to congestion, oedema, inflammation, amyloid infiltration, or tumour formation are excluded from the definition. The suffix—megaly is used to denote a large organ or tissue regardless of its cause, e.g. cardiomegaly is enlargement of the heart, splenomegaly is enlargement of the spleen, etc.

It is important to realize that those hyperplasias due to a specific stimulus exist only for so long as that stimulus is applied. When it is removed, the hyperplasia ceases and the tissue tends to revert to its normal size.

Although the concept of hyperplasia is traditionally a morphological one, it must never be forgotten that the increase in size of the organ is accompanied by a corresponding increase in function. Nowhere is this more apparent than in hyperplasia of the endocrine glands.

Hyperplasia in the endocrine glands. In endocrine hyperplasias there is enlargement of the gland (or glands, as the case may be). Sometimes this enlargement is diffuse, but in many instances it is circumscribed and discrete. The nodules so formed are often labelled adenomata. In secreting epithelia generally the line of demarcation between hyperplasia and benign neoplasia is so tenuous that a distinction is often purely arbitrary.

Parathyroids. The parathyroid glands show hyperplasia in response to a persistent hypocalcaemia (see secondary hyperparathyroidism, p. 298). In primary hyperparathyroidism the stimulus for the hyperplasia is unknown.

Thyroid. Thyroid hyperplasia is sometimes the result of prolonged stimulation by pituitary thyrotrophic hormone (see p. 621. As a primary idiopathic condition it occurs in Graves's disease (p. 623).

Hyperplasia of the endocrine glands is described in greater detail in Chapter 39.

Hyperplasia in the target organs of the endocrine glands. *Breasts.* Hyperplasia of the epithelial tissue and surrounding specialized connective tissue is a normal feature of the female breast at puberty, during pregnancy and lactation, and to a lesser extent towards the end of each menstrual cycle.

In *mammary dysplasia,* also called cystic hyperplasia of the breast and 'chronic mastitis', there is considerable epithelial hyperplasia, and cysts often develop. It is quite a common condition, and causes discomfort as well as nodularity of the breast substance. Hormonal imbalance is presumed to be the cause, but its nature is obscure.

Prostate. Senile enlargement of the prostate is due to epithelial hyperplasia as well as an increase in the fibromuscular element. The condition is common over the age of 60 years, and is erroneously called 'benign prostatic hypertrophy' or 'adenomatosis of the prostate'. It is an important cause of urinary obstruction, and surgical treatment is often necessary to relieve back-pressure effects on the bladder and kidneys. The cause is unknown, but is probably hormonal in nature.

Hyperplasia of skin. Hyperplasia of the epidermis is a feature of many skin diseases. It may be caused by a wide range of physical 'irritants' acting for a long time, e.g. scratching. The corn on the toe caused by the friction of an ill-fitting shoe is a good example of hyperplasia of a covering epithelium in response to damaging trauma. Hyperplasia may also be induced by viral infection, e.g. the common wart (verruca vulgaris). papilloma virus.

Hyperplasia of bone marrow. Pronounced hyperplasia is seen in the haematopoietic tissue when there is a stimulus for blood cell production. The erythroid series is affected in hypoxia and in many types of anaemia, e.g. pernicious anaemia. In infection it is the white-cell precursors which are affected. The cellular marrow extends into the long bones of the adult (normally filled with fatty marrow), while in childhood extramedullary foci of haematopoiesis may occur in the liver, spleen, and other organs.

Hyperplasia of the RE system and lymphoid tissue. Both undergo hyperplasia in chronic infection. This accounts for the enlargement of the spleen (*splenomegaly*) and lymph nodes (*lymphadenopathy*).

Hyperplasia in relationship to chronic inflammation

As noted previously hyperplasia is sometimes a feature of longstanding chronic inflammation (p. 139).

In the skin hyperplasia may affect the epithelium or the connective tissue. Epithelial hyperplasia may be seen at the edge of chronic ulcers. Another example is *keratoacanthoma* (molluscum sebaceum), in which there is an exuberant downgrowth of hyperplastic epithelium which extends as far as the level of the sebaceous glands. The surrounding dermis shows an inflammatory reaction. It may be almost impossible to differentiate this condition from an early invasive squamous-cell carcinoma; the natural history, however, is quite different, for the keratoacanthoma grows rapidly and then involutes spontaneously after a few months, finally healing with scarring. The nature of this lesion is quite obscure, and it has in the past often been misdiagnosed as cancer.

The *granuloma pyogenicum* is another curious skin lesion in which there is such a profuse proliferation of blood vessels and fibroblasts that the elevated nodule which is produced closely resembles a haemangioma. The lesion is misnamed, for it is not granulomatous nor is it inflamed unless as a secondary event following ulceration of the covering epidermis due to local trauma. Pyogenic granulomata often grow rapidly for a time and can easily be mistaken for a malignant tumour or a spindle-cell naevus (juvenile melanoma, see p. 384). The pyogenic granuloma that arises from the free gingiva is probably an exaggerated inflammatory lesion associated with gingivitis. Like its cutaneous counterpart, it is extremely vascular but it is always heavily infiltrated with polymorphs. The lesion is particularly common in pregnant women (*pregnancy tumour*).

In the oral mucosa chronic inflammation may likewise cause epithelial or connective tissue hyperplasia. Multiple warty epithelial overgrowths may occur, apparently as a result of the irritation from an ill-fitting denture (*papillomatosis*).[2,3] Chronic inflammation may produce hyperplasia of the connective tissue so that fibrous nodules are formed. These are sometimes called 'fibromata', or if pedunculated, *fibro-epithelial polyps*. An *epulis* is a nodule on the gingiva, and most examples are due to connective-tissue hyperplasia induced by inflammation. Sometimes the fibrovascular proliferation and giant-cell formation is so marked that the lesion resembles a giant-cell tumour of bone.[4] It is called the *peripheral giant-cell reparative granuloma* (*giant-cell epulis*) (Fig 21.1).

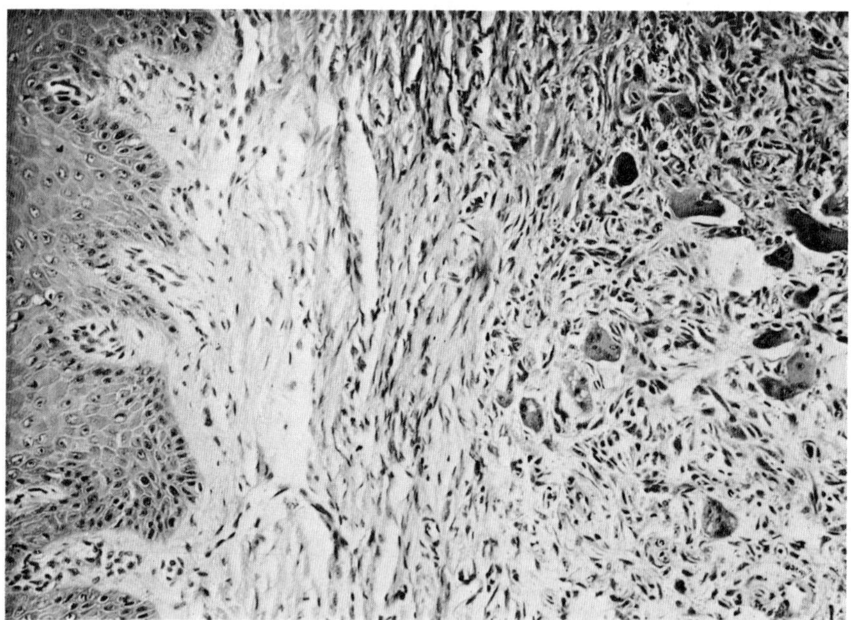

Fig. 21.1 Peripheral giant-cell reparative granuloma. There is a heavy infiltration of foreign-body giant cells in a stroma of collagen and spindle-shaped cells. This is situated in the subepithelial connective tissue of the gingiva, and is separated from the overlying epithelium by a narrow zone of fibrous tissue. × 100.

Pseudoneoplastic hyperplasia

Reference has been made to the difficulties in distinguishing nodular hyperplasia from benign neoplasia, particularly in the endocrine glands, the prostate, and the breast. From a practical point of view the distinction is unimportant since both processes are benign. There are, however, many examples of hyperplasia in which the mass of cells produced closely resembles a malignant tumour. Experience has taught that they are benign, since they either resolve spontaneously or respond to simple treatment. Their importance lies in their recognition, for a mistaken diagnosis can result in grave therapeutic errors. Almost any tissue can show such lesions, and only a few examples will be described.

Pseudomalignant connective tissue hyperplasia

Pseudolymphoma. Pseudolymphoma of the skin[5] appears as nodules of lymphoid tissue which histologically closely resemble the nodular type of lymphocytic lymphoma (p. 347). Unlike the latter, however, the cutaneous lesion never becomes systematized nor develops into an overtly malignant process. Similar pseudolymphomata are described at other sites, e.g. orbit,[6] rectum, and mediastinum.[7] A persistent inflammatory reaction to an insect or tick bite can closely mimic a cutaneous lymphoma.

Pseudosarcomatous nodular fasciitis[8] affects the subcutaneous tissues, commonly of the arm. There is rapid growth of a highly vascular mass which diffusely infiltrates the surrounding tissues. Many mitoses are present in its spindle-cell component, but in spite of the malignant microscopic appearance the lesion is benign in its behaviour.

Pseudomalignant epithelial hyperplasia

Marked hyperplasia of the epidermis which gives an appearance of dermal invasion by squamous cells is seen from time to time in a great variety of chronic skin lesions ranging from fungal granulomata and insect bites to basal-cell carcinoma. The lesion is commonly called *pseudoepitheliomatous hyperplasia* and at times differentiation from squamous-cell carcinoma is not possible, especially when small biopsy specimens alone are available for study.

Pseudoepitheliomatous hyperplasia is well shown in the keratoacanthoma described on page 313. It is also seen over a *myoblastoma,* a somewhat controversial lesion found most often on the tongue and occasionally in the skin. It is composed of very large polygonal and strap-shaped cells, the cytoplasm of which contains coarse eosinophilic granules. The tumour is now thought to be derived from Schwann cells rather than muscle, and the cause of the overlying epithelial hyperplasia is unknown.

Hypertrophy

Definition. Hypertrophy is the increase in size of an organ or tissue due to increase in size of its constituent specialized cells. Pure hypertrophy without accompanying hyperplasia occurs only in muscle, and the stimulus is almost always a mechanical one.

Hypertrophy of smooth muscle. Any obstruction to the outflow of the contents of a hollow muscular viscus results in hypertrophy of its muscle coat. It is seen in the *bladder* when there is prostatic hyperplasia, and in any part of the *gut* above an obstruction, e.g. a stricture or a carcinoma. The *myometrium* of the uterus shows tremendous hypertrophy during pregnancy, and the stimulus, although partly mechanical, is also a hormonal action of oestrogen.

Hypertrophy of cardiac muscle. Although the heart of the newborn child weighs only 30 g, it is believed that no further muscle cells are produced. The fibres increase in size tenfold by the time adult life is reached. Any demand for an increased work-load leads to hypertrophy of the fibres of the chamber affected. The stimulus is probably the stretching which results from the additional strain, and the ability of the heart to respond in this way constitutes a part of the cardiac reserve (p. 521). Hypertrophy is best seen in the left ventricle (Fig. 21.2). Systemic hypertension, aortic valvular disease, and mitral regurgitation are the common causes.

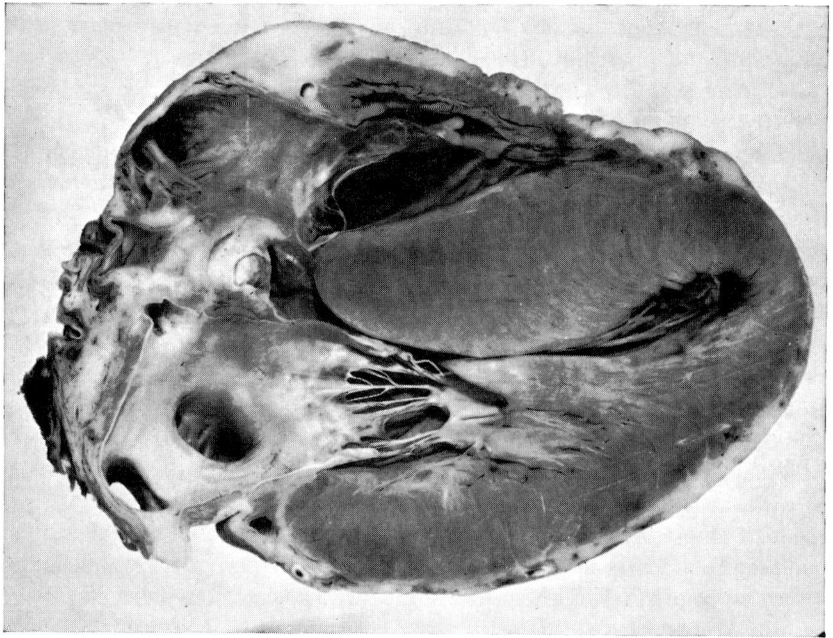

Fig. 21.2 Hypertrophy of the heart. The muscle of the left ventricle is greatly thickened. The cause of this hypertrophy is systemic hypertension. (C20.3. *Reproduced by permission of the President and Council of the Royal College of Surgeons of England.*)

Hypertrophy of skeletal muscle. The village blacksmith's brawny arms provide a simple illustration of hypertrophy due to mechanical stimulus.

DIMINISHED GROWTH

Nomenclature. *Agenesis* is a failure of development of an organ or tissue (p. 377). *Hypoplasia* is a state of imperfect development resulting in a small under-developed organ. *Aplasia* has been used in the context of extreme hypoplasia (short of agenesis), but in practice it is better to restrict the use of this term to the condition seen in the bone marrow (see aplastic anaemia, p. 461). *Atrophy* is the acquired diminution in size of an organ due to a decrease in size or number of its constituent elements. Only in muscle is a decrease in size the major factor. In all other instances the number of cells is also reduced. This is brought about by the periodic destruction of some of the cells, but as the process occurs insidiously and sporadically, the actual necrosis is not apparent (see below). A failure to replace lost cells is also a factor in the pathogenesis of atrophy in labile tissues, e.g. the bone marrow. By custom atrophy of the marrow is called *aplasia,* and if not too marked the word *hypoplasia* is used by some authorities. Unfortunately both these terms are used in a different connotation as noted above. It is evident that the nomenclature is illogical and confusing.

Atrophy

The cellular basis of atrophy

In tissues composed of labile cells, and to a lesser degree stable cells also, there is a constant loss of mature elements and their replacement by the mitotic activity of their fellows. The mechanism of this destruction of old cells is usually not obvious, since coagulative necrosis is not a feature of normal tissues.

Recently the concept of *apoptosis* (derived from the Greek and meaning 'dropping off' or 'falling off') has been introduced to describe the process by which cell numbers are reduced physiologically and also in some pathological conditions.[9, 10] The cell condenses, apparently due to the loss of water, to form a pyknotic nuclear mass surrounded by a variable amount of cytoplasm in which the organelles are still easily recognizable. This is called an 'apoptotic body'. Apoptotic bodies are phagocytosed by histiocytes and neighbouring epithelial cells, in which they are incorporated in lysosomes where they are digested, finally to form small, dense residual bodies (see p. 19). Apoptotic bodies derived from the epithelial cells lining free mucosal surfaces are also shed directly to the exterior.

Apoptosis, unlike coagulative necrosis, is not attended by an inflammatory reaction. The lysosomal residual bodies soon disappear, possibly by exocytosis. The process seems to be involved in the cell turnover in many healthy adult tissues. It is probably also responsible for the focal elimination of cells during normal embryonic development. Pathologically it is prominent in untreated malignant tumours, and it participates in some types of therapeutically induced tumour regression.

In cells undergoing atrophy there are abundant secondary lysosomes (autophagocytic vacuoles) and some residual bodies. There is often evidence of apoptotic bodies also. This explains the progressive cell depletion in atrophy without evidence of frank coagulative necrosis.

The physiological death of cells described above has also been called 'necrobiosis', but apoptosis would seem to be a preferable term.

Physiological atrophy

There are numerous examples of structures which are well developed at a certain period of life but which subsequently undergo atrophy or involution. Many *fetal structures,* e.g. the notochord, branchial clefts and thyroglossal duct, completely disappear before birth, while others such as the ductus arteriosus atrophy early in postuterine life. From adolescence onwards the lymphoid tissue in the body undergoes atrophy, and is partially replaced by fat. After the menopause and in old age there is atrophy of the gonads, and as age advances most tissues take part in a generalized atrophy that finally terminates in death.

Pathological atrophy

Pathological atrophy may be generalized or local.

Generalized atrophy. *Starvation atrophy.* All tissues of the body show atrophy during prolonged starvation. The *cachexia* of malignant disease is in many instances largely dependent upon an inadequate food intake.

Atrophy is most marked in the adipose tissues and in muscle. The brain is least affected. The heart in extreme cases may be reduced to a third of its normal size, and appear brown due to the lipofuscin in its fibres (*brown atrophy of the heart*).

Senile atrophy. This is the marked accentuation of the process of physiological atrophy of old age. Brown atrophy of the heart is especially prominent in senility, and other organs, e.g. the liver and spleen, may also show a lipofuscin accumulation in their cells. This substance, also called 'wear-and-tear pigment', is produced in the cells by the oxidation of fats.

Endocrine atrophy. Hypopituitarism leads to atrophy of the thyroid, adrenal cortex, and gonads. Rarely the whole body becomes stunted and the patient cachectic (see Simmond's disease).

Atrophy of bone (osteoporosis) is described in Chapter 37.

Local atrophy. *Ischaemic atrophy.* This is a local form of tissue malnutrition in which hypoxia is superimposed. With gradual vascular obstruction the parenchyma of many tissues undergoes atrophy, and this is followed by fibrous replacement. Cerebral atrophy is a feature of cerebral atherosclerosis, and the subsequent neuronal loss with replacement gliosis plays an important part in the atrophy of the cortex and the intellectual impairment of old age.

Pressure atrophy. This is a variant of ischaemic atrophy. It follows pressure on a solid organ, the vessels of which are progressively occluded by compression. It is the capillaries that suffer the most, and damage is caused both by malnutrition and hypoxia. In this way the capsule around a benign tumour or a cyst is formed (p. 324). Some of the best examples of pressure atrophy are seen in relation to bone.

Disuse atrophy. The best examples are seen in the locomotor system and in the exocrine glands. The atrophy of bone, ligaments, and muscles that follows joint immobilization must always be borne in mind when limbs are encased in plaster. It also occurs when joints are ankylosed, or movement is prevented by pain; the atrophy around rheumatoid and tuberculous arthritis is particularly marked. Following the loss of teeth there is atrophy of the supporting alveolar bone.

When the duct of a secreting gland is suddenly and completely blocked, the parenchyma undergoes atrophy, e.g. after total obstruction of a ureter, a salivary duct, or the pancreatic duct. It is interesting to recall that it was this method of producing pancreatic atrophy which was employed by Banting and Best in the isolation of insulin.

Neuropathic atrophy. This term is loosely applied to the atrophy of a limb which follws nerve lesions. It has two components. Motor paralysis leads to atrophy of the muscles as well as to a more generalized disuse atrophy. Sensory loss may also

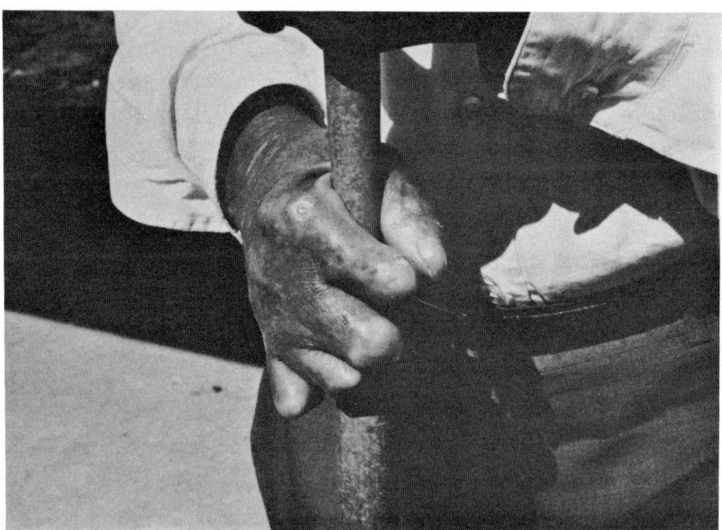

Fig. 21.3 Neuropathic atrophy of fingers. This is a photograph of the hand of a victim of lepromatous leprosy. Note the severe trophic changes involving the skin of the fingers as well as the destruction of the phalanges and soft tissues of the fingers, which are thereby shortened by a concertina effect. Nails are still present at the tips of the fingers. This type of leprosy is associated with involvement of nerves causing a symmetrical peripheral neuropathy. In addition, there is infiltration and destruction of the tissues by bacteria-laden macrophages.

prevent use of the limb, and lead to disuse atrophy. Direct damage due to unnoticed trauma and infection may sometimes be an additional factor (Fig. 21.3).

Whether there is a specific 'neuropathic atrophy' of tissues that is unrelated to either disuse atrophy or direct trauma is disputed. In amphibia, the usual regeneration after an amputation does not occur if the limb is first denervated. Indeed, the stump may be absorbed, so that amputation of even a finger may result in complete resorption of the limb.[11] This nervous influence, whether for regeneration or for maintenance of structural integrity, is called *trophic*, or more specifically, *neurotrophic*.

Idiopathic atrophy. There are examples of atrophy in which no cause is evident. In some instances, for example adrenal atrophy causing Addison's disease (p. 625), an autoimmune basis has been suggested. In other cases presenile change or inherited defect is possible.

ABNORMALITIES OF CELLULAR DIFFERENTIATION

Metaplasia

Metaplasia is a condition in which there is a change in one type of differentiated tissue to another type of similarly differentiated tissue. The importance of the word differentiated should be noted, because its use excludes tumour formation as a form of metaplasia. Metaplasia may occur in both epithelial and connective tissues.

Epithelial metaplasia

Squamous metaplasia. Many types of epithelium are capable of changing to a stratified squamous variety which may undergo keratinization. It often appears to be the result of chronic inflammation. For instance, squamous metaplasia may occur in the gallbladder and urinary bladder when these organs are chronically inflamed, especially if in addition stones (calculi) are present. It is also seen in the bronchi in chronic bronchitis and bronchiectasis (Fig. 21.4).

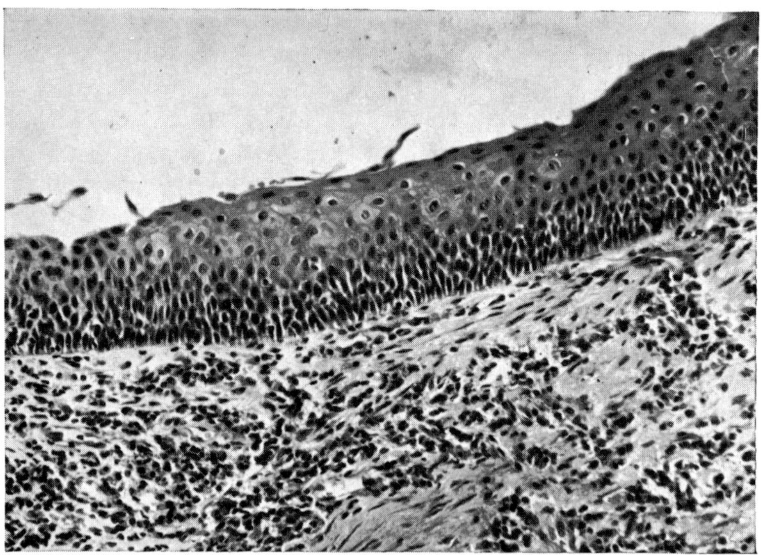

Fig. 21.4 Squamous metaplasia of bronchial epithelium. The normal pseudo-stratified columnar ciliated respiratory epithelium has been replaced by a stratified squamous epithelium. × 200.

Keratinization and the formation of a granular layer may occur in the mobile oral mucous membrane if it is subjected to repeated trauma.* Such a white lesion must be distinguished from other white lesions in which dysplasia is a feature (p. 370).

While in these examples 'chronic irritation' appears to be the cause of the metaplasia, there is one condition in which squamous metaplasia is common, but in which irritation plays no part. This is *hypovitaminosis A*. Squamous metaplasia is widespread, being found in the nose, bronchi, and urinary tract. Squamous epithelia show hyperkeratinization which is manifested in the 'toad-skin' appearance of the exposed skin. There is also conjunctival hyperkeratosis, or *xerophthalmia*, and this may be complicated by corneal ulceration and infection leading to loss of sight.

Columnar metaplasia. Squamous epithelium rarely shows metaplasia to a columnar type. It is occasionally seen in the lining of a periodontal cyst. (p. 301).

Specialized columnar epithelium may change to a more simple type. The conversion of the pseudostratified columnar ciliated respiratory epithelium to a

* Keratinization is found normally in the attached gingiva and in the mucosa overlying the hard palate.

simple mucus-secreting columnar type is commonly seen in chronic bronchitis and bronchiectasis, and is a factor in predisposing patients with these conditions to bronchopneumonia.

Connective tissue metaplasia

Osseous metaplasia. Whether fibroblasts can produce osteoid tissue or not is largely a matter of how one defines 'fibroblast' and 'osteoblast'. The two cell types certainly exhibit great morphological similarity, and before the appearance of the intercellular substance, whether fibrous tissue or osteoid, they cannot be distinguished. 'Fibroblasts' do not normally produce osteoid, but under some conditions they may be regarded as undergoing metaplasia to 'osteoblasts'. Bone then makes its appearance. An alternative explanation is that the osteoblasts are derived from primitive stem cells.

Osseous metaplasia is occasionally seen in scars, and also in the fibrous tissue adjacent to any area of dystrophic calcification—cystic goitres, caseous foci in the lung, etc.

Changes in mesothelium. The mesothelial cells lining the pleura and peritoneum may change to an epithelial type, columnar or even squamous. This is rare, but is important because such cells cast off into the pleural cavity may be mistaken by the unwary cytologist for cancer cells.

Tumour metaplasia. See p. 355.

Other cellular dystrophies

Dystrophy may be defined as a disorder, usually congenital, of the structure or function of an organ or tissue due to its perverted nutrition. In its widest sense it includes agenesis, atrophy, hypertrophy, and metaplasia, but in practice the term is usually applied to those disorders which do not readily fit into any of these other categories. The alternative term dysplasia* may also be used for such an abnormal development of tissue, although strictly it should be applied to developmental disorders only. Dyscrasia* literally means a bad mixture (of the four humours), and is now used by haematologists to describe any blood disorder of uncertain aetiology.

One of the best examples of a dystrophy is the lesion found in pernicious anaemia. Although the abnormal nuclear maturation found in the red-cell precursors in this disease led Ehrlich to describe them as megaloblasts, it was not realized at that time that other cells showed similar changes. Examination of the cells of the gastric, buccal, nasal, vaginal, and other mucosae has revealed certain nuclear abnormalities presumably caused by vitamin-B_{12} deficiency. The changes include pleomorphism, giant polyploid nuclei, and large nucleoli. These observations have an important application: the exfoliative cytologist must avoid mistaking these cells for malignant cells in sputum, gastric washings, urine, etc. The premature greying of the hair and the degeneration of the spinal cord indicate that pernicious anaemia is more than merely a haematological disorder.

Many special dystrophies involving muscle, bone, cornea, retina, etc. have been

* The Greek derivation of these words is as follows: Dys—bad or difficult; Krasis—a mingling; Plasis—a forming.

described, but these are outside the scope of this book. It must be reiterated that the term dystrophy has no specific intrinsic meaning, but like dysplasia is used to describe a lesion whose nature is not understood and for which the author can find no other more appropriate name. In recent years dysplasia has acquried a specific meaning when applied to epithelium—most commonly that of the cervix uteri. It is used to describe a type of hyperplasia which is thought to progress to *carcinoma-in-situ* in some cases and later to invasive cancer (p. 370). But dysplasia is also used in other instances, e.g. fibrous dysplasia of bone and mammary dysplasia, in which there is no suggestion of incipient neoplastic change.

In this chapter many different perversions of cell growth have been described. The one thing they all have in common is that they are self-limiting and reversible if the stimulus is removed. In the following chapter neoplasia is considered. Here the perversion of cell growth persists even when the stimulus that produced it is eradicated.

REFERENCES

1. Post J, Hoffman J 1968 Cell renewal patterns. New England Journal of Medicine 279: 248
2. Donohue W B 1957 Palatal papillomatosis. Journal of the Canadian Dental Association 23: 523
3. Waite D E 1961 Inflammatory papillary hyperplasia. Journal of Oral Surgery 19: 210
4. Lucas R B 1976 Pathology of Tumours of the Oral Tissues, 3rd edn. Churchill Livingstone, Edinburgh, p 271
5. Lever W F, Schaumburg-Lever G 1975 Histopathology of the Skin, 5th edn. Lippincott, Philadelphia, p 708
6. Hogan M J, Zimmerman L E 1962 Ophthalmic Pathology, 2nd edn. Saunders, Philadelphia, p 765
7. Anagnostou D, Harrison C V 1972 Angiofollicular lymph node hyperplasia (Castleman). Journal of Clinical Pathology, 25: 306
8. Mackenzie D H 1972 The fibromatoses: a clinicopathological concept. British Medical Journal, 4: 277
9. Kerr J F R, Wyllie A H, Currie A R 1972 Apoptosis: a basic biological phenomenon with wideranging implications in tissue kinetics. British Journal of Cancer, 26: 239
10. Leading Article 1972 Apoptosis. Lancet 2: 1011
11. Thornton C S 1968 Amphibian limb regeneration. Advances in Morphogenesis, eds Abercrombie M, Brachet J, King T J Vol 7, Academic Press, New York, p. 2–5–249

22

Tumours

Introduction

The concept that tumour growth is a distinctive clinical and pathological entity has been evolving for many centuries. At first the term 'tumour' was applied to any swelling, and the use of the suffix -oma became established to denote such a lesion; even today this relic of the past persists in the use of names like haematoma, hamartoma, tuberculoma, and granuloma. In time the swellings of known aetiology, especially the infective ones, were excluded from the classification of tumours, and there was left a group of swellings of unknown cause apparently produced by the unrestrained growth of the individual's own cells. It appeared that these cells were no longer subject to the normal mechanisms controlling their growth, and had become independent. The trite definition of a tumour as 'an autonomous parasite' embodies this concept, but we cannot define a tumour on this basis because we are ignorant about the normal mechanisms of control, and therefore cannot be certain when a cell has escaped from them.

Although the excessive growth of cells is often manifested by the production of a tumour mass, this is not invariable. Sometimes the migration of cells outside the normal confining limits outweighs the bulk of the abnormal proliferation. In this case no 'tumour' as such exists—an excellent example is to be seen in the diffuse infiltrating carcinoma of the stomach (p. 548). *Neoplasm,* which literally means new formation or new growth, is a more suitable term. It implies that there is an abnormal type of growth which may be evident not only in the intact animal but also when the cells are grown in culture.

TYPES OF TUMOUR

Classification according to the tissue of origin (histogenetic classification). Since tumours are formed as a result of the overgrowth of cells, it is logical to name them according to the tissue of origin. The basic subdivision of the body into epithelium and connective tissue is reflected in the recognition of two major groups of tumours: those derived from epithelial cells and those derived from connective tissue. Furthermore, within each group there are many subdivisions, just as there are many different types of epithelium and connective tissue.

Classification according to behaviour. An equally important classification is based upon the behaviour of the tumour cells. In some neoplasms the cells always appear to maintain contact with one another, and never wander off into the surrounding tissues nor invade lymphatics or blood vessels. These tumours remain localized, never spread, and are therefore called *innocent,* or *benign.* This contrasts with *malignant* tumours, in which the neoplastic cells invade the surrounding tissues and enter natural tissue spaces such as the lumina of lymphatics and blood vessels. Frequently groups of tumour cells break off, and the resulting tumour emboli become lodged at some distant site, grow, and thereby produce *secondary deposits,* or *metastases.* Between these two extremes of behaviour a third group of *intermediate tumours* is found.[1]

BENIGN OR INNOCENT TUMOURS

General considerations and effects

The cells which constitute this type of tumour show no tendency to invade the surrounding tissues. Instead, the excessive accumulation of cells produces an expanding mass which causes two local effects:

Pressure atrophy. Adjacent parenchyma undergoes pressure atrophy while the more resistant connective tissue survives to form a fibrous *capsule.* The tumour is therefore *well-circumscribed,* and is not intimately connected with the surrounding tissue except for those points of entry of the vascular supply. Benign tumours are fairly easy to excise surgically, and provided local removal is complete, they do not recur. A benign tumour within the skull or vertebral column, however, can produce serious effects by pressure.

Obstruction. A benign tumour may obstruct a natural passage and cause extensive damage. Obstruction of a bronchus leads to collapse of the lung and bronchopneumonia. A tumour of the intestine may produce intestinal obstruction.

Gross characteristics

Encapsulation. This is a characteristic feature when the tumour is situated in a solid organ or tissue (see above).

Shape. Benign tumours are usually rounded, but the shape may be moulded by the distribution of surrounding structures. A particular arrangement of fascia may make a tumour ovoid.

Size. Although benign tumours are usually smaller than their malignant counterparts, they may at times attain enormous proportions. The largest tumour in the museum of the Royal College of Surgeons of England is a fibroma of the kidney weighing 37 kg (82 lb)! A malignant tumour would have killed the patient long before reaching this size.

Ulceration and haemorrhage. These features are rare except in certain surface growths.

Rate of growth

The rate of growth of a benign tumour is generally slow. It is often erratic, and growth may cease after a period. Enormous tumours are therefore uncommon.

Hormonal effects

Benign tumours of endocrine tissue may produce excessive quantities of hormone which can have far-reaching and sometimes fatal effects. A tumour of the β cells of the islets of the pancreas may secrete so much insulin that the blood sugar level falls precipitously, and symptoms of hypoglycaemia occur. These are characterized by convulsions and mental disturbances, as the neurons require a constant supply of glucose. Tumours of the APUD cells are considered in Chapter 39 together with tumours of other endocrine glands.

Microscopic appearance

The arrangement of the cells of a benign tumour closely resembles that of the parent tissue. The tumours are therefore described as being *well differentiated.* The cells themselves tend to be regular in size, staining, and shape. Mitotic figures are scanty, and when present are of normal type. The tumour cells are supported and nourished by a network of host connective tissue which consists predominantly of blood vessels, fibroblasts, and a varying amount of collagen. It is called the *stroma,* and although an intimate part of the tumour, it is not itself involved in the neoplastic change.

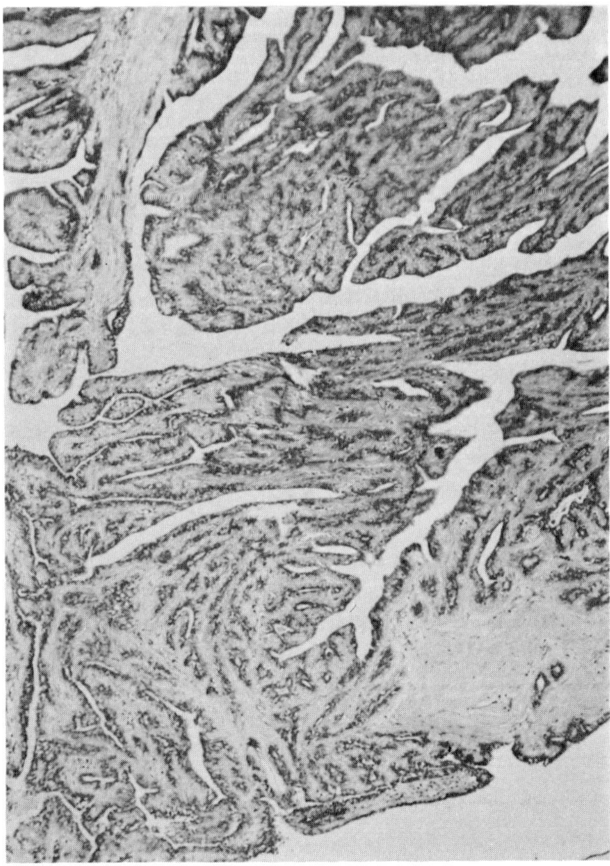

Fig. 22.1 Intraductal papilloma of breast. This is a portion of a complex columnar-cell papilloma in a breast duct. The central stromal core is prolonged into an extensive framework which is surmounted by neoplastic epithelium. × 40.

Benign epithelial tumours

These are of two main types. Benign neoplasia of a surface or lining epithelium produces a warty tumour, or *papilloma* (Fig. 22.1). In a compact gland (e.g. breast) the tumour is embedded in the tissue, and is called an *adenoma.*

Papillomata

Papillomata may occur on any epithelial surface. Some have a broad base and are described as *sessile,* while others become pedunculated and may be called *polyps,* a morphological term applied to any pedunculated mass attached to a surface and not necessarily neoplastic.

Papillomata are supplied by a core of connective tissue stroma containing blood vessels, lymphatics, and nerves. This is covered by a profuse neoplastic epithelium, composed of either stratified squamous, transitional, or columnar cells, according to that from which it has arisen. The cells show a regular arrangement, and the basement membrane is intact unless there is distortion due to inflammation. The epithelial cells are entirely restricted to the surface, and do not show invasion.

Stratified squamous-cell papilloma. Papillomata occur on the skin and other stratified squamous epithelial surfaces, e.g. the tongue and buccal mucosa. There is always *acanthosis,* i.e. a proliferation of the prickle-cell layer, and in the case of cutaneous papillomata there is often excessive keratin formation (*hyperkeratosis*) also. These lesions are described in greater detail in Chapter 40. Squamous-cell papilloma is a common tumour of the mouth, and is not infrequent in the larynx.

Transitional-cell 'papilloma'. This type of tumour occurs throughout the urinary passages, and has characteristic, delicate, finger-like processes, or fronds, which give it the appearance of a sea anemone. Bleeding is quite common and leads to haematuria. Multiple lesions are the rule, and recurrence is common after their removal. Hence these lesions are best regarded as malignant from a practical point of view regardless of their histological appearances.

Columnar-cell papilloma. This tumour occurs on any surface covered by columnar epithelium, for example in the colon. Papillomata are also to be found in cystic adenomata (see below).

Adenomata

Adenomata are composed of dense masses of acini lined by exuberant epithelium which may be columnar or cuboidal in shape. They occur in the salivary glands, pancreas, kidney, ovary, and the endocrine glands. They may also arise in the small glands which open on to epithelial surfaces; thus adenomata originate in sweat and sebaceous glands in the skin and the mucous glands of the mouth and respiratory tract.

Intestinal adenomata tend to become polypoid, and in the hereditary condition of *polyposis coli* thousands of tumours are present. Malignant change is almost inevitable, and the patient dies of cancer of the colon. In a related condition, *Gardner's syndrome,* colonic polyposis is found in association with sebaceous cysts, osteomata of the face and skull, and multiple fibromata. This too is inherited as a dominant trait and terminates in colonic cancer.

A rather similar condition is the *Peutz-Jeghers syndrome,* in which multiple polyposis of the stomach and intestine (small and large) is associated with a brownish pigmentation peppered around the lips and mouth and sometimes in the skin elsewhere (Fig. 22.2). The polyps are not prone to become malignant, unlike those of polyposis coli; indeed, they are probably hamartomatous rather than neoplastic.

Cystadenoma. Sometimes adenomata form elaborate spaces into which papillary ingrowths of neoplastic epithelium occur. These *papillary cystadenomata* are most common in the ovary, but may also be found in the salivary glands and kidneys.

Fibro-adenoma. The common tumour in the breast of young women is the fibro-adenoma. It consists of epithelial and connective tissue elements, both of which are considered to be neoplastic.

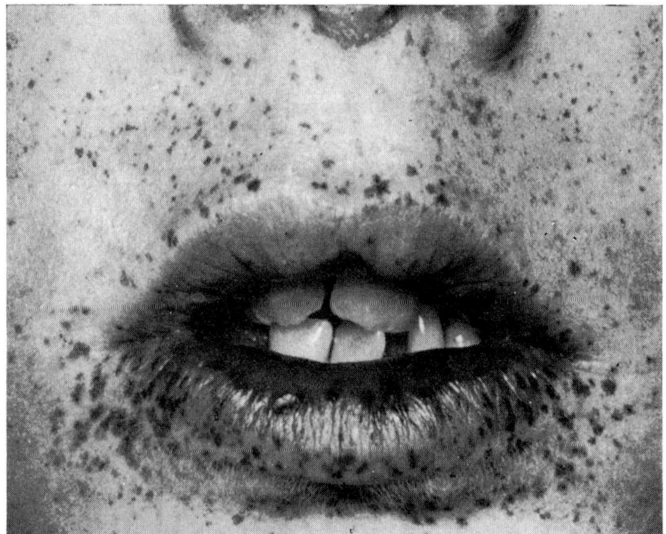

Fig. 22.2 Peutz-Jeghers syndrome. The multiple, circumoral, brown macules are well shown. The pigmentation is due to melanin. (*From Sheward J D 1962 British Medical Journal 1:921.*)

Benign connective tissue tumours

Benign tumours of connective tissue are usually composed of cells which closely resemble the parent tissue. They are supported by an excellent stroma from the adjacent connective tissues, and there is a characteristic tendency to merge with this stroma. The neoplastic cells are not nearly so well demarcated from the stroma as are those of epithelial tumours. The tumours are named according to the cell of origin, e.g. fibroma from fibroblast, osteoma from osteoblast, myoma from muscle, etc.

Fibroma. Fibromata are not very common tumours. They consist of circumscribed collections of fibroblasts between which there is a variable amount of collagen. Hard fibromata have much collagen, whereas the softer variety is predominantly cellular. They are found in many sites, e.g. stomach, ovary, gingiva, etc. Fibromata also occur in bones (p. 596).

There are a number of curious proliferative conditions of fibrous tissue, grouped as the *fibromatoses,* in which histological assessment of malignancy is difficult.[2] In *nodular fasciitis,* which affects the subcutaneous tissues and deep fascia, there is rapid growth of a highly vascular mass which diffusely infiltrates the surrounding tissues. Mitoses can be quite numerous, but although the histological picture may suggest malignancy, the lesion behaves in a benign manner. Nodular fasciitis is most frequently encountered in the arms, but can occur in any situation, e.g. the cheek or neck.

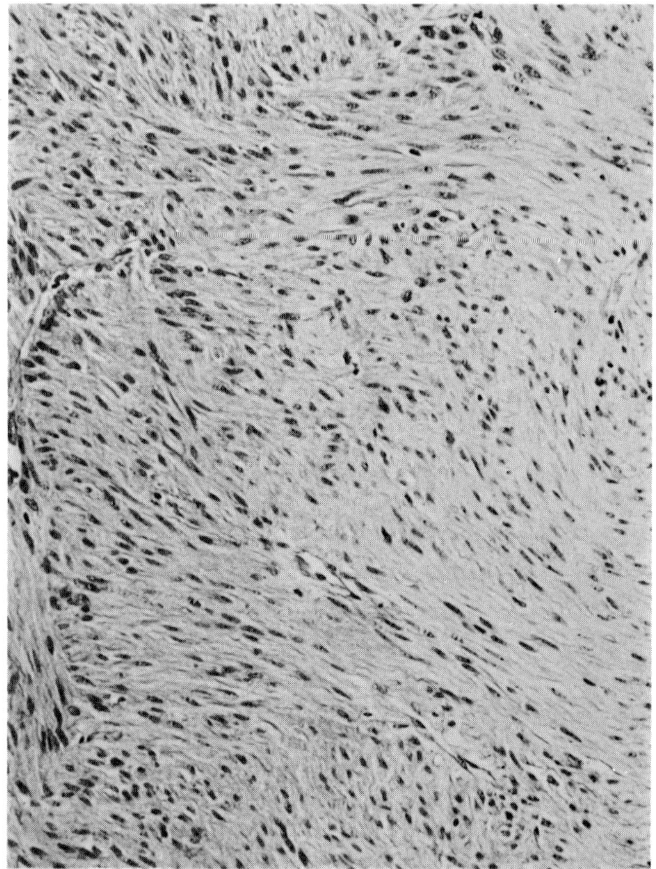

Fig. 22.3 Leiomyoma of stomach. The tumour consists of sheaves of elongated, spindle-shaped smooth-muscle cells arranged in interlacing whorls. × 100.

Myxoma. This is an uncommon tumour of connective tissue consisting of scattered stellate cells disposed in an expanse of connective-tissue mucin in which there is a network of reticulin fibres. Its histological and biochemical features resemble those of Wharton's jelly, which is found in the umbilical cord of the mature fetus.

The myxoma may be found in the jaw (where it is probably of odontogenic origin) and arising from the interatrial wall of the heart and from soft tissues, usually in association with striated muscle and neighbouring tissues. In appearance it is well circumscribed, oval or spherical, and of translucent grey colour. Its cut surface is glistening and slimy, and it may exude a mucoid material. It probably arises from a fibroblastic cell that has not differentiated enough to produce collagen but is capable of forming acid mucopolysaccharides. Alternatively it may be of primitive mesenchymal origin.

Myoma. Tumours of muscle are of two types: from smooth muscle (leiomyoma) and striated muscle (rhabdomyoma).

Leiomyoma. This is the commonest of all tumours, being found in the uteri of about 20 per cent of women over 30 years of age. Leiomyomata of the skin, stomach, and intestine are also not uncommon. Usually they are small and often multiple. A leiomyoma is composed of whorls of smooth muscle cells interspersed among which there is a variable amount of fibrous tissue (Fig. 22.3). In due course the muscle element may be replaced by fibrous tissue, and the *fibroleiomyoma* (or fibroid) is produced. Such a tumour may undergo cystic change, or else it may be the seat of dense calcification. On section the whorled interlacing pattern of glistening white fibres resembling watered-silk is characteristic.

Rhabdomyoma. Benign rhabdomyomata are exceedingly uncommon.

Neurofibroma.[3] The neurofibroma is now thought to arise from Schwann cells rather than fibroblasts. It causes a diffuse, fusiform enlargement of a nerve, and is composed of spindle cells arranged in flowing streams with a varying amount of intervening reticulin and collagen. Nerve fibres pass through the tumour, and myxomatous change is not infrequently present. The tumours may be solitary, and can occur on a spinal nerve root or a peripheral nerve. When multiple, they constitute a major feature of von Recklinghausen's disease. Whether all the nodules in this disease are true neoplasms is debatable—it may be more reasonable to regard them as hamartomatous in origin (see p. 387).

Schwannoma.[3] This tumour is usually solitary, and may arise from any cranial or peripheral nerve. It is encapsulated and appears to arise focally on a nerve trunk, so that the nerve itself is stretched over the tumour rather than running through it, as in the neurofibroma. A common site for schwannomata is the auditory nerve, and they may be bilateral. Microscopically, the tumour is very similar to a leiomyoma, the whorled arrangement of spindle cells being common to both. Often the spindle cells have a palisaded, or regimented, appearance with all the nuclei being aligned in one strip and the clear cytoplasm of the cells in an adjacent strip (Fig. 22.4).

Lipoma. This common tumour is composed of adult adipose tissue. It is usually subcutaneous, but may be retroperitoneal or subserosal. Oral lipomata are uncommon.

Chondroma and **osteoma** are considered in Chapter 37.

MALIGNANT TUMOURS

General considerations

The cells of a malignant tumour infiltrate and erode the surrounding tissue. Normal cells are enveloped and destroyed, and the tumour edge is therefore ill-defined. Complete excision by surgery is correspondingly difficult, and even if the tumour is removed with much surrounding normal tissue, malignant cells often

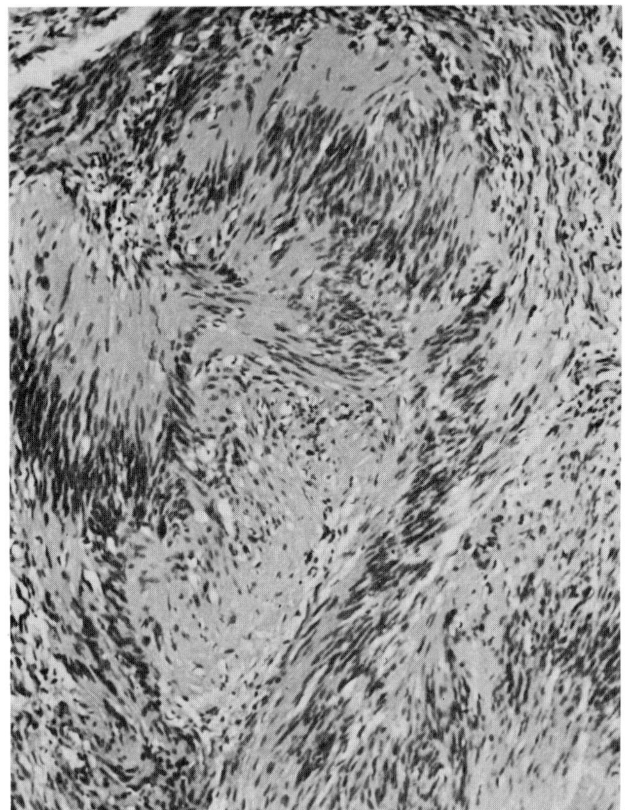

Fig. 22.4 Schwannoma. Note the palisaded, or regimented, appearance of the long, spindle-shaped cells; their nuclei form a continuous sinuous column, and on each side there is a similar column composed of clear cytoplasm. × 200.

remain behind, and their continued growth results in a *local recurrence.* In malignant tumours the invading cells spread in the planes of least resistance: finger-like processes extend outwards from the main tumour mass, and this growth produces a fanciful resemblance to the silhouette of a crab, hence the term *cancer,* which is derived from the Latin word meaning a crab. It is generally applied to all malignant tumours. *A carcinoma is a malignant tumour of epithelial cells, while a sarcoma is one derived from connective tissue.*

Embolic spread of tumour cells is responsible for the production of distant metastases. *Local invasion and embolic spread are the two characteristics of malignant tumours.* Both are probably related to the reduced cell adhesiveness which is a fundamental characteristic of cancer cells, and is evident not only *in vivo* but also in tissue culture—the cells growing out of the explant do not resist mechanical separation as well as do those of normal tissue. The power to invade and spread combined with the capacity for progressive growth make the term malignant particularly suitable for this type of tumour. Death is inevitable in untreated cases, except for those very rare, though well-documented, cases of *spontaneous regression,* in which proven cancers have disappeared of their own accord.[4, 5]

Gross characteristics

Lack of encapsulation. Malignant tumours have no limiting capsule, because the cells actively infiltrate the adjacent tissues. In certain rapidly growing tumours (e.g. metastases in the liver) cell division exceeds infiltration, and the tumour by its expansive growth may give a false impression of encapsulation. Microscopy, however, always reveals infiltration.

Shape. This is irregular in outline and diffuse in definition.

Size. Malignant tumours are usually larger than their benign counterparts.

Ulceration and haemorrhage. As would be expected from the destructive property of cancer, these are common features. *Any ulcer which fails to heal within a few weeks should always be regarded as malignant until proved otherwise.* In the mouth exfoliative cytology may be used to aid in the diagnosis of suspicious lesions[6] (p. 370).

Rate of growth

Malignant tumours usually undergo a rapid and steady increase in size. This can be of diagnostic importance; for example, if a shadow on a lung or bone radiograph is known to have remained stationary in size for many months, it is unlikely to be due to a malignant tumour.

Microscopic features

Microscopically several important features should be noted. The tumour tissue may resemble the parent tissue to a considerable extent, but the similarity is not as great as with benign tumours. Differentiation is not so well developed, and recognition of the tissue of origin is often difficult or even impossible; tumours which show little or no differentiation are called *undifferentiated.* At one time it was thought that normal differentiated cells could become neoplastic and revert to a more primitive state and appearance. This process of 'dedifferentiation' is nowadays discredited. Primitive cell-forms are ascribed to a basically primitive cell origin with a subsequent failure of normal differentiation. Neoplastic cells do differentiate, but frequently the differentiation is abnormal and does not conform to that found normally in the tissue. To describe a tumour as poorly differentiated is probably inaccurate, but it is a common practice and means that to the observer the neoplastic cells are making little attempt to resemble the structure of those found normally in the tissue.

Malignant tumours usually show much mitotic activity. The synthesis of DNA prior to division results in nuclear enlargement and hyperchromatism. This together with the formation of cells with abnormal numbers of chromosomes accounts for the irregularity in size and shape (*pleomorphism*) and staining which is so characteristic of malignant tumours. Mitoses are not only numerous, but sometimes also abnormal, and the number of chromosomes may diverge from the normal 46. Triradiate mitoses with the formation of three daughter cells are particularly characteristic of malignancy. No single, constant change in chromosome form or number is characteristic of malignancy. However, in a few tumour types an abnormality of a particular chromosome has been reported. The best-known example is the Philadelphia chromosome that is found in chronic myeloid leukaemia.

Anaplasia is a term which was introduced to describe new cells which deviated from the normal and resembled those of embryonic tissue. It is now generally restricted to those cellular changes which are found in malignant tumours. Thus a tumour which shows a high degree of anaplasia is poorly differentiated, and has frequent and bizarre mitoses and cells that are pleomorphic and have prominent nucleoli (see Fig. 22.9).

Effects of malignant tumours

Malignant tumours produce their ill-effects in a large number of ways:

Mechanical pressure and obstruction. Like benign tumours, malignant growths press on adjacent structures and cause obstruction to natural passages. A carcinoma of the colon soon leads to intestinal obstruction. Collapse of a lung and bronchopneumonia are often the features which first call attention to a carcinoma of the bronchus.

Destruction of tissue. In addition, malignant tumours, both primary and secondary, infiltrate and destroy tissue. This is well illustrated in bone where destruction may be so marked that pathological fractures occur, and replacement of the marrow results in anaemia.

Haemorrhage. Malignant tumours which involve any surface usually ulcerate and bleed. Repeated bleeding causes anaemia, and occasionally the erosion of a large artery leads to a massive fatal haemorrhage. This may happen when a carcinoma of the tongue involves the lingual artery. *Clinically unexplained bleeding from any site should be treated seriously, as it is a common symptom of cancer.* Haemoptysis is common in lung cancer, haematuria in urinary cancer, and vaginal bleeding, especially after intercourse, in cervical cancer.

Infection. All ulcerative cancers are bound to undergo secondary bacterial infection, and this aggravates the clinical condition. Infection also follows obstruction to the urinary or respiratory passages, e.g. bronchopneumonia occurs in lung cancer, and cystitis and pyelonephritis in cancer of the prostate. Cancer of the mouth interferes so much with swallowing that in due course there is inhalation of food and saliva into the respiratory passages. It is not surprising that suppurative bronchopneumonia is the commonest cause of death in this condition.

Starvation. In cancers of the mouth, oesophagus, and stomach there may be a direct nutritional effect due to the failure of food intake.

Pain. In advanced malignancy pain may be severe. It occasions anxiety and leads to insomnia.

Anaemia. Anaemia is common and may be due to chronic blood loss, malabsorption of essential dietary components, or bone-marrow replacement. Often, however, the cause is obscure.

Cachexia. The emaciated appearance of patients with advanced cancer is characteristic, but it is not uncommon for patients to remain obese. The cause of the loss of weight and the generalized body atrophy in cancer has given rise to much speculation. At one time a toxic product of necrotic tissue was postulated, but this has never been substantiated. The present tendency is to attribute cachexia to secondary factors, e.g. starvation, haemorrhage, infection, liver damage, etc.

In advanced malignancy there is usually *pyrexia,* a raised ESR, and a neutrophil leucocytosis, quite apart from any secondary infection. The pathogenesis is obscure.

Hormonal effects. Malignant tumours of the endocrine glands occasionally produce effects due to an excessive production of hormones. This is less common than with benign tumours.

Carcinomatous syndromes.[7,8] A variety of syndromes have been reported in association with neoplasms which are not explicable in terms of infiltration either by the primary tumour or its metastases. *Muscle weakness* and *skin eruptions* are two such examples. Sometimes a patient exhibits signs and symptoms referable to the *nervous system* (weakness, signs of intracranial tumour, etc.) and yet at necropsy no nervous involvement by tumour is found. *Venous thrombosis* sometimes leading to fatal pulmonary embolism, is an inexplicable complication of some neoplasms, especially carcinoma of the pancreas. Another curious phenomenon is the *hormonal effects* produced by tumours of non-endocrine origin.[8,9] Thus *hypoglycaemia* is seen in some mesotheliomata, and *Cushing's syndrome* may occur in cancer of the lung. The latter tumour may also be associated with *clubbing of the fingers,* and sometimes the joints are so swollen that rheumatoid arthritis is closely simulated. Hyponatraemia is another effect of oat-cell carcinoma.

Two other hormonal effects should be noted: polycythaemia in association with renal-cell carcinoma and hyperthyroidism in association with hydatidiform mole and choriocarcinoma.[10]

The mechanism of these curious syndromes is the production by the tumours of a hormone or hormone-like substance. Thus hyponatraemia is due to the production of antidiuretic hormone, and hyperthyroidism is caused by a specific thyrotrophic hormone secreted by molar tissue. The Cushing syndrome is probably caused by the secretion of ACTH, since adrenocortical hyperplasia is usually present. An increasing number of syndromes are being described, and it seems that almost any tumour can produce any hormone. Cancer of the lung seems to be particularly adept at this perverted behaviour; in addition to the syndromes already noted, hypercalcaemia has been described as the result of parathyroid-hormone-like secretion. Gynaecomastia can result from the production of gonadotrophin, and marked hyperpigmentation is seen when there is excessive secretion of melanocyte stimulating hormone. The latter syndrome has been particularly ascribed to carcinoma of the pancreas. The carcinoid syndrome and other features of tumours of the APUD system of cells are described on pages 554 and 627.

The ectopic secretion of various substances by tumours, once a clinical curiosity, is now becoming one of the most rewarding studies in cancer. Not all these secretions are hormones, and therefore do not necessarily produce a clinical effect. But their presence in the blood can be a useful marker, not so much in the diagnosis of cancer as in its follow-up after therapy. For instance, alpha-fetoprotein is secreted by some hepatomata and teratomata, whereas carcino-embryonic antigen (CEA) is secreted by a number of carcinomata, especially of the gastrointestinal tract. A rise in the level of these proteins may be the first herald of a recurrence many months before clinical relapse becomes apparent. This interval may afford an opportunity for the clinician to try cytotoxic or other therapy while the recurrence is still small.

Spread of malignant tumours[11]

Direct invasion and embolization are the two methods of spread and must be examined in detail.

Direct spread

The direct infiltration of the surrounding tissues means that the microscopic edge of the tumour extends beyond what is macroscopically apparent. Infiltration along tissue planes and septa is well shown in cancer of the breast, and in this way the tumour becomes *attached to the skin and deep fascia* (Fig. 22.12). Evidence of local invasion of a tumour is an important clinical sign, for it is tantamount to a diagnosis of malignancy.

Invasion of lymphatics. Carcinoma, but not sarcoma, shows a particular
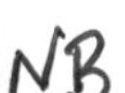
tendency to invade lymphatic vessels at an early stage, and the cells may grow as a long, ever-extending cord (Fig. 22.5). The process is called *lymphatic permeation,* and the lymphatic obstruction which it produces can cause lymphatic oedema.

Invasion of arteries and veins. This is a common event, and may lead to thrombosis and obstruction. It is frequent in lung cancer because so many large vessels are readily accessible to the tumour.

Spread by metastases

Groups of cells may become detached, travel in some natural passage to a distant site, become implanted, and finally grow to produce secondary deposits, or *metastases.* Spread *via* the lymphatics, blood vessels, and serous cavities are the most important examples.

Lymphatic spread. Detached groups of tumour cells in an invaded lymphatic are swept into the draining regional lymph nodes. If the cells survive and grow, the node soon becomes replaced by the tumour, and further spread occurs to the next group of nodes by way of the efferent channel. This is a familiar event in the course of carcinoma and melanoma, but is rare in sarcoma. A blockage of lymphatics results in a reversal of lymph flow in other vessels, and metastases may appear in unexpected lymph nodes. This is known as *retrograde embolism,* and the best-known example is the involvement of the left cervical nodes in gastric cancer. This is due to obstruction of the thoracic duct near its entry into the left subclavian vein, so that lymph is diverted up to the neck.

Blood spread. The occurrence of blood-borne metastases is the feature of malignant disease which is responsible for death in most cases. It is also the factor which limits the surgical and radiotherapeutic treatment of cancer.

At first sight the mode of production of secondary tumours is easy to understand. Malignant cells invade small venules, become detached, and are then carried by the blood stream to some distant site where they reach a capillary network. There the emboli become impacted, and the cells proliferate and develop into secondary tumours. A second method of blood-borne metastasis is by way of the lymphatics, for all the lymph eventually drains into the venous circulation.

As would be expected, one of the commonest sites of metastasis for most tumours is the lung. Likewise, primary tumours arising from an area drained by the portal vein regularly metastasize to the liver. Purely mechanical factors would

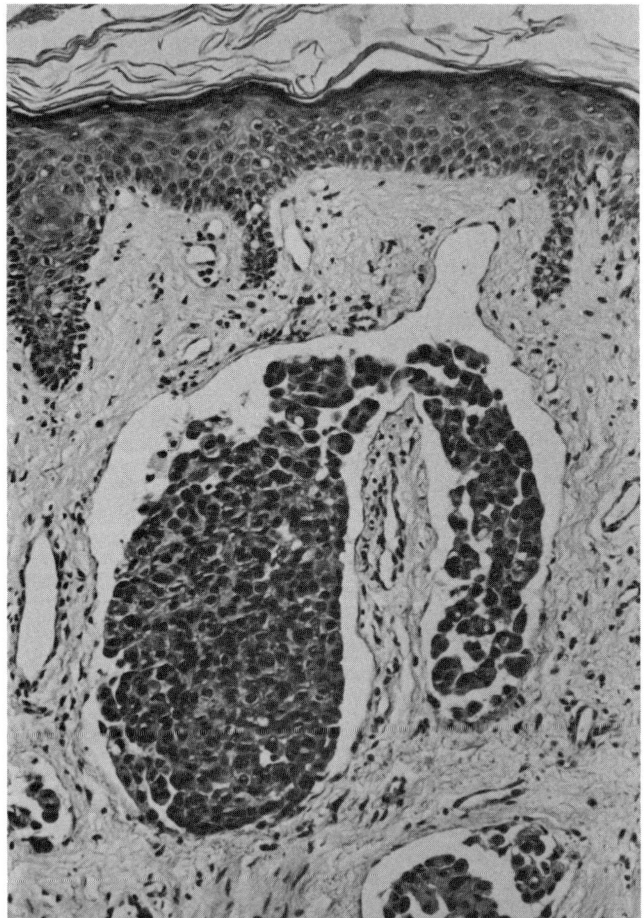

Fig. 22.5 Lymphatic permeation of cancer. This is a section of skin showing dilated lymphatic vessels filled with spheroidal carcinoma cells arranged in solid cords. There was an advanced carcinoma of the breast. × 200.

appear to account for this distribution, but closer examination makes such an explanation inadequate.

Many tumours, e.g. of the breast and kidney, give rise to metastases not only in the lungs, but also in the liver, bones, and other organs, and such systemic metastases sometimes occur in the absence of apparent lung deposits. It is possible that these are really present, but have been missed because of an inadequate *post-mortem* examination by the pathologist. Alternatively the cells may have been able to pass through the lung capillaries and become arrested elsewhere, or else there may be a direct venous communication between the primary and secondary sites, e.g. prostate and pelvic bones.

The distribution of secondary tumours might be expected to be related to the blood supply, but this is not the case. Cardiac and skeletal muscle have an abundant blood supply, and yet are rarely the site of metastases. The spleen likewise is not commonly involved. The liver, on the other hand, is frequently studded with secondary tumours regardless of the site of the primary.

There is considerable evidence that malignant cells often reach the blood stream but that most of them die. Only a selected few are able to take root to grow into secondary deposits. What factors govern this are poorly understood. The 'seed' may be widespread, but only where the 'soil' is suitable does growth occur. Some examples of this *selective metastasis* must now be examined.

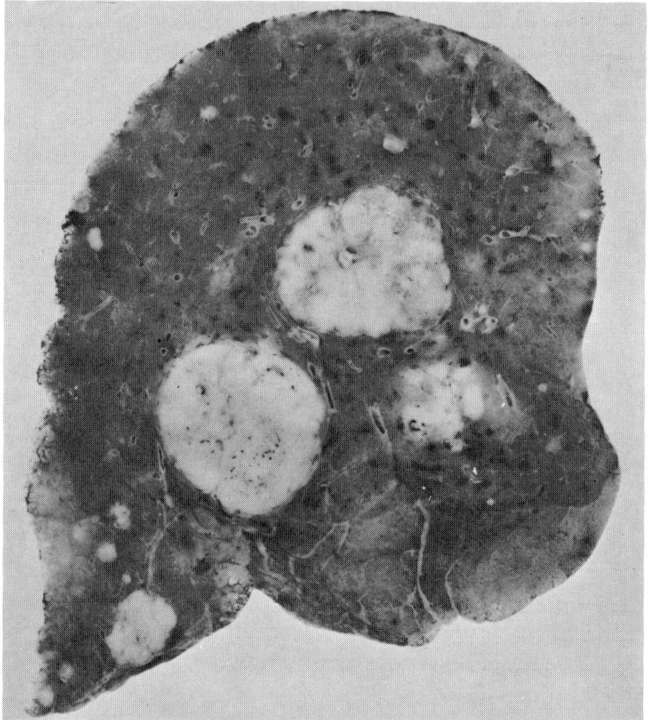

Fig. 22.6 Metastatic carcinoma of lung. Note the circumscribed white deposits. Primary lung cancer infiltrates the surrounding tissue much more obviously. The primary tumour in this case arose from the breast. (R47.3. *Reproduced by permission of the President and Council of the Royal College of Surgeons of England.*)

1. *Liver.* The commonest organ in which blood-borne metastases occur is the liver, for this organ appears to afford an excellent environment for the growth of tumour cells.

2. *Lung.* This is the next most common site for metastases (Fig. 22.6).

3. *Bone.* Carcinomata of the breast, lung, prostate, kidney, and thyroid quite frequently produce bony metastases.

4. *Brain.* Carcinoma of the lung is notorious for the frequency with which it metastasizes to the brain.

5. *Adrenal glands.* These are frequently the site of secondary deposits of cancer of the lung and breast.

Experimental work on mice suggests that selective metastasis is related to the nature of the tumour cells rather than to the soil. The transplantable B16 melanoma metastasizes to many organs, including the lungs. If a metastatic lung tumour is grown in tissue culture, harvested, and reinjected intravenously into a group of mice, an increased number of lung metastases is obtained. Repetition of the cycle—lung metastasis, tissue culture, reinjection into mouse, lung colonisation, etc—results in a strain of B16 melanoma that forms significantly more lung metastases than the original tumour. A strain of melanoma that metastasizes to the brain can be obtained by a similar procedure. Hence it appears that the original tumour is heterogeneous and contains subpopulations of cells, each differing in their potential to form metastases in a particular environment. This conclusion has been confirmed in another way. Clones of the original tumour can be obtained by tissue culture derived from single cells. When injected into groups of mice, each clone gives rise to widely different numbers of metastases in various organs, indicating that the original uncloned tumour contains subpopulations, each differing with regard to malignancy and metastatic potential. Thus the behaviour of a particular human tumour may in part be related to the time taken for a particular malignant clone to become the dominant tumour cell.[12]

Transcoelomic spread. When a malignant tumour invades the serosal layer of a viscus it causes a local acute inflammatory response. This results in the formation of a serous exudate into the cavity. Haemorrhage into the fluid is common, and therefore *the presence of a blood-stained effusion into a serous cavity should always raise the possibility of malignancy.* Tumour cells may break off and float *free* in the fluid, where they can be detected by the cytologist. They may alight on to other sites in the cavity and form the basis of secondary seedling growths. Such transcoelomic spread is seen in the pleural cavity with cancer of the lung, and in the peritoneum with cancer of the stomach and ovaries.

Staging of tumours

The extent to which an individual tumour has spread can be depicted by assigning it to a particular stage. The criteria used for staging cancers of various organs differ, but a typical example is as follows:

Stage 1. Tumour confined to the organ of origin.
Stage 2. The growth involves the local lymphatic nodes.
Stage 3. Tumour extends to distant lymphatic nodes.
Stage 4. Blood-borne metastases present.

The assessment of the stage is done on clinical grounds aided by histological examination of any available tissue (e.g. lymph nodes if the tumour has been excised), radiology, and other specialized techniques for the detection of tumour in the liver, brain, etc. The method is necessarily inaccurate, but nevertheless this is a useful calssification because it is related to the prognosis. Thus with carcinoma of the tongue stage 1 tumours have an average 5-year survival-rate of over 40 per cent, while tumours of stages 2 to 4 have a 5 per cent 5-year survival-rate.[13]

Dormant cancer. A difficulty about staging is the tendency for some metastases to appear many years after the primary tumour has been successfully removed. Such patients may remain well for 10 to 25 years, and then suddenly develop multiple secondary deposits, despite the absence of a local recurrence. It is assumed that the tumour cells were present in the body during the entire period, but for unknown reasons remained dormant. Factors that predispose to the phase of renewed growth after a period of dormancy are intercurrent illness, psychological trauma, and physical injuries. Carcinoma of the breast and kidney and melanoma of the eye are tumours notorious for this tendency towards dormant metastases.

Malignant epithelial tumours

These are called carcinomata, and are the commonest of all malignant tumours. This is probably because epithelium is a much more labile tissue than connective tissue (p. 000). Three types of carcinoma may be recognized:

1. *Squamous-cell carcinoma*
2. *Carcinoma of glandular epithelium*
3. *Transitional-cell carcinoma.*

Squamous-cell carcinoma

These tumours arise at any site normally covered by stratified squamous epithelium—skin, mouth, oesophagus, etc. They account for 90 per cent of all malignant oral tumours. At other sites they may occur as a result of tumour metaplasia, or possibly neoplasia in an area of squamous metaplasia, e.g. salivary gland, lung, and urinary tract.

Macroscopic types. Two are usually described:

The papillary (or exophytic) carcinoma appears as a warty outgrowth with an infiltrating base; this type may arise in a papilloma.

The nodular (or endophytic) type produces a hard, nodular mass beneath the surface, and shows more rapid infiltration and dissemination. Both types usually ulcerate to form a typical *carcinomatous ulcer.* This has a raised, craggy, rolled edge which is fixed to surrounding skin and deeper structures. The base is composed of white necrotic tissue, which is usually friable and bleeds easily.

Histological type. In considering the histological structure of a squamous-cell carcinoma it is necessary first to understand its formation (Fig. 22.7).

Formation. When epithelium shows malignant propensities, there is a progressive proliferation of the prickle-cell layer. This is sometimes so irregular that, even before the cells actually break through the basement membrane, they have the microscopic features of malignancy. To this condition the name *carcinoma-in-situ* is applied (p. 370).

The criterion of truly invasive carcinoma is the destruction of the basement membrane by masses of malignant cells, which then stream down into the deeper connective tissue and muscle. As they proceed they tend to break up into separate groups or columns. These clumps may comprise hundreds of cancer cells, or else only a few. In the most anaplastic tumours there may be no attempt at any splitting up, and the tumour mass proceeds in one diffuse sheet.

As the tumour infiltrates it destroys the tissue with which it comes in contact, and this is replaced by a fibrous stroma.

Nearly all malignant tumours excite an inflammatory reaction around them; lymphocytes are particularly numerous. It is generally accepted that they play a part in restricting invasion. Once ulceration of the surface occurs, there is a more acute type of response due to secondary bacterial infection.

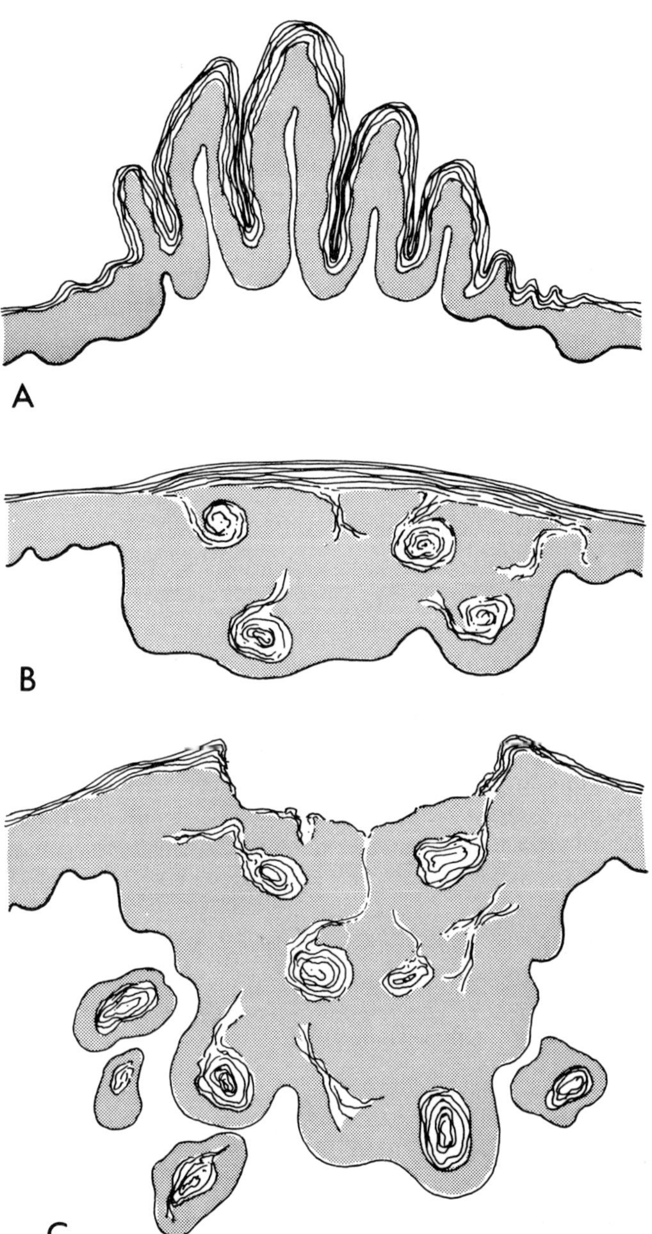

Fig. 22.7 Three types of neoplasia of a keratinizing squamous stratified epithelium, e.g. epidermis.
(A) Benign neoplasia results in an excessive production of regular epithelium, which is thrown into a complicated, folded structure in order to be accommodated. This formation is called a *papilloma.* The epidermal cells mature in an orderly way from the basal cells to the superficial squames.
(B) In *carcinoma-in-situ* there is excessive growth of epithelium, which thereby becomes thickened (acanthosis). Maturation of the cells is disorderly; foci of keratinization are found within the epidermis instead of being present only on the surface (dyskeratosis).
(C) In *carcinoma* the atypical epithelial cells break through the basement membrane and invade the underlying tissues. (*Drawings by Margot Mackay, Department of Art as Applied to Medicine, University of Toronto.*)

In those carcinomata which break up into discrete columns, each individual clump may then differentiate partly or completely to resemble the normal epithelium from which it has arisen.

Differentiation. Squamous-cell carcinomata vary considerably in the degree of differentiation which they show. When differentiation is good, *epithelial pearls* (also called *keratin,* or *horn, pearls*), or *cell nests,* are formed: these are groups of cells, which by differentiating produce a central whorl of keratin (Fig. 22.8).

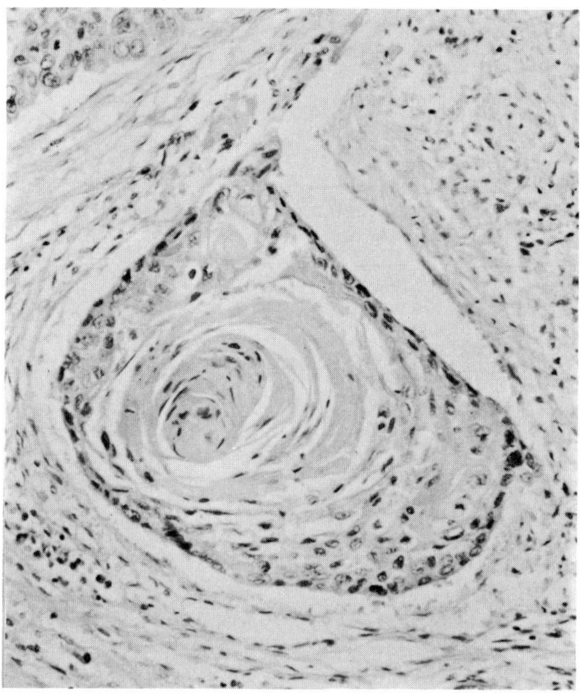

Fig. 22.8 A cell nest or epithelial pearl. This is a group of cells from a well-differentiated squamous-cell carcinoma. In the centre of the group the cells have differentiated so well that they resemble stratum corneum with keratin in the midst. × 380.

Surrounding this there are prickle cells, and sometimes a stratum granulosum is recognizable. A basal-cell layer is not well formed. In this way there is a fairly accurate reproduction of the upper layers of normal keratinizing stratified squamous epithelium. The cells are usually fairly uniform in size and shape, their nuclei are evenly staining, and mitoses are scanty. On the whole spread is slow. The skin is the commonest site, but sometimes well-differentiated cancers occur in the oral cavity and bronchus.

The more undifferentiated tumours contain no keratin, although groups of prickle cells may still be recognizable.

Highly undifferentiated, or anaplastic, tumours show no attempt at prickle-cell formation. There is a diffuse sheet of neoplastic cells supported by a scanty, vascular stroma. No attempt at forming groups of cells is recognizable. The cells themselves show great pleomorphism, and mitotic figures abound—some of these are bizarre. Tumour giant cells may be present (Fig. 22.9). It may be impossible

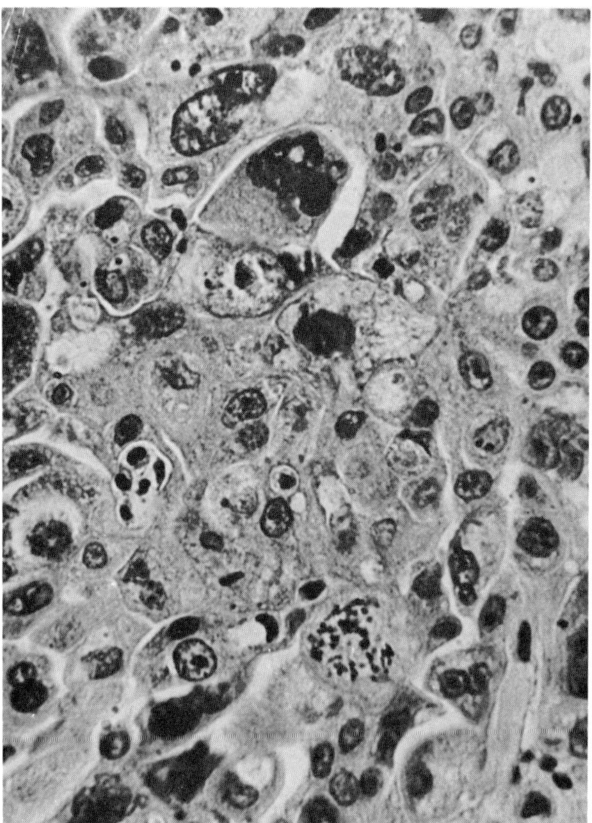

Fig. 22.9 An anaplastic tumour. This section shows the main features of malignant cells—pleomorphism, irregularity in size and staining capacity of the nuclei, giant forms, and an abnormal mitotic figure. ×570.

to distinguish the tumour from a sarcoma. This type of tumour is usually found in the mouth, bronchus, and cervix.

Variations of squamous-cell carcinoma

Transitional-cell papillary carcinoma. Some squamous-cell carcinomata of the pharynx and lung have a papillary structure, and are composed of a transitional type of epithelium similar to that of the urinary passages. It is better not to call this type of tumour transitional-celled, as it simply causes confusion.

Verrucous carcinoma. This papillomatous well-differentiated tumour occurs in the mouth, larynx, and genital region. It is noteworthy for having a very good prognosis. It is best regarded as a tumour of intermediate type since metastasis rarely occurs.

Spindle-cell, squamous-cell carcinoma. Occasionally the cells of a squamous-cell carcinoma are fusiform or spindle shaped. This is a very undifferentiated type of tumour, and generally arises in an area of radiodermatitis.

Grading. Histological grading as described by Broders is of some help in assessing prognosis. Four grades are recognized, according to the degree of differentiation.

Grade 1. More than 75 per cent cell-differentiation.
Grade 2. 50–75 per cent cell-differentiation.
Grade 3. 25–50 per cent cell-differentiation.
Grade 4. Less than 25 per cent cell-differentiation.

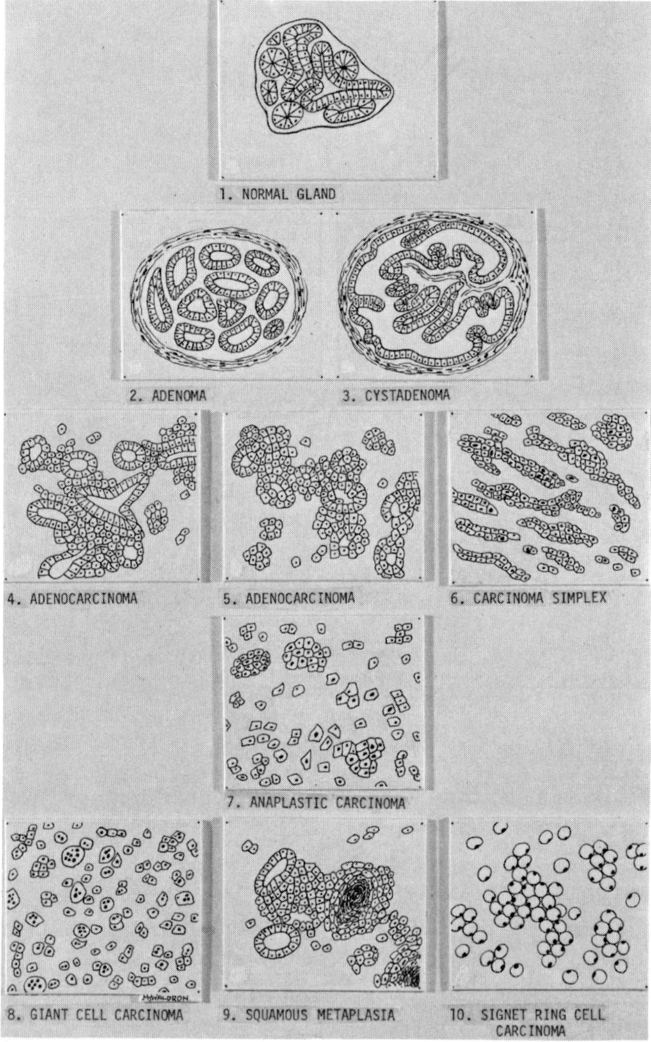

Fig. 22.10 Tumours derived from glandular epithelium. The normal gland (1) is contained within a sheath of connective tissue. Benign neoplasia results in the formation of an adenoma (2) with well-differentiated structure and encapsulation. Cystic dilatation of acini and complicated infolding of the epithelium produce a cystadenoma (3). The remainder of the tumours are malignant. The adenocarcinomata show some tubular differentiation which may be good (4) or poor (5). Lack of differentiation results in a carcinoma simplex (6). The most anaplastic tumours form a sheet of loosely attached cells (7). Giant-cell forms may predominate (8). These anaplastic tumours may be difficult to distinguish from sarcomata, melanomata, and tumours of squamous epithelial origin. Abnormal differentiation results in squamous metaplasia (9) or the formation of signet-ring cell carcinoma (10).

Grading on a numerical basis is seldom used because it is time-consuming, and in any case the assessment is subjective.

It is more helpful to define three grades—well-differentiated, poorly-differentiated, and undifferentiated. Although many exceptions are found, the higher the grade the worse is the prognosis, but the more radiosensitive is the tumour.

Some authorities are not convinced that grading is of any great help in the individual case. Certainly the site of the tumour is of great importance. A grade 1 squamous-cell carcinoma of the skin has an excellent prognosis, while in the lung the outlook is poor. Similarly, a grade 4 tumour of the cervix has a much better prognosis than a similar tumour of the lung or pharynx.

Carcinoma of glandular epithelium

These tumours arise from surface, secreting epithelia as well as from underlying glands. They may arise from columnar-cell papillomata and adenomata.

The pattern of invasion of neoplastic epithelium beneath the basement membrane into the deeper tissue is similar to that already described; in this case the groups of cancer cells, instead of producing keratin, tend to arrange themselves into acinar structures containing a central lumen into which secretion pours. The cells surrounding this lumen may be columnar, cuboidal, polygonal, or spheroidal (Fig. 22.10).

The well-differentiated cancers show excellent acinus formation, which mimics normal glandular structure. These tumours are called *adenocarcinomata* (Fig. 22.11).

In less well-differentiated tumours there are merely clumps of cells surrounded by a stroma, and no attempt at central cavitation to produce acini. To this type of cancer the names *carcinoma simplex,* spheroidal-cell, or polygonal-cell carcinoma are applied. It is seen most commonly in the breast, where the cancer clumps are often surrounded by a dense fibrous stroma. Often there is acinus formation elsewhere in the tumour.

The most undifferentiated tumours have diffuse, sheet-like arrangements typical of anaplasia. Distinction from squamous-cell cancers or even sarcomata or amelanotic melanomata is sometimes very difficult. Electron microscopy may be of assistance in resolving this difficulty (p. 355).

Mucoid cancer. The cells of a carcinoma derived from glandular epithelium may contain demonstrable mucus. Sometimes there is so large an accumulation of mucus in the cytoplasm that the nucleus is compressed on to the cell wall. This type of cell is called a *signet-ring cell.* If mucus secretion is marked, the tumour is called a mucoid cancer. Often the stroma contains large lakes of mucus in which there are disintegrating malignant cells. It is a mistake to regard these tumours as degenerate, for they are often highly malignant despite their acellular appearance.

Transitional-cell carcinoma

These tumours occur in the renal pelvis, ureter, and bladder. They are often papillomatous in appearance, but differ from papillomata in having a broader base and showing invasion.

Stromal reaction in carcinoma

The reaction of the invaded tissue to carcinoma cells varies; its growth may be so

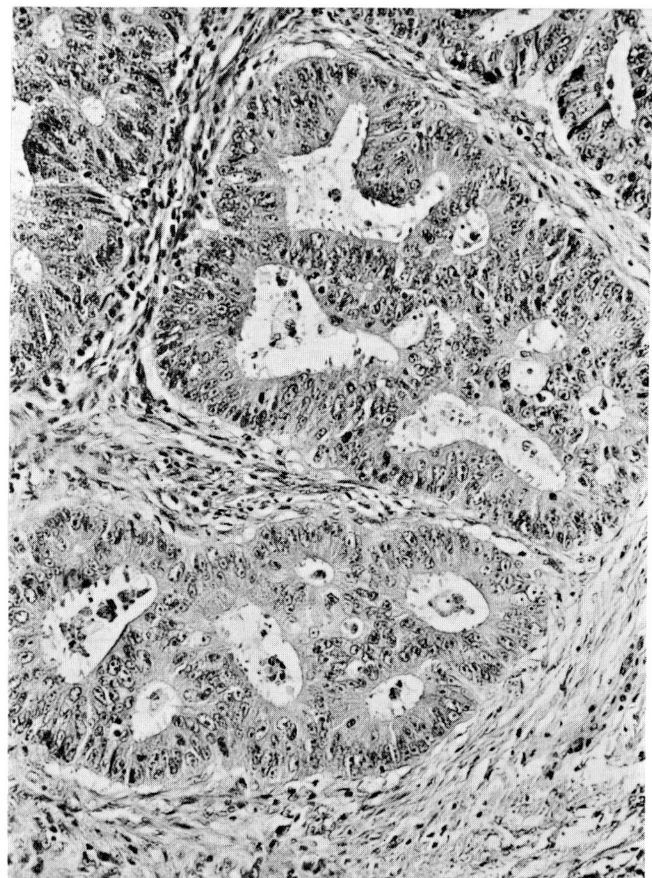

Fig. 22.11 Columnar-cell adenocarcinoma. This is a well-differentiated adenocarcinoma of the stomach. It consists of large, well-formed acini containing secretion, and is lined by exuberant columnar cells. It is infiltrating the muscle diffusely. × 80.

stimulated that a hard, fibrotic (*scirrhous*) type of tumour is produced. Most breast cancers are of this type (Fig. 22.12). The dense fibrosis appears to be associated with a contracting tendency, which is ill understood. In the breast there is an accompanying retraction of the nipple and dimpling of the skin. Eventually a stony fixation to the chest wall ensues.

Scirrhous tumours are also commonly found in the stomach and colon. The contraction causes a 'purse-string' deformity, and obstruction of the lumen follows.

When a tumour has little stroma in relation to cell bulk it is soft or brain-like, and is described as *medullary,* or *encephaloid.* Some cancers of the stomach and colon are of this type, and ulceration and bleeding occur rather than early intestinal obstruction.

Malignant tumours of connective tissue

These are called *sarcomata.* They are much less common than carcinomata, and

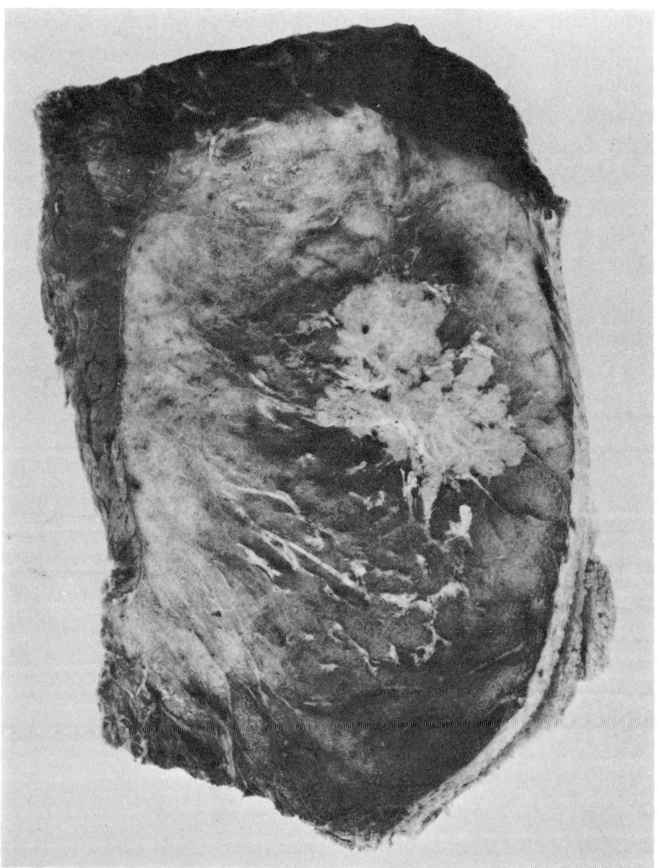

Fig. 22.12 Carcinoma of breast. This is a typical scirrhous carcinoma. Its outline is irregular and badly defined, for it extends sinuously into the surrounding fibro-fatty tissue. (EB10.1. *Reproduced by permission of the President and Council of the Royal College of Surgeons of England.*)

unlike them, they occur at all ages. While carcinomata tend to be arranged in discrete cellular clumps surrounded by a variable amount of stroma, sarcomata are always disposed in diffuse sheets, in which the neoplastic cells merge inseparably into the stroma.

On the whole sarcomata spread more rapidly than carcinomata, and the prognosis is correspondingly more grave. Early blood-borne metastases are the rule, and the lungs are often riddled with secondary deposits. Lymphatic involvement is very much less common than with carcinoma.

Fibrosarcoma. Fibrosarcomata are not encapsulated, and the cells show the cytological features of malignancy—pleomorphism and mitotic activity. Nevertheless, a well-differentiated fibrosarcoma shows considerable cellular regularity and collagen formation, and in practice the distinction from fibroma can be very difficult. Poorly-differentiated tumours show little or no collagen formation, and are then called *spindle-cell sarcomata*. They may be indistinguishable from other anaplastic sarcomata (e.g. leiomyosarcoma, neurofibrosarcoma, liposarcoma, etc.) or even anaplastic carcinomata.

Haemorrhage and necrosis are common features of most sarcomata, because the stroma is delicate and the vascular supply inadequate to meet the demands of the tumour.

Osteosarcoma. This is a common form of sarcoma, and is described in connexion with the section on bone (p. 597).

Liposarcoma. This is one of the commoner types of sarcoma. It arises usually from the deeper connective-tissue planes of the limbs, especially the thighs, and has considerable invasive potentialities. It metastasizes rather late. Histologically it consists of malignant lipoblasts which may assume giant proportions. A conspicuous tendency is the production of myxomatous tissue, which may overshadow the lipomatous element of the tumour.

Malignant tumours of blood vessels. *Angiosarcoma* is a rare tumour which usually arises in the soft tissues including those of the oral cavity, and consists microscopically of poorly-formed vascular channels lined by atypical endothelial cells. *Kaposi's sarcoma* is quite common in certain areas, particularly Eastern Europe and Eastern and Southern Africa. It commences as red or purple areas of discoloration of the lower legs, appearing to arise multicentrically and affecting both legs and later the arms. In time the lesions become more nodular, and may later ulcerate. After some years new lesions develop elsewhere; it may affect the oral cavity and internal organs. Microscopically the early macular and papular lesions closely resemble granulation tissue, but later the lesions become more solid, as atypical spindle cells proliferate and produce a more obviously sarcomatous picture. The presence of clefts containing blood between spindle cells is particularly striking.

Tumours of the stem cell and its derivatives[14]

The neoplastic lesions of these cells are the *lymphomata* and the tumours of the *haematopoietic tissues.*

Lymphomata. These are all malignant, and since they vary considerably in their clinical course, many attempts have been made to classify them so that behaviour might be related to histological type. There is no agreed classification and the nomenclature is confusing. Hence it is often impossible to compare the results of treatment in one centre with those of another. The lymphomata are the most common form of malignant tumour after the carcinomata. They arise from the cellular elements of the lymph nodes and bone marrow, and unlike other types of sarcoma, they spread rapidly to other lymph-nodes, eventually becoming systematized. The spleen, liver, and bone marrow are extensively infiltrated, and deposits are also present in the lungs and other organs. Another difference from other types of sarcoma is their extreme radiosensitivity; dramatic remissions follow radiotherapy. Sometimes a localized lesion may be cured, but unfortunately recurrence and systematization are the rule.

In the classification most widely used at present, Hodgkin's disease, clinically the most important lymphoma, is separated from the others because of its distinctive histological features. The remaining 'non-Hodgkin's lymphomata' are classified according to the predominant cell type involved, whether lymphocytic or histiocytic, and according to whether the neoplastic cells are disposed in distinct nodules or in a diffuse manner. A nodular disposition is associated with a better prognosis than is a diffuse one but, as will be pointed out later, there is increasing doubt about the true nature of the neoplastic histiocytes found in the lymphomata (including Hodgkin's disease). The great majority may well be transformed lymphocytes. The nodular lymphomata may become diffuse as the disease progresses, but the diffuse ones never become nodular. The lesions therefore always tend to become more malignant.

The following lymphomata are described:[14]

Histiocytic lymphoma—nodular or diffuse.

Lymphocytic lymphoma—nodular or diffuse. Each may be poorly, moderately, or well differentiated.

Lymphoma, mixed cell type—nodular or diffuse.

Hodgkin's disease. The subdivisions are described later.

Histiocytic lymphoma. This tumour, also called reticulosarcoma or reticulum-cell sarcoma, is a disease of later life that generally commences in one particular group of lymph nodes. Sometimes the tonsil or small bowel is the site of the primary lesion. The disease soon spreads to involve the spleen, liver, bone marrow, lungs, and other sites. Histologically the normal architecture of the affected lymph nodes is obliterated by the invasion of large, pale, histiocytic cells. Many mitoses, areas of necrosis, and capsular invasion are conspicuous features. In some tumours the cells are very pleomorphic; in others the cells appear primitive and resemble stem cells. This tumour is called a *stem-cell sarcoma.*

Lymphocytic lymphoma. This tumour is commonly called a *lymphosarcoma,* a term which is deprecated by many experts in the field but which may retain its place by virtue of common usage. The neoplastic cells can vary in differentiation and resemble mature lymphocytes (*lymphocytic lymphosarcoma*) or immature lymphoblasts (*lymphoblastic lymphosarcoma*). An intermediate group can also be recognized. Lymphocytic lymphoma is about twice as common as histiocytic lymphoma and affects a similar age group. Clinically the two are indistinguishable. Histologically the architecture of the lymph node is destroyed by sheets or nodules of uniform neoplastic lymphocytes. Indeed, destruction of the normal structures is an important diagnostic feature in helping to decide whether a particular lymph node is affected by a lymphoma or merely a reactive inflammatory process. With one exception lymphomata are uncommon tumours of the oral cavity. The exception is the *Burkitt tumour* (Fig. 22.13), a lymphoma occurring extensively in low-lying, moist regions of Central and West Africa.[15] It is peculiar in being almost exclusively confined to children between the ages of 2 and 14 years, and affecting the jaws (especially the maxilla), ovaries, retroperitoneal lymph nodes, and kidneys. The usual mode of presentation is as an enormous facial swelling with loosening of the neighbouring teeth.

Lymphoma, mixed-cell type. The lymph-node architecture is destroyed by neoplastic lymphoblasts and histiocytes. It differs from Hodgkin's disease in that there are no Sternberg-Reed cells.

Hodgkin's disease. This is the commonest lymphoma, and attacks young and middle-aged adults predominantly. The affected lymph nodes are replaced by a characteristically pleomorphic mass of cells, the most important of which are neoplastic histiocytes. These vary in size and shape, and include in their number giant cells with double, mirror-image nuclei and prominent nucleoli (*Sternberg-*

Reed giant cells, Fig. 22.14). The other cells present comprise lymphocytes, plasma cells, neutrophils, and often many eosinophils. There is a tendency to fibrosis, and sometimes to necrosis. Hodgkin's disease usually manifests with a localized enlargement of lymph nodes, but sometimes constitutional symptoms such as intermittent fever (Pel-Ebstein fever), wasting, and itching of the skin predominate. This is liable to occur especially when the abdominal nodes are primarily involved.

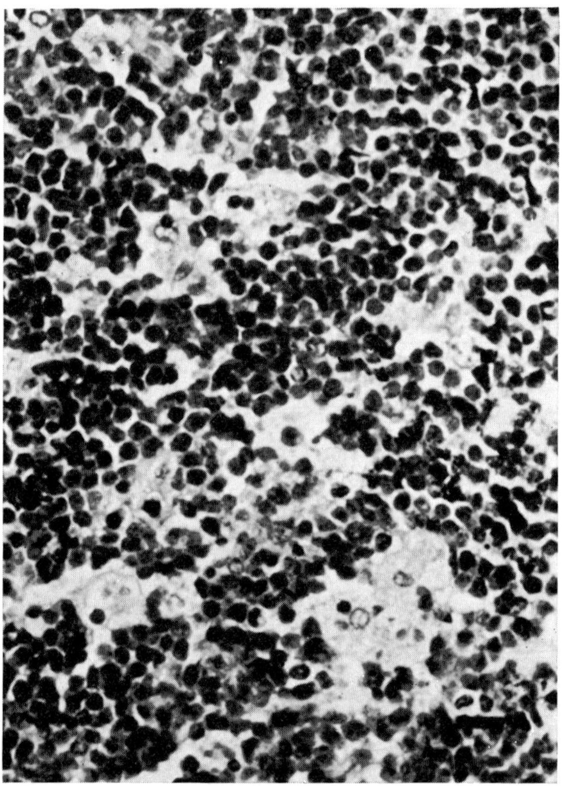

Fig. 22.13 Burkitt's tumour. Note the uniform lymphocytes, interspersed among which are large histiocytes. This is the 'starry-sky appearance' stressed in Burkitt's tumour, though seen in other lymphocytic lymphomata also. × 400.

The prognosis of Hodgkin's disease has been related to histological appearances: four types are recognized.[16,17] In the *lymphocytic predominant type,* Sternberg-Reed cells are scanty and lymphocytes are plentiful. The disease is much less malignant than the pleomorphic type described above, now described as the *mixed cellularity type.* It remains localized for a long time, and is amenable to local treatment such as radiotherapy. A nodular variant (*nodular sclerosing Hodgkin's disease*) also has a relatively good prognosis. The end stage of Hodgkin's disease, and therefore one that has the worst prognosis, is the *lymphocytic depletion type,* which is characterized by a paucity of lymphocytes with either diffuse fibrosis or else a proliferation of atypical Sternberg-Reed cells.

The prognosis of Hodgkin's disease is also related to the extent of the disease and a system of staging has been evolved. It ranges from stage I, where there is involvement of the lymph nodes of one region, to stage IV, in which there is widespread disease.

Other generalized lymphomata. Although the majority of conditions in which there is a malignant proliferation of the stem cell and its derivatives can be placed in one of the categories already described, there are a number of rare

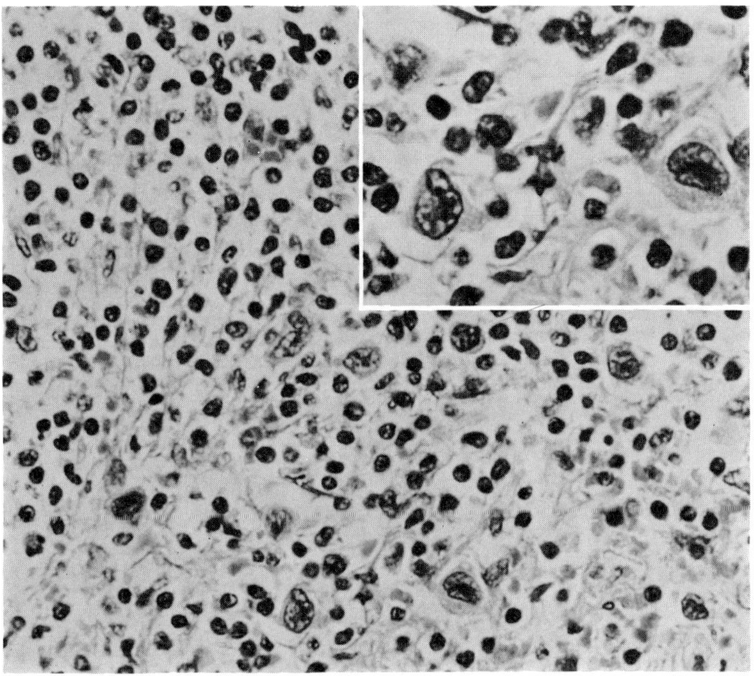

Fig. 22.14 Hodgkin's disease. This is the mixed cellularity type. In addition to the neoplastic macrophages there are several typical Sternberg-Reed giant cells. There is also an infiltration of lymphocytes, plasma cells, and a few granulocytes. ×250.
At the top right-hand corner there is an insert of a field showing two Sternberg-Reed cells. ×320.

diseases which appear to be separate entities. For these the concept of *malignant reticulosis* can be retained. Waldenström's macroglobulinaemia may be cited as an example, for there is a widespread proliferation of cells which are 'plasmacytoid'—cells which are neither lymphocytes nor plasma cells.

A new classification of the lymphomata.[18,19] Lukes and his colleagues have recently suggested that the majority of lymphomata are derived from transformed lymphocytes. Using B-cell and T-cell markers, they have concluded that many lymphomata are derived from transformed B lymphocytes. The two major exceptions are Hodgkin's disease and mycosis fungoides,* and in these diseases the neoplastic 'histiocytes' are actually transformed T lymphocytes. The

* Mycosis fungoides is a primary lymphoma of the skin that pursues a prolonged course before it finally involves internal organs. It is a distressing condition; for many years the patient has to endure the presence of many skin lesions that ultimately evolve into fungating tumours. Persistent itching is a major feature.

Sternberg-Reed cell is a polyploid transformed T lymphocyte rather than a histiocyte.

This new classification must await confirmation before it is generally adopted. It has the merit of combining functional studies with the purely cytological description of the established classifications of the lymphomata.

Malignant conditions of the haematopoietic tissues. The most important are the *leukaemias,* in which the malignant cells are found circulating in the peripheral blood, and *multiple myeloma,* in which the marrow is replaced by a plasma-cell tumour. These conditions are discussed in Chapters 30 and 37 respectively.

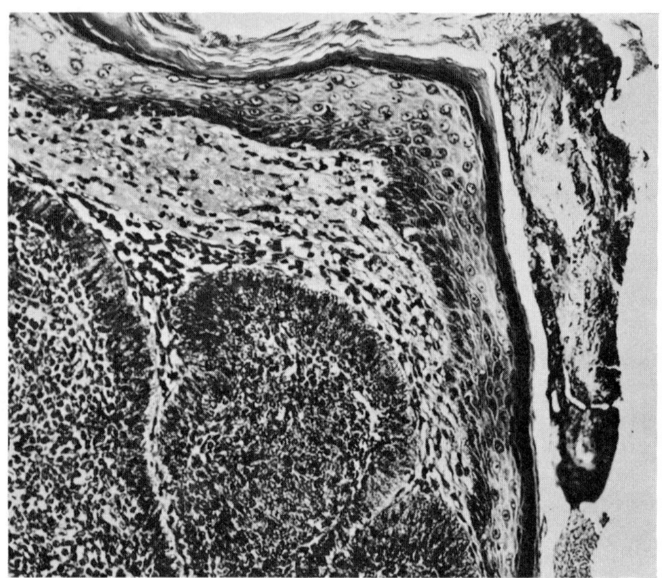

Fig. 22.15 Basal-cell carcinoma. Beneath the epidermis there is a solid mass of basal-cell carcinoma. The cells adjacent to the dermal stroma are arranged at right angles to it in the form of a palisade. × 200.

INTERMEDIATE TUMOURS

In their behaviour this group of tumours lies between the benign and the malignant groups. Local invasion occurs, therefore the tumours cannot be regarded as benign. Nevertheless they do not show the steady inexorable growth pattern of true malignant tumours. The victims do not inevitably die of the disease if left untreated.

Several types of tumour may be considered under this somewhat controversial group of intermediate tumours, a term coined by Morehead.

Locally malignant tumours

The *rodent ulcer, or basal-cell carcinoma,* is a typical example of this group. Local invasion is prominent, but metastasis is so rare that it can for practical purposes be ignored.

The tumour is found most frequently on the skin of the face, and appears as an indurated ulcer with a hard, rolled, pearly border. Microscopically the dermis is infiltrated by groups of small round or fusiform cells with prominent darkly-staining nuclei. The layer of cells at the edge of each clump is usually arranged in the form of a palisade, and resembles the germinative layer of the normal epidermis (Fig. 22.15). Indeed, this tumour probably arises from these basal epidermal cells. It differs from squamous-cell carcinoma in that if the cells tend to show differentiation, it is into adnexal structures—hair follicles, sweat glands, or sebaceous glands—but not into cells of the surface epithelium.

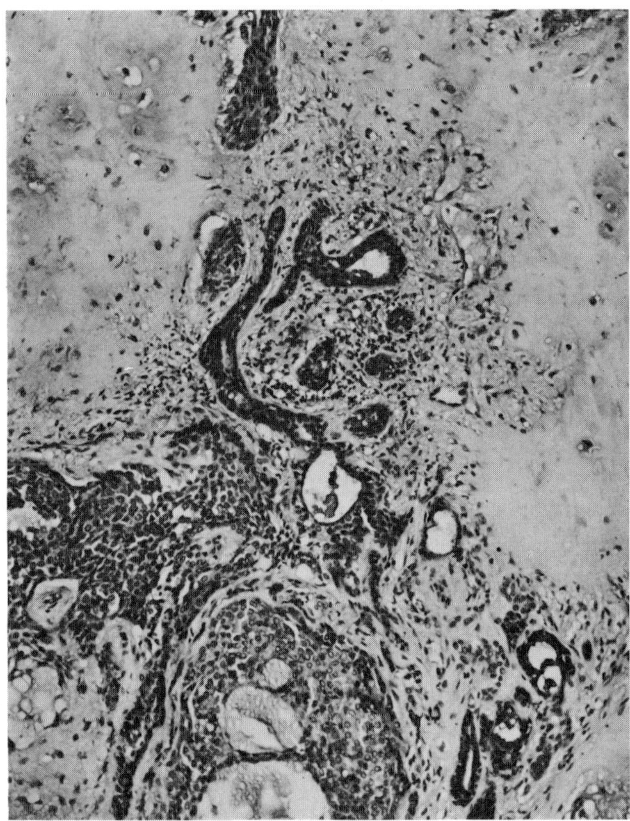

Fig. 22.16 Pleomorphic salivary gland tumour ('adenoma'). There are columns of epithelial cells, some arranged in ductules, surrounded by a dense, rather acellular stroma which resembles hyaline cartilage. ×110.

The basal-cell carcinoma shows progressive local invasion and destruction of tissue. Growth is usually very slow, and it is common to find small tumours in patients who have had the lesion for several years. On rare occasions basal-cell carcinoma exhibits a relentless course of local invasion, and it may destroy the nose and eye; finally it can penetrate the scalp and lead to fatal meningitis.

The ameloblastoma is also a locally malignant tumour (p. 387).

Tumours of erratic behaviour

Other tumours are known in which local invasion occurs, and occasionally distant metastases are produced. Usually, however, the distant metastases are small and do not shorten life. These tumours are of erratic behaviour, and a good example is the *pleomorphic salivary gland tumour.*

Pleomorphic salivary gland tumour. These tumours are found most commonly in the parotid gland, but may arise from other salivary glands and also

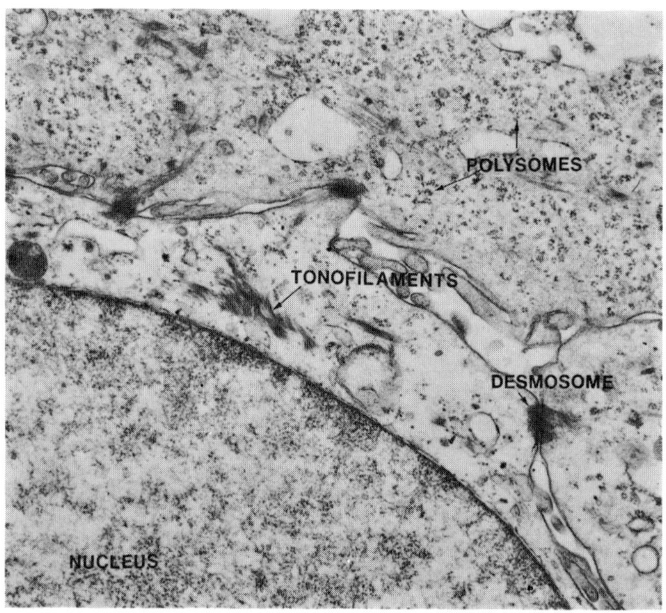

Fig. 22.17 Squamous-cell carcinoma of nose. A 50-year-old man developed a polypoid lesion of the nose. This was excised, and the specimen reported as consisting of inflammatory tissue. However, the lesion recurred, and a biopsy revealed a vascular lesion with many spindle cells consistent with a diagnosis of spindle-cell sarcoma. Electron microscopy showed typical features of an epithelial tumour. The figure shows several tight junctions with desmosome formation. In the cytoplasm tonofilaments are present as well as numerous free ribosomes, which are grouped as polysomes. The tumour was therefore regarded as a spindle-cell squamous-cell carcinoma. × 27 500. (*Photograph by courtesy of Dr Y C Bedard.*)

the mucous glands of the oral mucosa, trachea, and bronchi. They consist of acini, cords, and thin strands of epithelial cells suspended in a stroma which often has a myxomatous appearance (Fig. 22.16). This was at one time regarded as true cartilage, and the tumour was called a 'mixed parotid tumour'. It is now realized that the mucoid appearance is due to a sero-mucinous secretion from the tumour cells into the stroma. True cartilage is very rarely found, and when it is present it is due to chondral metaplasia of the stroma.

The tumour may appear well encapsulated, but the capsule is often infiltrated by lateral extensions of growth. Simple enucleation is likely to be followed by recurrence. Furthermore, obvious local invasion may sometimes occur. Occasionally distant blood-borne metastases are encountered, even in tumours which appear 'benign' microscopically.

Mucoepidermoid carcinoma. This tumour commonly arises in the parotid gland. It consists of cells that show both mucus formation and areas of squamous differentiation. An abundance of mucous cells is found in tumours of low-grade malignancy; these grow slowly and rarely metastasize. Extensive squamous differentiation and anaplasia are found in tumours of high-grade malignancy; in these widespread metastasis is likely to occur. As with the pleomorphic salivary gland tumours, clinical behaviour cannot reliably be predicted from the microscopic appearances.

Adenoid cystic carcinoma. This tumour also occurs in the parotid gland, but more frequently arises in the other major salivary glands or from the mucosal

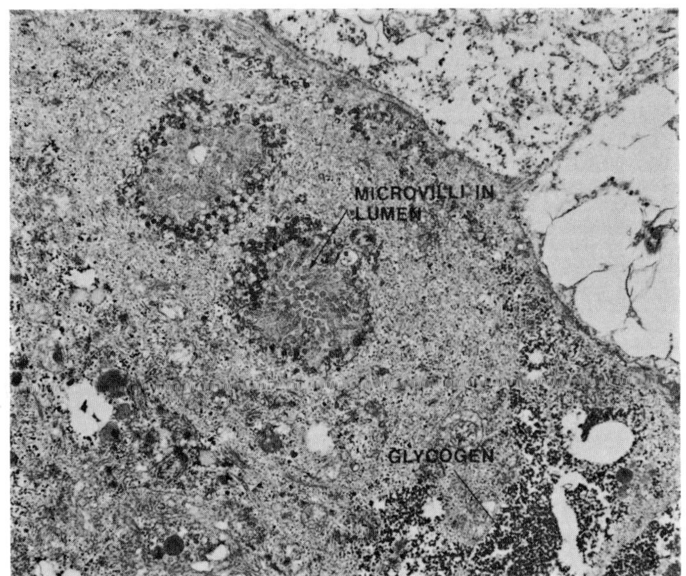

Fig. 22.18 Carcinoma of the breast. A 65-year-old woman developed enlarged axillary lymph nodes, and biopsy revealed an anaplastic tumour. Lymphoma was considered to be the most likely diagnosis, but electron microscopy revealed intracellular lumina with microvilli. This is a feature of poorly-differentiated glandular carcinoma. A blind biopsy of the ipsilateral breast of this patient showed infiltrating lobular carcinoma. Note the presence of numerous glycogen granules. × 14 000. (*Photograph by courtesy of Dr Y C Bedard.*)

glands of the nose, mouth, pharynx, or respiratory tract. The tumour consists of columns or clumps of cells which often contain a central cavity containing PAS-positive material. A cribriform pattern is common. The tumour is locally invasive and tends to recur unless widely excised. In some locations this is technically difficult, e.g. in the trachea. Hence in this situation the prognosis is poor. Lymph-node metastases and blood-borne spread ultimately occur in some cases.

There are a number of other tumours which show a similar erratic behaviour (e.g. carcinoid tumours of the intestine, see p. 554), but they are uncommon and will not be described here. It will, however, be appreciated that as regards behaviour there exist tumours which range from those which may be called completely benign, which never invade and never metastasize, to those which are called malignant and which always invade and always metastasize.

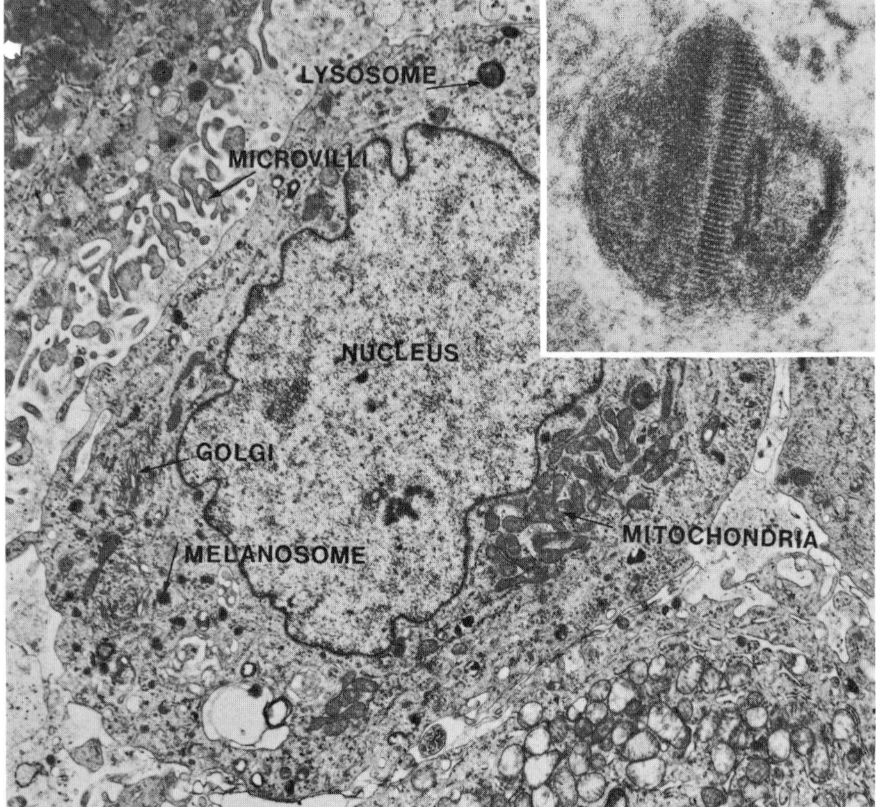

Fig. 22.19 Malignant melanoma. A 16-year-old boy developed enlargement of the inguinal lymph nodes, and biopsy revealed an anaplastic tumour consistent with anaplastic carcinoma, lymphoma, or malignant melanoma. No melanin could be demonstrated by silver staining. Electron microscopy revealed cytoplasmic structures (mel), which on high magnification (inset) show the characteristic banding of melanosomes that is visible before the extensive deposition of melanin obscures this detail. On reviewing the patient's history it was found that a 'mole' had been removed from the leg two years previously. This had been reported as a benign naevus, but in fact was a malignant melanoma. × 11 000. Insert × 143 000. (*Photograph by courtesy of Dr Y C Bedard.*)

Difficulties in tumour classification

The difficulties encountered in the classification of neoplasms are those which are inherent in the classification of any condition of unknown aetiology. No single classification is wholly satisfactory. By examining tumours from different aspects various subdivisions are possible. While some classifications are more useful than others, none is more correct than the other. Histogenetic and behavioural characteristics form the basis of our present classification, but nevertheless certain difficulties are encountered. Those connected with behaviour have been considered. Difficulties encountered with histogenesis may be considered under five headings:

Endothelium and mesothelium. The flattened lining cells of the serous spaces, like the pleural cavity, and the endothelial cells of blood vessels are sometimes regarded as epithelial, but in fact the tumours which are derived from them usually behave as connective-tissue tumours, and are commonly classified as such.

Undifferentiated tumours. A second difficulty in the histogenetic classification is the occurrence of tumours so poorly differentiated that their cell of origin defies recognition. Such anaplastic tumours are given names which are descriptive of the appearance of the cells. Large-cell, small-cell, pleomorphic-cell, giant-cell, spindle-cell, and oat-cell, are all self-explanatory terms when applied to tumours.

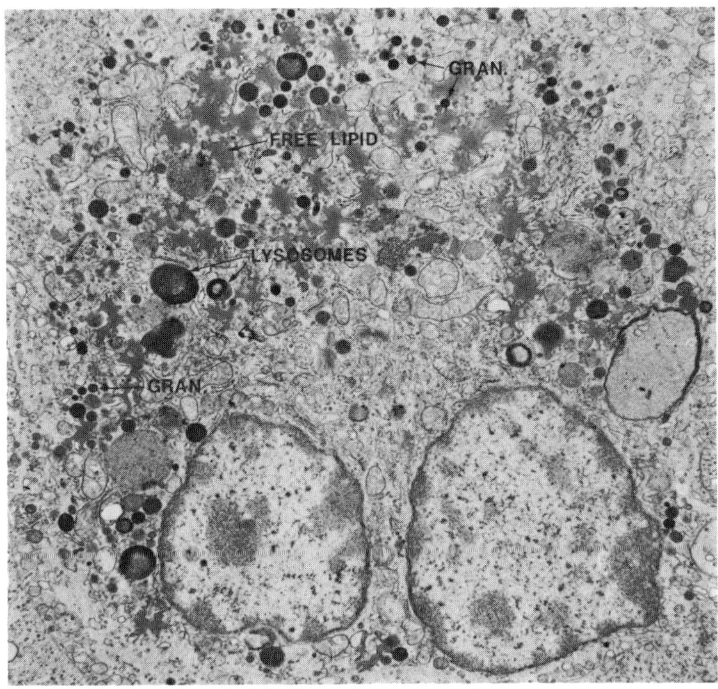

Fig. 22.20. Oat-cell carcinoma of the lung. A 45-year-old woman developed features of Cushing's syndrome, and a scalene lymph-node biopsy revealed an anaplastic tumour consistent with the diagnosis of oat-cell carcinoma of the lung. The electron micrograph of the tumour shows typical neurosecretory granules. Note also the presence of free lipid and lysosomes, some of which contain myelin figures. × 14 000. (*Photograph by courtesy of Dr Y C Bedard.*)

Electron microscopy is sometimes of help in determining the origin of a tumour: the presence of desmosomes and the formation of basement membrane adjacent to cells indicates an epithelial origin (Fig. 22.17). The formation of intracellular lumina suggests a glandular origin (Fig. 22.18). The presence of melanosomes indicates that an anaplastic tumour is a malignant melanoma (Fig. 22.19). On the other hand, the presence of neurosecretory granules points to an origin from cells of the APUD series (Fig. 22.20).

Tumour metaplasia. A further difficulty arises when tumour cells differentiate in a direction other than that of the parent tissue; thus sometimes a tumour of glandular epithelium shows differentiation towards a keratinizing squamous-cell type. Such a tumour would be called a squamous-cell carcinoma, although it is of glandular origin (see carcinoma of lung, p. 542).

Melanoma. A fourth difficulty is the histogenetic classification of tumours arising from cells whose precise origin is disputed. The best example of this is the *melanoma* of the skin (p. 382).

Placental and embryonic tumours. Finally certain tumours arise from cells which are not normally present in the adult body. Three groups can be recognized:

1. *Tumours of placental origin,* e.g. choriocarcinoma
2. *Tumours of germ-cell origin,* e.g. teratomata
3. *Tumours of embryonic origin.* These tumours arise from cells which, although present in the developing embryo, should normally have disappeared by the time of birth. They are considered in Chapter 24.

An outline of the present classification of tumours is shown in Table 22.1. It is evident that it is far from satisfactory, but since we have little useful basic knowledge regarding the nature of neoplasia this is hardly surprising. There is not even a satisfactory definition of a neoplasm, although that given by Willis is useful:[20] '*A tumour is an abnormal mass of tissue, the growth of which exceeds and is uncoordinated with that of the normal tissue, and persists in the same excessive manner after cessation of the stimuli which evoked the change.*'

It seems certain that the continued growth of tumours is quite useless, and the neoplastic response to a stimulus has no survival value in the evolutionary process. When it is remembered that most tumours occur during the post-reproductive years this is not altogether surprising.

Table 22.1 Classification of tumours

Tissue of origin	Behaviour		
	Benign	Intermediate	Malignant
Epithelium			
1. *Covering and protective epithelium*			
(*a*) Squamous	Squamous-cell papilloma		Squamous-cell carcinoma
(*b*) Transitional	Transitional-cell papilloma		Transitional-cell carcinoma
(*c*) Columnar	Columnar-cell papilloma		Adenocarcinoma
2. *Compact secreting epithelium*	Adenoma. If cystic, cystadenoma or papillary cystadenoma		Adenocarcinoma. If cystic, cystadenocarcinoma
3. *Other epithelial tumours include*		Basal-cell carcinoma Salivary and mucous gland tumours Carcinoid tumours (argentaffinoma)	
Connective tissue			
Fibrous tissue	Fibroma		Fibrosarcoma
Nerve sheath	Neurofibroma		Neurofibrosarcoma
Fat	Lipoma		Liposarcoma
Smooth muscle	Leiomyoma		Leiomyosarcoma
Striated muscle	Rhabdomyoma		Rhabdomyosarcoma
Synovium	Synovioma		Malignant synovioma
Cartilage	Chondroma		Chondrosarcoma
Bone			
Osteoblast	Osteoma	Giant-cell tumour	Osteosarcoma
Mesothelium	Benign mesothelioma		Malignant mesothelioma

Tissue of origin	Behavoiur		
	Benign	Intermediate	Malignant
Blood vessels and lymphatics	? Benign haemangioma and lymphangioma		Angiosarcoma
Meninges	Meningioma		Malignant meningioma
Specialised connective tissue			
Neuroglia and ependyma	Astrocytoma; oligodendroglioma; ependymoma*		
Chromaffin tissue	Carotid body tumour		Malignant carotid body tumour
Lymphoid and haematopoietic tissue	Benign lymphoma e.g. of rectum and skin		Lymphocytic lymphoma Histiocytic lymphoma Hodgkin's disease Multiple myeloma Leukaemias
		Myeloproliferative disorders†	
Melanocytes			Malignant melanoma
Fetal trophoblast	Hydatidiform mole		Choriocarcinoma
Germ cell			
(*Totipotential cell*)	Benign teratoma		Malignant teratoma Seminoma
Embryonic tissue			
(*Pluripotential cell*)			
Kidney			Nephroblastoma
Liver			Hepatoblastoma
(*Unipotential cell*)			
Retina			Retinoblastoma
Hind-brain			Medulloblastoma
Sympathetic ganglia and adrenal medulla	Ganglioneuroma		Neuroblastoma
Pelvic organs			Rhabdomyosarcoma (sarcoma botryoides)
Embryonic vestiges			
Notochord			Chordoma
Enamel organ		Ameloblastoma	
Parapituitary residues		Craniopharyngioma	
Branchial cyst			Branchiogenic carcinoma
Hamartoma			
Melanotic	? Benign melanoma		Malignant melanoma
Angiomatous	? Benign angioma		Angiosarcoma
'Exostoses' and 'ecchondroses'			Chondrosarcoma
Neurofibromatosis	Neurofibroma		Neurofibrosarcoma
Tuberous sclerosis	Glioma		Malignant glioma.

NOTE. Any malignant tumour may be so undifferentiated that it must be classified on a histological basis, e.g. carcinoma simplex, spindle-cell sarcoma, etc.

* These tumours are difficult to classify. The common types are locally malignant, but some also metastasize within the central nervous system. Rarely, and most often in children, they appear to be benign.

† These include polycythaemia vera, haemorrhagic thrombocythaemia, and myelosclerosis (see p. 463).

GENERAL READING

Ackerman L V, Rosai J 1974 Surgical Pathology, 5th edn. Mosby, Saint Louis
US Armed Forces Institute of Pathology: Atlas of Tumor Pathology. Many fascicles have been published, and each covers the tumours of a particular organ or system. Series 1 and 2, Washington, DC, 1949–1976.

REFERENCES

1. Morehead R P 1965 In: Human Pathology, McGraw-Hill, New York, p 181
2. Mackenzie D H 1972 The fibromatoses: a clinicopathological concept. British Medical Journal 4:277
3. Fisher E R, Vuzevski V D 1968 Cytogenesis of schwannoma (neurilemoma), neurofibroma, dermatofibroma, and dermatofibrosarcoma as revealed by electron microscopy. American Journal of Clinical Pathology 49:141
4. Boyd W 1966 The Spontaneous Regression of Cancer, Thomas, Springfield, Illinois
5. Everson T C, Cole W H 1966 Spontaneous Regression of Cancer, Saunders, Philadelphia
6. Cahn L R 1965 Oral exfoliative cytology. British Journal of Oral Surgery 2:166
7. Azzopardi J G 1966 Systemic effects of neoplasia. In: Harrison C V (ed) Recent Advances in Pathology, 8th edn. Churchill, London, p. 98–184
8. Leading Article 1976 Ectopic secretion by tumours. British Medical Journal 1:1300
9. Ellison M L, Neville A M 1973 Neoplasia and ectopic hormone production. In: Raven R W (ed) Modern Trends in Oncology, 1: Part I, Butterworth, London p 163
10. Leading Article 1976 Hyperthyroidism of hydatidiform mole. British Medical Journal 1:179
11. Willis R A 1973 The Spread of Tumours in the Human Body, 3rd edn. Butterworth, London, 417 pp
12. Nicholson, G L 1979 Cancer metastasis. Scientific American Vol 240, No 3, 50
13. Lucas R B 1976 Pathology of Tumours of the Oral Tissues, 3rd edn. Churchill Livingstone, Edinburgh, p 145
14. Anderson W A D (ed) 1977 Pathology, 7th edn. Mosby, St Louis, 2:1526 et seq.
15. Berard C et al. 1969 Histopathological definition of Burkitt's tumour. Bulletin of the World Health Organisation 40:601
16. Lukes R J, Butler J J 1966 The pathology and nomenclature of Hodgkin's disease. Cancer Research 26:1063
17. Lukes R J, Butler J J, Hicks E B 1966 Natural history of Hodgkin's disease as related to its pathologic picture. Cancer (Philadelphia) 19:317
18. Lukes R J, Collins R D 1975 New approaches to the classification of the lymphomata. British Journal of Cancer 31, supplement No 11, 1
19. Leading Article 1975 Classification of lymphomata. British Medical Journal 3:4
20. Willis R A 1967 Pathology of Tumours, 4th edn. Butterworth, London, p 1

23

The aetiology and incidence of tumours

Introduction

In spite of a vast amount of research into the cause of cancer, the essential difference between the neoplastic and the normal cell is unknown. Insofar as the human being is concerned, much is known about the incidence of particular tumours. Careful observations have established that some types of malignancy are particularly common in groups who are subjected to abnormal *occupational* or *environmental* factors. This has led to the recognition of various chemical and physical agents which are responsible, and which are called *carcinogenic agents.* A large number of these is now known.

On a more intimate level hereditary factors have been studied by observing certain families which are known to bear the trait of neoplastic diseases.

The experimental side of cancer research concerns the artificial production of tumours in animals. As in the human, *chemical, physical,* and *hereditary factors* have been investigated, and in addition it is possible to study tumours by transplanting them from one animal to another. This work has led to the recognition that cell-free extracts can on occasion induce tumour formation, and that *viruses* appear to be responsible.

Although there are many known causes of cancer in animals, most human tumours arise spontaneously in response to an unknown stimulus. In a few instances human neoplasms can be attributed to some tangible preceding cause.

THE ORIGIN OF TUMOURS

The mode of origin of a tumour is still not completely understood. An early theory introduced by Cohnheim in 1875 was that tumours arose from 'cell rests' sequestered during embryonic life, that underwent neoplastic change many years later. This theory may explain the development of the germ-cell tumours and the embryonic tumours of infancy, but there is no evidence that the common adult tumours arise from cell rests, the very existence of which has not been proved.

The current evidence suggests that most tumours arise from a **single clone of cells**, or perhaps only a few such clones, that have undergone malignant transformation. This evidence is derived from the following sources:

(1) In the monoclonal gammopathies, described in Chapter 29, of which multiple myeloma is the typical example, there is good evidence that a single clone

of B lymphocytes (which have developed into plasma cells in the case of multiple myeloma) have become malignant, and by metastatic spread as well as local proliferation have crowded out the many normal clones of immunoglobulin-forming B lymphocytes. These neoplastic cells produce only one type of immunoglobulin molecule, and so can be easily identified.

The same argument applies to those tumours of B lymphocyte origin which, although not producing a circulating immunoglobulin, nevertheless have a specific cell-surface immunoglobulin. Chronic lymphatic leukaemia is a good example.

(2) According to the Lyon hypothesis, one of the X chromosomes in each cell of a female becomes inactivated early in fetal life*. This random inactivation may affect either the maternal or paternal X chromosome, and the progeny of the cell inherits this change. The enzyme glucose-6-phosphate dehydrogenase (G6PD) is coded for by a gene on the X chromosome, and in Black populations two allelic forms, called A and B, are commonly found. Some 40 per cent of Black females are heterozygous, so that extracts of blood, skin, and other tissues contain a mixture of enzyme types A and B. It is apparent that if only one type of enzyme, whether A or B, is found in an extract of a tumour from a person whose normal tissues contains both types, the inference is that the tumour arose from a single clone of cells.

On the basis of G6PD typing a clonal origin has been demonstrated for many tumours both benign and malignant.

This emphasis on a clonal derivation does not mean that many tumours develop from a transforming event affecting only a single cell. It is probable that successive waves of neoplastic clones emerge during the course of malignancy, but that one particular clone dominates and forms the overwhelming mass of tumour by the time the condition is clinically evident. In some tumours there is a strong suggestion of two separate clones of cells that have independently undergone malignant transformation. The evidence does, however, indicate that most tumours grow by the proliferation of one or a few 'committed' cells rather than by continuous recruitment of normal cells through the horizontal transmission of some oncogenic factor. At present the search continues for a usable X-linked polymorphism in White populations.

If it appears that most tumours arise from one or a few clones of cells, there is also compelling clinical evidence that many tumours tend to arise on a restricted area of tissue which is called a **field of growth**. The field of growth theory is based on the frequency of origin of multiple tumours on a restricted site and for apparently recurrent tumours to develop near the site of removal of a primary tumour. It is exceptional for a whole field of growth to become malignant; much more usually there are circumscribed foci of neoplasia on it, developing no doubt from individual clones of cells that have undergone transformation.

* This hypothesis was put forward by Mary Lyon, and it is called *lyonization of the X chromosome*. The inactivated chromosome replicates later than the other chromosomes during the mitotic cycle, and its descendants follow the same pattern. Since the two chromosomes may carry different sets of X-linked genes, there may be patchiness of a visible characteristic transmitted thus, e.g. coat colour in an animal. Women heterozygous for glucose 6-phosphate dehydrogenase deficiency, an X-linked dominant characteristic, possess two races of red cells, one normal and the other enzyme deficient, and it is the latter that undergo haemolysis.

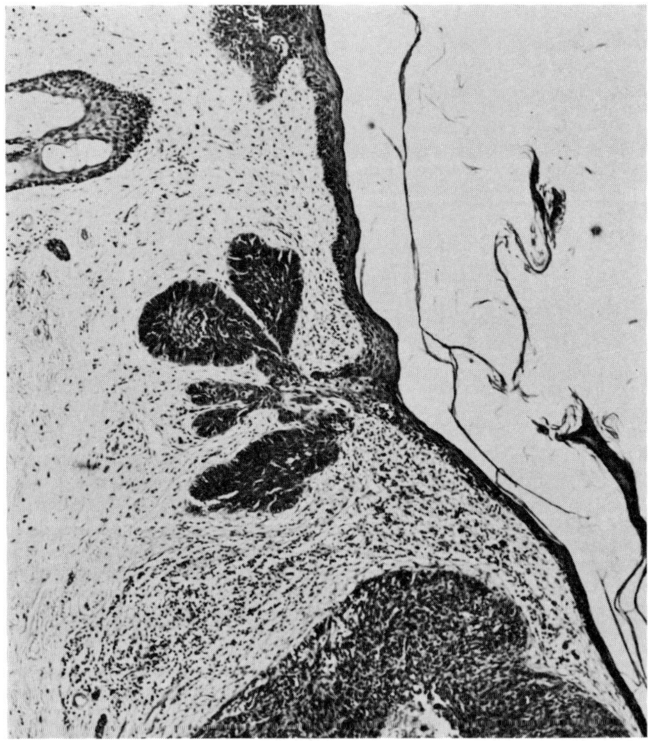

Fig. 23.1 Multifocal origin of basal-cell carcinoma. The mode of origin of the tumour as a downgrowth from the basal-cell layer is apparent, and its resemblance to an embryonic hair follicle is quite marked. The surrounding epidermis is normal, but at the edge of the section there is part of a much larger basal-cell carcinoma. × 100.

Clinical support for the field of growth concept comes from two observations:

(1) The tendency for *multiple tumours* to arise in a restricted area of tissue (Fig. 23.1).

(2) The frequency of *recurrences* appearing near the area where a primary tumour had been completely removed.

Multiple Primary Tumours. There are many examples:

Multiple squamous-cell and basal-cell carcinomata of the face.

Multiple papillary carcinomata of the ureter and bladder.

Oral cancer. Multiple primary tumours appear in about 10 per cent of patients with oral cancer. Carcinoma of the mouth is also associated with primary squamous-cell carcinoma elsewhere, for instance in the larynx, oesophagus, or lung.

Polyposis coli (Fig. 23.2).

Cancer of the liver supervening on cirrhosis is often multicentric.

Leiomyomata of the uterus.

Recurrences of Tumour. The origin of a recurrent tumour following in the wake of an excised one is something difficult to decide. Malignant tumours infiltrate so insidiously that a group of cells may be left behind to form the origin of a new tumour mass. Nevertheless, there are many good examples of recurrent

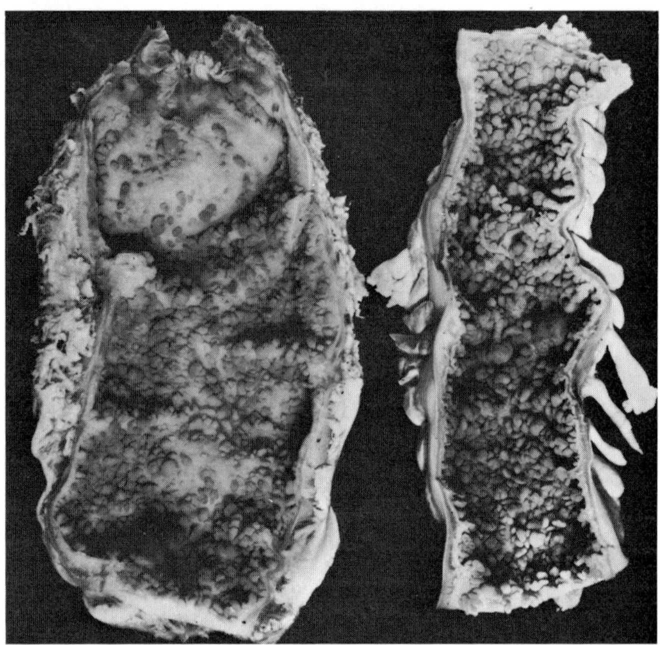

Fig. 23.2 Polyposis coli. The mucosa of the descending colon and rectum is studded with polyps, some of which are pedunculated and others sessile. The bowel wall and the intervening mucosa are normal. None of the polyps shows macroscopic evidence of malignancy. (A74.4. *Reproduced by permission of the President and Council of the Royal College of Surgeons of England.*)

tumour occurring in an adjacent area of the field of growth. Such recurrences may be seen following the removal of carcinoma of the tongue in dysplastic leukoplakia. Thus the field of growth concept of tumour formation has important surgical consequences. Only complete excision of the entire field can ensure that no further tumours will develop.

Factors known to produce cancer. The three factors generally recognized as causes of human neoplasia are:

External carcinogenic agents—chemical and physical agents.

Hereditary predisposition.

Chronic disease, usually of an inflammatory nature.

Two additional factors have to be considered, *hormones* and *viruses.*

External carcinogenic agents[1,2]

Chemical carcinogens

It has been known since the eighteenth century that those people whose occupation brings them into contact with coal tar or mineral oil are liable to develop carcinoma of the skin. The chemicals concerned are *aromatic polycyclic hydrocarbons*, and credit is due to the Japanese workers Yamagiwa and Ichikawa, who were the first to produce skin cancers in rabbits by painting their ears with tar. The next step was the isolation of the actual chemical substances in tar which were responsible for carcinogenesis. The first pure carcinogen to be discovered, by Kennaway, was the hydrocarbon *1:2:5:6-dibenzanthracene.* Subsequently *methylcholanthrene, 3:4-benzpyrene*, and many others have been isolated. The important agent in human cancer of this type is 3:4-benzpyrene.

A recently discovered occupational hazard is adenocarcinoma of the nasal sinuses occurring in *hardwood furniture makers.* This association has been noted in the High Wycombe area of Buckinghamshire. Apparently it is the inhaled dust that contains the carcinogenic factor, but its nature is still not known.[3]

The *aromatic amines* have been found to be carcinogenic. Their importance stems from the fact that workers in the aniline-dye industry are particularly liable to develop bladder cancer. The carcinogen concerned is *2-amino-1-naphthol*, a substance which is excreted in the urine, being formed in the body from aromatic amines, chief among them being β-naphthylamine, used in the dye, rubber, and cable industries. This is an example of *remote carcinogenesis*, since the agent, though taken by mouth, produces its effects in the urinary passages.

Another chemical agent that has recently proved to be carcinogenic is *vinyl chloride* (CH_2CH_2Cl).[4] This, as the monomer, is a gas at normal temperatures and pressures, but in its liquefied form under pressure readily polymerises into polyvinyl chloride, a white, solid plastic which is widely used. There is a greatly increased incidence of angiosarcoma of the liver in those working with vinyl chloride monomer.

Certain *natural foodstuffs* carry a carcinogenic hazard. The mould *Aspergillus flavus*, which contaminates ground-nut meal, produces a toxin, *aflatoxin*, which is a powerful liver carcinogen. This may well explain why this type of cancer is so prevalent in Africa.[5] The *nitrosamines* cause liver cancer in rats; these chemicals can be formed in the stomach from nitrites present in the diet, e.g. in processed meat. The nitrosamines, like many carcinogens, do not act directly on their target cells to produce cancer. They are metabolized by the cells, in this case the hepatocytes, and some metabolic product is the actual carcinogenic agent. Its nature has yet to be determined.

Genetic influence in chemical carcinogenesis. An important feature of experimental carcinogenesis is that animals react specifically. Many fruitless years were spent trying to induce coal-tar cancers in rats and dogs, animals which are almost completely resistant. Furthermore, dissimilar strains of animals respond differently. Thus the administration of a particular carcinogenic substance to different strains of animals will produce differing effects. In some there may be no tumour formation at all, while others may show tumours of various organs.

Physical carcinogenic agents

The important relationship between ionizing radiation and cancer is considered in detail in Chapter 25. Ultraviolet radiation exerts its harmful effect in the form of strong sunlight continually acting on the exposed skin of fair-complexioned people. Farmers in Australia and South Africa, sailors, and others habitually exposed to the elements, tend in later life to develop multiple lesions on their faces and hands (*actinic*, or *solar, keratoses*), and these sometimes develop into squamous-cell carcinomata. *Basal-cell carcinoma* is also more common in this group of people, as is *carcinoma of the lip.*

The latent period in carcinogenesis

An important factor notable in all occupational and environmental cancers is the long latent period which elapses from the time of application of the agent to the time of the first appearance of the tumour. This may vary from 5 to over 20 years, and it is evident that there is ample time for the initiating stimulus to be completely forgotten by the patient. The same latent period is also evident in experimental work on animals, although here it is measured in weeks or months rather then years.

The precancerous state: initiation and promotion

During the early years of experimental coal tar carcinogenesis it was noticed that the skin of an animal which had been painted with tar was particularly liable to develop tumours at the site of any wound subsequently inflicted on the painted area. The concept arose that carcinogenesis was a two-stage phenomenon. The application of a carcinogen to the skin produced a change which was called *initiation*, such that when any part of the area was subsequently wounded or damaged by a second agent, which was called a *promoter*, a tumour developed at the site of injury. In addition to trauma itself, non-specific irritants such as croton oil, chloroform, etc. were found to be efficient promoting agents.

Skin which had been initiated frequently showed no histological evidence of the change. Initiation could be demonstrated only by the subsequent development of tumours following the application of a promoting agent. Experimental evidence indicated that initiated skin could remain in this state of precancer for long periods. When this concept is applied to occupational cancer, the long latent period between leaving employment and the development of the tumour becomes more readily understandable.

Hereditary predisposition

It is doubtful whether there is any significant hereditary predisposition to most of the common types of cancer, for statistical surveys among relatives of cancer patients have not yielded convincing evidence of an increased incidence of tumours in them. Cancer of the breast is somewhat more common in the relatives of affected women than in the population at large.

There are, however, a number of uncommon neoplastic diseases which are inherited.

The trait of *polyposis coli* is transmitted as an autosomal dominant. Multiple adenomata of the colon usually first manifest themselves at puberty (Fig. 23.2). They are not present at birth. By the time the patient reaches the age of 30 years, multiple colonic cancers appear. Life is seldom prolonged over the age of 40 years. Gardner's syndrome is also associated with an increased incidence of colonic carcinoma (p. 326).

Xeroderma pigmentosum is inherited as an autosomal recessive trait. The skin is abnormally susceptible to the effects of sunlight, and multiple squamous-cell and basal-cell carcinomata develop on the exposed parts. Death usually occurs within the first decade.

The mechanism of xeroderma pigmentosum has now been elucidated.[6]

Ultraviolet light gives rise to dimer formation between neighbouring thymidine radicles in DNA, and when such DNA replicates, the dimer causes a mutation. In normal cells there are enzymes that can excise the dimer and replace it by the correct nitrogen bases. In xeroderma pigmentosum one such enzyme is lacking, and the disease is an inborn error of metabolism.

The inherited susceptibility to the action of carcinogen in experimental work has been mentioned previously.

Chronic disease as a cause of cancer

Chronic irritation

Although commonly cited as a cause of cancer, a concept of chronic irritation is too vague to have much meaning nowadays. It is extremely doubtful whether physical irritation acting alone can ever produce cancer, though it may certainly promote a tumour in a field already initiated by a carcinogenic substance. There are, however, a number of chronic diseases which may from time to time be complicated by malignancy. These are called precancerous lesions.

Precancerous lesions

A precancerous lesion is any condition in which cancer is more liable to develop than in the normal tissue. The following examples should be noted:

Chronic ulcers. The sinuses of chronic osteomyelitis, and old burn scars occasionally give rise to squamous-cell carcinoma.

Syphilitic glossitis has been regarded as an important precursor of oral cancer. The glossitis was often associated with dysplastic leukoplakia on the tongue and elsewhere in the mouth, and this condition often proceeds to malignancy. But whether the leukoplakia was due to syphilis, or whether the syphilis was merely a coincidental lesion is not certain. Syphilitic glossitis, like many other tertiary lesions of this infection, is now so rarely encountered that the controversy is unlikely to be settled.

Ulcerative colitis. About 4 per cent of all cases eventually develop carcinoma.

Cirrhosis of the liver. Primary liver-cell cancer is usually superimposed on a previous cirrhosis. Liver cancer is extremely prevalent in African races and also among the Chinese and Japanese. This is undoubtedly due to the high incidence of cirrhosis, and is not dependent upon racial factors.

The Plummer-Vinson syndrome is associated with postcricoid carcinoma (pp. 450).

Paget's disease of bone is occasionally complicated by osteosarcoma.

Malformations. There are a number of *hamartomatous lesions* which occasionally become malignant, for example neurofibromatosis.

A *congenitally abnormal organ*, e.g. an imperfectly descended testis, is more liable to malignancy than is a normal one.

Hormones and neoplasia

The early observations that oestrogens were a factor in the causation of cancer of the breast in mice led to widespread speculation that such a mechanism was applicable to the human being. However, it soon became evident that in mice other more important factors are operative, namely *genetic predisposition* and the *Bittner virus*. So far as the human is concerned, there is little evidence that hormonal imbalance is responsible for the production of any tumour, except under very unusual circumstances. Thus enormous doses of oestrogen (as secreted by granulosa-cell tumours of the ovary) may lead to endometrial and breast cancer. Vaginal cancer has been reported in young girls whose mothers were given oestrogen during the pregnancy in which they were fetuses.[7]

Hormone-dependent tumours. If hormones cannot be directly incriminated in the aetiology of human cancer, they are undoubtedly of great importance in maintaining the growth of some tumours. These are called the *hormone-dependent tumours*, and the best example is *carcinoma of the prostate*.

Both the normal prostatic epithelium and the carcinomata derived from it are dependent for their integrity upon a supply of testosterone. If patients with carcinoma of the prostate are castrated, there is often a dramatic relief of symptoms and regression of the tumour and its metastases. Nowadays large doses of stilboestrol are given, and surgical castration is unnecessary. The relief may last for at least 5 years, and, as many of the patients are over 70 years of age, some succumb to intercurrent illness before the cancer loses its hormone dependency and once more pursues its progressive course.

Carcinoma of the breast is another tumour which manifests hormone dependence in some patients. The picture is, however, complicated, because the tumour may depend upon ovarian, adrenal, or pituitary hormones. Nevertheless, in some patients the removal of the ovaries, adrenals, or pituitary produces a marked but temporary remission. In other cases the administration of oestrogens or testosterone may have an ameliorative effect.

Viruses and neoplasia[8,9]

Tumour-producing (oncogenic) viruses are arousing much interest, for an increasing number of animal tumours are proving to have a viral aetiology. The first such tumour was fowl leukaemia (Ellerman and Bang, 1908) and it was followed by fowl sarcoma (Rous 1911), rabbit papilloma (Shope, 1932), renal adenocarcinoma in frogs (Lucké, 1934), and mammary carcinoma in mice (Bittner, 1936). The last agent is an RNA retrovirus (see below), and is transmitted from the mother to its offspring in the milk, but the tumour does not occur until the female mice attain maturity, since oestrogens must first act to produce breast development.

Gross (1951) isolated the virus of mouse leukaemia, and in 1953 a second unrelated virus was found in his material. This was remarkable in that it produced tumours in many species of mice, rats, hamsters, and other animals. Furthermore many types of tumour were produced. The salivary glands were especially vulnerable, but tumours of the connective tissues, breasts, and kidneys were also encountered. This agent is now called the *polyoma virus*, and is widely distributed in nature, apparently lying latent in many mice. Certain human and simian *adenoviruses* are oncogenic in baby hamsters, as is also a virus than can be cultivated from the monkey-kidney tissue used in the preparation of poliomyelitis vaccines.

In order to establish the viral aetiology of a tumour it is necessary to transmit the lesion by bacteriologically sterile, cell-free filtrates to other animals. It has also been found that some oncogenic viruses, notably polyoma virus, induce changes in cells grown in tissue culture. This phenomenon, *cell transformation*, is indicated by a rapid proliferation of the cells with copious irregular mitotic activity, and when they are transplanted into animals they exhibit malignant propensities. Some tumour viruses contain DNA and others RNA, and both can transform normal cells into genetically stable cancer cells.

The DNA oncogenic viruses

In an infection with DNA oncogenic viruses, the cell undergoes transformation, and infective virus can no longer be detected. The viral DNA becomes incorporated into the cell's genome and replicates with it; mRNA of viral type is produced, and subsequently viral-type protein is synthetized by the cell. One early product is the *T-antigen*, which is found in the nucleus of infected cells. Another is the *tumour-specific transplantation antigen*, which is present on the cell's surface. The situation is not unlike that of lysogeny in bacteria, when bacteriophage may remain latent in the organismal DNA during a temperate phase.

The RNA oncogenic viruses

The RNA oncogenic viruses, called *oncoviruses* (alternatively called *oncornaviruses*) are one of three genera within the family of *retroviruses*.[10,11] These are single-stranded, RNA-containing, enveloped viruses that are characterized by the occurrence of *RNA-dependent (or directed) DNA polymerase*, also called *reverse transcriptase* (the first syllables of these two words are the origin of the word retrovirus), within the virion. The enzyme transcribes the viral RNA into *DNA provirus*, which is then integrated with the DNA of the chromosomes of the host cell. This process is of great theoretical interest in being a reversal of the usual sequence of DNA control of RNA and protein formation in the cell (see pp. 23 and 246). The provirus encodes for further viral RNA, and free virus particles are released from the infected cells. These can then infect adjacent cells, and the tumour can grow by local recruitment. It follows that if a tumour is transplanted from one animal to another, the transplanted tumour soon becomes replaced by tumour cells of host origin.

Oncoviruses contain a *group-specific (gs) antigen* which is common to the viruses that infect a particular species of animal. Thus mammalian oncoviruses have a common gs antigen distinct from that of avian viruses. It has been found that the gs antigen can be a component of the normal cells in the appropriate species, and that its presence is determined by a dominant autosomal gene. This remarkable finding has led to a number of hypotheses. Perhaps infective virus could be generated by apparently uninfected cells. Possibly the DNA provirus exists in all normal cells as part of a normal gene pool—the so-called oncogene. Another possibility is that informational transfer from DNA to RNA, and back to DNA, is a normal process. Disruption of this transfer mechanism, e.g. by radiation or chemical damage, could result in an alteration of the genetic information encoded in a cell during its lifetime.

It is important to realize that the mere presence of a virus in a cancer is no indication of its causal role. Cancers frequently harbour *passenger viruses*, which lie latent and play no part in the neoplastic growth.

It is not certain whether oncogenic viruses merely initiate cells which then pursue an independent course of neoplasia (as with chemical agents), or whether the presence of the virus (perhaps in an unrecognized form) is necessary for the continued propagation of the tumour.

At present much research is being done in investigating a viral aetiology for certain human tumours. The essential criterion, the inoculation of suspected viruses into human beings, is clearly impracticable. So far the neoplasm in man which seems most likely to have a viral origin is the Burkitt tumour (p. 347). The *Epstein-Barr virus* is closely associated with it (p. 265), for patients always have a high titre of antibodies to this herpesvirus, which is also associated with infectious mononucleosis. Perhaps a combination of chronic lymphoreticular hyperplasia due to recurrent malarial infection and an assault by this virus produces the Burkitt tumour. This suggestion would help to explain the sharp geographical distribution of the tumour.

Patients with nasopharyngeal carcinoma also have a high titre of antibodies to the EB virus, but as with the Burkett tumour the relationship is not understood.

Virus particles, similar electronmicroscopically with the Bittner factor, have been found in human breast-cancer cells. Indeed, there is also considerable biochemical evidence that human tumours contain viral RNA, but the precise relationship of this to the tumour remains to be determined.[12,13]

Finally women with carcinoma of the cervix uteri have a higher incidence of herpex-simplex antibodies than do normal women.[14] Once again the relationship is not understood for the association may be coincidental—there is an increased incidence of both cervical cancer and herpes infection in women who have frequent intercourse, particularly if with different partners. Cancer of the cervix is common in prostitutes and almost unknown in nuns.

Multiple factors as a cause of neoplasia

Although the simple two-stage mechanism in the formation of tumours (see initiation and promotion, p. 364) is now less clear in the light of more recent evidence, it is nevertheless true that the production of tumours involves several different factors. This is called *cocarcinogenesis*.

Oestrogens will promote cancer in mouse breast which has been initiated either by application of hydrocarbons or by infection with the Bittner virus. Radiation will induce leukaemia in mice due to the fact that a leukaemia-producing virus is apparently lying latent in the animals. The disease is then transmissible by the virus. The Shope papilloma virus will produce malignant tumours in rabbits when the skin has been tarred beforehand. There is a similar two-stage mode of carcinogenesis in respect of remotely acting agents. Croton oil produces cancer in the skin initiated by the oral administration of the powerful carcinogenic compound 2-acetylaminofluorene. It is no wonder, what with the long latent periods involved and the multiplicity of agents which may be concerned, that the cause of many human cancers remains unknown.

Early malignant lesions

In the human subject the question of early malignant change is of great importance, for it is at this stage that complete eradication of the disease is easiest. In recent years a number of interesting lesions involving epithelial surfaces has been recognized. In these areas there is atypical epithelial proliferation with the cells showing the microscopical changes usually associated with malignancy. They vary in size and shape, have large, darkly-stained nuclei, and show an increased amount of mitotic activity. The cells tend to lose their polarity, and lie haphazardly in relationship to one another. In stratified squamous epithelium there may be foci of abnormal keratinization within the area of cell proliferation, and this is called *malignant dyskeratosis*. Cellular pleomorphism, atypical mitotic activity, and other features of *dysplasia* may become so marked that the epithelium gives the impression of malignancy even though the cells have not broken through the basement membrane and invaded the underlying tissues. To this condition the names *carcinoma-in-situ* or *intra-epithelial carcinoma* are applied (Fig. 23.3).

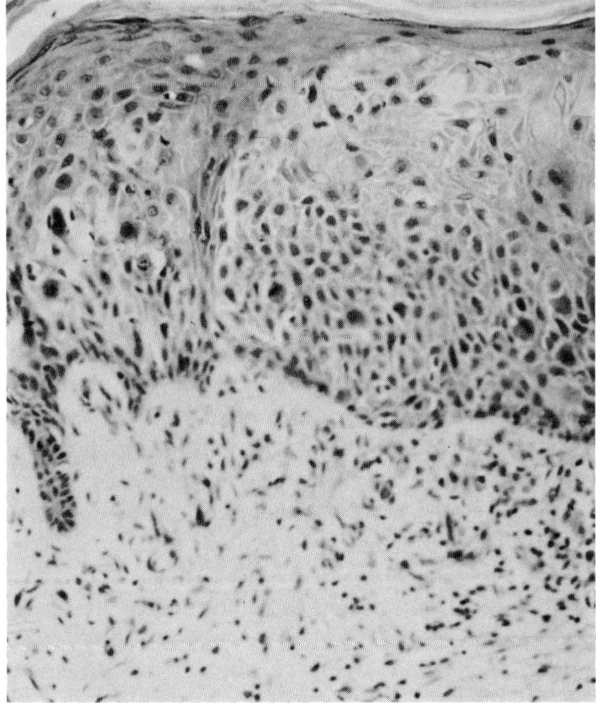

Fig. 23.3 Carcinoma-in-situ. This is a skin biopsy from a case of Bowen's disease. The cells are pleomorphic, and the orderly arrangement of the upper layers of the prickle-cell layer is disrupted. A number of cells have large, darkly-staining nuclei, and elsewhere in the section there were mitotic figures. There is a heavy lymphocytic infiltration in the dermis. Serial sections of the block failed to show any evidence of invasion. ×200.

Carcinoma-in-situ has been described in most epithelia, and it is encountered most typically in the stratified squamous covering epithelium of the skin, mouth, and cervix. Some clinical examples are worth noting:

Bowen's disease of the skin. This occurs in the middle-aged and elderly, and appears as discrete, red plaques which are sometimes mistaken for superficial basal-cell carcinoma, or resistant chronic dermititis or psoriasis. Any area of the skin may be implicated. Invasive carcinoma may finally ensue, sometimes after many years.

Actinic, or solar, keratosis. All gradations of changes are seen varying from mild atypicality of the epithelial cells to *carcinoma-in-situ* and on occasions invasive squamous-cell carcinoma. This rarely metastasises, but it is advisable to treat all senile keratoses.

Erythroplasia of Queyrat. This is a rare condition which usually involves the penis and appears as a red, velvety plaque of *in-situ* carcinoma. It can also occur in the oral mucosa.

Leukoplakia with dysplasia.* This appears as dead-white shiny plaques on a mucous membrane. The mouth and tongue are commonly affected, and the vulva is another favourite site. Microscopically the epithelium shows all degrees of cellular atypicality ranging from mild dysplasia to *carcinoma-in-situ.* Invasive squamous-cell carcinoma may develop, especially in the vulva.

Dysplasia of the cervix uteri. Dysplasia of the cervical epithelium is common, and may vary from mild atypicality to *carcinoma in-situ.* The study of this condition has been greatly aided by the technique of exfoliative cytology.

Exfoliative cytology

When cancer involves a lining epithelium, some of the neoplastic cells are shed on to the surrounding surface. If the surface is internal these cells are trapped in the secretions of the part, and are ultimately discharged to the exterior. Bronchial carcinoma cells may be coughed up in the sputum, gastric carcinoma cells may be aspirated in the gastric juice, and cervical carcinoma cells may be shed into the vaginal secretions. In recent years much progress has been made in recognizing clumps of cancer cells in such secretions, and sometimes this allows the early diagnosis of malignant disease. The technique was pioneered by Papanicolaou, and has been applied especially to the study of cervical cancer ('Pap smear').

It is often assumed that the onset of malignant change is a sudden event, but exfoliative cytology has shown that in the case of the cervix uteri this is certainly not so. There is considerable evidence that the first change in the epithelium involves certain cellular abnormalities which have been called *dysplasia*. The nuclei are enlarged, show variation in size and shape, and are hyperchromatic (*dyskaryosis*). The epithelium is not as abnormal as has been described in *carcinoma-in-situ.* Nevertheless, a dysplastic epithelium is thought to progress to a state of *carcinoma-in-situ* and finally to one of true invasive squamous-cell

* The term leukoplakia is often used clinically in its literal sense to describe any white plaque on a mucosal surface. This may include candidiasis, epithelial naevi, simple keratosis due to trauma, dysplasia, carcinoma, and lichen planus, as well as other less common conditions. To some pathologists the term implies a dysplastic condition that will in due course progress to invasive cancer. Hence the term should never be used without qualification.

carcinoma. The whole process is apparently drawn out over a long period, probably in the order of 10 years. Routine cytological examinations will detect early lesions, which although not cancerous themselves, are thought to progress to invasive, killing cancer. The same situation applies in the mouth. All suggestive or atypical lesions should be smeared to detect the presence of abnormal cells. If these are found, biopsy should be carried out. Dysplastic epithelium may be watched and treated, but if *carcinoma-in-situ* is present, excision of the whole lesion is indicated.

Incidence of certain tumours

Cancers of the skin

Geographical factors. The incidence of basal-cell and squamous-cell cancers of the exposed parts of fair-skinned people living in the tropics has already been noted. A more localized example of a geographical incidence of skin cancer is encountered in the *Kangri cancer of Kashmir*. The Kangri, a charcoal-heated basket, is carried close to the skin of the abdomen, and its continued use is often accompanied by carcinoma of the abdominal skin. It is probable that the carcinogenic agents in the fumes initiate the tumour, and the heat of the basket acts as a promoting agent.

Occupational factors. The industrial hazards of exposure to ionizing radiations and polycyclic hydrocarbons are now largely of historic interest, since strict public health regulations have been introduced.

Hereditary predisposition. Xeroderma pigmentosum has already been noted.

Chronic skin lesions have already been described as precursors of squamous-cell cancer. The prolonged ingestion of arsenic compounds sometimes leads to squamous-cell cancers.

Cancer of the lip

This is commonest in elderly, pipe-smoking, agricultural workers; sunlight probably initiates the tumour and the heat of the pipe promotes it to activity.

Cancer of the mouth

Geographical factors. Oral cancer is very common among some communities in South-East Asia who indulge in the habit of *betel chewing*. The quid which is kept in the mouth for long periods of time consists of betel nut, spices, tobacco, lime, and buyo leaves. It is probably the betel that is the carcinogenic agent. Cancer of the buccal aspects of the cheek and lower jaw is the usual site, but the tongue may also be involved. Another peculiar habit associated with oral cancer is *reverse cigar smoking* which is practised in parts of India, Sardinia, and Latin America. The lighted end of the cigar is held in the mouth, which is burned in consequence. Cancer of the palate and tongue may ensue.

Chronic disease. Oral cancer has been attributed to hot foods, alcohol, and chronic dental disease, but there is no convincing evidence that this is true. Tertiary syphilis with leukoplakia was said to be an important predisposing factor in the past. Women with the Plummer-Vinson syndrome show an increased incidence of oral cancer.

Cancer of the lung

The alarming increase in incidence of bronchial cancer in recent years has focused much attention on the problem. There can be little doubt that *heavy tobacco smoking* predisposes to lung cancer, and that the danger is greater in cigarette users than in pipe smokers. Another factor of undetermined importance is atmospheric pollution with soot and smoke. It probably acts together with tobacco smoking in producing lung cancer.

In certain *industries* cancer of the lung can be attributed to the inhalation of radioactive substances, nickel, chromium, or asbestos. This last produces pleural mesothelioma as well as squamous-cell lung cancer.

There is no evidence that chronic inflammatory diseases such as tuberculosis and bronchiectasis are precancerous.

Nature of the cancer cell

Changes in appearance. The pleomorphism and bizarre appearance of cancer cells have already been described in detail. There is, however, no constant variation characteristic of all malignant cells.

Changes in chemical content. No definite change in the DNA or RNA composition of malignant cells has yet been described. Extensive investigation of the enzyme contents of malignant cells has shown that tumour cells tend to contain the same enzymes as do the parent tissue, but that the quantity is usually reduced. So far no specific change has been found.

Antigens.[15–17] There is considerable evidence that some tumours are deficient in antigens. Tumours tend to grow as allogeneic homografts and heterografts under conditions where normal tissues would not. It is tempting to think that this lack of antigenicity might be a factor in allowing malignant cells to penetrate freely into tissues where normal cells are not allowed to proceed.

On the other hand, some tumours induced by hydrocarbons and viruses develop new transplantation antigens. Tumours induced by hydrocarbons are capable of manifesting antigenicity in the strain of origin, so that the host become resistant to a challenge of the same tumour. The antigens are individual for the particular tumour. With virus-induced tumours the new transplantation antigen is tumour-specific, and is the same for all tumours produced by the particular virus. Anti-viral antibodies are also produced. Some tumours produce new antigens which are not transplantation antigens and their detection can be used as an aid to diagnosis. Thus some carcinomata of the colon produce an antigen normally only found in the fetus (called *carcino-embryonic antigen*), and this antigen together with its antibody can be detected in the plasma.[18,19] It is interesting that carcinogens, both chemical and viral, are more potent in immunologically inadequate hosts, e.g. the newborn mouse.

It has been suggested that the cell-mediated immune response has been evolved to act as a defence against the development and growth of malignant tumours. Thus it is common to find a lymphocytic infiltrate around an early malignancy, e.g. a melanoma or squamous-cell carcinoma of the skin. Destruction of tumour cells by sensitized T cells can be demonstrated in experimental tissue culture systems, but whether this can occur *in vivo* is unclear. Nevertheless, the attractive *immunological surveillance* function of lymphocytes that was at one time popular has come under considerable criticism. There is certainly an increased incidence of tumours in the immunological deficiency syndromes and after immunosuppression for homografts, but the majority of the tumours are lymphomata.

Circulating immunoglobulins can be demonstrated against tumour antigens, but experimentally these can have diverse effects. They may *enhance* tumour growth (perhaps by interfering with T-cell function), or they may destroy tumour cells by activating complement. Thus there is abundant evidence of an immune response to tumour antigens, but the relationship of the antibodies to tumour progression, regression, or dormancy is complex and not understood. Attempts to increase patients' immunity to their own tumours have been made by injecting BCG and other agents. The results have generally been disappointing.[20, 21]

Changes in behaviour. *In vivo.* Progressive growth is characteristic of neoplasia. Malignant tumours invade and metastasize. Even so the phenomena of dormancy and regression indicate that some tumours undergo phases of retrenchment.

Inappropriate secretion. This is a common phenomenon. Epidermal cells can produce mucus, as in Paget's disease, and respiratory epithelial tumours can form keratin (see metaplasia, p. 355). The inappropriate secretion of hormones is described on page 333. Tumour cells may revert to activities normally seen only in their parents during embryonic life. The formation of carcino-embryonic antigen has been noted on page 372. Another example of considerable practical importance is seen in cancer of the liver. *Alpha-fetoprotein* is a globulin which normally forms about 50 per cent of the total plasma proteins of the fetus.[22] Its formation ceases in the third trimester, and it is therefore absent from the serum at birth. In 50 to 79 per cent of cases of hepatoma α-fetoprotein reappears in the plasma, and its presence has proved to be a useful diagnostic test.

In vitro. Malignant cells do not, on the whole, grow nearly so well as cells from normal tissues. However, a few lines of cancer cells have so adapted themselves to cell culture that they are now well established and grown in many laboratories; the HeLa cell is a good example. Such cells lack the alignment of normal cells grown in tissue culture, and tend to heap up into several layers. Normal cells (with the exception of lymphocytes and haematopoietic cells) form monolayers, and will grow only on a firm surface such as glass or solid agar: they are described as *anchorage dependent*. Growth ceases if the concentration of cells becomes too high, a phenomenon described as *contact inhibition of growth*. Normal cells also need an unidentified factor present in normal serum for their growth. Virus-transformed malignant cells are less anchorage dependent, and will grow in soft agar. They show less contact inhibition of growth and require little or no serum factor. Finally, normal cells have a finite life-span, whereas some neoplastic cells have acquired the property of indefinite life provided suitable growth facilities are provided either in tissue culture or in a host animal.

This brief survey of the properties of cancer cells is sufficient to indicate that although there are often many points of difference from the normal, there is no single characteristic by which they can be recognized. Perhaps it is wrong to expect that this should be so. The well-documented morphological features of cancer cells are of great importance to the cytologist and diagnostic histologist, but researches into cell metabolism have been essentially sterile both as regards a reliable cancer test and the elaboration of an effective chemotherapeutic agent. Studies of the antigenic composition and the *in-vitro* behaviour of tumour cells may perhaps yield more fruitful results.

It is humiliating to reflect that the vast majority of tumours in man arise with no apparent cause and appear to develop spontaneously. While some geographical factors are suggestive and a few occupational hazards have been successfully unmasked and controlled, there is still no indication as to the fundamental abnormality in cancer or the nature of its progressive growth.

Control of cancer

The most successful approach to the control of cancer at the present time lies in its prevention. The many known physical and chemical carcinogenic agents have already been described, and their avoidance can appreciably reduce the incidence of cancer. A second method of cancer prophylaxis is the treatment of known precancerous lesions. In the previous chapter a point of view has been expressed that cancer must be defined and diagnosed in terms of its invasive behaviour. The observations on the development of uterine cancer have led us to believe that the invasive tumour is the final development of a sequence of precancerous lesions. These lesions are sometimes reflected in the abnormal appearance of the cells, and, in the cervix, they can be detected and treated with relative ease. Cancer of the cervix uteri is therefore a preventable disease, and the same almost certainly applies to cancer of the oral cavity and tongue. Unfortunately in other organs the outlook is less bright. There is as yet no means of detecting the early stages of cancer of the breast, stomach, or colon. All three are extremely common tumours.

It is to be hoped that future discoveries will throw fresh light on the nature of neoplastic growth, so that more efficacious and less mutilating procedures may be developed to deal with the disease. At the present time there is much information regarding animal tumours but remarkably little concerning cancer in humans.

REFERENCES

1. Goldblatt M W 1958 Occupational carcinogenesis. British Medical Bulletin 14: 136
2. Ryser H J-P 1971 Chemical carcinogenesis. New England Journal of Medicine 285: 721
3. Hadfield E H 1970 A study of adenocarcinoma of the paranasal sinuses in woodworkers in the furniture industry. Annals of the Royal College of Surgeons of England 46: 301
4. Leading Article 1976 Vinyl chloride: the carcinogenic risk. British Medical Journal 2: 134
5. Leading Article 1975 More on the aflatoxin-hepatoma story. British Medical Journal 2: 647
6. Leading Article 1974 Xeroderma pigmentosum. Lancet 1: 792
7. Leading Article 1974 Vaginal adenocarcinomas and maternal oestrogen ingestion. Lancet 1: 250
8. Epstein M A 1971 The possible role of viruses in human cancer. Lancet 1: 1344
9. Allen D W, Cole P 1972 Viruses and human cancer. New England Journal of Medicine 286: 70
10. Fenner F J, White D O 1976 Medical Virology, 2nd edn. Academic Press, New York, p 170
11. Fenner F 1976 Classification and Nomenclature of Viruses. Second Report of the International Committee on Taxonomy of Viruses. S Karger, Basel
12. Leading Article 1972 Viruses and human breast cancer. Lancet 1: 359

13. Axel R, Schlom J, Spiegelman S 1972 Presence in human breast cancer of RNA homologous to mouse mammary tumour virus RNA. Nature, London, 235: 32
14. Leading Article 1976 Herpesvirus and cancer of uterine cervix. British Medical Journal 1: 671
15. Klein G 1968 Tumour-specific transplantation antigens. Cancer Research 28: 625
16. Klein G 1968 Summary: antigens of chemically induced tumors; and search for tumor-specific antigens in other human cancers. Cancer Research 28: 1354
17. Prehn R T 1968 Tumor-specific antigens of putatively nonviral tumors. Cancer Research 28: 1326
18. Zamcheck N, Moore T L, Dhar P, Kupchik H 1972 Immunologic diagnosis and prognosis of human digestive-tract cancer: carcinoembryonic antigens. New England Journal of Medicine 286: 83
19. Mach J-P, Jaeger P, Bertholet M-M, Ruegsegger C-H, Loosli R M, Pettavel J 1974 Detection of recurrence of large-bowel carcinoma by radioimmunoassay of circulating carcinoembryonic antigen (CEA). Lancet 2: 535
20. Leading Article 1975 Immunological control of cancer. Lancet 1: 502
21. Leading Article 1976 Immunostimulation. Lancet 2: 349
22. Smith J B 1970 Alpha-fetoprotein: occurrence in certain malignant diseases and review of clinical applications. Medical Clinics of North America 54: 797

24

Developmental anomalies: Developmental tumours and tumour-like conditions

Introduction

It is incredible that in the course of a few months, a single cell, the fertilized ovum, can proliferate and differentiate into the complex system of organs and tissues that constitute the mature organism. Minor variations are so common that the differences which result are regarded as normal. More serious errors in development result in the production of various malformations which are usually apparent at birth, but which may develop at any time during the growing period of childhood and adolescence. Gross abnormalities may be incompatible with life, and these result in abortion, stillbirth, or neonatal death.

Causes of developmental anomalies

Developmental anomalies may occur either as a result of genetic errors or be due to environmental factors.

Genetic errors. These have been described in Chapter 3. Chromosomal abnormalities should always be looked for when developmental anomalies are present.

Environmental factors. It is becoming increasingly obvious that many external agents are capable of causing serious developmental anomalies. These *teratogenic agents* have the most severe effects when they act *in utero.*

Infection.[1] Transmission of infection from the mother to the fetus may cause severe damage. The first trimester of pregnancy is the most dangerous time, as it is during this period that rapid division and differentiation occur. Rubella has acquired a particularly evil reputation: deformities occur in as many as 25 per cent of babies born to mothers who have had this infection during pregnancy.

Drugs.[2] A notorious tragedy occurred around the period of 1960, when pregnant women who had taken the sedative thalidomide gave birth to grossly deformed babies[3,4] The thalidomide is dangerous during the crucial period from 37 to 54 days after the first day of the last menstrual period.[5] The most common anomalies were absence of limbs or parts of limbs, haemangiomatosis of the upper lips and nose, and malformations of the alimentary tract, heart, and genito-urinary system.

Cytotoxic agents also produce malformations, and the use of large doses of *progesterone* can produce genital deformities in female infants.

An even more serious hazard to fetal development is *maternal alcoholism.*[6]

Expectant mothers who consume large amounts of alcohol tend to give birth to infants that are short and below average weight. There is often hypoplasia of the maxilla with prominence of the forehead and lower jaw, short palpebral fissures, microcephaly, and mental retardation. Other defects are also described, and it is evident that excessive amounts of alcohol in the fetal blood constitute a very real teratogenic hazard.

It is obviously wise to avoid the use of all drugs during pregnancy, especially during the first three months.

Ionizing radiations (p. 397).

Rhesus incompatibility, i.e. haemolytic disease of the newborn (p. 454).

It is to be hoped that abnormalities due to external agents will become less frequent as knowledge about the factors involved is acquired.

Types of malformation

Although it is a somewhat artificial subdivision, it is convenient to consider the types of malformation under separate headings:

Failure of development. There may be complete failure of development of a part (*agenesis*), or the part may remain rudimentary (*hypoplasia*) and never attain a full mature size. In the rare condition of anodontia there is agenesis of the dental lamina and complete absence of all the teeth. Congenital absence of a few teeth (partial anodontia) is more common. Both these conditions may be associated with a general defect of ectodermal structures affecting the hair, nails, and sebaceous and sweat glands (ectodermal dysplasia).

Failure of fusion. During development many structures normally fuse, and

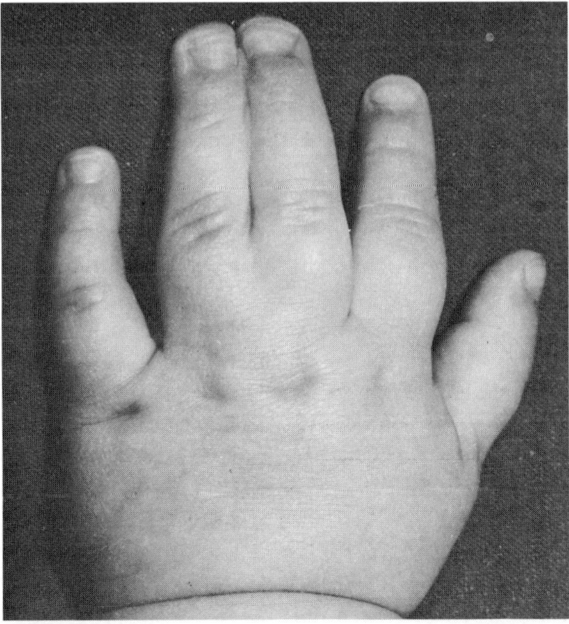

Fig. 24.1 Syndactyly. The third and fourth fingers of the hand are completely fused. (*Photograph by courtesy of Mr V. S. Brookes.*)

a failure to do so results in an abnormality. A cleft of the lip and palate occurs as a result of failure of fusion of the globular portion of the median nasal process with the lateral nasal and maxillary processes.

Failure of separation. A good example of this is the webbing which may persist between the digits (Fig. 24.1).

Failure of canalization (atresia). Various channels in the body may fail to canalize, e.g. oesophageal atresia and imperforate anus.

Ectopia. Sometimes organs and tissues are found in abnormal sites. This is called ectopia, heterotopia, or aberrance. Aberrant adrenal tissue may be found on the surface of the kidney and gonads, and an ectopic testis may be encountered in the abdominal cavity, the perineum, or the pubic area. Ectopic thyroid may be found in the tongue in the region of the foramen caecum, and in some cases no thyroid tissue may be present in its normal situation.

Heteroplasia. Sometimes there is an anomalous differentiation of a particular tissue in an organ. For instance, sebaceous glands may be found in the buccal mucosa (Fordyce spots). This is called heteroplasia, and must be distinguished from metaplasia, in which the alteration of the tissue occurs after normal differentiation has taken place. Heteroplasia implies that the abnormal differentiation is a primary affair.

Local gigantism. Sometimes there is simple overgrowth of an organ or tissue, e.g. an enlarged digit or limb in neurofibromatosis, and this is rather dubiously called 'hypertrophy'. It is in fact better called local gigantism, because the organ has never been normal in relation to the remainder of the body. In true hyperplasia and hypertrophy the part is initially normal in size and subsequently undergoes enlargement (p. 000).

Supernumerary organs. Additional, or supernumerary, teeth may be present; likewise additional digits may occur (polydactyly).

Hamartomata

A *hamartoma* is a tumour-like malformation in which the tissues of a particular part of the body are arranged haphazardly, usually with an excess of one or more of its components. The term was coined by Albrecht in 1904, and is derived from the Greek word *hamartion,* a bodily defect. The concept it embodies is of great importance, for a large number of common lesions fall into the general category of hamartomata.

A well-known example of hamartoma is the isolated cartilaginous mass not infrequently found in the substance of a lung (Fig. 24.2). This is composed of areas of hyaline cartilage separated by clefts lined by respiratory epithelium. There is no true capsule between the lesion and the surrounding lung. It is evident that this lesion contains several different elements, but that all of these are normally found in the lung. It would appear that it is a malformation derived from a developing bronchus, for all the tissues of a bronchus are present in it, though they are grossly misaligned and there is an excess of cartilage.

It is very important to distinguish between this type of lesion and a teratoma, which is a true tumour. In a hamartoma: (a) the tissues present are those specific to the part from which it arises, and (b) the lesion has no tendency towards excessive growth. There is no capsule around a hamartoma, as its growth proceeds

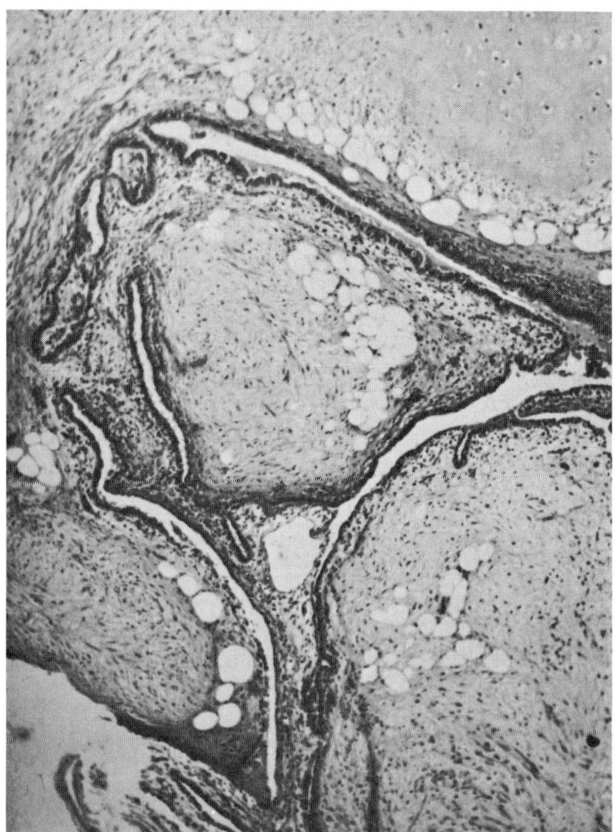

Fig. 24.2 Hamartoma of lung. There are masses of connective tissue intersected by deep clefts lined by respiratory epithelium. In the connective tissue there are areas of adipose tissue, and at the top there is a mass of hyaline cartilage. ×55.

pari passu with that of its surroundings. There is no question of pressure atrophy and therefore no connective-tissue condensation.

It should be noted that many hamartomata are given 'tumour-sounding' names. These are so much part and parcel of histopathological nomenclature that they are bound to persist, e.g. angioma, benign melanoma, and chondroma of the lung.

Vascular hamartomata. The very common haemangioma is a hamartomatous malformation and not a true tumour. The commonest site is the skin, where it forms a variety of *naevus*, a word used to describe any type of developmental blemish of the skin. A noteworthy feature of angiomata is their tendency towards multiplicity. They may be accompanied by angiomatous involvement of internal organs as well as being a component of a more generalized disorder. Several characteristic syndromes have been described, and a number of these will be noted, since they involve the head and neck and are likely to come to the attention of the dentist.[7]

Spider naevus. The characteristic morphology of the cutaneous spider naevus is due to the presence of a central pulsating arteriole which leads to a leash of radiating capillaries. The lesion blanches on pressure. Spider naevi may develop during childhood, but most commonly they occur in the course of chronic liver disease—usually cirrhosis. Spider naevi may also occur on the mucous membranes, but their 'spider' morphology is less evident than those on the skin.

Telangiectatic naevus. Persistent dilatation of the skin capillaries produces the characteristic *port-wine stain.* The condition is generally evident at birth, and commonly affects the face and oral mucosa in the distribution of the trigeminal nerve. It is usually unilateral. Apart from its cosmetic significance, it may be associated with vascular anomalies of the meninges and eye; this is called *encephalotrigeminal angiomatosis,* or the *Sturge-Weber syndrome.* Hemiparesis on the side opposite to the lesion, convulsions, and mental defect are due to hypoxia of the underlying cerebral cortex.

Strawberry, or capillary, haemangioma. This lesion is usually present at birth or during the first month of life as a well-defined lesion on the face (Fig. 24.3). It increases in size, often quite rapidly. Spontaneous regression with scarring usually occurs, but surgical treatment may be required for cosmetic reasons or for delayed

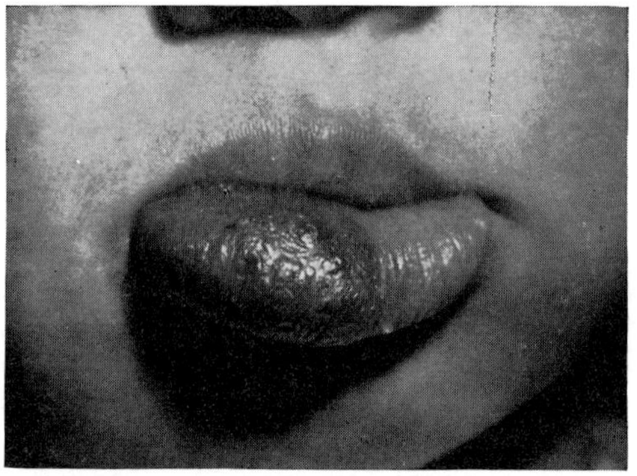

Fig. 24.3 Haemangioma of lower lip. (*Photograph supplied by Mr G. S. Hoggins.*)

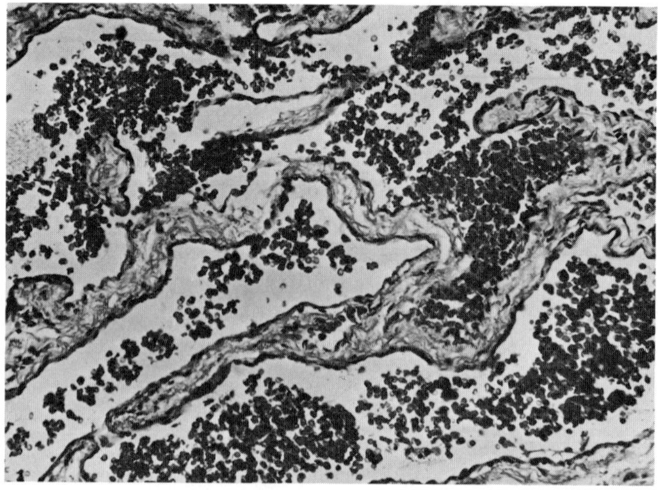

Fig. 24.4 Haemangioma. This is a cavernous haemangioma, and it consists of extensive vascular spaces enclosed in loose strands of endothelial-lined connective tissue. × 200.

regression. The strawberry naevus is predominantly composed of capillary-sized vessels, but it may be of mixed capillary-cavernous type.

Cavernous haemangiomata (Fig. 24.4) are less well circumscribed, and tend to extend more deeply into the subcutaneous tissues. They may occur on the lips, tongue, and bone. Bone involvement by haemangiomata should be suspected if there is early eruption of teeth in that area (Figs. 24.5 and 24.6). If these teeth are extracted, there may be uncontrollable haemorrhage.

Hereditary haemorrhagic telangiectasia (Osler-Rendu-Weber disease). This disease is inherited as an autosomal dominant trait, and generally becomes apparent at puberty or somewhat later. Multiple telangiectases develop on the skin, being particularly conspicuous on the face and lips. The mucous membranes are invariably involved, and bleeding can occur from any site; thus bleeding from the nose (epistaxis) may be the first symptom. Arteriovenous malformations may occur in the lungs and other internal organs.

Ataxia telangiectasia. This syndrome, which occurs in young children, is characterized by an immunological deficiency affecting both T and B lymphocyte systems, recurrent respiratory infections, cerebellar ataxia, and the presence of telangiectases first evident on the conjunctiva and later on the ears and the butterfly area of the face. The disease is inherited as an autosomal recessive trait,

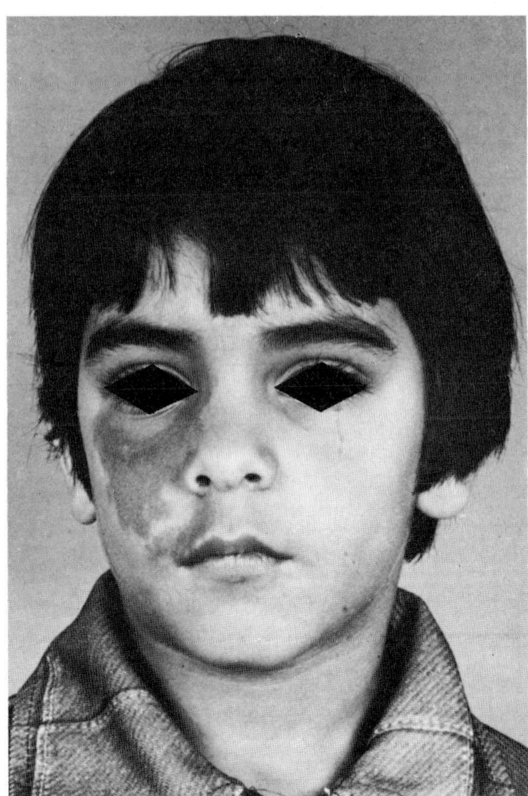

Fig. 24.5 Haemangioma affecting the skin of the right side of the face in the region of the maxilla.

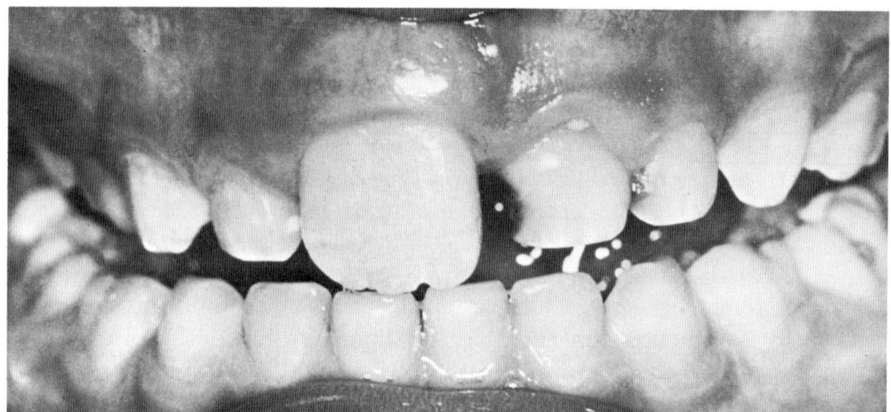

Fig. 24.6 This comes from the same case as Fig. 24.5. There has been early eruption of the central incisor on the side affected by the haemangioma, which suggests bone involvement of the maxilla.

and death usually occurs by adolescence either from infection or a malignant lymphoma.

Microscopically haemangiomata consist of poorly-demarcated, non-encapsulated masses and leashes of vascular channels, which are sometimes capacious, and described as *cavernous,* (Fig 24.4), and at other times narrow and well formed (*capillary haemangioma*).

True tumours of blood vessels—angiosarcomata—are known, but are uncommon (p. 346).

Another type of vascular hamartoma is the lymphangioma. A well-known example is the cystic hygroma of infancy, which forms a characteristic swelling in the neck. It infiltrates the vital surrounding structures so intimately that its complete removal is seldom possible.

Melanotic hamartomata. The common mole, also called a *melanotic naevus* or a *naevocellular naevus,* of the skin is another example of a hamartomatous malformation (Fig. 24.7). The parent cells, the melanocytes, are believed to originate in the region of the neural crest and to migrate to the epidermis with the peripheral nerves. Here they become incorporated among the cells of the basal layer. An excessive accumulation of these cells, which are then called *naevus cells,* leads to the formation of the melanotic naevus. The cells are shed into the dermis during childhood. Naevus cells remaining in the basal layer of the epidermis are prone to undergo phases of proliferation, called *junctional activity,* but by the age of 30 years all the cells should be embedded in the dermis. Such a naevus is described as *intradermal* (Fig. 24.8). If some of the cells are still attached to the epidermis, the naevus is *compound* (Fig. 24.9), and if there is no dermal migration at all, the naevus is called *junctional.* It is the junctional element of a naevus that is liable to spurts of proliferation (junctional activity), whereas an intradermal lesion is inert. Junctional activity is of little significance during childhood, but in adult life any marked degree is to be regarded with suspicion, as it may be the first indication of neoplastic change.

Naevocellular naevi, unlike many other hamartomata, do occasionally become malignant. Lesions on the extremities and genitalia, and especially under the nails are most liable to this change.

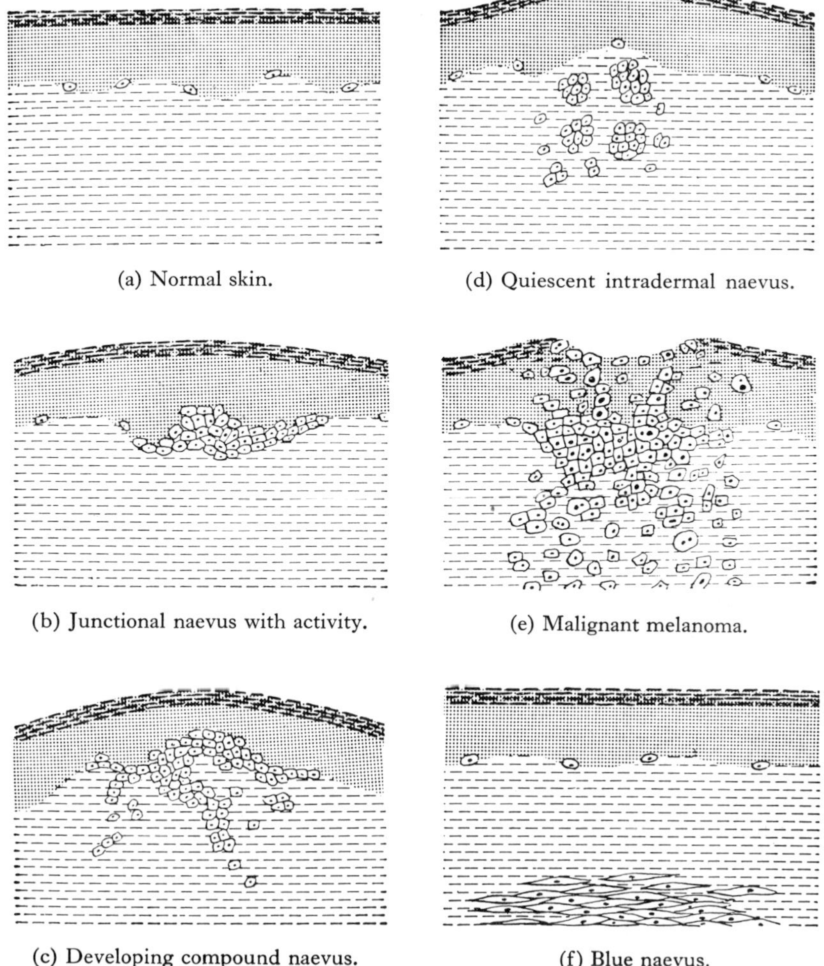

(a) Normal skin.
(d) Quiescent intradermal naevus.
(b) Junctional naevus with activity.
(e) Malignant melanoma.
(c) Developing compound naevus.
(f) Blue naevus.

Fig. 24.7 Sketches to show the various types of melanotic naevi: the only cells drawn are melanocytes and naevus cells. In the normal skin melanocytes are present only in the basal layer of the epidermis. A focal proliferation of these cells produces a junctional naevus (b) which may be regarded as a stage in the development of a compound and intradermal naevus. Such junctional activity is of little importance in a young person, but in an adult is to be regarded as dangerous; (c) shows the formation of a compound naevus by the invasion of the dermis by melanocytes. When the junctional activity regresses, the naevus cells remain in the dermis as an intradermal naevus (d); (e) shows a malignant melanoma which in addition to junctional activity, shows invasion of the epidermis as well as the dermis and deeper structures. Atypicality of the cells serves as a further distinguishing feature from the compound naevus, which an early malignant melanoma may resemble. (f) The strap-like naevus cells situated deep in the dermis impart the colour to the blue naevus.
(a) Normal skin.
(b) Junctional naevus with activity.
(c) Developing compound naevus.
(d) Quiescent intradermal naevus.
(e) Malignant melanoma.
(f) Blue naevus.

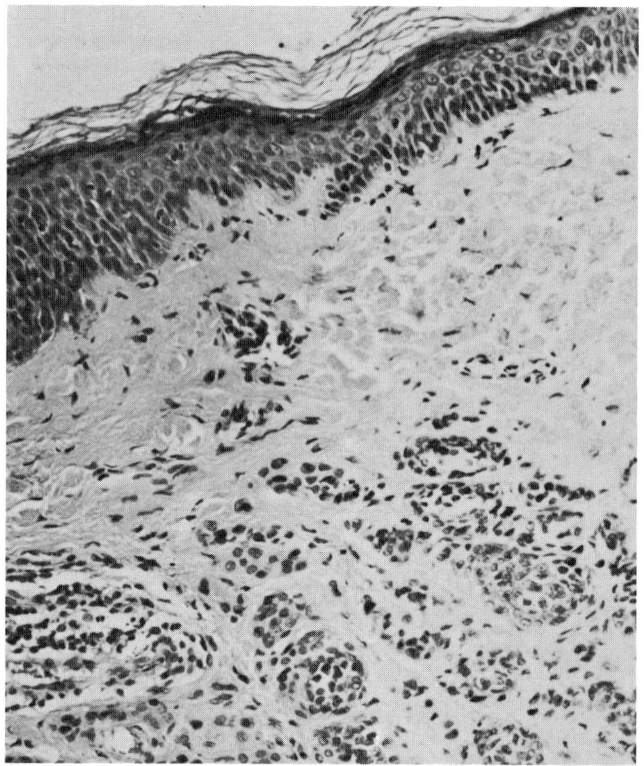

Fig. 24.8 Intradermal naevus. There is a focal accumulation of naevus cells in the deeper layer of the dermis, but they are well separated from the overlying epidermis. × 130.

Spindle-cell naevus of Spitz. This is a type of naevus, usually compound, which occurs in young people, and because of its rapid growth imitates a malignant melanoma. Histologically the predominant cell type is spindle-shaped or epithelioid, and the presence of mitoses can easily lead to a diagnosis of malignant melanoma. The lesion is usually not pigmented, but is vascular. The spindle-cell naevus is entirely benign, and its old name 'juvenile melanoma' is misleading.

The blue naevus. This type of naevus shows focal accumulations of dendritic melanocytes in the dermis, and has a different mode of formation to that of the common naevocellular naevus. The blue naevus is generally present at birth, and appears blue because the pigment is situated entirely in the dermis. A localized nodular form of the lesion is called a *common blue naevus.* Sometimes the naevus is diffuse and produces a wide area of hyperpigmentation that somewhat resembles a tattoo. When the eye and surrounding skin are involved, this is called the *naevus of Ota.* It is quite common to find a similar type of lesion at birth over the sacral region in the Oriental races. This *Mongolian spot* differs from the blue naevus described above in that it invariably fades as the baby grows up.

Malignant melanoma.[8,9] If a naevocellular naevus is becoming malignant it increases in size and changes in colour, usually becoming darker, but it may also fade in some areas. It tends to become itchy and may bleed. Microscopically there is marked junctional activity, and the malignant cells are seen to invade not only

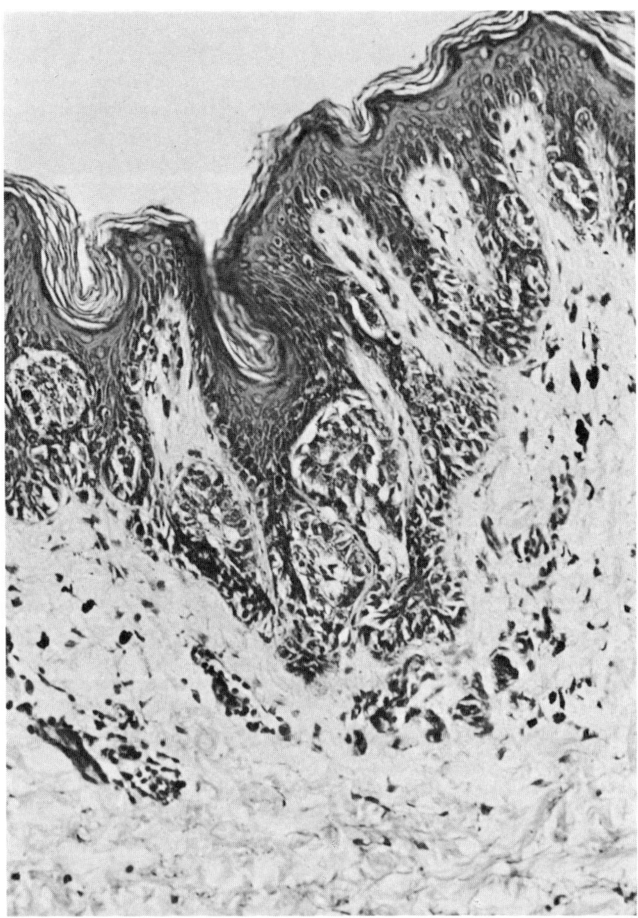

Fig. 24.9 Junctional naevus. There are considerable aggregations of naevus cells in contact with the basal layer of the epidermis, but there is no evidence of invasion of the epidermis. × 100.

the dermis but also the superficial layers of the epidermis, which is destroyed, hence the ulceration and bleeding. A lymphocytic reaction around the lesion is characteristic, and probably represents an immunological response to the developing malignant cells.

The cells of a malignant melanoma show the usual characteristics of tumour cells (Fig. 24.10). They vary in size and shape, and their nuclei are irregular and darkly staining. Mitotic activity is invariable, and tumour giant cells are often present. Usually both the primary tumour and its metastases are well pigmented, but sometimes there is almost complete absence of melanin (amelanotic melanoma).

The commonest site for malignant melanoma is the skin, and it has often been assumed that the majority of tumours arise in pre-existing naevi. This has been questioned by some investigators who believe that over 90 per cent arise *de novo,* and that the risk of malignancy occurring in a naevus has been greatly exaggerated

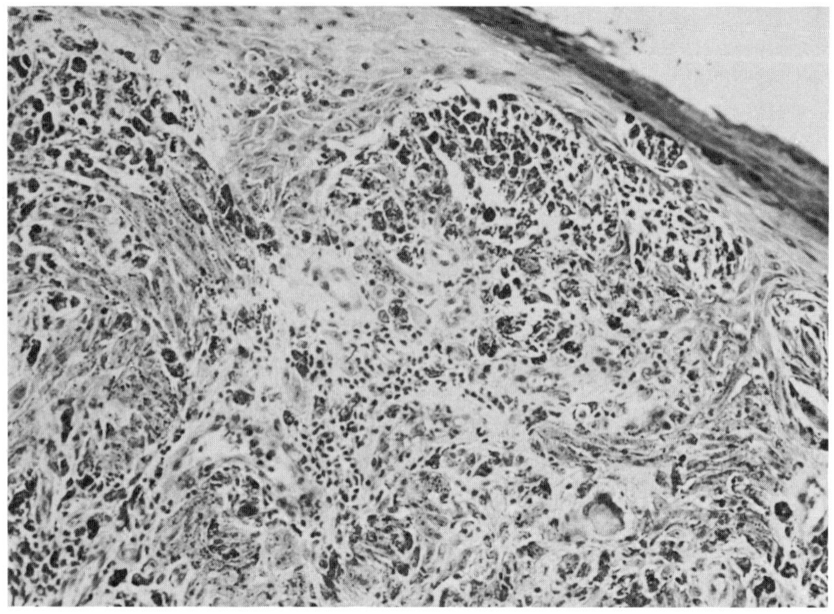

Fig. 24.10 Malignant melanoma. The dermis is diffusely infiltrated by pleomorphic tumour cells, some of which are pigmented. The epidermis is considerably thinned, its deeper layers having been destroyed. Adjacent to this area there was extensive ulceration. × 100.

in the past. This conflict of opinions has not yet been resolved. Three types of melanoma are recognised:

Nodular melanoma. Tumour cells stream into the dermis and invade the epidermis. There is early invasion of local lymphatics, and widespread lymphatic and blood-borne metastases are the rule. Regardless of treatment the prognosis is bad.

Superficial spreading melanoma. This type is flat and shows irregular pigmentation; in due course nodules may appear. Microscopically the epidermis is invaded and disorganised by melanoma cells, and later the dermis is invaded. The prognosis is better than in the nodular type.

Lentigo-maligna melanoma. A lentigo maligna, or Hutchinson's freckle, appears as a flat, pigmented macule on the cheek of an elderly person. Microscopically the basal layer of the epidermis contains an increased number of atypical melanocytes, so that the lesion may be regarded as a type of *in-situ* malignancy. After a number of years some patients develop invasive melanoma, which usually leads to the lesion becoming crusted, ulcerated, or nodular. The prognosis is good in this type of melanoma.

Other sites of primary melanoma are the uveal tract of the eye and the juxtacutaneous mucous membranes of the mouth, nose, anus, vulva, and vagina.

Skeletal hamartomata. The common solitary exostosis which grows out from the epiphyseal cartilage of a long bone is a good example of a cartilaginous hamartoma. It stops growing after puberty, when it completely ossifies. The rare condition of multiple exostoses, inherited as an autosomal dominant trait, is a generalized hamartomatous disorder involving many bones. The condition is also called *diaphysial aclasis.*

Dental hamartomata. The *odontome* is a malformation of all the dental tissues. As odontomes are composed of enamel, dentine, and cementum, they are termed composite, and there are several types. The compound composite odontome consists of a number of very small calcified structures which resemble teeth and are called denticles. The complex composite odontome consists of an irregular mass of calcified dental tissues. The odontome may replace a tooth in the arch, or it may be additional to the complete dentition and have arisen from a supernumerary anlage.

Generalized hamartomatous dysplasia. *Neurofibromatosis* (*von Recklinghausen's disease*) is a well-known condition, inherited as an autosomal dominant trait, in which there is a widespread hamartomatous overgrowth of nerve-sheath tissue. Histologically the lesions closely resemble the tumours described as neurofibromata. The condition may be associated with regional gigantism, which, if the face is affected, produces gross deformity. There may also be café-au-lait spots on the skin, and characteristically freckles are present in the axillae. A neurofibromatous lesion may undergo sarcomatous change.

Persistence of vestigial structures

In the course of development may parts which are of immense importance to the embryo undergo obliteration by the time of birth. If this does not happen, these normally vestigial structures persist and may lead to subsequent trouble. The two most important complications are *neoplasia* and *cyst formation.*

Neoplasia

Developmental anomalies occasionally form the basis for subsequent tumours. This may occur in a number of ways:

The embryonic tumours of infancy. Tumours may arise from primitive undifferentiated cells which are normally present only during embryonic life. The cells may persist into postnatal life and become neoplastic. Such tumours are most common during infancy, although they occasionally occur in later life. The tumours are highly malignant. It would seem that a portion of an organ undergoes a perversion of development to form a neoplasm instead of the normal parenchyma of the part. A good example is the *nephroblastoma* (*Wilms's tumour of the kidney*). Many of these tumours are undifferentiated and are composed of small darkly-staining cells, but sometimes the malignant nephroblasts show differentiation into tubular epithelial structures as well as forming recognizable connective tissue elements. Such tumours are therefore called mixed.

Other tumours of this type arise from the retina (*retinoblastoma,* Fig. 24.11), hind-brain (*medulloblastoma*), and sympathetic ganglion cells and adrenal medulla (*neuroblastoma*). Histologically they resemble each other closely.

Tumours developing in hamartomata. This has already been discussed.

Tumours arising from vestigial remnants. *Ameloblastoma.* This is a cystic tumour of the jaws which grows slowly and is locally malignant. Both in behaviour and in structure it resembles the common basal-cell carcinoma quite closely. It usually occurs in the mandible, and is seen most often in young adults. It consists

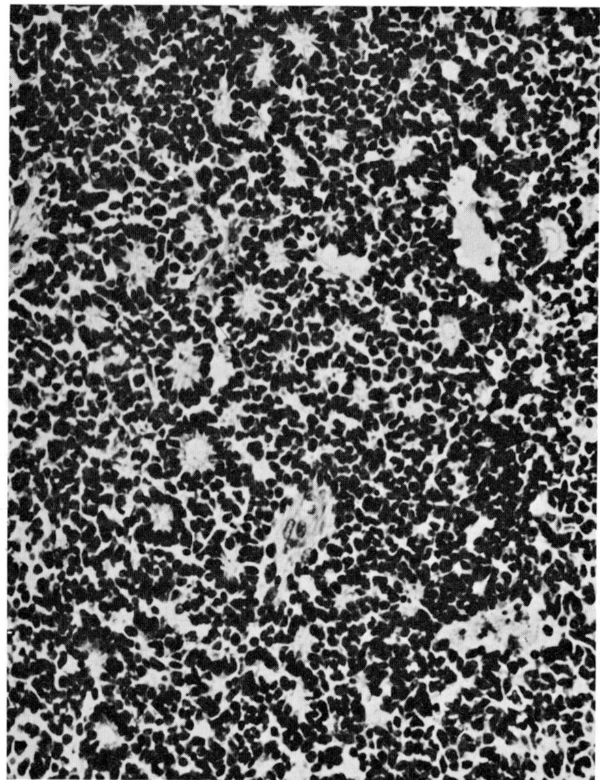

Fig. 24.11 Retinoblastoma. The tumour is composed of small, darkly-staining, fusiform cells arranged in rosette formation. In some of the rosettes there is a central cavity. × 150.

of round or angulated clumps of epithelial cells. In the centre of these aggregations there is often an open meshwork resembling the stellate reticulum of the enamel organ. Between the cells there is an accumulation of fluid which gives rise to the cystic appearance typical of this tumour (Fig. 24.12). Other tumours in this group are rare. The *chordoma* arising from the notochord and the *craniopharyngioma* arising from residues of Rathke's pouch may be cited as examples.

Tumours arising from ectopic organs and tissues. Ectopic tissues are particularly liable to neoplastic transformation. Malignancy in ectopic testes is the most important example.

Teratomata.[10] These are tumours consisting of multiple tissues foreign to the part from which they arise. The common sites are the ovary and testis. Rarely teratomata are found in the mediastinum, retroperitoneal tissue, and intracranially. Testicular teratomata are composed of cystic spaces lined by a variety of different types of epithelium and a connective tissue element which usually contains cartilage, lymphoid tissue, and primitive mesenchyme. The tumour, which affects young men, is highly malignant, and rapidly metastasizes both by the lymphatics and the blood stream. On the other hand, ovarian teratomata are usually well differentiated and benign, and are encountered chiefly in young and middle-aged women. They are usually cystic, and the wall is lined by stratified

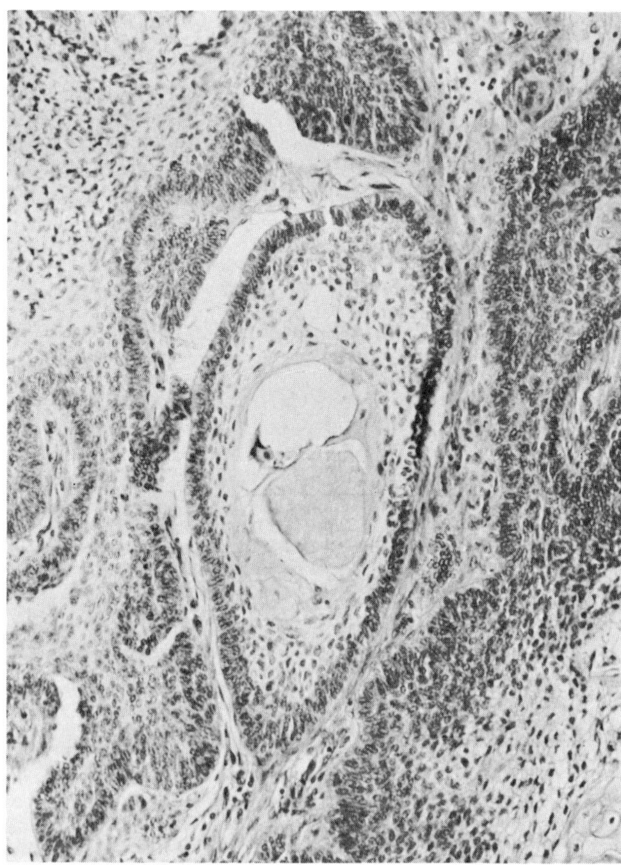

Fig. 24.12 Ameloblastoma. The tumour consists of aggregations of small epithelial cells, the outer layers of which form a palisade as is found in the basal-cell carcinoma. In the midst of the central clump there is an open meshwork reminiscent of the stellate reticulum of the developing tooth germ ('enamel organ'). × 100.

squamous epithelium and contains sebaceous glands and hair follicles. The cyst is usually filled with a greasy mass of sebaceous material in which there is matted hair. There is often a nodule in the wall, called the umbo, which contains a variety of structures such as bone, teeth, thyroid tissue, brain, etc. The tumour is therefore truly mixed in type (Fig. 24.13).

The origin of teratomata has long been disputed. The current view is that they arise from germ cells. The germ cells first appear in the embryo in the wall of the yolk sack, from where they migrate to the genital ridge on the posterior abdominal wall. They become incorporated into the developing gonad, but it is believed that some cells remain behind or stray from their final path, and come to rest at various sites along the posterior wall of the embryo near the midline. If these cells remain viable they later give rise to tumours in just these situations. Hence, teratomata are found in the retroperitoneal area, the sacral region, and the mediastinum, and around the pineal gland; the greatest number, of course, are in the gonads. Since the cells may be regarded as totipotential, it is to be expected that virtually any

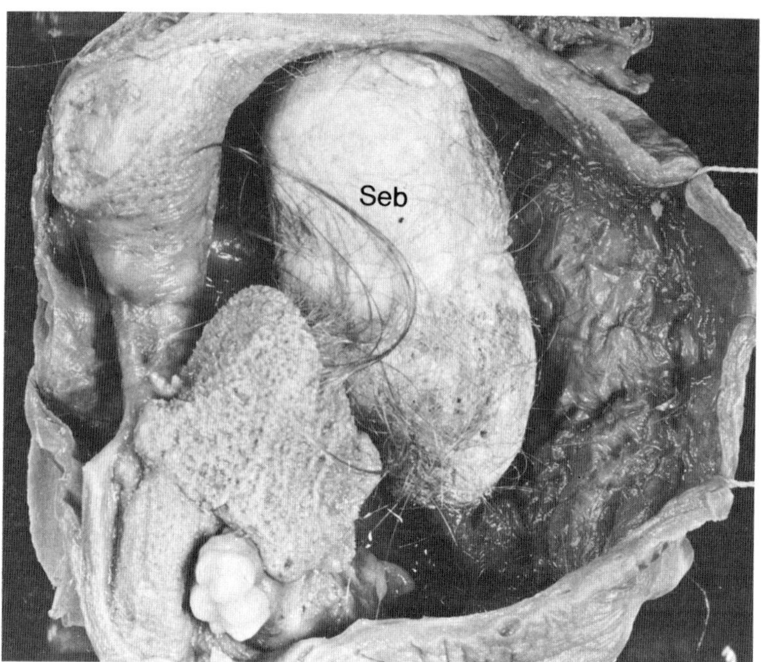

Fig. 24.13 Teratoma of ovary. For five years the patient had had occasional episodes of abdominal pain. At the age of 32 she experienced a particularly severe attack, which led to her being admitted to hospital. A rounded swelling was palpated in the abdomen above the pubis, and a cystic ovarian tumour was removed at laparotomy.

The specimen shows the opened cyst. It is lined by skin, and on one side a mass projects into the cavity. This is covered by spongy skin containing numerous sebaceous glands, and from it is growing a tuft of hair. The mass contains bone in which a number of teeth are partially embedded, one of which is clearly shown in the photograph. Another mass of tissue (Seb) contains hair but is otherwise lying free in the cyst cavity. It consists largely of sebaceous material and desquamated keratin. *(Photograph of specimen by courtesy of the Boyd Museum, University of Toronto.)*

type of tissue can be found in a teratoma, particularly if it is well differentiated and benign.

CYSTS

It is appropriate to end this chapter with an account of the types of cyst, for many of them have a developmental basis.

The word *cyst,* derived from the Greek *kustis* a bladder, means a *pathological fluid-filled sac bounded by a wall.* The fluid may be secreted by cells lining the wall or it may be derived from the tissue fluid of the area. It is often clear and colourless, but it may be turbid and thick, or contain shimmering crystals of cholesterol. By common usage a cyst does not contain frank pus or blood—in these circumstances the terms abscess or haematoma are employed.

Where the cyst wall is lined by an epithelium, this layer may be derived from developmental residues such as the epithelial rests of Malassez in the periodontal ligament or epithelial residues lying in planes of embryonic fusion. On the other hand it may arise from a normal anatomical structure, such as the cells lining the ducts and acini of an exocrine gland. Often the stimulus which provokes the epithelial proliferation is unknown, as for instance in cysts arising in planes of embryonic fusion like the globulo-maxillary cyst. Sometimes chronic inflammation is a factor, as in the development of the *periodontal cyst* (also called *apical* or *radicular cyst*), the commonest of the odontogenic cysts. Here the chronic inflammation in the periapical tissues of a dead tooth stimulates the epithelial rests of Malassez to proliferate and line the liquefied apical granuloma, thus forming part of the wall of the cyst, the contents of which are turbid and characteristically contain cholesterol crystals, which are a product of tissue breakdown.

The classification of cysts is difficult, but the most practical one is based on the pathogenesis of the lesion.

1. *Developmental.* See below.
2. *Inflammatory,* e.g. the periodontal cyst.
3. *Degenerative,* e.g. cystic changes in goitres, in solid tumours like the uterine myoma (fibroid), and in other pathological lesions like fibrous dysplasia of bone. The basic change is necrosis which is almost always ischaemic in origin. A degenerative cyst may occur in vascular disease, as in brain cysts following cerebral infarction, or in a tumour or other lesion with inadequate blood supply. The necrotic debris subsequently becomes liquefied.
4. *Retention,* e.g. a ranula, which is a cystic dilatation in the submandibular or sublingual gland formed as a result of obstruction of its duct. The name refers to the frog-like swelling produced—*ranula* is Latin for a little frog.
5. *Implantation.* See epidermoid cyst, page 126.
6. *Hydatid,* a parasitic cyst, found usually in the liver and lungs, due to the proliferation and expansion of the larval form of the canine tapeworm *Echinococcus granulosus.*
7. *Hyperplastic,* e.g. mammary dysplasia.
8. *Neoplastic,* e.g. cystadenoma of the ovary and cystic teratoma.

Developmental cysts. These may arise from ectopic tissues or from the persistence of vestigial remnants.

Ectopia of various tissues. In ectopia there is a dislocation of tissue into a neighbouring area, where it often becomes cystic. A good example is the *dermoid cyst,* which is due to the sequestration of a piece of skin beneath one of the lines of fusion of the various embryonic body processes. Dermoid cysts occur most commonly in the subcutaneous tissue of the face, usually near the angle of the orbit. Another site is under the tongue (sublingual dermoid). A dermoid cyst is lined by stratified squamous epithelium, and in its wall there are hair follicles, sebaceous glands, and sweat glands. It contains a thick, greasy material consisting of keratin produced by the epithelial lining and sebum secreted by the sebaceous glands. Matted hair is also often present. Unlike a teratoma, it does not include other tissues in its wall.

Persistence of vestigial remnants. Examples of this type are the branchial and thyroglossal cysts. A branchial cyst develops from a persisting portion of the cervical sinus; it is lined by stratified squamous epithelium and is surrounded by lymphoid tissue. Some odontogenic cysts are also due to the persistence of paradental remnants, e.g. the dentigerous cyst which surrounds the crown of an unerupted tooth, of either the regular or the supernumerary dentition. It is formed by the accumulation of fluid between the layers of the enamel epithelium or between the epithelium and the tooth crown.

REFERENCES

1. Brown G C 1966 Recent advances in the viral aetiology of congenital anomalies. Advances in Teratology, 1, 55, *loc cit*
2. Smithells R W 1966 Drugs and human malformations. Advances in Teratology, ed. Woollam D H M, 1, 251. London Logos Press
3. Leading Article 1962 Thalidomide and congenital malformations. Lancet, 1 : 307
4. Leading article 1962 Thalidomide: part 2. Lancet, 1 : 336
5. Lawrence D R 1973 Clinical Pharmacology, 4th edn., pp. 667–670. Churchill Livingstone, Edinburgh
6. Clarren S K, Smith D W 1978 The fetal alcohol syndrome. New England Journal of Medicine, 298: 1063
7. Bean W B 1958 Vascular Spiders and Related Lesions of the Skin. Blackwell, Oxford
8. Levene A 1972 Moles and melanoma: the pathological basis of clinical management. Proceedings of the Royal Society of Medicine, 65: 137
9. Mihm M C, Clark W H, From L 1971 The clinical diagnosis, classification and histogenetic concepts of the early stages of cutaneous malignant melanomas. New England Journal of Medicine 284: 1078
10. Brown N J 1976 Teratomas and yolk-sac tumours. Journal of Clinical Pathology, 29: 1021

25

The effects of ionizing radiation

Introduction

The ever-increasing use of radioactive substances in both industry and medicine has made the study of radiation damage of great practical importance. On the human body the effects of radiation vary from local tissue necrosis to genetic damage, cancer, and death. With such a perplexing array of effects it is little wonder that the ionizing radiations are regarded with fear and amazement. As their physical nature is so well understood, it might be expected that the mechanisms involved and the damage which they produce would be equally explicable. Such, however, is not the case.

The basic action of ionizing radiations is to produce changes in the structure of the atoms through which they pass. Such changes in turn lead to secondary events in molecules, cells, tissues, and finally in the individual as a whole. These events will be examined in turn, but with so many steps it is not surprising that there are many gaps in our knowledge of the pathogenesis of radiation damage.

Physical and chemical considerations

The energy of the absorbed radiation gives rise to the following changes:

1. Ions and free radicles are formed
2. There is excitation of molecules
3. Secondary electrons are generated, and these produce changes similar to (1) and (2) in adjacent areas.

The net effect is that molecules become more reactive and chemical changes ensue. Large biological molecules like DNA and proteins could be affected by two separate processes:

Direct action. Energy absorbed in the molecule itself may lead to chemical change, e.g. denaturation of a protein.

Indirect action. Alternatively chemical change may be induced in a large molecule as a result of the action of an adjacent ion or radicle, e.g. $OH^{\bullet}$ and $HO_2^{\bullet}$ radicles are formed from water. Powerful oxidizing agents, e.g. H_2O_2 are formed particularly when the radiation is performed in the presence of oxygen.

It is generally supposed that ionizing radiations produce a type of biochemical lesion, but if this is so its nature has so far eluded detection.

EFFECTS ON THE CELL[1]

Although it would be desirable to explain the cellular damage in terms of the known physico-chemical changes, it must be admitted that this is not yet possible. The effects of radiation on cells in culture may be summarized:

1. Immediate death of the cell occurs with very heavy dosage, i.e. 10 000 r* or more. This effect occurs regardless of the stage of mitosis and is called *interphase death.* It is also seen in very sensitive cells, e.g. small lymphocytes, with moderate dosage.
2. DNA synthesis is inhibited.
3. Mitosis is delayed, usually due to a prolongation of the G_2 phase (see p. 29).
4. DNA synthesis may occur unrelated to cell division so that giant-cell forms are produced. Giant fibroblasts are seen in irradiated skin.
5. When mitosis does occur in irradiated cells, abnormalities such as chromosome breaks may occur. At this stage the cell may die. Nevertheless, a cell may go through several mitotic cycles before death finally occurs.
6. The growth rate may be slowed down even in sublethally irradiated cells.
7. Fractionated doses of radiation do not produce a strictly cumulative effect. Hence there appear to exist intracellular mechanisms whereby radiation damage can be reversed or 'repaired'.
8. The sensitivity of cells to damage varies according to the stage in the cell cycle when the radiation is given. Maximum sensitivity occurs in most cell-types during mitosis itself. Cells are relatively resistant during most of the G_1 phase, but radiosensitivity returns during the late G_1 and early synthetic (S) phases. They are most resistant during the late S and early G_2 phases.

Two main theories have been put forward to explain the cellular damage:

The target theory supposes that the injury is due to damage in some specific sensitive spot in the cell. Attractive as it may be to visualize a chromosome or an organelle as a target, there is in fact very little to support this theory.

The poison theory proposes that the ionization leads to the production of poisonous substances, usually powerful oxidizing agents, which then cause the damage. There is considerable evidence that oxidizing substances are formed in irradiated tissue. Thus chemicals with a reducing action (e.g. cysteine) will give some degree of protection against ionizing radiation. Furthermore, if cells are irradiated in the absence of oxygen, they are 2 to 3 times more resistant. This is probably because free oxygen is necessary for the production of oxidizing substances by ionizing radiation. This observation is of some importance in clinical radiotherapy, because many areas of a tumour are relatively hypoxic and might conceivably be less sensitive to damage during irradiation therapy.[2]

EFFECTS ON THE INTACT ANIMAL

This most important aspect of radiobiology is also the most difficult. A feature which is outstanding is the remarkable *delay* in the appearance of radiation lesions.

* The letter r signifies roentgen, a commonly used measurement of radiation. One roentgen is that amount of radiation which under specified conditions produces in 1 ml. of air at NTP, one electrostatic unit of electricity of either charge.

The actual damage caused by radiation must be almost instantaneous, and yet the effect may not be apparent for days, months, or even years. Experiments with amphibians help to explain this phenomenon. Frogs can be given a dose of radiation which will kill them within 6 weeks. If the irradiated animals are kept at 5°C, they remain alive for several months, but on being warmed up die within 6 weeks, like the control animals kept at normal temperature.[3] The experiment indicates that radiation damage manifests itself only when cells are active. This lends strong support to the concept that a biochemical lesion is produced. Such a lesion is not in itself harmful, but produces effects when cellular activity commences. This goes some way in explaining two of the phenomena of radiation damage:

1. **Relative sensitivity of cells.** In the human the germinal cells of the ovary are the most sensitive. Then in sequence follow the seminiferous epithelium of the testis, lymphocytes, the erythropoietic and myeloid marrow cells, and the intestinal epithelium. Least sensitive are nerve cells and muscle cells. This order to some extent parallels the rate of cell division seen in the various tissues; thus neurons never divide, while epithelial tissue, especially that of the intestine, shows constant mitotic activity.

2. **The chronic nature of radiation lesions.** When tissue is irradiated, several phases of damage occur. This is probably because different tissues have different rates of division and metabolic activity, and therefore exhibit damage at different times. Hence an irradiated area shows changes which persist for many weeks or even months and have the characteristics of chronic inflammation, even after a single exposure.

When considering the action of radiation on any tissue, two main effects must be borne in mind.

The primary effect of radiation on the tissue concerned.

The secondary effect, which is due to damage to adjacent tissues. The most important example of this is the damage to vessels which, by causing thrombosis or endarteritis obliterans, leads to ischaemia. Some authorities attribute much of the beneficial effects of radiotherapy in cancer to this mechanism.

The effect of irradiation on individual tissues

Skin. Following a single exposure to ionizing radiation, redness (erythema) appears after about 10 days, and the skin shows all the features of acute inflammation. Pigmentation is increased, giving the skin a red dusky colour. With heavy dosage necrosis occurs, and ulceration results. Healing is often very slow, and ulceration may recur; even when healed the scar may break down after trivial injury so that chronic ulceration with much surrounding fibrosis is frequent. With lower dosage the blood vessels show endarteritis obliterans. The hair follicles and accessory glands are much more sensitive to radiation than is the less active surface epithelium. With a dosage of above 700 r these structures undergo necrosis, and do not regenerate. The delaying effect on wound healing is described in Chapter 8.

Gonads. The ovary and testis are particularly susceptible, and with a dosage of over 500 r the germinal cells are destroyed and permanent sterility results.

Lungs. Irradiation of the lungs produces inflammatory changes which culminate in fibrosis. This is sometimes seen as a complication of radiotherapy for lung, breast, and oesophageal cancers.

Bone. Irradiation of bone produces inflammatory changes which may persist for years, and are punctuated by episodes of painful radionecrosis. If the jaw is involved, radionecrosis is often precipitated by the extraction of teeth and complicated by infection. Doses of over 1000 r inhibit growth at the epiphysis, an effect of importance in children. Thus the coincidental irradiation of the mandibular condyle during the ill-advised treatment of an angiomatous hamartoma may lead to cessation of growth with consequent hypoplasia of the mandible.

Total body irradiation

The effects of total body irradiation depend on the dosage, and have been studied in people involved in atomic explosions. It is convenient to describe the effects of total body irradiation under two headings—those occurring during the first two months (immediate), and those occurring later.

Immediate effects

Although no hard-and-fast rules can be given, three groups of cases may be recognized:

Very heavy dosage (over 5000 r single exposure) produces severe effects due apparently to direct damage to the brain. Death occurs within a day or two following shock, convulsions, and coma.

Moderate dosage, 800 to 5000 r single exposure. Loss of appetite, nausea, and vomiting develop soon after irradiation, the reasons for which are not known. The symptoms usually abate, only to recur some 2 to 3 days later with intractable severity. This latter episode of vomiting is accompanied by severe diarrhoea due to necrosis of the intestinal epithelium. This is called the *gastrointestinal syndrome,* and usually results in death from dehydration and shock.

Low dosage, under 800 r single exposure. Initial nausea and vomiting are less severe, and the subject may then appear to make a complete recovery. Two or three weeks later the results of bone-marrow aplasia become apparent. The serious effects of irradiation during this *haematological phase* are due to damage to the haematopoietic tissues.

Blood changes following irradiation. *Lymphocytes.* Lymphopenia is the earliest blood change of total body irradiation, and is most marked after a day or two.

Granulocytes. The total granulocyte count falls after about a week, and may reach very low levels by the second to sixth weeks. This predisposes to infection, e.g. of the mouth and lungs.

Platelets. After a few days the number of platelets drops dramatically, and is very low by 4 weeks. This leads to a haemorrhagic tendency which may manifest itself either as trivial petechial haemorrhages into the skin or other organs, or as severe, possibly fatal, intestinal or pulmonary bleeding.

Red cells. Because the primitive, or erythroblastic, cells are highly radiosensitive and the mature red cells are resistant, the effect of bone-marrow aplasia on the peripheral count is delayed. The anaemia is of gradual onset and maximal at 6 to 8 weeks.

Late effects of total body irradiation

Those exposed to a sublethal dose may show the following after-effects:

The carcinogenic effect. It has been realized since the beginning of the century that tumours may develop after the application of ionizing radiation. The first case, a carcinoma of the skin, was reported in 1902, and subsequently *squamous-cell cancers of the skin* of the hands have been frequently seen in x-ray workers. This also occurred in dental surgeons who held films in position in the mouth. It is important for all those who use x-rays to avoid unnecessary exposure to radiation.

Another danger of exposure to ionizing radiation is the development of *leukaemia.* A high incidence of this disease has been recorded in the survivors of the Nagasaki and Hiroshima atomic explosions and in patients with ankylosing spondylitis treated with radiotherapy. However, the hazard of modern diagnostic radiology is slight.

Osteosarcoma has been reported to follow local irradiation years after the treatment of benign or inflammatory bone lesions. The tumour has also followed the injection or ingestion of radioactive substances, such as radium and mesothorium, which are stored in the bones.

Genetic effects. The ability of ionizing radiation to increase the rate of mutation is well established in micro-organisms, plants, and animals. In somatic cells this effect is probably not important, but in the germ cells it is of potential significance, since the new factor is handed down to subsequent generations. It may have a profoundly deleterious effect, since most mutations are harmful.

RADIOTHERAPY

The destructive effects of ionizing radiations on living cells, particularly those in an active state, have led to their widespread use in the treatment of malignant disease. Nowadays radiotherapy plays an important part in the curative treatment of some primary cancers, as well as in the palliation of those which have already metastasized, and are beyond the scope of surgical excision.

Factors influencing response

Tumours differ widely in their reaction to radiotherapy, and it is only after treatment has been commenced that the response can be assessed. However, some guide to the probable local results of treatment may be given by consideration of the following factors:

Tissue of origin. The relative sensitivities of normal tissues are often reflected in the radiosensitivities of the tumours derived from them. Thus lymphocytic lymphoma, like the parent lymphocyte, is very radiosensitive. Fibrosarcoma, however, like the fibroblasts from which it is derived, is radioresistant.

Degree of differentiation and mitotic activity. It is generally taught that within any tumour group the most undifferentiated tumours are also the most radiosensitive. As a generalization this is true, but nevertheless it is found that the histological appearances of an individual tumour are no sure guide to the results obtained in practice. It is found, for instance, that well-differentiated squamous-cell carcinomata of the skin and tongue frequently respond very well.

The tumour bed. The nature of the stroma supporting a tumour is probably important. If it is avascular as the result of previous irradiation, the tumour is more resistant. This may well be attributable to hypoxia. Some authorities maintain that the connective tissues have a restraining effect on the growth of the tumour. If excessive irradiation is given, the results are said to be much worse than if a modest dose is given, because under these circumstances the tumour bed itself is destroyed. It seems quite certain that all tumour cells are not destroyed by radiotherapy, and that the cure of the patient is related to some other destructive mechanism on the growth of the tumour.

Nature of the individual tumour. Certain tumours respond extremely well, for example most basal-cell and squamous-cell carcinomata of the skin. On the other hand, squamous-cell carcinoma of the lung generally responds poorly. It is evident that tumours of similar histological appearance in different organs may react very differently to irradiation. The reason for this is not known.

Cure rate

The *cure rate* to be expected from radiotherapy must, as with surgical treatment, be considered in relation to the general properties of the tumour. Many malignant conditions, for example lymphoma, cannot be considered as local diseases, and although a tumour mass may respond remarkably well to treatment, the disease progresses sooner or later to its inevitable end. Oat-cell carcinoma of the lung is a similar example.

Radiotherapy is often effective as a palliative treatment. It can reduce the size of a tumour mass and produce relief of symptoms. This is well seen in mediastinal tumours producing obstruction to the great vessels. Radiotherapy may also control haemorrhage from a bleeding tumour, and help to clear up a fungating carcinoma of the breast. Pain from bony metastases may be alleviated. Slowly-growing tumours, like cancer of the breast and Hodgkin's disease, can sometimes be held in check for long periods, and the patient given several years of useful life. It may well be that radiotherapy and surgery are both forms of palliation which allow the body to retard the growth of the tumour. Depending on whether the malignant cells stay dormant for a short or long period, one may speak of a five-year cure, ten-year cure, etc. There is increasing evidence, however, that on some occasions a thorough eradication of malignant cells is effected by the combined action of therapeutic measures, whether surgical excision, ionising radiation, or cytotoxic drugs, on the one hand, and the natural defences of the body on the other. In these cases the patient's life-span is no shorter than that of a healthy control, and we may speak with growing confidence of a complete cure.

GENERAL READING

Alexander P 1957 Atomic Radiation and Life, A simple account of ionising radiations and their effects. Penguin, Harmondsworth, 239 pp

Bacq Z M, Alexander P 1961 Fundamentals of Radiobiology, 2nd edn, Pergamon Press, Oxford, 555 pp. Both this and the first edition (1955, Butterworth, London) should be consulted for details on specific aspects of radiobiology

Cronkite E P, Bond V P 1960 Radiation Injury in Man, Thomas, Springfield, Illinois, 200 pp

Glasser O, Quimby E H, Taylor L S, Weatherwax J L, Morgan R H 1961 Physical Foundations of Radiology, 3rd edn, Pitman Medical, London, 503 pp

Mole R H 1960 The toxicity of radiation. In: Recent Advances in Pathology—7 ed. Harrison C V, Churchill, London, pp 339–383

Rubin P, Casarett G W 1968 Clinical Radiation Pathology, Vol. 2, Saunders, Philadelphia, pp 518–1057

Warren S 1970 Radiation carcinogenesis. Bulletin of the New York Academy of Medicine, 46:131

REFERENCES

1. Little J B 1968 Cellular effects of ionising radiation. New England Journal of Medicine, 278:308 and 369
2. Leading Article 1972 Hyperbaric oxygen and radiotherapy. British Medical Journal, 2:368
3. Patt H M, Swift M N 1948 Influence of temperature on the response of frogs to X irradiation. American Journal of Physiology, 155:388

26

The general reaction to trauma: haemorrhage and shock

Following major trauma there ensues a complex series of changes from which scarcely any tissue of the body escapes. The nervous system responds promptly with an increased outflow of autonomic impulses. There is an immediate outpouring of catecholamines from the adrenal medulla, while the other endocrine glands respond more slowly: stimulation of the hypothalamus leads to an increase in the secretion of ACTH from the pituitary gland, which in turn results in adrenocortical overactivity. These changes assist the injured animal to withstand trauma; in fact, there is little doubt that the adrenalectomized animal is less equipped to withstand infection and trauma than is the normal.

One very obvious early effect of trauma involves the circulatory system. When the trauma is severe, a state develops from which recovery may not occur; this is called *shock*, and is characterized by inadequate perfusion of the tissues, hypotension, and depression of general metabolic activity.

If the patient survives, there ensue metabolic changes that terminate in complete recovery. This is called the period of *convalescence.*

For descriptive purposes therefore it is convenient to consider the response to injury under three headings:

The metabolic changes.
The circulatory changes.
Shock.

THE METABOLIC CHANGES[1]

These changes may be considered under the following headings:

The early, or ebb, phase.
Convalescence: (*a*) *Catabolic phase.*
(*b*) *Anabolic phase.*

The early or ebb phase

The early response to injury is termed the low flow, or ebb, phase. After severe injury it is an accompaniment of the state of shock. It is characterized by a reduction in the metabolic rate, a reduced body temperature, and an increased output of catecholamines from the adrenal medulla (see Table 26.1). The increased blood level of catecholamines has several effects:

1. There is increased glycolysis in the liver.

2. Lactic acid is released from the muscles and is converted into glucose in the liver (Cori cycle). The result of all this is hyperglycaemia and possibly glycosuria.

3. A reduction in insulin secretion promotes gluconeogenesis in the liver, and this contributes to the hyperglycaemia.

4. Catecholamines have a lipolytic effect, and fatty acids are released from the adipose tissues. The blood level of fatty acids is therefore raised. The metabolic acidosis that accompanies this ebb phase in shocked patients is considered on page 421.

Table 26.1 Metabolic changes following injury*

	Low-flow phase	High-flow phase
Metabolic rate	↓	↑
Body temperature	↓	↑
Catecholamine output	↑	Normal or slightly ↑
Blood insulin level	↓	↑
Blood glucose	↑	Normal or slightly ↑
Blood lactate	↑	Normal or slightly ↑
Blood fatty acid	↑	↓

**Modified from Ryan N T* 1976 Metabolic adaptations for energy production during trauma and sepsis. Surgical Clinics of North America 56: 1073

Convalescence

Assuming that the patient survives the initial phase and does not die of shock, there ensues a period of metabolic upset that has been termed the *high-flow phase*, or simply the *flow phase.* This has two components: (*a*) a *catabolic phase*, which is characterized by excessive protein breakdown and a negative nitrogen balance, followed by (*b*) an *anabolic phase*, during which the body's stores are replenished. These important metabolic changes are highly complex and are incompletely understood. They have been studied extensively both in animals and the human subject.

The catabolic phase

During the catabolic phase there is increased glucose production in the liver (Table 26.1). This gluconeogenesis is fed by lactate, pyruvate, and alanine and other animo acids derived from muscle, which are used as substrates. The breakdown of muscle components, particularly the proteins, for use in energy generation leads to muscular atrophy and a consequent loss of weight. The nitrogen of the metabolized amino acids is excreted as urea, and the body enters a phase of negative nitrogen balance. The duration of this nitrogen loss varies with the extent of the trauma: after a minor surgical procedure it may last only a day or two, but with severe burns it can continue for 10 days or more. Fractures cause more disturbance than might be supposed from the clinical condition; suppuration may prolong the catabolic state for weeks. The following points should be noted:

1. The nitrogen loss cannot be abolished by increasing the protein intake; any extra protein in the diet is broken down and the extra nitrogen excreted. There is therefore no point in forcing patients to ingest protein during this phase.

2. The administration of carbohydrate does reduce the nitrogen loss very considerably.

3. Protein starvation prior to injury depletes the protein reserve of the body, and virtually abolishes the nitrogen loss.

4. Patients with Addison's disease and adrenalectomized animals do not show any post-traumatic nitrogen loss.

During the catabolic phase there is an increased production of insulin two or three times above normal. Nevertheless, the tissues appear to be resistant to the action of insulin, and gluconeogenesis is stimulated by the unopposed action of cortisol. The relative lack of insulin activity is the probable mechanism whereby amino acids are released from muscle. There is, however, sufficient insulin activity to inhibit lipolysis; hence fatty acids are not released from the adipose tissues, and while the muscles waste as a result of protein loss, the adipose tissues remain intact. This contrasts to the situation encountered in simple starvation.

Mechanism of the protein loss. The following should be noted:

1. The metabolic effects of injury are closely simulated by the effects of glucocorticoids.

2. The adrenal glands are known to enlarge following injury.

3. There is an increased secretion of adrenal cortical hormones after trauma.

4. Adrenalectomized animals do not show this nitrogen loss.

It would therefore not be unreasonable to assume that excessive adrenal function explains the loss of nitrogen, but that this is not the case is shown by the finding that adrenalectomized animals (and human subjects) on a constant maintenance dose of cortisol still show the same negative nitrogen balance when subjected to trauma. It would therefore appear that adrenal hormones are necessary for this metabolic change but do not directly produce it. It may be that they play a permissive role, but the increase in cortisol production is not the direct mechanism involved in the metabolic changes.

Other metabolic changes. *Sodium and water metabolism.* During the early period after trauma the urine volume diminishes owing to an increased secretion of ADH, and sodium is retained by the kidneys as a result of increased aldosterone secretion. This phase of sodium retention is a little shorter than the catabolic phase; it has been held that this is obligatory, and that the body is defenceless against overdosage, because it cannot excrete sodium and water (see p. 423).

There is a later return of sodium to the urine; unless there was excessive administration during the oliguric phase, its excretion is little increased.

Potassium metabolism. A negative balance occurs during the initial phase, and is most marked on the first day. Because potassium is intracellular, it is presumed to be liberated at the same time as protein is metabolized.

Other changes. There is an increased urinary excretion of *creatine* (derived from the muscles), *phosphate*, and *sulphur*. This occurs *pari passu* with the nitrogenous and potassium excretion, and is due to cellular breakdown.

Vitamin C is retained, its excretion in the urine being dramatically reduced. A scorbutic state may develop despite this careful guarding of the ascorbic-acid stores. *Riboflavin*, on the other hand, is excreted in excess.

During this catabolic phase there is a marked loss of weight. A moderate *pyrexia* is invariable, and is not due to concomitant infection.

The haematological changes are a moderate neutrophilia accompanied by a lymphopenia and eosinopenia. There is also a thrombocytosis (see p. 482). An interesting feature of severe trauma is the development of a progressive normocytic, normochromic anaemia. This is not due to iron deficiency; it may be that there is deficient haemoglobin synthesis during a period of general protein breakdown. Sludging may accentuate this anaemia (see p. 409).

The anabolic phase

The final stage of convalescence is characterized by a positive nitrogen balance and a resynthesis of muscle protein. The changes noted during the catabolic phase are reversed, and the body returns to normal.

THE CIRCULATORY CHANGES

The changes in the circulation are seen to their best advantage following acute haemorrhage; this will therefore be described first.

HAEMORRHAGE

Haemorrhage is defined as the escape of blood from the vascular system. The extravasated blood may escape to the exterior or it may remain internal.

Types of haemorrhage

External. Blood may be coughed up (*haemoptysis*), passed in the urine (*haematuria*), vomited (*haematemesis*), or be passed in the faeces either as fresh blood or, if from higher up in the intestinal tract, as a black, partially digested mass (*melaena*).

Internal. Small flat haemorrhages, less than 2 mm in diameter, are called *petechiae*, or *purpuric spots*; they are usually found in the skin and mucous membranes. A larger, more diffuse, haemorrhagic area is called an *ecchymosis*. A *haematoma* is a discrete pool of blood, usually clotted, in a tissue. Collections of blood in natural spaces are named anatomically, e.g. *haemothorax* (in the pleural cavity), *haemopericardium*, *haemoperitoneum*, *haemarthrosis* (in a joint cavity), etc.

Causes of acute haemorrhage

Trauma. Penetrating wounds involving the heart or large vessels may result in the very rapid loss of large quantities of blood.

Abnormalities in the blood-vessel wall. *Inflammatory lesions* may cause weakening of a vessel wall, usually arterial, with subsequent rupture. Aneurysmal dilatation may occur before the final rupture. The inflammation need not always be infective, e.g. polyarteritis nodosa.

Neoplastic invasion. Haemorrhage is a frequent terminal event in carcinoma of the tongue, and is due to rupture of the lingual artery; superimposed infection is a major factor in the weakening of the wall.

Other vascular diseases. Atheroma, either with or without aneurysmal dilatation, is the most common cause. Aneurysms due to trauma or persistent friction, e.g. subclavian aneurysm due to cervical rib, also fall into this category.

High blood pressure within the vessels. Systemic hypertension may precipitate haemorrhage at sites of arterial weakness. Raised venous pressure with varicose-vein formation, e.g. in the oesophagus, is another important cause of severe haemorrhage.

Effects of acute haemorrhage

The vascular system contains about 5 litres of blood, which is kept in motion by the action of the heart so that all the tissues are adequately perfused. The amount of blood reaching any area is determined by two factors—the *calibre of the arterioles supplying it* and the *blood pressure.*

The capacious venous system acts as a reservoir for the blood, and therefore when a small quantity is lost, an increase in venous tone reduces the capacity of the circulatory system, so that there is no reduction in the volume of blood reaching the heart (the venous return). Therefore there is no reduction in the cardiac output. When a larger volume of blood is suddenly withdrawn, this reserve mechanism is inadequate. The venous return is diminished, the cardiac output falls, and with it the amount of blood available for perfusing the organs. It is therefore not surprising that the next response to haemorrhage is a series of reactions designed to restore the blood pressure.

Restoration of blood pressure and redistribution of blood[2]. *Mechanism.* The fall in blood pressure is detected by the pressure-sensitive carotid sinus and the other baroreceptors, and these reflexly initiate a sympathetic outflow from the central nervous system (Fig. 26.1). The effect is a *vasoconstriction* of the arterioles of the *skin*, *kidneys*, and *splanchnic area* by direct action, as well as indirectly *via* the adrenal medulla, which is stimulated to secrete adrenaline and noradrenaline. The lowered blood pressure acts on the juxtaglomerular apparatus and causes the kidney to release renin (p. 478). There is therefore an over-all increase in the peripheral resistance. The blood pressure is restored, and the blood flow to the brain, heart, and respiratory muscles remains almost unaltered. However, the areas affected by arteriolar vasoconstriction tend to suffer; for example the *skin* is cold and pale, the *kidneys* show a reduced urinary output (oliguria), and the *salivary glands* cease to secrete. Thus the vasomotor response to acute haemorrhage causes a *redistribution of blood*, a mechanism which may be regarded as an emergency measure designed to keep the essential organs supplied.

Restoration of blood volume. During the first few hours after a haemorrhage extravascular fluids pass into the blood stream, the volume of which is thereby restored. This is easily demonstrated by following the haemoglobin level. Immediately after a sudden haemorrhage the *haemoglobin level is normal.* During the next 8 hours it falls as dilution occurs, and this process is largely complete by the end of 48 hours. At this stage therefore the haemoglobin level is a good guide to the extent of the previous blood loss. This transfer of extracellular fluid to the blood stream appears to be the result of the reduced capillary hydrostatic pressure which follows the arteriolar vasoconstriction. The osmotic pressure of the plasma due to its protein content is now greater than the hydrostatic pressure, and fluid is drawn into the blood until a balance is achieved (p. 425). Complete restoration of the plasma volume is dependent upon replacement of the lost plasma proteins.

These enter the circulation *via* the thoracic duct, and are primarily contributed by the liver.

Changes in the blood. Within a few minutes of bleeding the clotting time is considerably decreased, and during the next few hours there is a considerable increase in the level of platelets and neutrophils, which persists for several days.

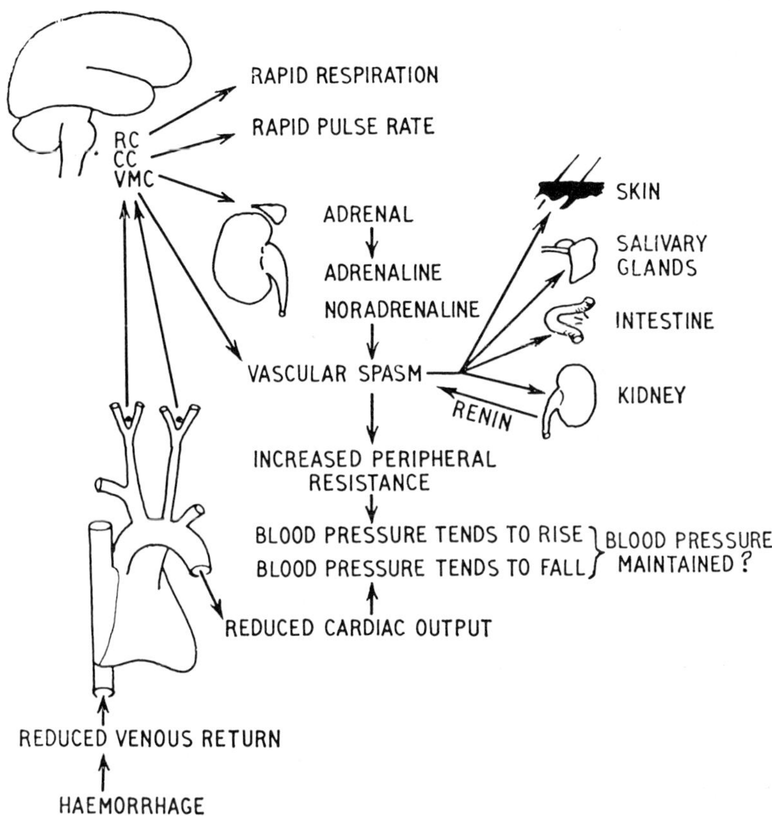

Fig. 26.1 The cardiovascular effects of sudden haemorrhage. RC (Respiratory Centre). CC (Cardiac Centre). VMC (Vasomotor Centre).

The restoration of the red-cell count is a much slower process, since the body has virtually no reserve store of erythrocytes. New red cells have to be manufactured, and a normal count is not attained until 4 to 6 weeks later.

The effects of acute haemorrhage depend upon both the volume and the speed with which the blood is lost. The normal adult can donate one pint (approx. 500 ml, or 10 per cent of the blood volume) with little discomfort. A sudden loss of 30 to 50 per cent may well be fatal; however, if spread over a day or so it can be tolerated. If the haemorrhage is so severe that the compensatory mechanisms are inadequate to maintain an adequate blood flow to vital organs, death ensues. This constitutes one variety of *shock*, a subject which will now be considered.

SHOCK[3]

Shock is the name given to a clinical state in which the patient has tachycardia (an increased heart rate), and is pale, ashen, and sweating. Two quite separate conditions have been included:

Vasovagal attack, primary shock, or syncope

Immediately following injury or loss of blood, a patient may feel nauseated. become giddy, and finally lose consciousness. Convulsions occasionally occur. The attack rarely lasts more than a few minutes, and causes no permanent damage. It is sometimes seen after quite trivial injury, e.g. the insertion of a needle, or even, in nervous individuals, at the suggestion of injury. The attack appears to be mediated by a vasomotor imbalance so that widespread vasodilatation occurs in the skeletal muscles. The blood pressure drops, the heart rate slows, and the cerebral blood flow diminishes so that consciousness is lost[2]. If the patient is laid horizontally, or attains that position spontaneously, recovery soon occurs. In rare cases death may occur—at least this is one suggestion for the rare cases of sudden death which occur unexpectedly, e.g. when introducing a needle into the pleural cavity or during an attempted abortion. It has been reported that syncope occurring during the induction of anaesthesia may be fatal if the anaesthetic is administered with the patient in the upright position, e.g. in a dental chair.

Secondary shock

This is a much more important condition, and it is best to restrict the unqualified term 'shock' to it. Shock is seen following many forms of injury; it may occur immediately, or there may be a period of comparative well-being before the characteristic features make their appearance. The patient lies still and apathetic, the temperature is subnormal, the skin cold and clammy, and the face ashen grey. Obvious cyanosis may be present. The blood pressure is low, and the pulse rapid and thready. Little or no urine is passed.

The clinical picture of shock may occur in a variety of conditions, and not surprisingly these have all been assembled under the all-embracing title of 'shock'. They are:

Loss of blood (haemorrhagic shock)
Post-traumatic
Loss of plasma, e.g. burns
Loss of fluid and electrolytes
Overwhelming infection
Cardiogenic shock
Anaphylactic shock.

The inclusion of so many divergent syndromes under one heading has tended to obscure our understanding of the condition. They all produce a similar clinical picture which is described as shock, but it is hardly to be expected that the mechanisms involved would be the same in each case. It should also be remembered that a state of shock frequently precedes death regardless of the cause, e.g.

electrocution, overdose of drugs, drowning, or following massive total body irradiation (p. 396). To attempt to understand 'shock' it is necessary to consider each cause separately.

Haemorrhagic shock. If following a large haemorrhage the compensatory mechanisms described on p. 404 fail to maintain the blood pressure, either as a result of their own inefficiency, or the excessive load placed upon them by a large haemorrhage, the patient enters into a state of shock. Recovery may occur spontaneously, or as a result of efficient treatment, e.g. transfusion; such shock is therefore said to be *reversible*. It sometimes happens that in spite of vigorous and efficient treatment the blood pressure continues to fall, the patient's clinical condition deteriorates, and death ensues. This is *irreversible shock*.

Traumatic shock. The circulatory changes which follow trauma are very similar to those following haemorrhage. Initial *syncope* may occur, to be followed shortly by secondary shock. The possible causes of the latter are:

Haemorrhage It is often not appreciated that injury, apart from causing external bleeding, leads to an extensive blood loss into the tissues. Thus in a closed fracture of the femur 4 pints of blood may be lost. It is obvious that the swelling of injured parts is produced either by extravasated blood or by inflammatory exudate, i.e. plasma.

In surgical operations it is very important to estimate the amount of blood lost so that it can be replaced. The amount on swabs can be estimated by weighing, or by extracting the haemoglobin and measuring it colorimetrically.

Toxins from damaged tissue have been postulated, but their importance has never been substantiated.

Infection of the wound. There is little doubt that the powerful exotoxins of the pathogenic clostridia exert a profound effect on the circulation. Gas-gangrene even in the absence of substantial traumatic damage causes a shock-like state which may result in death.

Endotoxic factor. Since the generalized Shwartzman phenomenon resembles shock, it has been suggested that following trauma the intestinal coliform organisms or their endotoxins enter the blood stream and cause a similar reaction. Nevertheless, this has not been substantiated as an important cause of human traumatic shock, although it is probably important in the severe shock which develops in patients with Gram-negative septicaemia (see below).

In summary, it seems that *blood loss is the most important factor in traumatic shock.*

Shock following burns. The severe shock which follows burning appears to be due to the tremendous loss of plasma in the inflammatory exudate. At a later stage infection with organisms, e.g. *Ps. aeruginosa*, may play a part. An important point of difference from haemorrhagic shock is that there is haemoconcentration rather than haemodilution.

Shock due to loss of fluid and electrolytes. Loss of fluid or sodium can lead to such depletion of the extracellular tissue fluids that, unless replacement therapy is instituted, a state of shock develops due to the inadequacy of the circulating plasma volume. This is seen in pyloric stenosis, intestinal obstruction, and cholera, and also in heat-exhaustion due to loss of salt and water in the sweat. As in the shock of burns there is haemoconcentration, and the increased viscosity of the blood further impedes the blood flow through the tissues.

In the examples of shock so far considered, it is believed that the capacity of the circulatory system is either normal or reduced. The major factor at fault is a diminished volume of circulating fluid. The term *hypovolaemic shock* is therefore often used. It is evident that a state of shock could also occur if the *capacity* of the circulatory system were to increase without a corresponding increase in blood *volume*. This certainly occurs in the transient vasovagal attack, and is probably the explanation of the shock in severe infections, e.g. septicaemia, and in the Shwartzman phenomenon. This type of shock is often called *peripheral vascular failure*, and is due to peripheral vasodilatation which produces pooling of blood. Often it seems that the blood accumulates in the splanchnic area.

Shock in infection. Shock is seen in a variety of infections. It is prominent in infections with toxic organisms, e.g. diphtheria and gas-gangrene, but it is also a feature of many other severe infections—pneumonia, peritonitis, etc. In recent years a new syndrome, *endotoxic shock* (bacteraemic or Gram-negative shock), has been recognized, and is caused by the sudden entry of Gram-negative organisms into the circulation. It is a complication of any coliform infection, but is usually seen as a sequel to urinary infection. There is a sudden onset of profound shock, and unless treated expeditiously this carries a high mortality. The condition bears some resemblance to the shock seen in the generalized Shwartzman reaction (p. 105).

The shock seen in infection is of complex pathogenesis: at least three factors should be considered:

Peripheral circulatory failure due to vasodilatation and pooling of blood, especially in the splanchnic area. This occurs in septicaemic plague, endotoxic shock, and probably in other infections and toxaemias.

Loss of fluid in the exudate. In gas-gangrene the profuse loss of protein-rich exudate is responsible for the haemoconcentration and reduction in blood volume.

Heart failure. Bacterial toxins, e.g. diphtheria toxin, may damage the myocardium, and an element of heart failure may further embarrass an already failing circulation.

Cardiogenic shock. Myocardial infarction, severe cardiac dysrhythmias, and the sudden accumulation of fluid in the pericardium may sometimes lead to a state of shock which resembles that following trauma. A low cardiac output with underperfusion of the tissues is the initial effect, but the resulting metabolic acidosis (see below) causes peripheral vasodilatation and pooling of blood.

Anaphylactic shock. See Chapter 13.

The metabolic upset during shock[4]

A patient in shock shows a profound *reduction in metabolic rate*, the nature of which is not well understood; it appears that there is a block in carbohydrate utilization. In spite of cutaneous vasoconstriction, and therefore a reduction in heat loss, *the body's temperature falls*. An important effect of shock is that the under-perfusion of tissues results in anaerobic glycolysis with the release of pyruvic and lactic acids into the circulation. There is therefore often a severe *metabolic acidosis* (see p. 421). It is evident that an important aspect of shock is that tissues are underperfused with blood. Indeed, it has been stated that 'shock is not merely a problem of blood volume, blood pressure, and anaemia, but essentially a problem of flow'. A factor to be considered in this respect is sludging.

Sludging

If the flowing blood of a shocked patient is observed, it will be seen that the red cells are clumped together. This differs from true agglutination in that the masses can be broken up, though with some difficulty. The original description of the phenomenon described the blood as being converted into a 'muck-like sludge'—hence the name *sludging*. The *cause* of this is an increase in the level of high-molecular-weight substances (e.g. fibrinogen) in the plasma and a reduction in

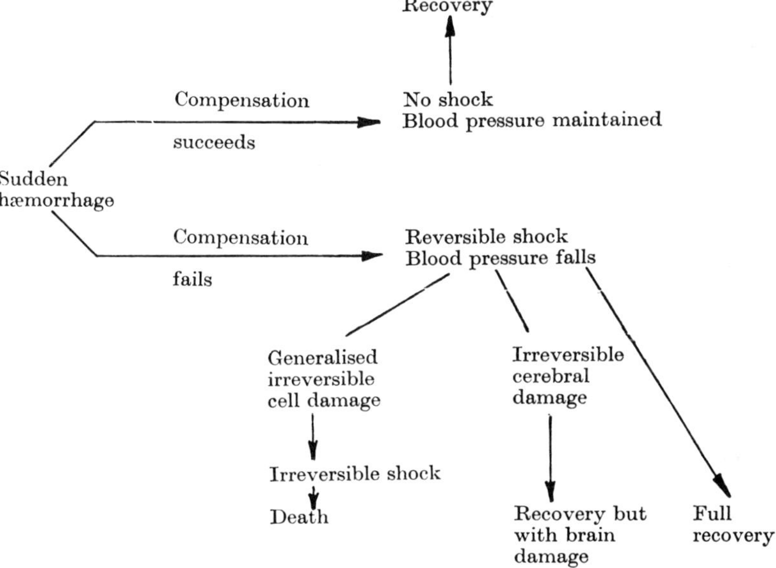

Fig 26.2 The possible end-results of a sudden haemorrhage.

the low-molecular-weight albumin. The ESR is increased (p. 436). The *effect* is to impede the blood flow through the tissues. Sludging can be prevented or reversed by the infusion of low-molecular-weight substances; for example dextran of MW 40 000 daltons has been used.

Irreversible shock

Some patients with shock recover either spontaneously or as a result of treatment. Others steadily deteriorate in spite of all efforts to save them and there has arisen a concept that there exists a stage from which recovery is impossible. This is called *irreversible shock* (Fig. 26.2).

The causes and the concept. These must now be examined:

Prolonged underperfusion of tissue. Although the selective vasoconstriction and redistribution of blood flow tide the patient over the initial period following injury, they may, if they persist, lead to permanent damage. The *kidney* is particularly vulnerable, and complete anuria may result. However, it is unlikely that this could kill the patient in as short a time as 24 to 48 hours, the duration of irreversible shock. Superadded *heart failure* and *liver damage* have also been suggested as important factors in making shock irreversible. Also the *metabolic acidosis* may induce vasodilatation and further lower the blood pressure. Whatever the mechanism, there is little doubt that the longer a patient remains in shock, the less likely is he to recover.

Infection. The toxaemia of severe infection may damage vital tissues and cause peripheral circulatory failure. This has already been described.

Inefficient treatment[5]. It is sometimes not fully appreciated that in hypovolaemic shock the appropriate fluid, whether blood, plasma, or electrolyte-containing fluid, must be poured into the circulation until the blood volume is adequate. The slow drip has no place in the treatment of massive haemorrhage! Large quantities must be given rapidly, and the only limiting factor is the occurrence of an increase in systemic venous pressure, which indicates that the heart is failing to deal with the venous return. A catheter attached to a manometer should therefore be placed in the jugular vein while transfusions are being given. More recently measurement of the left atrial pressure has been regarded as a more reliable guide.

Patients in shock are very susceptible to the action of depressant drugs like morphine and anaesthetic agents, and may easily be killed by overdosage. Alcohol induces cutaneous vasodilatation, and adds to the hypotension and hypothermia already present. It therefore should not be given to shocked patients.

Damage to vital organs. An injured patient may have sustained damage to some vital organ, e.g. a laceration of the brain or bleeding into the pericardium. Unless relieved death will ensue—apparently from the mysterious 'shock'.

Conclusion. There are many features about shock which we do not understand. Nevertheless, vigorous, well-designed treatment can save many cases. 'Shock' is not a diagnosis which should be accepted unqualified; it indicates that something is wrong—a low blood volume, metabolic acidosis, sludging, arterial desaturation, renal failure, pericardial haemorrhage, etc., all of which may be diagnosed and treated. With severe injury, in old age, and in the chronic sick, death may be inevitable, but the diagnosis of irreversible shock can be made only *post mortem.*

SUMMARY

The changes that occur in the wounded animal from the time of injury to the return to complete health are highly complex.

During the first few hours the response is concerned largely with circulatory adjustments, the aim of which appears to be the maintenance of an adequate blood supply to vital organs. Energy production is reduced, and the body's temperature falls. Thus the animal needs little food, and is spared the necessity of hunting. During the catabolic phase of convalescence fluid and sodium are retained to help maintain the circulation; in addition, they are needed for the inflammatory exudate around the wound. Energy is now provided by the protein stores, which are also used to build the new tissues during repair and regeneration. As convalescence proceeds and the wounded area heals, so the animal becomes fit enough to resume its search for nourishment. Protein catabolism ceases, and energy is produced from ingested food; the depleted stores are replaced, and health is restored.

REFERENCES

1. Ryan N T 1976 Metabolic adaptations for energy production during trauma and sepsis. Surgical Clinics of North America 56: 1073
2. Dickinson C J, Pentecost B L 1974 In Clinical Physiology, Campbell E J M, Dickinson C J, Slater J D H 4th edn, p. 69. Blackwell, Oxford
3. Shires G T, Carrico C J, Canizaro P C 1973 Shock. Saunders, Philadelphia
4. Baue A E 1976 Metabolic abnormalities of shock, Surgical Clinics of North America 56: 1059
5. Walt A J, Wilson R F 1975 Treatment of shock, Advances in Surgery 9: 1

27

Temperature regulation: fever and hypothermia

Introduction

One of the most important developments in the higher animals is the evolution of mechanisms whereby a constant environment is maintained for its constituent cells. This fixity of the internal environment has been well recognized since the time of Claude Bernard. Temperature regulation is an important aspect of homeostasis, which in the case of the human being and other warm-blooded mammals has attained a high degree of efficiency. Cellular activity, involving as it does numerous chemical reactions largely dependent upon enzymatic activity, is very susceptible to changes in temperature. On the other hand, some of the energy released during cell metabolism is emitted as heat. Indeed, the temperature of highly active organs, like the brain and heart, would rise were it not for the cooling effect of the blood stream which carries away the excess heat, and distributes it to those areas where it can be dissipated to the atmosphere, viz. the skin and the mucosa of the upper respiratory tract.

It is probable that the development of a reliable temperature-regulating mechanism has contributed considerably to the biological supremacy of the warm-blooded group of animals.

The normal body temperature

Methods of measuring. Body temperature is usually measured with the thermometer placed under the tongue, or else in the axilla, groin, or rectum. Of these readings, those obtained from the axilla and groin show the widest variation, and are generally regarded as being least reliable. This is hardly surprising, since the surface skin temperature fluctuates widely, and may approximate to that of the external environment. The rectal temperature is highest, being about 0.3°C (1°F) higher than the arterial temperature. It is said to be the least responsive to changes in the arterial temperature. Thus, if warm saline is infused into a vein, the rise in blood temperature is reflected in an elevation of the sublingual temperature but not that of the rectum. The sublingual temperature taken with the lips closed is therefore held to be the most reliable guide to the arterial temperature.

Normal variation. The normal temperature taken in this way is 36.8°C (98°F), with a range of 36.1°C to 37.4°C (97°F to 99.3°F). The maximum temperature is generally attained at about 6 p.m., while it is at its lowest at about 3 a.m. In women there is an elevation of the temperature during the middle of the menstrual cycle; its onset is thought to herald ovulation and is probably caused by the action of certain steroid hormones.

Mechanism of temperature regulation[1]

The constancy of the body's temperature is maintained by balancing the amount of heat gained with that lost.

Sources of heat. The major source of heat is from the body's metabolic activity. Heat production under fasting conditions with the individual at complete mental and physical rest is called the *Basal Metabolic Rate* (*BMR*).This ranges from 1400 to 1800 calories per day. Under active conditions additional heat is produced by *exercise* and the *ingestion of food*, especially protein. Fever itself affects the BMR, a rise of 1°C in body temperature increasing it by about 10 per cent.

Sources of heat loss. Heat is lost from the blood as it perfuses the skin—evaporation of sweat, conduction, and convection all play a part. Since the blood supply to the skin is regulated by the autonomic nervous system, the latter plays a dominant role in the maintenance of a constant body temperature. Some heat is also lost from the respiratory tract, and in animals this can be increased by panting.

The temperature regulating mechanism

Mechanisms are present for both increasing and decreasing the body's temperature. These come into play in response to impulses from the temperature-sensitive receptors. These receptors are situated both centrally within the nervous system and peripherally, mainly in the skin. A change of as little as 0.2°C can activate the compensatory mechanisms.

The central receptor. Situated in the anterior part of the hypothalamus, in the *preoptic area,* is a group of nerve cells that are sensitive to the temperature of the arterial blood reaching them. When the temperature of the blood changes, impulses pass from this area to other parts of the hypothalamus. There are two main areas: (1) an anterior *heat-losing centre,* which when stimulated leads to changes in the remainder of the body, causing increased heat loss, and (2) a posterior *heat-promoting centre*, which when stimulated leads to increased heat production and conservation (Fig. 27.1).

Peripheral temperature receptors. The heat-regulating mechanism is also influenced by impulses received from the peripheral receptors mainly in the skin. The peripheral receptors are of greatest importance when the body's temperature falls. Impulses then pass to the posterior centre in the hypothalamus and lead to conservation of heat.

Mechanism of decreasing body temperature. When the body's temperature tends to rise, there is a withdrawal of sympathetic vasoconstriction activity, the skin becomes warm, and heat is lost. The subject feels hot and may remove clothing, retire to the shade, or take other appropriate action. If this regulating mechanism does not suffice, the heat-losing centre initiates *sweating* from the eccrine glands. Evaporation of this fluid requires heat, but an additional effect of sweating is the local release of bradykinin from the glands. This induces further vasodilatation and heat loss.

Mechanism for increasing body temperature. The heat-promoting centre acts mainly through the sympathetic division of the autonomic nervous system. Cutaneous vasoconstriction reduces the amount of heat lost from the skin, and blood diverted to the internal organs is insulated from the exterior by the subcutaneous fat. Furthermore, as the skin becomes cooler, the subject feels cold and may take appropriate voluntary action such as putting on extra clothing.

An important effect of increased sympathetic activity is generalized *increase in muscle tone.* This alone can increase heat production by 50 per cent: the mechanism

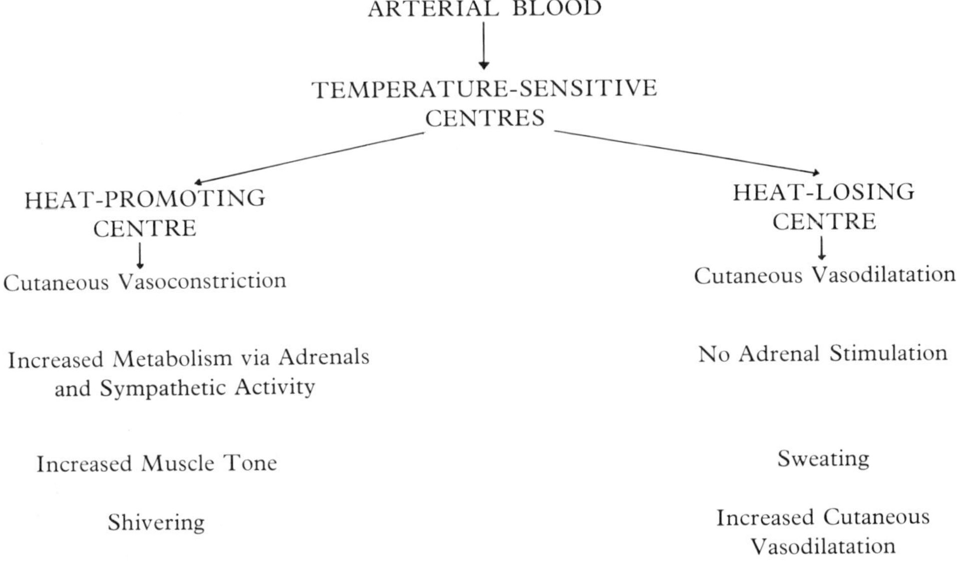

Fig. 27.1 Diagram to illustrate the principal heat-regulating mechanisms.

appears to be related to a partial uncoupling of oxidative phosphorylation. The increased sympathetic outflow causes an increased output of adrenaline and noradrenaline from the adrenal glands. Together with the increased sympathetic tone, these hormones increase the metabolic rate of cells by a mechanism that is not well understood.

If these mechanisms are inadequate, muscle tone increases to the extent that stretch reflexes are elicited and *shivering* commences. As one group of muscles contracts, so a stretch reflex of the antagonistic group is set in motion and initiates a fresh stretch reflex of the first group. This continuous shaking can increase the rate of heat production several fold

Fever[1,2]

Fever, also called *pyrexia,* may be defined as an elevation of the body's temperature consequent upon a disturbance of the regulating mechanism. When the temperature reaches or exceeds 40.5°C (104°F) the condition is called *hyperpyrexia.* Fever occurs under the following conditions:

Causes of fever

Heat-stroke. A rise in body temperature normally occurs during severe exercise when the heat-eliminating mechanisms cannot keep pace with the excessive heat production in the muscles. When the environment is hot and humid, even mild exercise may cause a marked rise in body temperature. This in turn increases the metabolic rate. Sometimes the heat-regulating mechanism breaks down under these circumstances, and the temperature rises to 41°C (106°F) or more. This is 'heatstroke', or 'sunstroke', and unless treated promptly the temperature may continue to rise, reaching 43°C (109°F) or more, a level at which the patient becomes comatose, and permanent brain damage ensues. Death is not uncommon.

Infection. Fever is a frequent accompaniment of infection by viruses, bacteria, and larger parasites. The pattern of the pyrexia is often characteristic of particular diseases, e.g. the sudden onset in influenza and the step-ladder rise in typhoid fever (Fig. 7.3).

Infarction. Fever is often seen in patients with myocardial infarction.

Tumours. Some tumours are particularly liable to produce pyrexia, e.g. Ewing's tumour of bone, renal carcinoma, and Hodgkin's disease.

Haemorrhage. This may be followed by fever, especially when it occurs into the gastrointestinal tract or the pleural or peritoneal cavities.

Brain damage. Cerebral haemorrhage and other intracranial lesions may disturb the central regulating mechanism.

Following injury. Fever occurs during the catabolic phase of convalescence.

Fulminating or malignant hyperthermia.[3,4] Although rare, this condition is of importance to practitioners whose patients are given a general anaesthetic. Most of the reported cases have followed the administration of halothane or suxamethonium. The pyrexia develops extremely rapidly, and unless vigorous cooling is employed, the temperature rises to very high levels, e.g. 43 to 44°C, and death occurs from cardiac arrest. In most cases the skeletal muscles develop increased tone, and this is presumably the source of the increased heat production. A predisposition to develop malignant hyperpyrexia is inherited in some families, and can be detected by finding an increased blood level of creatine phosphokinase (CPK).

Miscellaneous conditions. Fever is a prominent, but unexplained, feature of many other conditions. Acute rheumatic fever, serum sickness, and gout may be cited as examples.

Clinical features

Of all the causes of pyrexia, infection is by far the most important. The development of fever in an acute illness like lobar pneumonia or malaria has been the object of most study. Three stages are described:

The cold stage. At the onset of illness there is a feeling of intense cold, peripheral vasoconstriction is manifested by pallor, and the patient starts to shiver. Chattering of the teeth completes this picture of the familiar *rigor*. The temperature rises, as does the blood pressure. There is usually a rise in pulse rate of 18 beats per minute for each 1°C rise of temperature (10 per 1°F).

The hot stage. As the temperature approaches its peak, the peripheral vasoconstriction relaxes and the patient feels dry and warm. Heat loss now balances heat gain, and the temperature remains constant. The 'thermostat' of the heat-regulating mechanism is still in control, but is geared to maintain the temperature at a level higher than normal. The extra heat produced is due to the raised metabolic rate caused by the fever. Should hyperpyrexia occur, this regulation may fail. During this phase the blood pressure falls.

The sweating phase. The temperature begins to fall, and the patient soon experiences a sensation of intense heat. Bedclothes are thrown off, sweating becomes profuse, and the temperature returns to normal. This is described as termination by *crisis.* If the pyrexia subsides slowly, as in typhoid fever, the termination is described as *lysis.*

The pathogenesis of fever

The intravenous injection of Gram-negative organisms produces a sharp rise in temperature. This appears to be due to lipopolysaccharide or polysaccharide substances which are called *bacterial pyrogens.* These are thought to act indirectly. They cause the polymorphs to release an *endogenous pyrogen* which acts on the heat-regulating centre. In the human there is evidence that a similar pyrogen can be released from monocytes as well as polymorphs. This helps to explain the pyrexia which occurs in infections with organisms that excite a mononuclear response and also fever in patients with agranulocytosis.

The bacterial pyrogens are heat stable, and are of importance because they can produce febrile reactions if present in the fluids used in intravenous therapy, which though sterile, may still cause a sharp rigor. Fluids used for injection purposes must be carefully prepared by distillation to ensure the exclusion of all bacterial products. Such *pyrogen-free fluids* must always be used.

The fact that fever often accompanies necrosis, e.g. in tumours and infarcts, suggests that dead tissue contains pyrogenic substances, and pyrogens similar to those of bacteria have been isolated.

Although recent work has shed some light on the mystery of fever, much has yet to be learned. It would be satisfying to believe that a rise in temperature in infection is a beneficial reaction designed to aid the body's defences. In viral infections this may be so, because fever stimulates the production of interferon (p. 254). However, with most infections there is little evidence that fever is beneficial. For the present we must regard the maintenance of normal temperature as an important homeostatic mechanism for the proper functioning of the body. Any departure from the normal is usually deleterious to well-being and can, if marked, be fatal.

Hypothermia

Hypothermia may be defined as a body temperature below 35°C. It is an important cause of death in cold climates, especially of infants and the aged, and it has been utilized as an adjunct to anaesthesia.

Hypothermia in infants

Newborn infants are particularly susceptible to cold, because of the relatively high ratio of surface area to body mass, the paucity of subcutaneous fat, and the low production of heat by physical means because of the inability to exercise or shiver. Furthermore, the thermoregulatory mechanism is relatively inefficient at birth and remains so for several hours.

During the first few weeks of life, infants need constant warmth, especially when ill, In cold countries open windows, lukewarm baths, and power cuts can cause inconvenience to adults but can be fatal to infants.

The early signs of cold injury are lethargy and difficulty in feeding. Indeed, the child has a still, serene appearance and the cheeks, nose, and extremities have a flush that deludes the onlooker into believing all is well. The cry is like a whimper, and the body feels cold. Later, bradycardia and oedema of the eyelids and extemities occur. In the worst cases, the subcutaneous fat becomes hard.

Hypothermia in adults

Hypothermia can occur in adults in a number of circumstances. Immersion hypothermia is one of the lethal factors in shipwreck. Hypothermia is an important complication of myxoedema and hypopituitarism, and it also occurs in patients with widespread eczema and generalized erythroderma. In widespread skin disease, the passive diffusion of water through the epidermis is greatly increased, and heat is lost both by evaporation and convection.

Spontaneous hypothermia is a well-recognized occurrence in old people—usually women—who live alone in poorly heated rooms and are poorly clothed. Undernutrition is often an additional factor; in persons who are in both calorie- and protein-deficient states, the basal metabolic rate is decreased. Hypothermia in the aged is sometimes a complication of senile dementia, or the effects of depressant drugs like alcohol and chlorpromazine that have dulled the mind. There is sometimes a severe precipating infection such as pneumonia.

The patient with hypothermia looks ill. There is a corpse-like chill of the body, and the rectal temperature can be as low as 21 °C (70°F). The skin is pale, and the subcutaneous tissue is pliant and doughy. The patient remains still; muscles are rigid, and shivering is absent. The tendon reflexes are sluggish, and there is bradycardia, sometimes with atrial fibrillation. Since peripheral oedema and puffiness of the eyelids are common, myxoedema may be simulated. Oliguria (diminished urine output) is common, respiration is depressed, and death often occurs from cardiac arrest.

It is easy to overlook hypothermia, both in infancy and adults. Clinical thermometers that register as low as 24°C (75°F) should be available and used if the circumstances raise the possibility of hypothermia.

Induced hypothermia

Some animals have acquired the ability to hibernate for long periods in a state of hypothermia as a useful adjunct to survival in winter. From experimental work carried out on small animals, it has been found that they can be cooled below 0°C (32°F) if they are made first to ingest propylene glycol. Mice can be kept in suspended animation for about 1 hour and then reanimated by artificial respiration and microwave diathermy. Larger animals do not tolerate this treatment so well and usually die within a few days. A lesser degree of hypothermia has been used as an adjunct to cardiac surgery. If the body's temperature is lowered, cardiac arrest can be tolerated for about 1 hour. The development of extracorporeal circulatory systems has allowed profound hypothermia to be used in open-heart surgery. In one method, the blood is cooled rapidly by passage through a heat exchanger and the circulation is maintained extracorporeally. At the temperature of 12.7 to 15°C (55 to 59°F), the circulation is stopped, and the heart is opened in a bloodless field. When the operation is finished, the blood is rewarmed, the heart is defibrillated and a normal circulation is restored. Extracorporeal circulations are now so efficient that hypothermia is less commonly used or is merely used as an adjunct to this procedure.

Local hypothermia

Extreme cold causes tissue damage; when the part is rewarmed, an acute inflammation follows and blisters occur. Direct damage to the capillaries is prominent, and vascular occlusion contributes to tissue necrosis. This type of cold injury is called 'frost bite', and in cold climates is not uncommon following accidental exposure to cold. Usually, the toes, fingers, ears, and nose are affected. Deliberate application of extreme cold (cryosurgery) is used therapeutically in surgical and dental practice. Liquid nitrogen is commonly applied to warts and other skin tumours. Various types of probes that are refrigerated by liquid nitrogen have been devised for applying cold to deeper tissues. They have been used to treat eye tumours as well as in intracranial surgery. At present, the use of cold is confined to special centres; the late effects are still being assessed.

GENERAL READING

Guyton A C 1976 Body temperature, temperature regulation and fever in Textbook of Medical Physiology, 5th edn. Saunders, Philadelphia, ch 72

Petersdorf R B 1974 Alterations in body temperature. In: Harrison's Principles of Internal Medicine, edited by Wintrobe M M et al. 7th edn. McGraw-Hill, New York, pp. 48–54

Petersdorf R B 1974 Chills and fever in Harrison's Principles of Internal Medicine,pp. 54–63, loc. cit

REFERENCES

1. Atkins E & Bodel P 1972 Fever. New England Journal of Medicine, 286: 27
2. Wood W B 1970. In: Infectious agents and host reactions (ed) Mudd S (The pathogenesis of fever). Saunders, Philadelphia, pp146–162
3. Leading article 1971 Malignant hyperpyrexia. British Medical Journal 3:441
4. Gordon R A, Britt B A, Kalow W 1973 International symposium on malignant hyperthermia, Thomas, Springfield

28

Disorders of the body's fluids: oedema

ACID-BASE BALANCE

General considerations[1–4]

During metabolism, acidic substances are produced in large amounts. The most important of these is carbonic acid (H_2CO_3), which is the inevitable product of aerobic tissue activity. During anaerobic activity lactic acid is produced; phosphoric, sulphuric, and other acids are formed in smaller quantities. These acids are formed within cells and pass to the extracellular tissues where they tend to increase the acidity. Nevertheless, cellular activity can take place only within a narrow range of acidity. The regulatory mechanisms by which this range is maintained are an aspect of homeostasis, which is of vital importance. In order to understand this process, it is essential to have a working knowledge of acids, bases, and buffers.

An acid is a molecule or ion that is capable of giving up a hydrogen ion (H^+, or proton). A base is a molecule or ion that is capable of receiving a hydrogen ion. Thus, in the equation

$$HB = H^+ + B^-$$

HB is an acid, whereas B^- is the base.

A strong acid is one that readily gives up its hydrogen ion. Thus, in the equation

$$HCl = H^+ + Cl^-$$

HCl is a strong acid and Cl^- is a weak base.
On the other hand, carbonic acid (H_2CO_3) is a weak acid:

$$H_2CO_3 = H^+ + HCO_3^-$$

The bicarbonate ion HCO_3^- is a strong base, because it accepts a hydrogen ion more readily than H_2CO_3 gives it up.

* The pH of a fluid is the negative logarithm of the hydrogen ion concentration of a solution. The form $[H^+]$ is used to denote hydrogen ion concentration. In pure water at 25°C the following relationship exists:

$$[H^+] \times [OH^-] = 10^{-14}$$

$$\text{That is, } [H^+] = [OH^-] = 10^{-7}$$

Hence, pH = 7.0. At 37°C pH 6.8 corresponds to neutrality.

Maintenance of the pH of the blood*

The normal blood pH ranges from 7.36 to 7.44. Survival is not possible outside the range of about 6.9 to 7.7. To prevent changes of pH as much as possible, the body is provided with a series of *buffer systems.* These are chemical systems that are capable of 'mopping up' excess hydrogen ions if the pH falls and of contributing hydrogen ions if the pH rises.

A physiological buffer consists of a mixture of a strong base and a weak acid; thus, in the dissociation equation

$$HB \rightleftharpoons H^+ + B^-$$

If B^- is a strong base, an excess of H^+ combines with it to form more of the weak acid HB.

The most important buffer in the extracellular fluids is the bicarbonate–carbonic acid combination.

$$H^+ + HCO_3^- \rightleftharpoons H_2CO_3$$

If hydrogen ions are added to plasma, more H_2CO_3 is formed. This passes to the lungs, dissociates, and carbon dioxide (CO_2) diffuses into the alveolar gas and is eliminated. The great importance of the bicarbonate ion lies not only in its buffering capacity but also in the extreme volatility of carbonic acid and the ease with which CO_2 is eliminated by the lungs.

Two other buffer systems in the extracellular fluids should be noted: monohydrogen phosphate and the plasma proteins:

$$H^+ + HPO_4^{2-} \rightleftharpoons H_2PO_4^-$$

$$H^+ + \text{Protein}^{n-} \rightleftharpoons \text{HProtein}^{(n-1)-}$$

An important means of buffering carbonic acid within the blood is found within the red cells, which contain not only haemoglobin, which acts as a buffer, but also the enzyme carbonic anhydrase, which accelerates the following reversible reaction:

$$CO_2 + H_2O \rightleftharpoons H_2CO_3$$

The carbonic acid then dissociates into bicarbonate and hydrogen ions:

$$H_2CO_3 \rightarrow HCO_3^- + H^+$$

The hydrogen ions are largely buffered by the haemoglobin:

$$H^+ + Hb^- \rightleftharpoons HHb$$

The excess bicarbonate ions then diffuse into the plasma in exchange for chloride ions, which diffuse into the red cells. In this way the bicarbonate level in the plasma rises.

It is evident that the acids that are produced in the body or are ingested are eliminated by two routes: *the lungs*, as described above; and *the kidneys* (the cells of the distal tubules secrete H^+ ions).

Abnormalities of the pH of the blood

An increase in the hydrogen ion concentration of the blood (pH less than 7.36) is called *acidaemia*, whereas a decrease (pH over 7.44) is called *alkalaemia*. Although the terms *acidosis* and *alkalosis* are sometimes used synonymously with acidaemia and alkalaemia, it is preferable to restrict them to descriptions of conditions in which there would be an appropriate change in pH if there were no compensatory mechanisms.

Respiratory acidosis and alkalosis

If there is hypoventilation of the lungs, CO_2 is retained and forms carbonic acid in the blood, which is a source of hydrogen ions. $[HCO_3]$ rises as well, but by a lesser amount. Hence, the pH of the blood decreases. This process is called *respiratory acidosis*. In like manner, if there is hyperventilation, excess CO_2 is eliminated, and both carbonic acid and bicarbonate are reduced in the blood causing an increase in the pH. This process is called *respiratory alkalosis*. It is evident that respiratory acidosis is directly related to hypoventilation of the lungs, with a resulting retention of CO_2 and a rise in the arterial P_{CO_2}. In respiratory alkalosis the reverse obtains and there is a drop in arterial P_{CO_2}. A measurement of the arterial P_{CO_2} is therefore an accurate and useful method of assessing the respiratory component of acid-base balance. See p. 527 for further discussion of P_{CO_2}.

Effects of respiratory acidosis. This condition results in vasodilatation, which is a direct effect of the raised arterial P_{CO_2}. This vasodilatation may cause a rise in intracranial pressure. The level of plasma bicarbonate rises and the plasma chloride drops proportionally.

Effects of respiratory alkalosis. Respiratory alkalosis is seen during hysterical hyperventilation, during work at high temperatures or at a high altitude, or during anaesthesia when muscle relaxants are used and excessively vigorous artificial ventilation is applied. Peripheral vasoconstriction causes pallor of the skin. The lack of stimulation of the respiratory centre by CO_2 causes a tendency toward respiratory arrest. *Tetany* is characteristic. This physiological response is identical with that seen in hypocalcaemia. The symptoms are those of increased neuromuscular excitability. The most characteristic is spontaneous spasms of the hand muscles so that the fingers are extended and the palm hollowed. Generalized convulsions can occur.

Metabolic acidosis and alkalosis

If an excess of hydrogen ions is introduced into the blood, as a result of either ingestion or the production of acidic substances, the bicarbonate of the plasma is replaced by chloride and other anions. There is a secondary fall in the P_{CO_2} to match this low concentration of bicarbonate, an effect produced by the low pH stimulating the respiratory centre and causing overventilation. This is *metabolic acidosis*. Excessive ingestion of sodium bicarbonate leads to a rise in both the $[HCO_3^-]$ and the pH of the plasma. This is *metabolic alkalosis*.

Metabolic acidosis. A fall in both pH and bicarbonate level of the plasma occurs under the following conditions: (1) *in shock* and *following a cardiac arrest*, when underprofusion of tissue leads to anaerobic metabolism and production of lactic acid (*lactic acidosis*); (2) *in severe diarrhoea*, when there is a great loss of bicarbonate in the faeces; (3) *in starvation* and *in uncontrolled diabetes mellitus*, when there is ketosis. The acetoacetic acid and β-hydroxybutyric acid provide the extra hydrogen ions, and (4) *in chronic renal disease*, and in conditions in which there is a failure of the distal tubules to excrete hydrogen ions (e.g., renal tubular acidosis).

Clinical effects. The classic symptom of metabolic acidosis is 'air hunger'. Respirations are deep, rapid, and sighing. This is a compensatory mechanism, because it lowers the P_{CO_2} and thereby causes a respiratory alkalosis that tends to reverse the metabolic acidosis.

As the plasma bicarbonate falls, so there is a corresponding rise in other plasma anions, particularly the chloride ions. In such cases there is a *hyperchloraemic acidosis.*

Severe metabolic acidosis causes grave neurological symptoms that culminate in death. The heart's action is impaired, and a state of shock with low cardiac output and hypotension ensues. Metabolic acidosis is thought to potentiate traumatic and haemorrhagic shock, and it is one of the contributory factors in the development of irreversible shock (see Ch. 26).

Metabolic alkalosis. Both blood pH and blood bicarbonate level rise in this condition. Metabolic alkalosis occurs when there is excessive ingestion of bicarbonate or when there is excessive loss of acid from the body. The most common cause of this is persistent vomiting, such as with pyloric stenosis, when the ensuing loss of acidic gastric juice causes the alkalosis.

Effects of metabolic alkalosis. Tetany may occur. A fall in plasma chloride compensates for the rise in bicarbonate level.

THE BODY'S FLUIDS

The compartments of body fluids[1]

About 72 per cent of the lean body weight consists of water. It amounts to 42 litres in a normal adult man weighing 70 kg, and of this two-thirds (28 litres) are intracellular, and the remaining third (14 litres) extracellular. The latter has two components: the extravascular *interstitial fluid* which comprises 11.2 litres, and the *plasma volume* which is 2.8 litres.

Fluid balance

The total water content of the body is maintained by balancing the fluid output with the intake. This important homeostatic mechanism is not completely understood, and a textbook of physiology should be consulted for the details. It may, however, be noted that fluid balance is controlled by three factors:

1. *Indirectly, by the mechanisms that regulate sodium balance.* Sodium cannot be retained without water.

Aldosterone secreted by the adrenal cortex has the effect of increasing sodium reabsorption by the distal tubule of the kidney, and thereby causes water retention.

Sodium reabsorption from the proximal tubule is dependent to a large extent on the total glomerular filtrate. When the volume is reduced, as in shock and heart failure, sodium absorption is more complete, and water is therefore also retained.

2. *The mechanisms that regulate the output of water by the kidney.*

The antidiuretic hormone (ADH) from the posterior lobe of the pituitary is important in this connexion. It acts by increasing water reabsorption from the collecting tubules of the kidney.

3. *Regulation of the water intake by the sensation of thirst.*

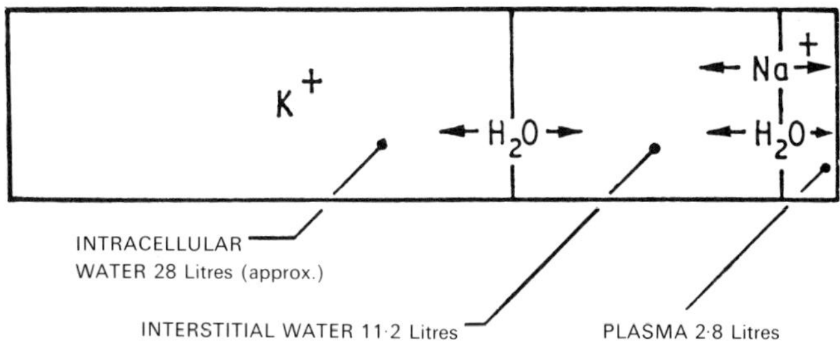

Fig. 28.1 Diagrammatic representation of the three compartments in which the body's water is accommodated. An excess or deficiency of water, which is freely diffusible, produces the greatest effects in the largest compartment, the intracellular one, whereas changes in sodium affect mainly the volume of the interstitial fluid.

Water is freely diffusible across the barriers which separate the various compartments (Fig. 28.1). The volume in each is preserved by the osmotic, electrochemical, and hydrostatic forces which are acting upon it. As far as osmosis is concerned potassium, phosphate, and protein are important in the intracellular compartment, while in the interstitial and intravascular spaces sodium, chloride, and bicarbonate have the greatest influence.

Water and sodium metabolism are so closely interrelated that it is convenient to consider them together.

Disturbances in water and sodium balance

Pure water deficiency. This follows the deprivation of water, e.g. in people who cannot swallow because of oesophageal obstruction or coma, and during enforced starvation. It is also seen in *diabetes insipidus*, which is due to a lack of ADH. Patients with this disease pass enormous quantities of urine, e.g. 20 litres per day instead of the normal 1 to 1.5 litres.

Effects. Since water can cross the membranes which separate the fluid compartments, they are all depleted. The largest compartment, the intracellular space, is the most severely affected, and the cellular dehydration causes intense thirst and eventually death.

Pure water excess. The converse condition, water intoxication, or cellular oedema, occurs when excess water is absorbed and retained. This may be seen in patients to whom too much water is given intravenously (as glucose solution), a situation particularly liable to arise during the postoperative period when water excretion is impaired and in acute renal failure (p. 568). The effects of water excess are serious. There is vomiting, muscle cramps, headache, convulsions, and sometimes death.

Combined salt and water deficiency. Salt, or salt and water, deficiency is seen when there is loss from:

The gastrointestinal tract, e.g. severe vomiting or diarrhoea,

The skin, due to prolonged excessive sweating (heat-exhaustion),

The kidney, e.g. following prolonged administration of diuretics for chronic heart failure.

Effects. The effect of salt deficiency is the undermining of the osmotic support of the extracellular fluid. The interstitial fluid volume is reduced in amount, and therefore the patient shows *dehydration.* The eyeballs are sunken, the skin wrinkled, the tongue dry and the face haggard. Thirst is often absent. Despite a compensatory vasoconstriction, the blood pressure is low and the veins are poorly filled. Little urine is passed, and there is a reduction in the plasma volume, which is evidenced by a rise in the packed cell volume and haemoglobin concentration (haemoconcentration). Unless relieved the condition rapidly terminates in circulatory failure.

Combined salt and water excess. This is another artificially induced condition, and is seen in patients with defective renal function who are given excessive amounts of saline solution, e.g. during the early postoperative period, or during the course of acute renal failure.

Effects. The fluid is distributed evenly throughout the extracellular compartment which therefore becomes expanded. The manifestations are those of increased venous pressure and oedema, both systemic and pulmonary; in due course pulmonary oedema will kill the patient.

Conclusion

It is evident from this brief account of electrolytes and acid-base balance that many abnormalities can occur in disease. With the aid of the modern clinical laboratory the abnormalities can be measured and appropriate treatment can be instituted. In acute illness, serial estimations are often necessary to assess the effects of treatment. The 'toxaemias' that once afflicted patients having cholera, dysentery, and intestinal obstruction with vomiting are no longer mysterious, untreatable agents of death. Instead, these conditions are now known to be diagnosable, treatable upsets of the internal environment of the body.

OEDEMA

Oedema may be defined as an excessive extravascular accumulation of fluid. In its usual context it is applied to the morbid accumulation of fluid in the interstitial tissues. It is particularly liable to occur in the various preformed serous sacs, giving rise to *ascites*, *hydrothorax*, and *hydropericardium*, as effusions into the peritoneal, pleural, and pericardial cavities are specifically called. When generalized, it is called *anasarca*, or *dropsy*. It is, of course, also possible to have intracellular oedema as in hydropic degeneration and in pure water intoxication, but for the remainder of this discussion only the interstitial type will be considered. It is necessary first to understand the normal mechanisms which regulate the distribution of fluid in the body.

Mechanism of normal control in the systemic circulation

Starling postulated that the movement of fluid between vessels and the extravascular spaces was determined by the balance of the hydrostatic and osmotic forces acting upon it (Fig. 5.1).

The forces tending to move fluid out of the blood vessels

The hydrostatic pressure in the vessels. This is generally accepted as 32 mm Hg at the arterial end of the capillary and 12 mm Hg at the venous end in the skin of the human subject at heart level.

The colloidal osmotic pressure, also called the oncotic pressure, of the interstitial fluid. Since the vascular wall is completely permeable to water and crystalloids, the only effective osmotic forces are those due to the colloids, mainly proteins. The interstitial fluids normally have a low protein content, and this is therefore not an important factor in the formation of the extravascular fluids under normal conditions. Furthermore those proteins which do escape into the tissue spaces are normally removed by the lymphatics.

The forces moving fluid into the blood vessels

The tissue tension. This is low (3 to 4 mm Hg). Tissue tension is important in relation to the distribution of oedema; for instance lax areas like the face, particularly around the eyelids, the ankles, sacrum, and scrotum, tend to accumulate fluid, while tense areas, like the palms and soles, are never the site of marked oedema. A rise in tissue tension is probably an important factor in limiting interstitial-tissue fluid formation in the legs under normal conditions and also in acutely inflamed parts.

The osmotic pressure (oncotic pressure) of the plasma proteins. The osmotic pressure of plasma proteins is about 25 mm Hg, and is due largely to albumin. Since the plasma proteins cannot normally pass through the vessel walls, the vascular permeability is important in regulating the distribution of fluids between the intravascular and the extravascular compartments. In the event of an increase in permeability, an exudate is formed which is rich in protein, e.g. in acute inflammation.

There are indeed two types of oedema:

An exudate, the accumulation of fluid due to an increased vascular permeability, such as occurs in inflammation—the fluid contains a high percentage of protein due to the increased vascular permeability.

A transudate, the accumulation of fluid due to a hydrostatic imbalance between the intravascular and the extravascular compartments, despite normal vascular permeability. It has a low protein content.

The importance of the lymphatics should not be forgotten. They form an elaborate network in most tissues, and their function is to drain away fluid and protein. The lymph is of considerably higher protein content than is the interstitial fluid itself.

The various factors involved in Starling's hypothesis are depicted in Fig. 5.1 (p. 73). It must be realized, however, that this merely represents an average state of affairs found in many capillaries at the level of the heart. Pressures in individual vessels show considerable variation.

Types of oedema

When considering the cause of any type of oedema, it should be realized that the process is usually due to a combination of factors. Starling himself appreciated this, and stated that dropsy was probably never due to a derangement of a single mechanism acting alone.

Oedema can be classified into local and generalized (widespread) types. The local oedemas are the simplest ones to understand because there are usually fewer factors involved in their production.

Local oedema

Acute inflammatory oedema (p. 73).

Hypersensitivity (allergic oedema). Oedema due to an increase in vascular permeability is present in all lesions of anaphylactic and immune-complex hypersensitivity. The oedema of anaphylaxis is widespread. Oedema is also seen in the acute inflammatory response of type-IV hypersensitivity.

Venous obstruction. A rise in venous pressure leads to an increase in capillary pressure, and the result is the formation of a transudate. This is seen in the legs following thrombophlebitis.

Lymphatic oedema. Extensive lymphatic obstruction can produce an oedema of rather high protein content, although not nearly as high as that of an exudate. Chronic lymphatic oedema stimulates an overgrowth of fibrous tissue, and in due course there is fibrous tissue and epithelial hyperplasia so that the affected part becomes grossly enlarged. If marked this is called *elephantiasis.* It is seen in the leg in filariasis due to the obstruction of the lymphatics by a nematode worm. A similar effect is sometimes caused by recurrent bacterial lymphangitis. Lymphoedema may occur in the arm, when the lymphatics of the axilla are obstructed by cancer of the breast or by the fibrosis which may follow radiotherapy.

Primary lymphoedema is a special variety of lymphatic oedema due to a malformation of the lymphatics of the lower limbs. Women are usually the victims. One type of primary lymphoedema is hereditary and congenital, and is called *Milroy's disease.*[5]

Generalized oedema

Cardiac oedema.[6] In right-sided and congestive cardiac failure there is a retention of sodium and water by the body as evidenced by an increase in body weight. The distribution of this fluid is influenced by gravity. When the patient is ambulant the legs are affected first, and swelling of the ankles is often the initial symptom; when recumbent the oedema appears in the sacral and genital areas. The oedema readily pits on pressure. The pathogenesis of cardiac failure is described in Chapter 32.

Renal oedema. *Acute glomerulonephritis.* Oedema is often the first symptom of this disease. It affects the face and the eyelids predominantly. There is no satisfactory explanation for this facial distribution. At one time it was thought that the oedema was due to damage to the blood vessels, but the more probable explanation is that it is due to heart failure which may follow the sudden rise in blood pressure seen in this condition.

Nephrotic syndrome. The outstanding feature of this is proteinuria with hypoproteinaemia. On Starling's hypothesis the diminished osmotic pressure of the plasma proteins can easily explain the generalized oedema, and this is undoubtedly an important factor. However, there are other considerations. A salt-free diet reduces the oedema, especially if combined with diuretics. It seems likely that salt and water retention, perhaps due to an oversecretion of aldosterone, is also important.

Chronic glomerulonephritis. The oedema is due to heart failure.

Famine oedema (nutritional oedema). The oedema that is seen after prolonged starvation is usually confined to the legs. At first sight it would seem to be explicable in terms of the marked hypoalbuminaemia which is usually present, but there is no close correlation between the level of the plasma proteins and the presence of oedema. The true explanation of famine oedema is not known. An important factor appears to be the loss of compact tissue, mostly fat, and its replacement by a loose connective tissue in which fluid can accumulate without a rise in tissue tension.

Marked oedema is a feature of *kwashiorkor*. This is described in Chapter 18.

Hepatitic oedema and ascites are considered in Chapter 35.

Unexplained oedema. Generalized oedema sometimes occurs in the absence of any known cause, and although such cases are uncommon, they indicate that factors other than those already discussed may operate even in the common types of oedema. A well-recognized condition is *cyclical*, or *periodic*, *oedema*, in which there are recurrent attacks of oedema involving skin, mucous membranes, joints, or even internal organs.[7] Usually the area involved is localized, and one type is called *angio-oedema*. One patient is recorded as having pain and swelling of the left hand on alternative Wednesdays, lasting one week, for 18 years! The immediate cause of the oedema appears to be an increase in vascular permeability, but the cause of this is not known.

One variety of angio-oedema is familial and associated with deficiency of the CI-esterase inhibitor of the complement system. How the attacks are precipitated is not clear but activation of the kinin system is probably involved.[8] Apart from skin and gut lesions, acute oedema of the larynx may occur and threaten life.

Pulmonary oedema. This is considered in Chapter 33.

Although dropsy has been recognized as a symptom of disease since the beginning of medical history, it is evident that the mode of its formation is complex. In patients under hypnosis it is sometimes possible by suggestion to produce oedema at the site of previous injury. The mechanism is completely unknown, and it is therefore no surprise to find that the mode of production of oedema in such simple conditions as acute inflammation and heart failure is incompletely understood.

REFERENCES

1. Campbell E J M, Dickinson C J, Slater J D H 1974 Clinical physiology, 4th edn. Blackwell, Oxford. See in particular, chapter 1, 'Body fluids' and chapter 5, 'Hydrogen ion (acid: base) regulation'
2. Davenport H W 1969 ABC of acid-base chemistry: the elements of physiological blood-gas chemistry for medical students and physicians, 5th edn. University of Chicago Press, Chicago
3. Robinson J R 1975 Fundamentals of acid-base regulation, 5th edn. Blackwell, Oxford
4. Siggaard-Anderson O 1975 The acid-base status of the blood, 4th edn. Williams and Wilkins, Baltimore
5. Leading article 1963 Milroy's disease and lymphoedema. British Medical Journal 2: 1483
6. Brod J 1972 Pathogenesis of cardiac oedema. British Medical Journal 1: 222
7. Leading article 1963 Periodic syndromes. Lancet 2: 563
8. Rosen F S, Austen K F 1969 The 'neurotic edema' (hereditary angiodema). New England Journal of Medicine 280: 1356

29

Some abnormalities of the plasma proteins

The plasma proteins form a heterogeneous group. They are worthy of study because they not only play an important role in the body's economy, but also, being readily accessible, can be extensively investigated. Changes in their concentration are often of great value diagnostically in clinical medicine.[1]

Separation of plasma proteins on the basis of physico-chemical properties

It should be appreciated that the plasma proteins have been separated and identified according to various physical and chemical characteristics. Their classification is therefore somewhat arbitrary and unsatisfactory. *Fibrinogen* is a protein which during coagulation forms an insoluble fibrin clot. When the remaining serum is half saturated with ammonium sulphate, a precipitate is formed which is composed of *globulin*. The protein which remains in solution is called *albumin*. The normal levels of these proteins are:

Albumin	40 to 57 g per litre
Globulin	15 to 30 g per litre
Fibrinogen	1 to 5 g per litre
Total	62 to 82 g per litre

Other physical characteristics have been used to separate further the plasma proteins.

Electrophoresis. If a mixture of proteins is placed in an electric field at an appropriate pH, there is movement of the individual proteins at different rates, dependent to a great extent on their size and charge. The test can be performed on filter paper, cellulose acetate strip, or starch gel, and after passing an electric current for a suitable time the separated proteins are stained with a simple dye, e.g. light green. Fig. 29.1 shows a typical electrophoretic separation of serum proteins. If the electrophoresis is performed in a gel, the separated fractions can be detected by adding suitable antibodies. This technique, know as *immunoelectrophoresis*, has revealed a great number of separate fractions which cannot be detected by simple electrophoresis (Fig. 29.2).

Solubility in water. The globulin fraction which is soluble in water is sometimes called the *pseudoglobulin*, while the insoluble portion is the *euglobulin*. Certain proteins precipitate out in the cold. These are called *cryoglobulins*.

Molecular size. Fibrinogen has a molecular weight of 400 000 daltons,

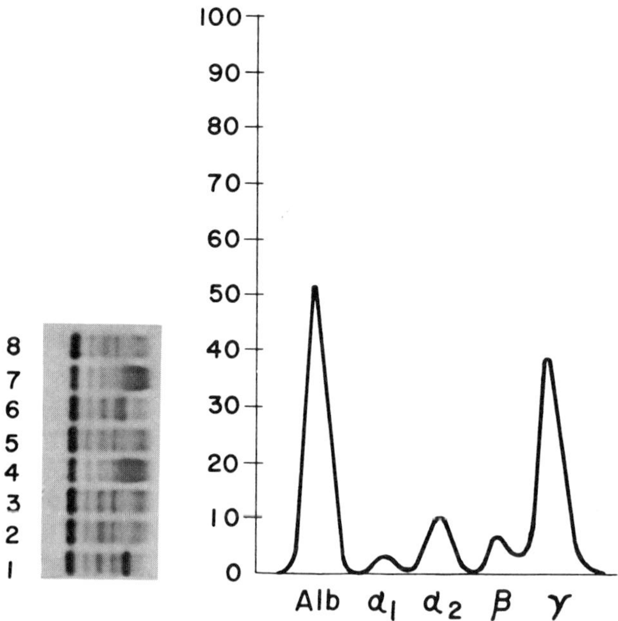

Fig. 29.1 Cellulose acetate electrophoresis of serum. On the left electrophoretic strips from 8 separate sera are shown. The anode is on the left, and the dense band that has moved furthest to the left is due to albumin. No. 8 is normal serum, whereas Nos. 4 and 7 show a diffuse increase in the γ-globulins; each shows the picture of a polyclonal gammopathy. No. 1 shows a dense band in the γ-globulin area; the density of the bands of strip No. 1 is depicted in graphic form on the right. The various serum proteins are in the same relative positions on both the strip and the graph. The sharp spike in the γ region is characteristic of a monoclonal gammopathy. (*Reproduced, with permission, from Hall C A 1976 Gammopathies. In: Halsted J A (ed) The laboratory in clinical medicine. Saunders, Philadelphia, p 493.*)

albumin 65 000 daltons, and the globulins range from 45 000 daltons to several million. The ultracentrifuge may be used to separate proteins on a basis of their molecular size (p. 153).

Functional groups. Another useful method of classifying plasma proteins is based upon their function. The following groups may be recognized:

1. *The proteins concerned with clotting*, e.g. fibrinogen, prothrombin, etc.
2. *The proteins concerned with fibrinolysis*, e.g. plasminogen
3. *Hormones*, e.g. hormones of the anterior lobe of the pituitary
4. *Enzymes*, for instance alkaline phosphatase
5. *Carrier proteins*. Many substances are carried in the blood bound to specific proteins—thus iron is bound by transferrin. Thyroxine and the corticosteroids of the adrenals are also bound to specific globulins. Albumin itself has an important carrier role; for instance it binds bilirubin, free fatty acids, sulphonamides, and many other drugs
6. *The immunoglobulins*
7. *The components of complement.*

Chemical composition. Some proteins contain lipid or carbohydrate. The former are called *lipoproteins*, and the latter *glycoproteins.*

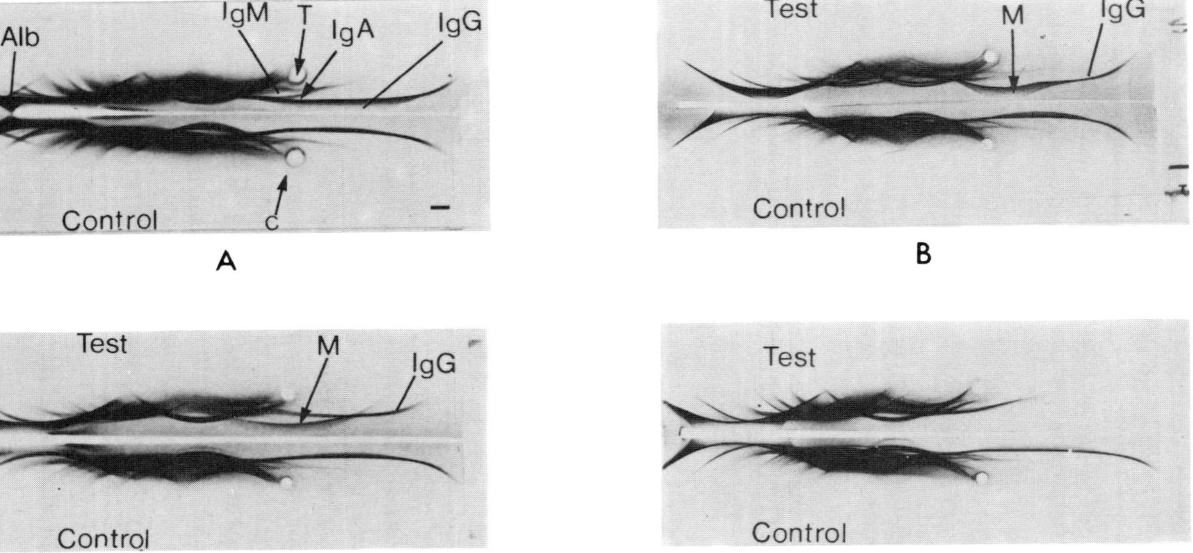

Fig. 29.2 Immunoelectrophoresis of serum. This method entails the separation of the proteins by electrophoresis in a gel, and then demonstrating each fraction by means of a precipitin reaction using an antibody.

Sera are placed in the two cups in a sheet of agarose gel. Test serum is in the upper cup 'T' and control serum in the lower cup 'C'. Albumin has a strong negative charge, and γ-globulin has a weak negative charge. The application of an electric field results in a tendency for the proteins to move towards the anode. Their actual movement, however, is determined not only by their molecular size and charge but also by a flow of water towards the cathode due to the phenomenon of electro-osmosis. This is due to a negative charge on the gel itself, and as the gel is fixed, so its tendency to move towards the anode actually results in a movement of water to the cathode. The weakly charged γ-globulins are thus carried towards the cathode.

The separated plasma components are demonstrated by placing antiserum to whole plasma down the central strip. From there the antibodies diffuse to form precipitin lines with each separated serum protein. A stain to accentuate these lines has been used.

A. The IgG band is heavier than that of the control and is closer to the central strip. Serum tested here was from a case of systemic lupus erythematosus with polyclonal hypergammaglobulinaemia. The IgA and IgM bands are well shown. *B*. An M-protein is present and distorts the normal IgG band (from a case of multiple myeloma with an IgG M-protein). *C*. An M-protein is present and is in the position of the normal IgA band; note how the normal IgG band crosses the M-protein (from a case of multiple myeloma with an IgA M-protein). *D*. Note the deficiency of the IgG band (from a case of congenital hypogammaglobulinaemia). (*Photograph by courtesy of Dr K C Carstairs.*)

It will be appreciated that any individual protein may be described in a variety of ways. Thus prothrombin is a globulin which is also a glycoprotein. Immunoglobulins are γ-globulins which may be of small molecular size (150 000 daltons) or in the macroglobulin range.

Source and fate of plasma proteins.[2,3] The principal plasma proteins are synthetised in the liver, the major exception being the immunoglobulins. The sites of metabolism are poorly defined. The liver and probably other organs are concerned with the breakdown of γ-globulin, and there is good evidence that albumin is secreted into the gastrointestinal tract, where it is broken down and its constituent amino acids reabsorbed.

Abnormalities of plasma proteins

There are three types of abnormalities of any protein group. The level may either be raised or lowered, or else an abnormal form of the protein may be present. The term *dysproteinaemia* indicates that there is an imbalance between the proportions of the various plasma proteins. It is generally used to describe the conditions in which the changes are marked, as when an M protein is present or a major component absent.

Albumin

The preponderance of albumin together with its low molecular weight make this protein an important factor in the maintenance of the non-crystalloid osmotic pressure in plasma. A low plasma albumin level therefore contributes to oedema formation (Chapter 28).

A low plasma albumin level is found whenever there is excessive loss from the plasma, e.g. in the nephrotic syndrome, with rapidly accumulating exudates, and with chronic loss of inflammatory exudate from the body such as from draining abscesses, extensive burns, and severe infected wounds. Protein-losing gastroenteropathy is an uncommon cause of hypoalbuminaemia which is due to loss of the protein into the intestine, and is associated with a variety of gastrointestinal lesions including gastric carcinoma, Crohn's disease and ulcerative colitis.[4,5] Clinically it is characterized by oedema and a low plasma albumin level, but with no obvious source of protein loss. During acute infections and following trauma or surgery the albumin level drops due to its increased metabolism. This drop is accompanied by a rise in the α-globulins (especially the α_2-globulin), fibrinogen and haptoglobin, and the appearance of C-reactive protein (see p. 434). This *acute reaction to stress* is non-specific, and is probably mediated by the release of adrenal hormones. It forms the basis for the erythrocyte sedimentation rate, which is discussed later.

The globulins[6]

The globulins include a wide array of plasma proteins. In some instances there is good evidence that the type of protein which occurs varies in different individuals—thus there are nine different types of transferrin. The type present in any individual is determined by genetic factors in much the same way as are the blood group antigens, and is an example of genetic polymorphism.

In clinical practice the globulin component which is most frequently estimated is the γ-globulin. This consists mostly of immunoglobulins. The normal level appears to be maintained by constant contact with micro-organisms. Thus, in the germ-free rat* the γ-globulin level is reduced to about one fifth of normal. When the intestinal flora of such animals is restored the plasma proteins return to normal.

Agammaglobulinaemia and hypogammaglobulinaemia. These are described in Chapter 12, since they are associated with various immunological deficiency states.

Hypergammaglobulinaemia. The immunoglobulins form the major component of the plasma globulins, and it follows that hyperglobulinaemia is invariably due to an increase in this fraction. Two main patterns are described:

Polyclonal gammopathy. This occurs whenever there is a prolonged and marked immune response, and is therefore common in chronic infections, e.g. tuberculosis, chronic osteomyelitis, lepromatous leprosy, and kala-azar. It is also a feature of certain diseases that have an autoimmune component, such as systemic lupus erythematosus and rheumatoid arthritis. Whether this is the explanation for the hypergammaglobulinaemia of hepatic cirrhosis, chronic active hepatitis, and sarcoidosis is not known. Hypergammaglobulinaemia occasionally develops in the absence of detectable disease and is then labelled idiopathic.

The electrophoretic pattern in these conditions is that of a broad-based elevation of the gammaglobulins as well as some increase in the beta and even the alpha fractions. There is an increase in many classes of immunoglobulin, and it is assumed that many clones of antibody-forming cells are involved, hence the term polyclonal gammopathy.

Monoclonal gammopathy. In some cases of hypergammaglobulinaemia there is a marked increase in the level of one of the major classes of immunoglobulin—IgG, IgA, IgM, IgE, or IgD—and furthermore it consists of either the κ or the λ variety. The supposition is that the globulin is produced by one particular clone of antibody-forming cells. Monoclonal gammopathy is usually associated with malignancy of the lymphoreticular system. The most common example is *multiple myeloma*, which is described elsewhere, but it is also seen in *Waldenström's macroglobulinaemia* and in a variety of other *malignant lymphomata* and occasionally other *malignant tumours*. The term M-protein (derived from *m*ultiple *m*yeloma, *m*acroglobulinaemia, *m*alignant lymphoma, and *m*alignant tumour) is therefore applied to the abnormal homogeneous protein which appears as a spike on electrophoresis in contrast to the broad-based increase seen in the polyclonal gammopathies (Fig. 29.1). Rarely an M-band consists of only light or heavy chains.

Hypergammaglobulinaemia generally presents as a symptomless biochemical abnormality which requires further investigation to uncover the primary cause. Sometimes, however, the plasma-protein abnormality may lead directly to secondary effects. In the *hyperviscosity syndrome* the presence of a high concentration of protein, especially a macroglobulin, increases the viscosity of the blood and impedes the peripheral circulation. This produces serious effects when

* A germ-free animal is one that has been specially reared under sterile conditions. Caesarian section is generally employed in the initiation of such a colony.

the retina and central nervous system are rendered ischaemic. *Cryoglobulinaemia* (the presence of a globulin in the blood that precipitates in the cold) may occur in hypergammaglobulinaemia, and the precipitation of the protein in the small vessels of the hands leads to ischaemic episodes (Raynaud's syndrome) when the limbs are exposed to cold. Cryoglobulins may consist of immune complexes. Abnormal proteins may interact and bind to other plasma components such as calcium, platelets, and the proteins of the clotting system. A *bleeding tendency* is thereby produced. Although M-proteins belong to the immunoglobulins chemically, they have little antibody activity. Indeed, the production of antibody immunoglobulin is often inhibited, and this is manifested as an *increased tendency to infection.* Multiple myeloma often terminates in this manner.

Multiple myeloma. The hypergammaglobulinaemia is due to the presence of an M-protein which is usually of the IgG class, but may be of the IgA, IgD, or IgE class. The tumour plasma cells manufacture this protein, and in addition often form an excess of the corresponding light chain, either κ or λ. This, being of low molecular weight (22 000 daltons), is excreted in the urine as *Bence-Jones protein* (p. 600). The myeloma protein is not itself excreted.

Macroglobulinaemia of Waldenström. This rare condition is characterized by anaemia, a high ESR and a tendency to the hyperviscosity syndrome and to haemorrhages from the mucous membranes, especially the gingivae, either spontaneously or following dental extraction. The condition runs a prolonged course, and appears to be a disease in which the lymphoreticular system manufactures excessive amounts of a homogeneous M-protein belonging to the IgM class.

Heavy-chain disease (Franklin's disease)[7,8]. This uncommon disease is characterized by painful enlargement of the lymph nodes of Waldeyer's ring, fever, splenomegaly, and recurrent bacterial infections. An odd feature is transient, though sometimes severe, oedema and erythema of the soft palate, similar to that seen in infectious mononucleosis. The disease resembles Waldenström's macroglobulinaemia in that it is a type of diffuse lymphoma, lacking the punched-out, tumour-like bony deposits so characteristic of myeloma. The abnormal cells produce a fragment of the γ heavy chain, and this abnormal protein is present both in the blood and urine.

Other types of heavy-chain disease have been described; in these either the α-heavy chain or the μ-heavy chain is involved.

C-Reactive protein

This protein is so named because it reacts as a precipitin with the C-polysaccharide of the pneumococcus. Described originally as occurring in human serum in cases of pneumonia, it is found also in infections due to other organisms, in rheumatoid arthritis, and following trauma. The significance of this is not known, but its appearance is closely related to a rise in the ESR.

The lipoproteins[9–11]

The major lipids of the blood are phospholipid, cholesterol and its esters, neutral fat (glyceryl triesters), and free unesterified fatty acid. Apart from the free fatty acid which is bound to albumin, the lipids are carried in the blood as complexes with each other and with special carrier proteins that are called *apolipoproteins* (or *apoproteins*). This latter group consists of at least six components chemically, and their characterization and classification is currently under review. Thus the lipoproteins can be classified according to their chemical composition. In addition, they may be classified according to their density as quantitated in the ultracentrifuge, and by electrophoresis. The following are the important groups of lipoproteins:

1. *Free fatty acid.* This is mostly combined with albumin. The fatty acid is derived from adipose tissue, and is the form in which lipid is transported from fat depots to the tissues.

2. *Chylomicrons.* These are particles, not over 0.1 μm in diameter, which on electrophoresis do not migrate from the point of their application. They have a high neutral-fat (triglyceride) content, and are formed in the intestine following the absorption of dietary fat.

3. *Low-density lipoproteins.* These are the β-lipoproteins, and contain much cholesterol.

4. *Very low-density lipoproteins.* This group is called the pre-β-lipoprotein fraction, and contains much triglyceride of endogenous origin.

5. *High-density lipoproteins.* This group migrates in the α fraction on electrophoresis.

Lipoprotein deficiency syndromes. Three conditions are known in which one or more lipoproteins are either absent or else in very low concentration. All are uncommon, and are usually detected biochemically by finding a low plasma cholesterol level which is a feature common to all three.

Tangier disease (familial alpha-lipoprotein deficiency).[12] In this rare disease, named after Tangier Island (in Chesapeake Bay) which was the home of the first recognized case, there is an absence of the normal high-density, α-lipoprotein fraction. Cholesterol is stored in the reticuloendothelial system, and this storage is responsible for the remarkable enlargement of the tonsils, which have a characteristic orange colour—a unique and virtually diagnostic sign. Disabling peripheral neuropathy may occur later.

Abetalipoproteinaemia.[13] This syndrome is characterized by steatorrhoea, crenation of the red cells, retinitis pigmentosa, and cerebellar ataxia. *Hypobetalipoproteinaemia* has also been described, and is symptomless.

The hyperlipoproteinaemias are a group of conditions which may be *primary* and presumably genetic since they tend to be familial, or they may be *secondary* to a wide variety of metabolic abnormalities such as obesity, diabetes mellitus, obstructive jaundice, and an imbalanced diet. Both groups can be subdivided into five types depending on the lipoproteins which are elevated. The hyperlipoproteinaemias are important because some types predispose to the development of atheroma, particularly of the coronary arteries. Lipid can also accumulate in RE cells to form localized deposits of foam cells in the skin and tendons. These are called *xanthomata*; a common example is seen in the eyelids of elderly people. Xanthomata in this situation are called *xanthelasmata*, and they may also occur in the absence of hyperlipoproteinaemia.

The erythrocyte sedimentation rate (ESR)

When a column of blood mixed with anticoagulant is allowed to stand vertically, the red cells steadily gravitate in a mass due to the fact that their density is greater than that of plasma. The speed at which the sedimentation occurs is dependent upon many complex factors, chief of which are the degree of rouleaux formation and the extent of sludging. Both these phenomena are related to the composition of the plasma rather than to any change in the red cells themselves. Any relative increase in the plasma content of high-molecular-weight substances is found to increase the ESR. Thus an increase in fibrinogen or globulin (especially the α and β fractions) has this effect; the 7S γ-globulins are the least effective. A raised ESR is particularly characteristic of macroglobulinaemia and multiple myeloma. Since albumin inhibits sedimentation, the ESR is increased in hypoalbuminaemia, e.g. in the nephrotic syndrome. An increased ESR is seen whenever there is tissue necrosis (e.g. myocardial infarction) and following trauma. The factors concerned are poorly understood, but usually there is an increase in the fibrinogen and α-globulin levels, while that of albumin tends to drop. Elevation of the ESR is therefore quite non-specific, but nevertheless the test is a useful investigation. The presence of a raised ESR must always be taken to indicate disease, although the slight rise caused by anaemia, and that normally present during pregnancy, should always be remembered.

The ESR is of value in following the course of a known disease, e.g. tuberculosis and rheumatoid arthritis.

There are several methods of performing the ESR, and a haematology text-book should be consulted for details. The Westergren method is probably the most satisfactory. A column, 200 mm high, of citrated blood is allowed to stand upright for 1 hour, and the upper level of the red-cell mass is then observed and its height from the top of the plasma recorded. Normally the drop is less than 15 mm in 1 hour for men, and less than 20 mm for women under the age of 50 years, and 20 mm and 30 mm respectively for those over that age.

AMYLOID[14,15]

Amyloid is an abnormal protein which is found deposited in various organs. When the deposits are extensive the condition is called *amyloidosis*.

Staining of amyloid. In H. & E. sections amyloid appears as a hyaline, eosinophilic, structureless extracellular material. There are three empirical staining reactions by which it may be recognized:

Iodine. This may be used either on the specimen itself or on a histological section. Amyloid is coloured mahogany brown, and since in this respect it resembles glycogen, the material was called starch-like, or amyloid, by Virchow. When the iodine is followed by acid, amyloid may turn dark blue.

Methyl violet. This is a metachromatic histological stain, for the amyloid changes the methyl violet from a violet to a rose pink colour.

Congo red. This is soluble in amyloid, and can therefore be used to stain sections. The amyloid stains an orange colour and when the stained slide is viewed in a polarizing microscope a characteristic green birefringence is imparted. Apart from electron microscopy, this is the most reliable method of identifying amyloid.

The dye is also used in a clinical test for amyloidosis. If a known quantity of Congo red is injected intravenously, its rate of disappearance from the plasma can be measured. When 60 per cent or more disappears within 1 hour and has not been excreted into the urine, amyloidosis can be diagnosed. Unfortunately, fatal anaphylactic reactions to Congo red have been reported, and the test is generally deprecated.

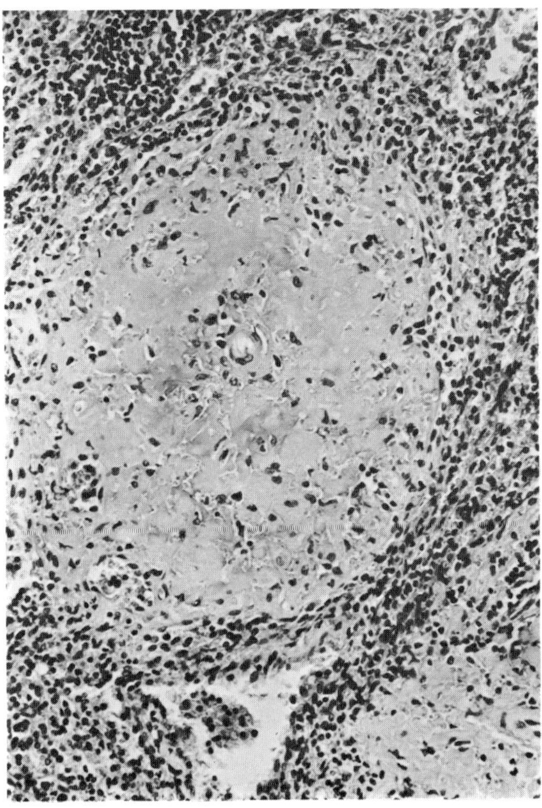

Fig. 29.3 Amyloidosis of spleen. The malpighian body is grossly enlarged, and is replaced by a mass of acellular amyloid. × 160.

Classification of amyloid disease

A classification according to associated clinical conditions is the most useful.

Secondary amyloidosis, is the commonest type of amyloid disease. It occurs in chronic infective conditions, especially where there is much necrosis or suppuration, e.g. chronic osteomyelitis, chronic empyema, caseous tuberculosis, and tertiary syphilis. It is also seen in rheumatoid arthritis, Hodgkin's disease, and occasionally in other malignant disease. The distribution of the amyloid is described as *typical*, and is found in the following sites:

Spleen. Amyloid is laid down in the walls of the malpighian arterioles, and the cut surface therefore presents a characteristic appearance of *sago spleen* with numerous scattered firm translucent nodules (Fig. 29.3). A diffuse type of amyloid spleen is also recognized, in which the amyloid is laid down in the walls of the sinuses.

Liver. The organ is enlarged, heavy, pale, and firm. The amyloid is laid down in the walls of the sinuses between the endothelium and the liver cells (Fig. 29.4).

Kidney. The organ is large and pale. The amyloid appears in the glomeruli, which may eventually be converted into hyaline masses. Proteinuria is severe, and the nephrotic syndrome follows.

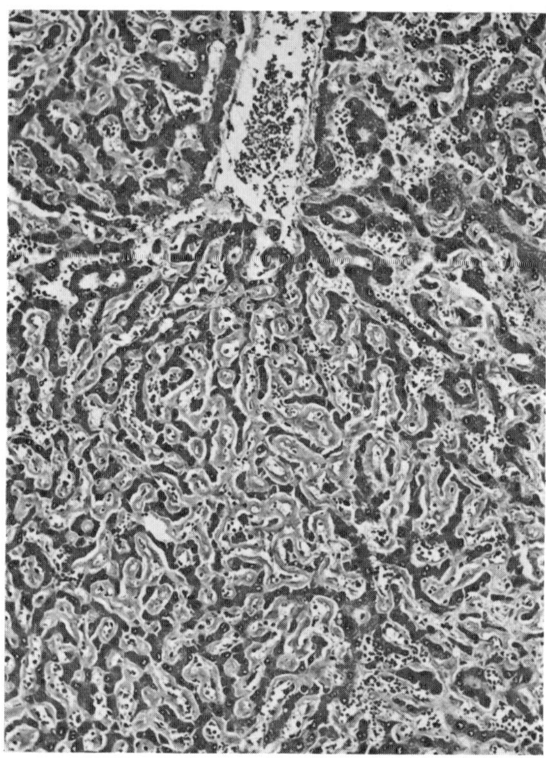

Fig. 29.4 Amyloidosis of liver. The amyloid is deposited in the space of Disse surrounding the sinusoids of the liver lobules. The liver cells adjacent to the amyloid are compressed, and show pronounced atrophy. × 120.

Other sites. Adrenals, lymph nodes, lung, and gut may all be affected. Deposits in the intestine may cause diarrhoea, and biopsy of the rectum is sometimes used as a diagnostic procedure. Amyloid is also laid down in the gingiva, and again biopsy may be employed to facilitate diagnosis.

Generalized amyloidosis is a well-known, complication of *multiple myeloma*, and in this it is quite often of atypical distribution as described below.

Primary amyloidosis. This occurs in the absence of any obvious cause. Its distribution may be typical as described in secondary amyloidosis, but more often it is *atypical* and involves the connective tissues of nerves and muscle, e.g. the heart, tongue, and gastrointestinal tract. The staining reaction is often atypical in that the specific stains may not all be positive.

Senile amyloid. Small deposits of amyloid are common in the heart and brain of elderly people and may be regarded as a normal feature of ageing. Occasionally the involvement of the heart may be sufficiently marked for it to cause heart failure.

Hereditary and familial amyloidosis. Several characteristic syndromes have been described but they are rare. Nevertheless, their existence serves as a reminder that the taking of a family history should never be neglected in a case of amyloidosis.

Localized amyloid. Deposits may occur in the form of localized masses, or 'tumours'. These are rare, and are generally found in the tongue, larynx, or bronchi. Amyloid may also be found in the stroma of certain true tumours, for example basal-cell carcinoma of the skin, medullary carcinoma of the thyroid, and calcifying epithelial odontogenic tumour.[16–18]

Effect of amyloid

The deposition of amyloid generally excites no inflammatory reaction, but there is atrophy of the parenchyma. In an organ with an abundant reserve like the liver this is of little functional significance, but in other situations, for example nerves and kidney, the effects may be severe. Renal failure is a common terminal manifestation of amyloidosis. An affected organ may become rigid and this is important if it has a mechanical function to perform, e.g. the heart and tongue. Affected vessels tend to bleed easily, and therefore repeated haemorrhages are to be expected. Since almost any tissue can be involved in amyloidosis, the clinical picture may be extremely varied and the diagnosis should always be kept in mind whenever one is confronted with an unusual case.

The nature and pathogenesis of amyloid[19, 20]

Amyloid is a protein with a β-pleated configuration but of no fixed composition. Electron microscopy reveals that it is composed of fibrils that have a characteristic appearance (Fig. 29.5). The fibrils are very insoluble and resistant to digestion. This insolubility has greatly hindered investigation into their chemical nature. Nevertheless, pure preparations of fibrils have been obtained, brought into solution, and subjected to detailed chemical analysis. Two major chemical types of amyloid have been identified.

Amyloid of immunoglobulin origin. The amyloid of primary amyloidosis, and that which accompanies multiple myeloma, consists of the light chains of immunoglobulin, or part of the light chain—always the amino-terminal fragment with the variable component of the polypeptide chain. Fibres with identical appearance and staining properties to that of native amyloid can be produced *in vitro* by limited proteolytic digestion of Bence-Jones protein—particularly of the λ type. The sera of patients with primary amyloidosis or multiple myeloma contain an M-protein with identical amino-acid sequence to that of the amyloid deposits in that particular patient. As might be expected, amyloidosis is more common in cases of myeloma with the λ type Bence-Jones protein than in those with the κ type. It should be noted that in amyloidosis of any type, all the deposits of amyloid present in a particular patient have the same chemical composition, but, of course, differ from the amyloid found in other patients.

Amyloid of unknown origin (AA). The amyloid of secondary amyloidosis has no amino-acid sequences in common with immunoglobulin, and is of unknown origin. It has a β-pleated configuration, and in any individual case there is a circulating plasma component, termed SAA, which is related in composition to the amyloid itself. This SAA may be a circulating precursor of the amyloid

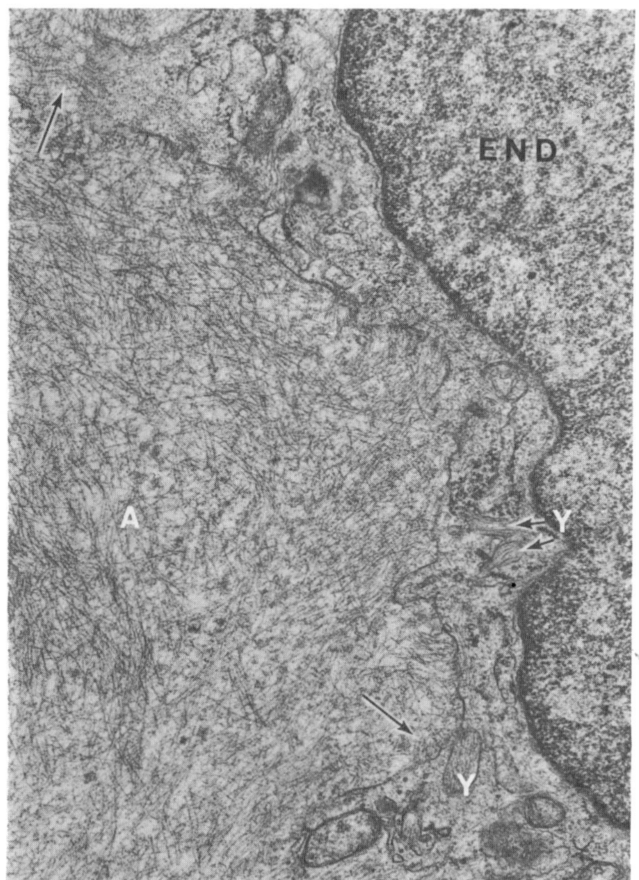

Fig. 29.5 Amyloid-laden rabbit spleen. The amyloid fibrils (A) fill most of the space near the endothelial cell (END), whose plasma membrane bears an intricate relationship to the fibrils, especially in the areas marked by arrows. In several areas (Y) fibrils appear to be intracellular. Osmium-fixed, Epon-embedded tissue, stained with lead citrate. × 24 000. (*From Cohen A S 1965 In: Richter G W, Epstein M A (eds) International review of experimental pathology, vol. 4. Academic Press, New York, p 159.*)

fibrils, and is found in all patients with amyloidosis. Indeed, it is found in all normal adults, but its concentration increases with age and also in some chronic diseases, for example tuberculosis, rheumatoid arthritis, and cancer. It has been found that the peptic digestion of many proteins, for example insulin, calcitonin, and glucagon, may yield products that *in vitro* will form typical amyloid fibres.

It is therefore probable that amyloid fibrils can be formed *in vivo* from a variety of polypeptide fragments, derived either from immunoglobulin or from some other protein. It may be that in a chronic destructive disease, such as osteomyelitis or tuberculosis, it is the tissue proteins themselves that provide the raw material for the formation of amyloid protein. It should be noted that some polypeptide fragments are more amyloidogenic than others: thus, as noted previously, the λ light chains form amyloid fibrils more readily than do the κ chains. Under some circumstances the formation of amyloid appears to be a local affair, and may be related to the partial breakdown of proteins by local reticuloendothelial cells. Thus the localized deposits of amyloid in medullary carcinoma of the thyroid may be derived from calcitonin.

In generalized amyloidosis it seems that an amyloidogenic protein, either immunoglobulin or SAA, is present in the blood-stream and is deposited in various sites. Even under these circumstances it is possible that the reticuloendothelial system plays some part, and the cells from this system could take up immunoglobulin antigen-antibody complexes, or other protein, and produce the necessary polypeptides for the formation of the amyloid fibrils of their characteristic β-pleating.

Although recent research has answered many of the questions that have raged over the composition and nature of amyloid fibres, many more questions remain unanswered. It is not known why amyloid deposition occurs in some patients and not in others, or why it occurs in some sites and not in others. It remains a possibility that amyloid is a normal constituent of the body, and that excessive accumulations occur as a result of its defective removal.

GENERAL READING

Putnam F W 1965 In The Proteins, 2nd edn Vol III, pp 153–267. Ed Neurath H, Academic Press New York & London

REFERENCES

1. Alper C A 1974 Plasma protein measurements as a diagnostic aid. New England Journal of Medicine 291 : 287
2. Haurowitz F 1961 In Functions of the Blood, p 527, ed Macfarlane R G, Robb-Smith A H T, Blackwell, Oxford
3. Rothschild M A, Oratz M, Schreiber S S 1972 Albumin synthesis. New England Journal of Medicine 286 : 748 and 816
4. Jarnum S 1963 Protein-Losing Gastroenteropathy., Blackwell, Oxford
5. Dawson A M 1965 In Recent Advances in Gastroenterology, p 126 (Protein-losing enteropathy), ed Badenoch J, Brooke B N, Churchill, London
6. Waldmann T A 1969 Disorders of immunoglobulin metabolism. New England Journal of Medicine 281 : 1170
7. Franklin E C 1970 Heavy-chain diseases. New England Journal of Medicine 282 : 1098
8. Franklin E C 1976 Some impacts of clinical investigation on immunology. New England Journal of Medicine 294 : 531
9. Fredrickson D S, Levy R I, Lees R S 1967 Fat transport in lipoproteins—an integrated approach to mechanisms and disorders. New England Journal of Medicine 276 : 34, 94, 148, 215 and 273
10. Lehmann H, Lines J G 1972 Hyperlipoproteinaemia classification : the optimum routine electrophoretic system and its relevance to treatment. Lancet 1 : 557
11. Leading Article 1971 Hyperlipoproteinaemias. Lancet 2 : 806
12. Fredrickson D S 1972 Tonsils, apolipoproteins and enzymes. New England Journal of Medicine 286 : 601
13. Ockner R K 1971 Abetalipoproteinemia : rarity and relevance. New England Journal of Medicine 284 : 848

14. Cohen A S 1967 Amyloidosis. New England Journal of Medicine 277 : 522, 574, and 628
15. Stirling G A 1975 In Recent Advances in Pathology, ed Harrison C V, Weinbren K, number 9, p 249., Churchill Livingstone, Edinburgh
16. Vickers R A, Dahlin D C, Gorlin R J 1965 Amyloid-containing odontogenic tumours. Oral Surgery, Oral Medicine, and Oral Pathology 20 : 476
17. Ranløv P, Pindborg J J 1966 The amyloid nature of the homogeneous substance in the calcifying epithelial odontogenic tumour. Acta pathologica et microbiologica scandinavica 68 : 169
18. Gardner D G, Michaels L, Liepa E 1968 Calcifying epithelial odontogenic tumour : An amyloid-producing neoplasm. Oral Surgery, Oral Medicine, and Oral Pathology 26 : 812
19. Katz A, Pruzanski W 1976 Newer concepts in amyloidogenesis. Canadian Medical Association Journal 114 : 872
20. Glenner G G, Page D L 1976 Amyloid, amyloidosis and amyloidogenesis. International Review of Experimental Pathology 15 : 2

30

Disorders of the blood

The formed elements of the blood are the red cells (*erythrocytes*), white cells (*leucocytes*), and *platelets*. In the fetus blood formation (*haematopoiesis*) occurs both in the bone marrow and in a few extramedullary sites such as the liver and spleen. After birth haematopoiesis is solely medullary.

THE RED CELLS

Development

The most primitive blood cell in the marrow is the stem cell, a large cell with abundant cytoplasm and a nucleus with several nucleoli. It is capable of forming erythrocytes, granulocytes, monocytes, megakaryocytes, and fibroblasts; under normal conditions it probably does not differentiate into cells of the lymphocyte series. If the stem cell is directed towards red cell formation it becomes smaller, its nucleus condenses, and its cytoplasm forms increasing amounts of haemoglobin. The first precursor cell is called a *pronormoblast*, which has nucleoli and whose cytoplasm has no haemoglobin. In the next cell type, the *normoblast*, nucleoli have been lost. Three stages are recognized—early, intermediate, and late—depending on the degree of haemoglobinization of the cytoplasm and the pyknosis of the nucleus (Fig. 30.2). Eventually the nucleus is extruded, and a mature red cell is left. These stages of development are indicated in Figure 30.1.

The mature cell

The red cell is a biconcave disc, and in blood films appears as a roughly circular cell. It stains red with the Romanowsky dyes used in haematology.* When young it contains rough endoplasmic reticulum, and this imparts a bluish tint to the cell. This is called *polychromasia*. If such a cell is stained supravitally with brilliant cresyl blue, the RNA stands out as a network, or reticulum, of fine blue strands, and the cell is called a *reticulocyte*. The proportion of reticulocytes to older red cells gives an indication of the activity of erythropoiesis. The *reticulocyte count* is normally 0.8 to 2.5 per cent in males, and 0.8 to 4.1 per cent in females. A rise in the reticulocyte count indicates increased red-cell formation. This occurs after:

1. Haemorrhage

* These include stains such as Leishman, Jenner, and Giemsa, and consist of a blended mixture of methylene blue and eosin.

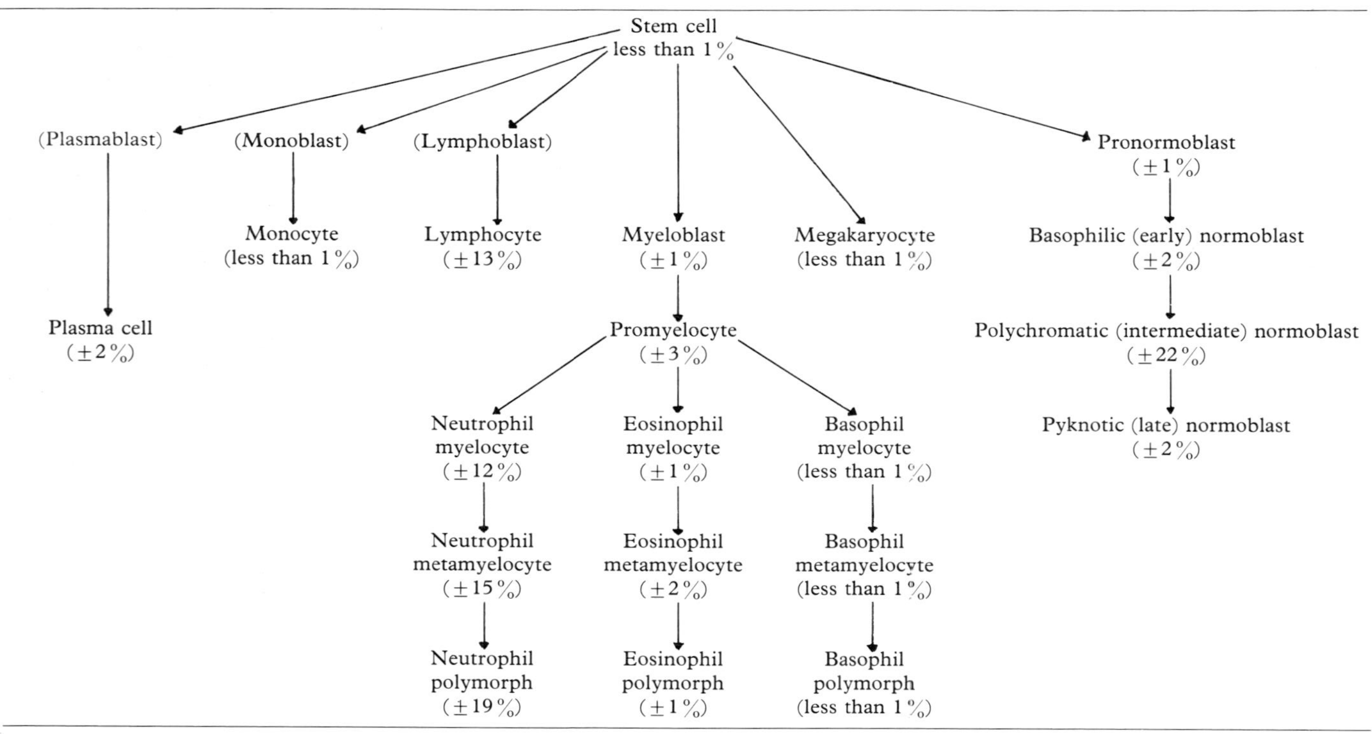

Fig. 30.1 The cellular constituents of the normal bone marrow.

2. Haemolysis
3. Successful treatment of an anaemia.

When erythropoiesis is much increased, nucleated forms also appear in the circulation. A good example is haemolytic disease of the newborn (Fig. 30.2).*

Examination of the red cell

The normal red cell count is 4.6 to 6.2 $\times$ 10^{12} per litre (4.6 to 6.2 million per μl or mm^3) in males, and the normal haemoglobin content is 14 to 18 g per dl. In women the red cell count is 0.5 $\times$ 10^{12} per litre less and the haemoglobin level 2 g per dl lower. The red cell count is high at birth, but drops precipitously within the first few months.

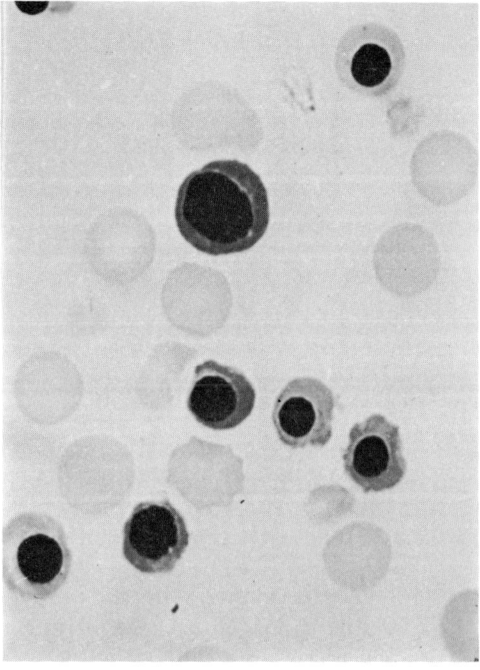

Fig. 30.2 Normoblasts in peripheral blood. The patient was an infant with haemolytic disease of the newborn due to rhesus incompatibility. One intermediate and six late normoblasts are shown. ×960.

A haemoglobin estimation is an essential examination to assess the presence and degree of anaemia. It is a simple and easily reproducible procedure, and is particularly useful if the laboratory is not equipped with an electronic cell counter for red cell estimations. The normal value is 14 to 18 g per dl. Another useful investigation is the *haematocrit* reading, or *packed cell volume*. In this test a thin, cylindrical, graduated tube is filled with blood and centrifuged for half an hour at 3000 revolutions per minute. In the adult male 40 to 50 per cent of the volume consists of red cells.

* An *erythroblast* is the collective name for any red cell precursor.

The experienced haematologist derives the most information about the red cell by inspecting a well-made, well-stained blood film. The normal red cell is described as *normocytic* and *normochromic*. If smaller than normal it is *microcytic*, and if larger, *macrocytic*. A cell cannot be over-haemoglobinized, and so there cannot be hyperchromia. If cells are poorly haemoglobinized, they look pale and are described as *hypochromic*; in a stained film they are easily recognized by their colourless centres, which may be so extensive that only a narrow rim of haemoglobin is left around them peripherally. In addition the cells may contain a small central aggregation of haemoglobin surrounded by the extensive colourless zone; these are called *target cells* (Fig 30.6). *Spherocytes* appear on a blood film as small, darkly staining cells. They are almost spherical in shape, and although the cells appear small, their volume is normal because of their increased thickness. *Burr cells*, or *acanthocytes*, are mature red cells which possess one or more spiky projections on their periphery. Burr cells are characteristic of those haemolytic anaemias in which mechanical trauma is believed to damage the red cells, e.g. microangiopathic haemolytic anaemia. They are also found in uraemia and abetalipoproteinaemia (p. 435).

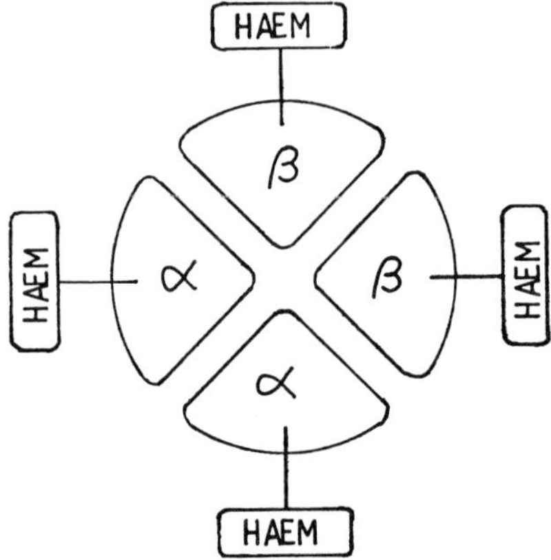

Fig. 30.3 Diagrammatic representation of haemoglobin. The four polypeptide chains of globin are labelled α and β. (*After Wintrobe M M 1967 Fig. 3.7 in Clinincial Hematology, 6th edn Lea & Febiger, p 139.*)

Marked variation in size of the population of red cells is called *anisocytosis*, and a marked variation in shape, *poikilocytosis*.

Haemoglobin

Haemoglobin is a conjugated protein. The molecule consists of four haem groups attached to the protein globin which in turn is composed of two pairs of polypeptide chains. Five types of chain are known—α, β, γ, δ, and ε. In haemoglobin A (Hb-A) the normal major component of adult human blood, the globin consists of two α chains and two β chains (Fig. 30.3). Fetal haemoglobin (Hb-F) is the type found in the fetus and during early infancy but not in the normal adult; it consists of two α chains and two γ chains. Other types of haemoglobin are known and an abnormal amount of them is formed in a group of conditions called the *thalassaemia syndromes.*

Another abnormality of the haemoglobin molecule can result from a genetic defect such that there is an abnormal sequence of amino acids in either the α or β chain of Hb-A. Sickle-cell anaemia (due to the formation of Hb-S) is the most important example of this type of defect (p. 46). The whole group of conditions in which there is an abnormality of haemoglobin, either quantitative or qualitative, is termed the *haemoglobinopathies.*

Requirements for red-cell formation

Apart from protein, which forms part of haemoglobin, the most important requirements are iron, folic acid, and vitamin B_{12}.

Iron. In its ferrous form (Fe^{2+}) iron is an integral part of haemoglobin. As seen in Fig. 30.4, the iron atom lies in the centre of the porphyrin structure composed

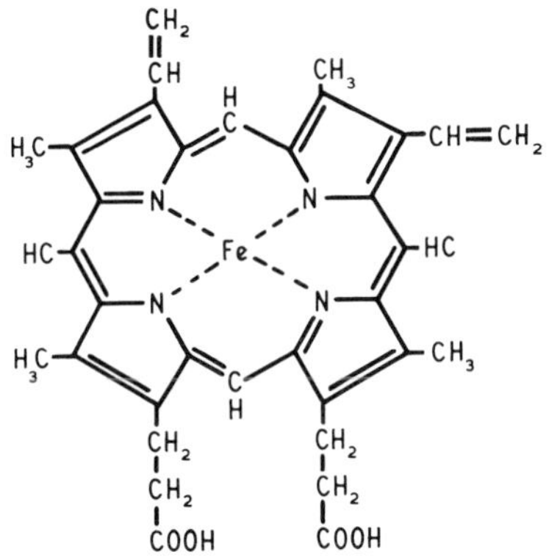

Fig. 30.4 The structural formula of haem. Note the protoporphyrin ring structure which is composed of four pyrrole rings joined by methene (=CH—) bridges.

of four pyrrole rings. Iron is absorbed from the food in an ionic form by the mucosal cells of the duodenum and upper small bowel. Here it combines, in ferric form (Fe^{3+}), with the iron-free protein *apoferritin* to form *ferritin*, the storage form of iron in the body. Ferric iron is absorbed as required into the blood stream and carried in combination with a globulin called *iron-binding protein*, *transferrin*, or *siderophilin.* The concentration of transferrin in the plasma is 1.2 g per litre, but more commonly transferrin is quantitated in terms of the total iron it will bind, the *total iron-binding capacity (TIBC) of the plasma*, which is normally 45 to 70 µmol per litre (250 to 400 µg per dl): the plasma is normally one-third saturated with iron. Iron is used for the synthesis of haemoglobin and myoglobin; it is stored in the RE system as ferritin.

Vitamins. The important group belong to the B complex—folic acid and vitamin B_{12}. Both are necessary for the proper development of the normoblast; without either (or both) the cell undergoes a perversion of development, remaining large, and retaining a delicate stippled pattern of chromatin instead of showing the nuclear pyknosis of a maturing normoblast. Such a cell is called a *megaloblast* (Fig. 30.5). Both vitamins are present in the diet and absorbed in the small bowel, but whereas folic acid is directly taken up, vitamin B_{12} cannot be absorbed unless bound to a complex mucoprotein secreted by the gastric mucosa. This substance is called *intrinsic factor*. It follows that the gastric secretion is essential for the absorption of vitamin B_{12}. Both vitamins are stored in the liver.

Other substances are required but their role is less well understood; they include copper, cobalt, and hormones, such as thyroxine, adrenal cortical hormones, sex hormones, and *erythropoietin*. The last is probably responsible for the erythropoiesis that occurs after hypoxia. It is formed in the kidneys and possibly in other organs also, and its plasma level is high in most anaemic states.

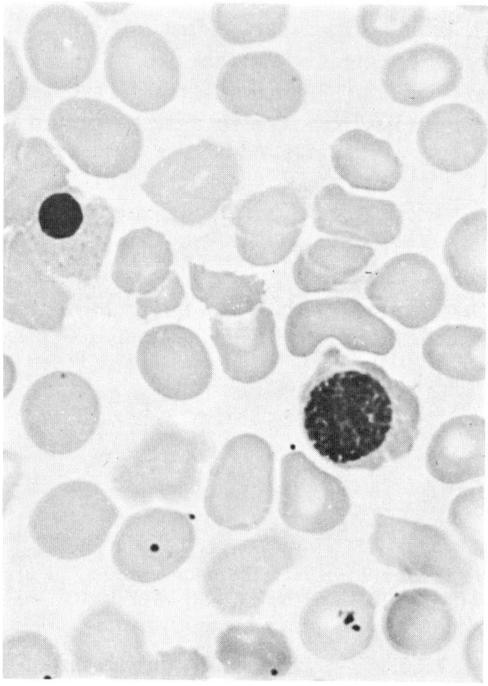

Fig. 30.5 A megaloblast. Note the large size of the cell and its stippled nuclear chromatin as compared with the much smaller normoblast and its pyknotic nucleus. The smear is from the marrow of a patient with pernicious anaemia. × 960.

Disposal of the red cell

The normal life-span of the red cell is about 120 days. The manner in which the effete red cells are destroyed is still uncertain. The process of ageing precedes and is responsible for eventual destruction, and it is possible that the cell undergoes fragmentation in the circulation prior to its ultimate removal by the RE cells of the liver, bone marrow, and spleen. In these cells the haemoglobin is broken down. The globin portion is released, degraded, and returned to the body's pool of amino acids. The iron portion of the haemoglobin is stored in the RE cells as ferritin, while the porphyrin nucleus is broken down to bilirubin which is excreted by the liver. Normally there is a mere trace of free haemoglobin in the plasma—any that does appear is immediately removed by combination with a globulin component of the plasma proteins called *haptoglobin*. If haemoglobin in excess of the haptoglobin binding capacity of the plasma is released, the free haemoglobin in the plasma is readily oxidized to methaemoglobin, which dissociates into haem and globin. The haem combines with *haemopexin*, a normal β-globulin of the plasma, and when this binding protein is exhausted its place is taken by albumin, which binds haem to form *methaemalbumin*. The haptoglobin, haemopexin, and albumin complexes are all metabolized in the RE system, principally in the liver, and none escapes into the urine. It is only when all these binding proteins are consumed that free haemoglobin appears in the blood (*haemoglobinaemia*) and urine (*haemoglobinuria*).

THE ANAEMIAS

Anaemia is defined as a condition in which there is a fall in the quantity of either red cells or haemoglobin in a unit volume of blood in the presence of a low or normal total blood volume. The normal blood volume is 5 litres, of which 2.8 litres is plasma and 2.2 litres red-cell mass. It might be expected that the blood volume would be reduced in anaemia owing to the decreased number of red cells, but in fact it is little altered as there is a compensatory rise in plasma volume.

The effects of anaemia are attributable to cellular hypoxia. At necropsy there is severe fatty change of the liver, heart, and kidneys, and death is usually attributed to heart failure. The classification of the anaemias is controversial, and the following scheme is recommended:

1. Acute posthaemorrhagic anaemia, which has been described on page 405
2. Iron-deficiency anaemia
3. Megaloblastic anaemia
4. Haemolytic anaemia
5. Anaemia of bone-marrow inadequacy.

The main clinico-pathological features of anaemia are as follows: *Pallor*, best detected in the conjunctiva, nail bed, or oral mucous membrane. Skin pallor, particularly of the face, is a deceptive sign. It may be absent in some patients with anaemia, and yet present in many pale-skinned healthy people.

Tiredness, easy fatiguability, and generalized muscular weakness are common symptoms; their pathogenesis, however, is not clear. Such symptoms are also common in psychoneurotic patients who are not anaemic.

Shortness of breath, and palpitations are common. They are related to tissue *hypoxia* and an increased cardiac output. *Heart failure* can occur.

Angina pectoris, intermittent claudication, and giddiness are due to tissue hypoxia in organs in which the blood supply is already impaired by arterial disease.

The basal metabolic rate is raised, and in severe degrees of anaemia *pyrexia* is quite common. The cause of this is unclear.

Iron-deficiency anaemia

Causes

Chronic blood loss. This is the most important cause, and is usually due to gastrointestinal bleeding from a peptic ulcer, tumour, or haemorrhoids. Excessive menstrual loss (menorrhagia) is another factor. Other important causes are *aspirin ingestion* leading to gastric erosions, and hook-worm infestation (*ankylostomiasis*).

Defective iron intake. This may be due to *dietary deficiency*, and is seen quite commonly in infants, pregnant women, and the elderly. It may also be due to defective absorption from the bowel in the *malabsorption syndrome*. This may follow intestinal lesions and also gastrectomy, which is often complicated by intestinal hurry.

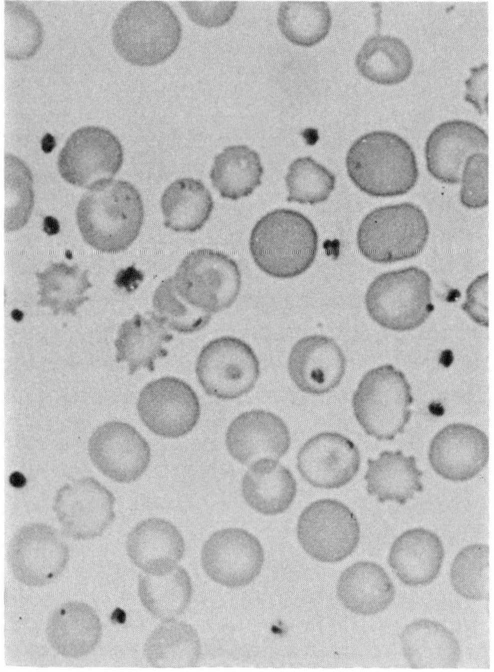

Fig. 30.6 Iron-deficiency anaemia. This film of peripheral blood contains red cells that are hypochromic. Quite a number show a target-like distribution of their haemoglobin. There are numerous platelets present. ×960.

The pathological effects

The pathological findings are seen in the peripheral blood and bone marrow. There is a moderate anaemia in which the red-cell count is relatively less reduced than the haemoglobin level. *The red cells are markedly microcytic and hypochromic*, and target cells may be present (Fig. 30.6). The reticulocyte count is normal or only slightly increased unless there has been a recent haemorrhage. The white cells and platelets are normal. The bone marrow shows normoblastic hyperplasia.

Other interesting features seen in some cases of chronic iron-deficiency anaemia are *koilonychia*—spoon-shaped, brittle, lustreless finger nails—and *oral manifestations*—angular stomatitis, denudation of the filiform papillae of the tongue, and dysphagia. These oral features together constitute the *Plummer-Vinson syndrome.**

* This syndrome was first described in 1906 by Paterson, and soon afterwards by Kelly; both were laryngologists. It should rightly be called the Paterson-Kelly syndrome.

Its relationship to iron deficiency is obscure. It is seen especially in anaemic, middle-aged women who have achlorhydria (the absence of hydrochloric acid in the gastric juice), and is sometimes complicated by oral and postcricoid cancer. Atrophic gastritis commonly complicates iron deficiency, and the achlorhydria further impedes iron absorption.

Megaloblastic anaemia

Megaloblastic anaemias are characterized by disordered DNA synthesis which results in megaloblastic erythroporesis in the bone marrow. In a great majority of cases they are due to a deficiency of vitamin B_{12} or folic acid, either alone or in combination. Rarely they are due to drug-induced or inherited disorders of DNA synthesis.

Causes

Dietary deficiency. This is quite common in under-developed countries, and the anaemia is due to a lack of folic acid.

Pregnancy. Pregnancy is sometimes complicated by anaemia which is also due to folic-acid deficiency either as a result of a poor diet or because of the extra demands of the fetus.

Gastric disease. The intrinsic factor of the stomach is necessary for vitamin-B_{12} absorption in the bowel, and therefore total resection of the stomach must in time lead to a vitamin-B_{12} deficiency anaemia. However, the most important example is *pernicious anaemia*, an idiopathic condition in which there is progressive atrophy of the gastric mucosa. The stomach fails to secrete pepsin, hydrochloric acid, and finally intrinsic factor itself. Pernicious anaemia is a familial disease, and it is of interest that many patients are of blood-group A. IgA autoantibodies against parietal cells and intrinsic factor are usually present in the patient's serum.

Intestinal malabsorption due to intrinsic disease of the small bowel usually affects folic-acid absorption more than it does vitamin-B_{12} absorption.

Drugs. Notably the *anticonvulsants* phenytoin sodium and primidone used in epilepsy, and the *antimetabolites* (e.g. methotrexate) used in the chemotherapy of cancer, antagonize folic acid and can cause a megaloblastic anaemia.

Inherited disorders of the DNA synthesis. The most important example is orotic aciduria, which is an inherited disorder of pyrimidine metabolism.

Pathological effects

The *peripheral blood* shows a severe anaemia in which the red-cell count is relatively more reduced than the haemoglobin level. The red cells are conspicuously *macrocytic* and *normochromic*; they show poikilocytosis and anisocytosis (Fig. 30.7). The reticulocyte count is usually not raised. Both the leucocytes and platelets are reduced in number. *The bone marrow is hyperplastic and contains many megaloblasts* (Fig. 30.5).

There is a mild element of haemolysis in this type of anaemia, and the plasma bilirubin is slightly raised. Ineffective erythropoiesis adds to the bilirubin load. The effects are those of a mild haemolytic jaundice (p. 563).

The other effects depend on the cause of the anaemia. Vitamin B_{12} is essential for the proper functioning of the central nervous system, and without it *subacute combined degeneration of the spinal cord* can occur. In this there is demyelination of the posterior and lateral colums of the cord. It occurs much less frequently in pure folic-acid deficiency.

In pernicious anaemia there is atrophy of the mucosa of the tongue with disappearance of the filiform papillae. This produces the characteristic raw, beefy tongue. Glossitis is also seen in sprue, but is not constant in the other megaloblastic anaemias.

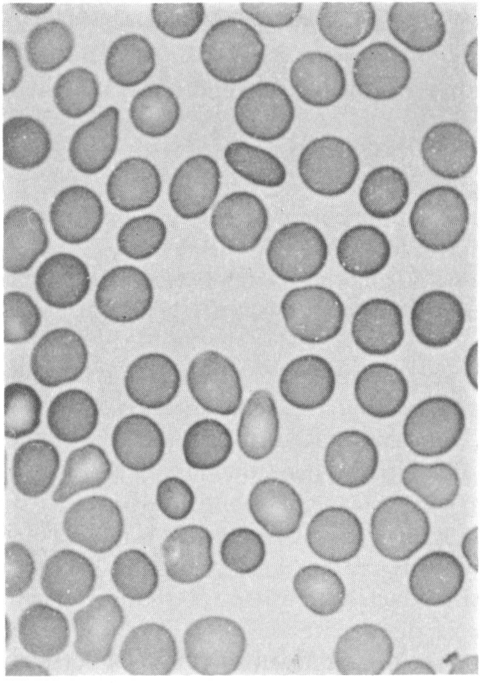

Fig. 30.7 Megaloblastic anaemia. This film of peripheral blood contains well-haemoglobinized red cells which show considerable variation in size and shape. Large forms (macrocytes) predominate. × 800.

Haemolytic anaemia

The term *haemolytic anaemia* is applied to those conditions in which there is an increased rate of red-cell destruction. This in turn stimulates red-cell formation which is manifested by a reticulocytosis. An increase in reticulocytes that occurs apart from haemorrhage or the treatment of an anaemia is nearly always due to increased haemolysis.

Causes

The increased haemolysis may be due either to abnormal red cells which are easily destroyed, or to a factor in the plasma which haemolyses normal red cells.

Corpuscular defects. The most important in Northern European races is *hereditary spherocytosis*, or *congenital acholuric jaundice*, in which there is a spherocytic malformation of the red cells. These are very liable to be trapped and destroyed in the spleen. Splenectomy is usually effective in allaying the anaemia while having no effect on the malformed cells.

The haemoglobinopathies. In Black populations the important congenital malformation is *sickle-cell anaemia.* Here the cells appear normal until deprived of oxygen, when they undergo bizarre sickling. This haemoglobinopathy is considered on page 46. Many other abnormal types of haemoglobin have been found. Thus Hb-C is encountered especially in West-African Blacks, and its presence leads to an anaemia less severe than sickle-cell anaemia.

The thalassaemia syndromes. β-thalassaemia major, or Cooley's anaemia, is most commonly found in the Mediterranean races; in it there is an inherited defect in the synthesis of the β chain of haemoglobin so that normal Hb-A is formed in inadequate amounts. As if to compensate for this there is an excessive formation of Hb-F. In homozygous individuals (β-thalassaemia major) the anaemia is severe; the red cells are grossly hypochromic and appear distorted and flattened (*leptocytes*). This type of cell is rapidly destroyed in the body, so that a severe haemolytic anaemia ensues. In β-thalassaemia minor, which is the heterozygous state, there is a mild anaemia, and the affected individuals have a tendency to develop gallstones. Other types of thalassaemia are known in which there is a defective synthesis of the α chain of globin.

Combinations of these haemoglobinopathies are quite common. The most important are sickle-cell-Hb-C disease, sickle-cell-thalassaemia, and Hb-C-thalassaemia. None of these conditions is as severe as sickle-cell anaemia or β-thalassaemia major.

Enzyme-deficient cells. The observation that certain Black Americans developed an acute haemolytic anaemia when given the antimalarial drugs pamaquine and primaquine, led to the discovery that their cells lacked the enzyme *glucose 6-phosphate dehydrogenase (G6PD).* G6PD deficiency is inherited as an incomplete dominant sex-linked trait, and affected individuals usually suffer no ill-effects unless they are given certain drugs. The antimalarials mentioned above are the most important, but the sulphones (used in the treatment of leprosy), sulphonamides, phenacetin, aspirin, and para-aminosalicylic acid can also precipitate acute haemolytic episodes. Once again the importance of iatrogenic disease is underlined. G6PD deficiency has also been found in Caucasians, especially those from the Mediterranean area, and furthermore other enzyme deficiences have also been found which cause haemolytic anaemia, either spontaneously or under the influence of drugs. The enzymes are those of glucose metabolism, and their normal function is important in maintaining the integrity of the red cell, particularly its haemoglobin content.

Extracorpuscular defects

Autoantibodies. Amongst the most important plasma factors acting on red cells are *autoantibodies.* Most occur idiopathically, but a few develop in the course of an infection, e.g. mycoplasmal pneumonia, a collagen disease, e.g. systemic lupus erythematosus, or a neoplasm, e.g. histiocytic lymphoma (reticulum-cell sarcoma) and Hodgkin's disease. Most autoantibodies are agglutinins.

Complete antibodies. Some antibodies, usually of the IgM class, can agglutinate red cells directly in saline suspension, and are called 'complete' antibodies. Most of these are not active at body temperature, but become powerful at colder temperatures. They are therefore called 'cold' antibodies. Although detected in the laboratory as agglutinins, *in vivo* their action leads to red-cell destruction. They cause a comparatively mild haemolytic anaemia, especially after exposure to the cold.

Incomplete antibodies. The more important autoantibodies do not agglutinate red cells in saline suspension. They are, however, adsorbed on to the red cells, which, if washed to remove extraneous protein, and then suspended in an anti-human-γ-globulin serum (obtained by immunizing a rabbit against human globulin), undergo immediate agglutination. This *antiglobulin test* is also known as the *Coombs test.* Antibodies which coat red cells in saline suspension are called 'incomplete antibodies', and most of them are IgG. *In vitro* they will agglutinate red cells suspended in 20 per cent albumin solution, but in practice the antiglobulin test is more sensitive. Most 'incomplete' antibodies act maximally at 37°C, and are therefore called 'warm' antibodies. *In vivo,* incomplete antibodies cause the cells which they coat to be destroyed. They therefore lead to a very severe type of haemolytic anaemia.

The level of complement in the plasma is lowered since haemolysis involves its activation and consumption. These anaemias are sometimes accompanied by falsely positive standard serological reactions of syphilis, due presumably to autoantibodies formed against normal lipid constituents of the body.

*Alloantibodies.** The blood-group antibodies can also cause haemolytic anaemia under certain circumstances. A good example is *Rh-haemolytic disease of the newborn (erythroblastosis fetalis)*, in which an Rh-negative mother, married to a Rh-positive man, produces an Rh-positive fetus. During the last part of pregnancy and especially during labour, a leak of fetal cells into the maternal circulation is quite common. The mother is thereby stimulated to produce Rh antibodies. An abortion can have a similar effect. While the first child escapes damage, future Rh-positive fetuses may be attacked by maternal anti-Rh antibodies which cross the placenta. The fetus develops a severe haemolytic anaemia with many nucleated red cells in its circulation (Fig 30.2)

An advance of great importance is the discovery that the administration of a gamma globulin containing incomplete anti-Rh of high activity can prevent the sensitization of Rh-negative mothers by Rh-positive fetal cells, provided it is given within 72 hours of delivery or abortion. The antibody probably suppresses the anti-Rh immune response by coating Rh-positive cells in the circulation, so that these are rapidly removed by the RE system. Alternatively, the antibody may, by combining with antigenic sites on the red cells, block any effective contact with antigen-sensitive cells. In this way antibody production is inhibited. The final alternative is that the antibody directly suppresses the immune response by acting upon the antigen-sensitive cells.

A Group-A or Group-B fetus may likewise be the victim of anti-A or anti-B antibodies from its Group-O mother. This is an uncommon event, because the

* An alloantibody is an antibody present in one member of a species, which is capable of reacting specifically with an antigen present in some other members of the same species (see p. 191). The term isoantibody was previously used in this connexion, but it has been discarded so that the terms now parallel those used in transplantation immunology.

naturally-occurring antibodies in the ABO system are of the IgM class and do not cross the placenta. Only when the mother produces sufficient quantities of IgG is there a risk of the fetus being affected.

Other important extracorpuscular factors that may lead to haemolytic anaemia are *organisms*, e.g. malarial parasites, *exotoxins*, e.g. the α-toxin of *Cl. welchii*, *drugs*, e.g. lead and sulphonamides, and *severe burns* which damage red cells locally.

Pathological effects of haemolytic anaemia

The peripheral blood shows an anaemia in which the red-cell count and haemoglobin level closely correlate. The red cells are normochromic and normocytic. The outstanding feature is a *marked reticulocytosis*, sometimes over 30 per cent. In specific types of haemolytic anaemia malformed red cells may be seen, e.g. target cells, spherocytes, and leptocytes. The red-cell fragility is increased in spherocytosis and decreased in leptocytosis. There is a leucocytosis in acute haemolytic anaemia, but the white-cell count drops to normal in chronic cases. The bone marrow shows marked normoblastic hyperplasia.

There is a moderate to severe haemolytic jaundice in most cases. When intravascular haemolysis occurs, as in some alloantibody and autoantibody reactions, there is also *methaemalbuminaemia* (p. 449) and even *haemoglobinaemia* with *haemoglobinuria*. The presence of free haemoglobin in the plasma may cause renal vasoconstriction and anuria, especially if the haemolysis has occurred as the result of an immunological reaction (p. 473).

Other pathological effects of chronic haemolytic anaemia are *gallstone (calcium bilirubinate) formation* due to the increased amount of bilirubin in the bile, and a *widening of the marrow cavities* of the bones with absorption of the compact cortex. This is due to the effect of increased, prolonged haematopoiesis. Some congenital haemolytic anaemias, e.g. hereditary spherocytosis and sickle-cell disease, are associated with *chronic leg ulcers*, but the connexion is not understood.

Anaemia of bone marrow inadequacy

Anaemia is a complication of many chronic diseases, e.g. rheumatoid arthritis, chronic suppuration, leukaemia, renal disease, and myxoedema. It is normocytic and normochromic, and is not attended by any significant reticulocytosis. It would appear that some deficiency or toxaemia impairs red-cell production, but the mechanism is not known.

Two other important types of anaemia that come into this category are those due to marrow aplasia (*aplastic anaemia*) and marrow replacement (*leucoerythroblastic anaemia*). They are considered later in the chapter.

POLYCYTHAEMIA

Polycythaemia is a condition in which the quantity of red cells is raised in a unit volume of blood in the presence of an increased total blood volume. It must be distinguished from haemoconcentration following plasma or fluid loss, in which the blood volume is reduced.

Polycythaemia may be *secondary* to chronic hypoxia, e.g. living at very great altitudes, chronic pulmonary disease, and cyanotic congenital heart disease. It is also seen occasionally in renal carcinoma—the tumour is presumed to secrete erythropoietin—and in Cushing's syndrome.

As a primary condition (*polycythaemia vera*) it is a neoplastic proliferation of the normoblastic element of the marrow. The red cell count may be increased to 10×10^{10} per litre (10 million cells per mm^3). There is usually a considerable increase in the white-cell and platelet counts, a change not occurring in secondary polycythaemia. These patients are usually middle-aged or elderly, of florid complexion, with enlarged spleens and livers, and are liable to succumb to thrombotic complications, e.g. mesenteric venous thrombosis, coronary thrombosis, etc. Peptic ulcer is another common complication.

THE WHITE CELLS

The important white cells are the granulocytes, lymphocytes, and monocytes.

Development

The precursor cell of the granulocyte series is the *myeloblast*, a cell which resembles the pronormoblast. As it matures it loses its nucleoli, and is then termed a *promyelocyte*. When specific cytoplasmic granules—neutrophil, eosinophil, or basophil—appear, the cell is called a *myelocyte*. The myelocyte nucleus becomes indented to form a *metamyelocyte*, and is ultimately drawn out into two or three discrete lobes joined by fine chromatin threads. This is the mature granulocyte, often called a *polymorphonuclear* (or polymorph) because of the shape of the nucleus. Most granulocytes are neutrophilic (fine lilac granules), but a few are eosinophilic (large red granules), and an occasional one is basophilic (very large blue granules).

The precursor cells of lymphocytes and monocytes are called *lymphoblasts* and *monoblasts*, but neither is normally present in appreciable numbers in the marrow. A few plasma cells are present in the marrow, but are not normally found in the peripheral blood. Figure 30.1 describes the composition of the bone marrow.

The normal white-cell count and its variations

The total white-cell count in the blood is 4000 to 11 000 per mm^3. The range of the differential count is:

Neutrophil polymorphonuclears	40 to 75 per cent (2.0 to 7.5 $\times 10^9$ per litre, or 2000 to 7500 per μl)
Eosinophil polymorphonuclears	1 to 5 per cent (0.05 to 0.4 $\times 10^9$ per litre, or 50 to 400 per μl)
Basophil polymorphonuclears	0 to 1 per cent (up to 0.1 $\times 10^9$ per litre, or 100 per μl)
Lymphocytes	20 to 45 per cent (1.5 to 4 $\times 10^9$ per litre, or 1500 to 4000 per μl)
Monocytes	3 to 7 per cent (0.2 to 0.8 $\times 10^9$ per litre, or 200 to 800 per μl).

The suffix-*cytosis* implies an excess of cells, e.g. *leucocytosis* indicates an increased white cell count, and *lymphocytosis* indicates an increase in the number of lymphocytes. The suffix *-penia* means a decrease in the relevant cells, e.g. *leucopenia* means a decrease in the number of white cells, and *lymphopenia* is a decrease in the number of lymphocytes. *Neutrophilia* is sometimes used as an alternative to neutrophil leucocytosis. Likewise *neutropenia* denotes a reduction in the total number of neutrophil polymorphs, and the term *agranulocytosis* is commonly used as a synonym. The figures in brackets in the range listed above indicate the absolute number of cells present. This is a more useful figure than the percentage. Thus, if there is a drop in the number of neutrophils, the percentage of lymphocytes increases—the condition called a *relative lymphocytosis*. The term, however, is misleading, since the actual number of lymphocytes can remain unchanged. The main variations in the white cell count are as follows:

Neutrophil leucocytosis (neutrophilia). This common condition is usually due to *infection by pyogenic organisms*, e.g. staphylococcal, pneumococcal, coliform, etc. Some non-pyogenic infections can also lead to a neutrophilia, e.g. plague, diphtheria, and anthrax.

Strenuous exercise, anaesthetics, and emotional stress all produce a transient rise in the number of neutrophils.

Other important causes are *massive tissue necrosis*, as following a myocardial infarct, *uraemia*, *acute gout*, *following severe haemorrhage and haemolysis*, *rapidly growing malignant tumours*, and *neoplastic disease of the marrow*, e.g. chronic myeloid leukaemia and polycythaemia vera.

At one time a classification of the maturity of neutrophils based on their nuclear segmentation was very much in vogue. Results were expressed in tabular form with the left-hand side of the page listing the most primitive cells and the more mature cells being on the right-hand side. Although this detailed counting is now obsolete, the term 'a shift to the left' is still useful in denoting an increase in the blood of young forms of polymorphs. In most of the causes of neutrophil leucocytosis listed above there is a shift to the left, and in extreme cases metamyelocytes and even myelocytes may enter the blood. This *leukemoid blood picture* can sometimes closely mimic leukaemia itself.

Neutropenia. This may occur in certain *infections*, such as typhoid fever and brucellosis. It is common during the prodromal period of viral disease and in chronic protozoal infection, e.g. malaria. Overwhelming infection of whatever cause also lowers the neutrophil count.

Other causes of neutropenia are some diseases associated with splenomegaly (*hypersplenism*), and also *pernicious anaemia*, *bone-marrow aplasia*, and *acute leukaemia*.

Regulation of the neutrophil count. The neutrophil count can be altered by two regulatory mechanisms:

1. Release of neutrophils from the reserves. Of the neutrophils in the blood stream, over half are in a 'marginated pool' adherent to the walls of blood vessels, particularly in the lungs. These can be released rapidly; their release accounts for the leucocytosis occurring during exercise and following the administration of adrenaline. The second reserve is in the bone marrow, where the number of neutrophils sequestered is about 10 times the total of the cells present in the blood.

The mechanism of their release is poorly understood, but various neutrophil-releasing factors have been described.

2. Increased production of neutrophils in the bone marrow. Granulocyte precursors can be cultured *in vivo* in semi-solid agar to form colonies, but this occurs only in the presence of stimulating substances. Such *colony-stimulating substances* have been isolated from various sources, e.g. macrophages, fibroblasts, and lymphocytes. An inhibitory granulocyte chalone has also been described. The role, if any, of these agents in the regulation of the neutrophil count in health or disease is not clear.

Lymphocytosis. An absolute lymphocytosis is not common. It is seen in *whooping-cough* and *infectious mononucleosis (glandular fever)*. In the latter disease the lymphocytes are atypical, and bear a resemblance to monocytes. The disease is an important cause of prolonged fever, and is not uncommon in young adults. Its cause is infective; a herpesvirus called the *Epstein-Barr virus (EB virus)* is incriminated, because after the disease there is invariably a high titre of antibodies against this virus in the serum. An interesting feature is the presence in the serum of antibodies which agglutinate sheep red cells to high titre (*Paul-Bunnell test*). There are other types of infectious mononucleosis that are part of cytomegalic inclusion disease and toxoplasmosis, and in these the Paul-Bunnell test is negative.

Another important cause of lymphocytosis is *chronic lymphatic leukaemia.*

Monocytosis. A rise in the monocyte count is seen typically in *protozoal diseases*, such as malaria, trypanosomiasis, and leishmaniasis. It may occasionally occur in *chronic bacterial infections* also, e.g. tuberculosis and *Strept. viridans* endocarditis. Another cause is *monocytic leukaemia.*

Eosinophilia. An eosinophilia is encountered in some *hypersensitivities of atopic type*, e.g. bronchial asthma, hay-fever, and urticaria. *Helminthic infections*, especially when the parasites are migrating through the tissues e.g. early schistosomiasis, trichinosis, and hydatid disease, and also filariasis, give rise to a marked eosinophilia. Intestinal worm infestation does not produce such a marked effect.

Eosinophilia is also seen in some skin diseases, e.g. pemphigus vulgaris and exfoliative dermatitis.

THE LEUKAEMIAS

Leukaemia is a condition in which there is a widespread proliferation of the leucocytes and their precursors throughout the tissues of the body, with a variable circulating component. The aetiology in man is unknown, and its course is nearly always fatal. It may follow exposure to ionizing radiations, and is much more common in victims of Down's syndrome than in the general population. In birds and mice the cause is viral (see pp. 366–367).

The classification of leukaemia depends on the rapidity of the disease process and the type of cell involved:

Chronic leukaemia	1. myeloid (myelocytic)
	2. lymphatic (lymphocytic)
Acute leukaemia	1. myeloid (myeloblastic)
	2. lymphatic (lymphoblastic).

The names in brackets allude to the predominant abnormal cell in the blood. Acute myeloid leukaemia has several variants, e.g. acute myelomonocytic leukaemia. Whether monocytic leukaemia is a distinct entity or merely represents one end of the morphological spectrum of acute myeloid leukaemia is uncertain, but it is known that the myeloblast and the monocyte have a common stem cell.

Chronic myeloid leukaemia

This is a disease usually of middle life. The outstanding haematological finding is an enormous leucocytosis, even up to 1000×10^9 per litre (1 million per µl). Nearly all of these are neutrophil polymorphs, metamyelocytes, and myelocytes, but there is also a significant increase in the eosinophils and basophils and their precursors. Myeloblasts are not numerous except terminally. If the leucocytes are grown in tissue culture, some show the abnormal Philadelphia chromosome (p. 51).

There is also a slowly progressive normocytic, normochromic anaemia and a gradual fall in platelet count. The bone marrow shows marked proliferation of the myeloid series of cells.

Clinically the patient has immense enlargement of the spleen and a lesser enlargement of the liver. Death usually occurs within 3 to 5 years, and may be heralded by an acute exacerbation in which the blood is flooded with myeloblasts.

Chronic lymphatic leukaemia

This is usually a disease of later life. There is marked lymphocytosis varying from 20 to 250×10^9 per litre (20 000 to 250 000 cells per µl). Most of these lymphocytes are mature, and any number of lymphoblasts in the blood is unusual. The polymorph element is reduced. There is a progressive normocytic, normochromic anaemia and thrombocytopenia. The marrow is less affected than in myeloid leukaemia, and it may show no changes at all initially. Later on it becomes replaced by lymphocytes.

The condition affects the lymph nodes primarily, and the patient usually presents with a generalized lymphadenopathy. Sometimes the tonsils are conspicuously affected, and occasionally there is bilateral salivary-gland enlargement. The spleen and liver are enlarged, but to a lesser extent than in myeloid leukaemia. Death usually occurs in 4 to 6 years, and is due to anaemia and secondary infection.

Acute leukaemia

The various types of acute leukaemia are best considered together, because it is often very difficult to distinguish between them either haematologically or clinically. In acute leukaemia the white-cell count can vary from less than 1×10^9 per litre (1000 per µl) up to 100×10^9 per litre (100 000 per µl). When there is a raised count the blood is flooded with primitive 'blast' cells. It is often difficult to be sure whether these are myeloblasts, lymphoblasts, or monoblasts. In some cases the presence of more mature forms helps in the diagnosis; for example, if there are also some myelocytes and polymorphs, the cells are probably myeloblasts, whereas if there are an appreciable number of lymphocytes, the primitive cells are probably lymphoblastic. In any case the number of mature polymorphs is always so small that there is an absolute neutropenia. In cases where the white-cell count is very low, nearly all the circulating leucocytic elements are primitive blast cells, and can be mistaken for lymphocytes by inexperienced workers. This type of leukaemia may be called 'subleukaemic'. A frankly 'aleukaemic leukaemia', in which there are absolutely no blast cells present in the blood, does occur but is very uncommon.

In acute leukaemia there is a rapidly progressive normocytic, normochromic anaemia and a severe thrombocytopenia. No matter how low the peripheral blood count, the marrow is crowded out with 'blast' cells except, of course, during a remission.

Acute leukaemia occurs at all ages. In childhood it is usually lymphatic, but in adult life the myeloid variety is more common. The monocytic variant of acute myeloid leukaemia is the least frequent and occurs most often in middle age. It is not possible to distinguish between them clinically. The onset is usually sudden, though there may have been a period of preceding malaise with obscure anaemia. The main features are high fever, a generalized bleeding tendency due to the thrombocytopenia, progressive anaemia, and necrotic infective lesions which are the result of the poor body resistance accruing from the absence of mature polymorphs (agranulocytosis). Oral and faucial lesions are prominent, and sometimes are the first symptoms which bring the patient for treatment. There is painful confluent ulcerative pharyngitis, stomatitis, and gingivitis. Gross gingival enlargement due to leukaemic infiltration is said to be particularly characteristic of the monocytic variant of acute myeloid leukaemia, but it can occur in the other varieties also.

Most patients die within 3 to 6 months, usually as a result of infection or bleeding into vital areas such as the central nervous system. Intensive modern therapy has increased the average survival period considerably. As many as 50 per cent of patients may survive 5 years, and perhaps one-third of children with acute lymphatic leukaemia can now be cured.

The morbid anatomy of leukaemia

There is a monotonous infiltration of leukaemic cells into numerous organs, which are enlarged, soft, and pale in colour. The lymph nodes, spleen, and bone marrow are particularly likely to be crowded out with the responsible cells. The liver is diffusely infiltrated throughout its sinusoids in chronic myeloid leukaemia, while in the lymphatic type it is the portal tracts which are mostly involved (Fig. 30.8). The bone marrow is pinkish-grey in colour, and extends down the shafts of the long bones. No organ is exempt, and massive local infiltrations are characteristic of the acute leukaemias. The other changes are those of diffuse haemorrhage and secondary infection.

MULTIPLE MYELOMA (MYELOMATOSIS)

Multiple myeloma is a condition in which a neoplastic proliferation of plasma-cell series occurs in the marrow. It is considered in Chapter 37.

The blood changes in myelomatosis are non-specific. There is usually a progressive normocytic, normochromic anaemia, but unlike leukaemia, it is unusual for the abnormal marrow cells to enter the circulation. There is likewise less tendency towards extramedullary collections of these cells.

BONE-MARROW APLASIA

When the marrow ceases to release mature elements into the circulation, there is a serious drop in the blood count and the condition is described as *aplasia of the bone marrow*. Sometimes the failure of division occurs at the 'blast' stage, in which

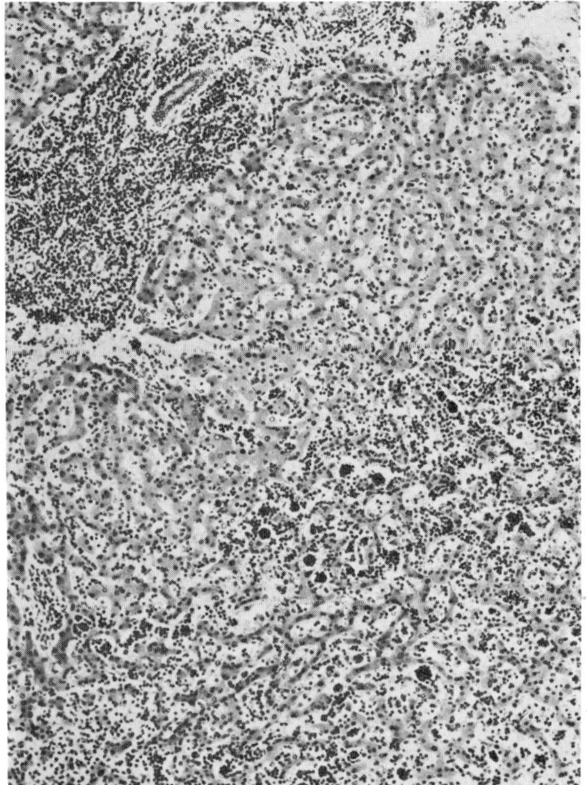

Fig. 30.8 Chronic lymphatic leukaemia. Note the dense infiltration of leukaemic cells especially in the portal tracts. There is a less dense infiltration in the sinusoids. × 100.

case no mature elements are present, but sometimes the failure in division occurs at the later stage of haematopoiesis. In this case the marrow is crowded with maturing cells, but few enter the peripheral blood. This is called 'maturation arrest'.

Aplasia of the marrow may involve all three elements, when it leads to diminution of all the cells of the blood (*pancytopenia*), or it may affect only one of the elements. Pure red-cell aplasia is very uncommon, but aplasia of the granulocytes, or *agranulocytosis*, is an important condition. Pure platelet aplasia probably does not occur.

Pancytopenia. Aplasia affecting all the elements of the marrow (aplastic anaemia) is usually due to an external agent, e.g. *ionizing radiations* or *drugs*, of which the most important are benzene, cytotoxic agents used in cancer chemotherapy, gold salts, and chloramphenicol. It is an occasional complication of *viral hepatitis*, and may be *idiopathic*, in which case it is important to rule out aleukaemic leukaemia by a careful study of the bone marrow. An occasional cause is *splenic overactivity* (see below).

Haematologically there is a normocytic, normochromic anaemia without any evidence of regeneration in the form of reticulocytes, a leucopenia with neutropenia, and a thrombocytopenia. The marrow is usually severely hypocellular, and those cells present are mostly lymphocytes. The prognosis is bad, and most cases die of infection or intractable haemorrhage. In maturation arrest the cellularity may be normal or even increased, and in these cases spontaneous recovery may occur.

Agranulocytosis. Aplasia of the white cells is a very serious complication of certain *drugs*, namely amidopyrine (an analgesic), thiouracil, phenylbutazone, chlorpromazine (a traquillizer), sulphonamides, pyribenzamine (an antihistamine), and troxidone (an anticonvulsant). It may follow ionizing radiations and cancer chemotherapy also, but is here part of a more widespread aplasia. Some cases are associated with splenic overactivity, and some are apparently idiopathic.

There is a profound leucopenia, and nearly all the white cells in the blood are lymphocytes. Red cells and platelets are unaffected. The marrow shows inhibition of white-cell production. The leucopenia leads to a serious deficiency in the body's defence mechanism, and ulcerative, infective lesions occur in the mouth and throat, lungs, gastrointestinal tract, and vagina. Death soon occurs from overwhelming infection, and the lesions all show a virtual absence of polymorphs. The cellular infiltration consists of lymphocytes and plasma cells.

Splenic overactivity (hypersplenism). The functions of the spleen as regards blood formation are ill-understood. It certainly is active in removing defective red cells from the circulation, and it possibly exerts an inhibitory effect on the formation of white cells in the marrow. It takes over the function of haematopoiesis when the marrow is destroyed, but normally plays no part in blood formation.

It sometimes happens that conditions leading to gross splenomegaly give rise either to *marrow aplasia* (of all, or of any of the three elements of the blood) or to *haemolytic anaemia*. If the spleen is removed, there may be a cure of the blood disorder even if the primary disease continues unabated. Apparently the enlarged spleen is overactive; it either inhibits marrow function or else has a directly destructive effect on the cells in the circulating blood. When it is associated with aplasia, hypersplenism produces a maturation defect rather than a depression in the earliest stages of haematopoiesis.

Sometimes the splenomegaly is primary, but more often it is secondary to some other condition, e.g. cirrhosis of the liver (when the whole condition is called Banti's syndrome), rheumatoid arthritis, Gaucher's disease, schistosomiasis, or leishmaniasis.

THE SYNDROME OF BONE-MARROW REPLACEMENT

The normal bone marrow is sometimes crowded out by foreign elements. The commonest is *tumour tissue* from skeletal metastases in cancer of the lung, breast, or prostate, or in cases of multiple myeloma. Sometimes the element is a *lipid-filled macrophage*, as in Gaucher's disease, *fibrous tissue* (myelosclerosis), or even *bone*, as in marble-bone disease of childhood, where there is a failure of replacement of osseous tissue by marrow spaces.

Bone-marrow replacement gives a typical blood picture of *leucoerythroblastic anaemia*. This consists of a normocytic, normochromic anaemia in which there are many nucleated red cells (normoblasts) in the blood. There is a moderate to considerable polymorph leucocytosis, and many myelocytes and metamyelocytes are also present in the blood. The main feature of this type of blood picture is thus the presence of both immature red and white cells in the circulation. The platelets may be reduced in number, and giant forms are sometimes present.

In longstanding cases the function of the marrow is assumed by the spleen and liver, and in both these organs there may be marked extramedullary haematopoiesis.

THE PLATELETS AND CLOTTING FACTORS

The normal platelet

The platelets are small discs, devoid of a nucleus but with fine intracellular granules. They are derived from the large polyploid *megakaryocytes* by a process of fragmentation of their cytoplasm.

The platelets are important in haemostasis because they readily adhere to damaged vessel walls and thereby prevent haemorrhage. Platelets thus adhere to surfaces and stick to each other, and these properties of *adhesiveness* and *aggregation* have been the subjects of much research because of their possible bearing on the cause of thrombosis (p. 479). Platelets synthetize a variety of prostaglandins, and they play a part in acute inflammation (p. 86) and in thrombosis (p. 481).

Platelet aggregation. Platelets aggregate immediately in the presence of adenosine diphosphate (ADP). This may be demonstrated *in vitro* by the addition of ADP to a platelet-rich preparation of plasma which is kept agitated. The aggregation can be detected by measuring the ensuing decrease in optical density. Adrenaline, noradrenaline, and 5-HT have a similar effect. *Thrombin* leads to aggregation, but only after a delay of 5 to 10 seconds. It probably acts by converting platelet adenosine triphosphate (ATP) to ADP.

Platelet adhesiveness. Platelets adhere to a variety of foreign surfaces, and the drop in platelet count when blood is passed through a column of glass beads has been used as an *in-vitro* method of measuring platelet adhesiveness. Platelets will also adhere to vascular endothelium if it is damaged mechanically, and to collagen, but not to pure fibrin.

Adherent platelets swell and release a variety of chemicals (*platelet release reaction*), including phospholipid (platelet factor 3, which plays a part in clotting), heparin neutralizing substance (platelet factor 4), 5-HT, and ADP. The last causes platelet aggregation and a small platelet thrombus is built up. This is unstable, and *in vivo* the platelets may break off and be released into the circulation as small emboli. Though clotting is not involved in the mechanism of platelet adhesiveness, the clotting system is soon activated by platelet factor 3, and by the activation of factor XII. Fibrin is formed, and this stabilizes the platelet thrombus.

Thus following injury, whether extensive or that caused by a pin-prick, the injured vessels are sealed by a mass known as a *haemostatic plug*. At first this consists of platelets, but soon this is consolidated by fibrin formation. Finally the entire aggregate contracts, probably due to the contractile protein in the platelets called *thrombosthenin*. Thrombin released during clotting causes further platelet deposition as well as fibrin formation. Defects in the intrinsic system of blood clotting, such as in haemophilia, do not prevent the formation of a haemostatic plug, and therefore the bleeding time is normal (p. 467). However, the plug is not stable and rebleeding occurs later. Serious bleeding can therefore follow the infliction of a wound such as that caused by dental extraction

It can be readily understood why a deficiency in platelets or in the clotting mechanism can lead to a bleeding tendency. The normal platelet count is 150 to 440 $\times$ 10^9 per litre (150 000 to 440 000 per µl) with an average of 250 $\times$ 10^9 per litre. It is raised after injuries and operations (especially splenectomy). A count below 100 $\times$ 10^9 per litre is designated *thrombocytopenia*.

The clotting mechanism

Blood clotting itself is a very complex mechanism (Fig. 30.9). In essence it consists of a conversion of *fibrinogen (Factor I)* to fibrin by the action of thrombin. This enzyme exists normally as an inert precursor *prothrombin (Factor II)*, which is activated to thrombin by *prothrombinase* which itself is generated by the interaction of activated Factor X (designated Factor Xa) with Factor V, platelet factor 3, and calcium ions (Factor IV). This sequence is called the *common pathway*, and can be initiated by two completely separate mechanisms, the *intrinsic (blood) system* and the *extrinsic (tissue) system*. (Figs. 30.9 and 30.10)

The intrinsic system. In the *intrinsic (blood) system*, contact with an abnormal surface leads to the activation of Factor XII to Factor XIIa. This activates Factor XI, and Factor XIa activates Factor IX. Factor IXa in conjunction with Factor VIII and platelet phospholipid, activates Factor X.

The extrinsic system. In the *extrinsic (tissue) system*, tissue damage results in the release of a tissue factor rich in phospholipid. It is called Factor III. This in conjunction with Factor VII activates Factor X, which, as already described, is involved in the production of prothrombinase *via* the common pathway.

The tissue factor is found in large amounts in the brain, extracts of which are used as a source of it in various laboratory tests, such as the prothrombin time. The venom of the Russell viper is also rich in it.

The two pathways of blood clotting are both important, for a derangement of either leads to a serious defect in haemostasis. The intrinsic system develops much more slowly that the extrinsic one, but both are initiated by tissue damage, either by releasing tissue factor or providing an abnormal surface. In both systems there is activation of Factor X, and from then on there is a final common pathway involving Factor V, platelet factor 3, calcium ions, prothrombin, and fibrinogen.

It should be noted that Factors II, VII, IX, X, XI, XII, and XIII are all

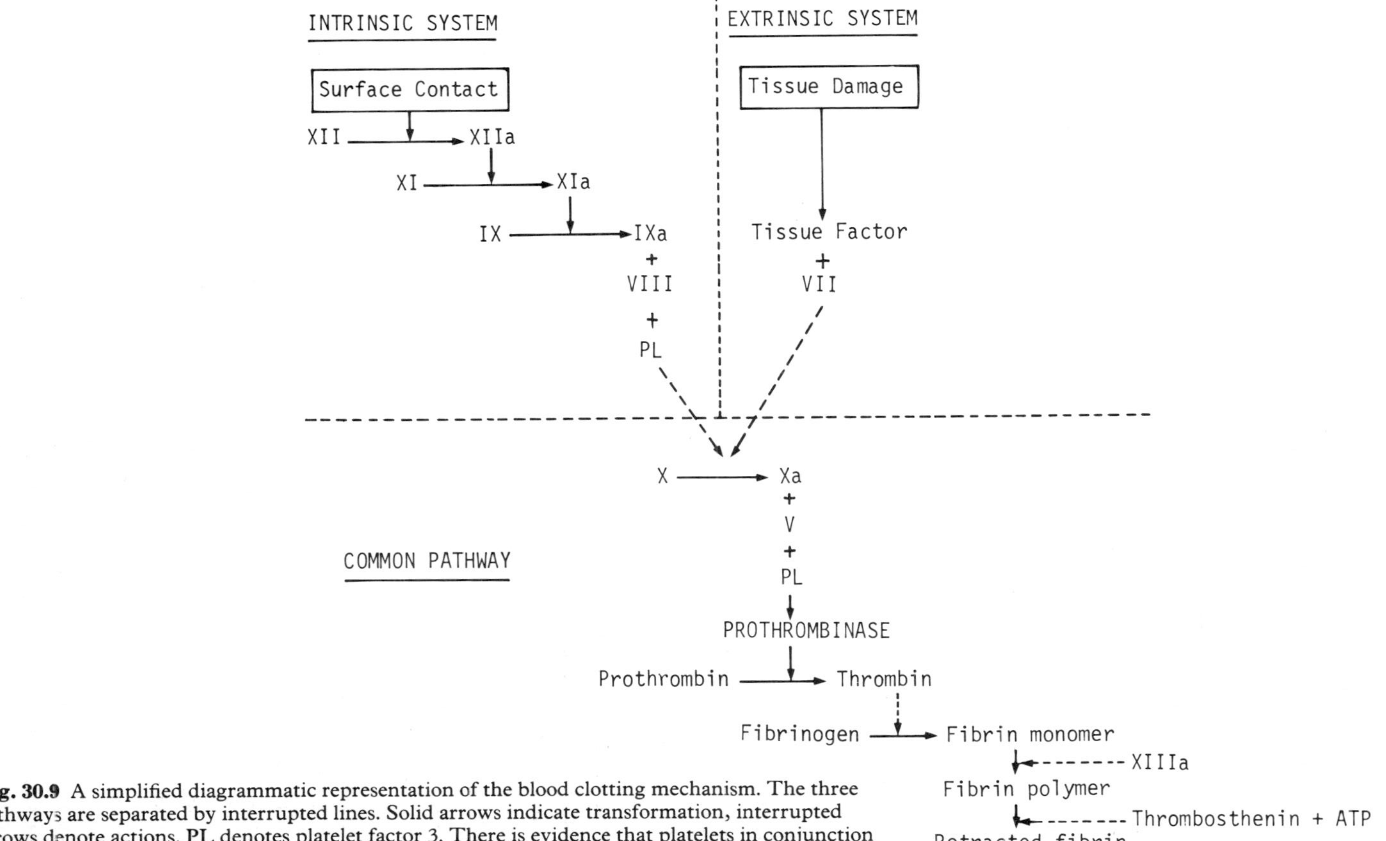

Fig. 30.9 A simplified diagrammatic representation of the blood clotting mechanism. The three pathways are separated by interrupted lines. Solid arrows indicate transformation, interrupted arrows denote actions. PL denotes platelet factor 3. There is evidence that platelets in conjunction with Factor XII can form a platelet 'tissue-factor' and thereby initiate the extrinsic system. The importance of this *in vivo* is debatable. Not shown in the diagram is the calcium which is required for most of the steps shown. (*After Marcus A J 1969 New England Journal of Medicine 280: 1213.*)

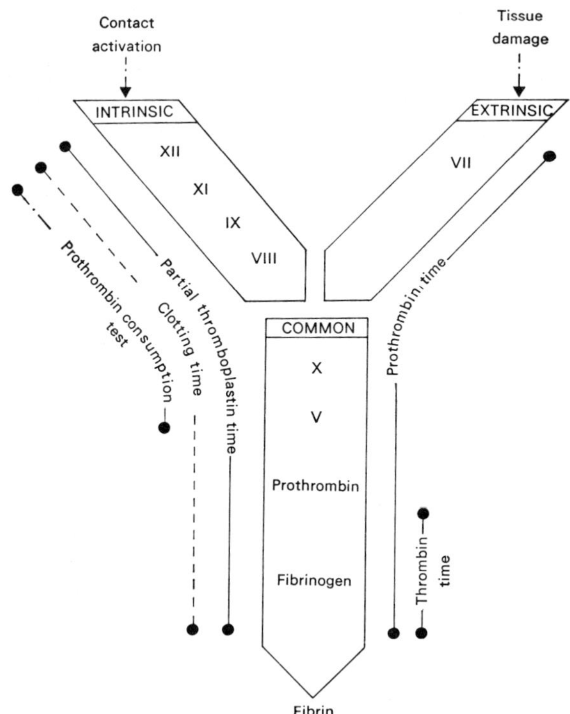

Fig. 30.10 The interpretation of screening tests of blood clotting. (*From Bithell T C, Wintrobe M M 1970 In Harrison's Principles of Internal Medicine, 6th edn Fig 62.3. McGraw-Hill, New York, p 323.*)

enzymes; they are of a class called *serine esterases.* Digestive enzymes and complement enzymes are also members of this class. Characteristically they are all stored as an inactive precursor, activated by a given stimulus, and then undergo a cascade-like activation. Thus the activation of the various factors involved in clotting is believed to follow a *cascade sequence*, many of the factors being substrates that are activated by a preceding enzyme.

The earliest phase of the intrinsic system is slow, but once thrombin is formed the process is greatly accelerated—indeed, there is a real cascade, for thrombin potentiates the activity of Factors V and VIII. It also causes platelets to aggregate and so increase the amount of lipid factor 3. This is called the *autocatalytic action of thrombin.* Interestingly, thrombin also destroys Factors V and VIII after potentiating their reactivity; in this way fibrin formation is stopped when a high concentration of thrombin has been achieved.

It should be noted that the plasma clotting factors (all globulins) are given Roman numerals. They are also given alternative names: Factor V *is labile factor*; Factor VII *is stable factor*; Factor VIII is *antihaemophilic factor*; Factor IX is *Christmas factor*; Factor X is *Stuart-Prower factor*; Factor XI is *plasma thromboplastin antecedent*; Factor XII is *Hageman factor*. The personal names refer to the surnames of the patients in whom a deficiency of the particular factor was first described. The latest factor described is *Factor XIII (fibrin-stabilizing factor)*, which converts soluble fibrin into insoluble, or stabilized, fibrin.

In order to prevent spontaneous intravascular clotting there are also natural anticoagulant mechanisms. The first natural mode of inhibition of intravascular clotting is the slowness of thrombin formation due to the exclusion of tissue factor and the almost complete absence of prothrominase, which is attributable to the stability of the various clotting factors. Once the vascular endothelium is damaged, there is a tendency for intravascular clotting to occur. This is counteracted by the presence of antithrombins which are described below. Fibrin once formed can be removed by the fibrinolytic system.

Antithrombins.

Fibrin, at one time called antithrombin I, is an antithrombin in that thrombin is adsorbed by the fibrin fibres.

Antithrombin III is by far the most important natural constraint to coagulation. It combines with, and inactivates, most serine esterases. This combination is enhanced by heparin. In fact, antithrombin III is the factor through which heparin exerts its effects, and for this reason is called the *heparin cofactor*.

Heparin is a sulphated mucopolysaccharide found in the granules of the mast cells. Its anticoagulant effects involve a preliminary interaction with plasma proteins called *heparin cofactors*. The most important of these is antithrombin III.

Fibrinopeptides (p. 84) also act as antithrombins.

The fibrinolytic system

Plasminogen is a normal plasma protein that can be activated in a variety of ways to produce the active fibrinolytic enzyme *plasmin*. The major activator of plasminogen is thought to be *kallikrein*, an enzyme that is itself present as an inert precursor form called *prekallikrein* (p. 84). Streptokinase probably acts by activating prekallikrein. The fibrinolytic system is activated under a wide range of conditions, e.g. exercise, stress, anaphylaxis, shock, as well as locally whenever fibrin is formed. One may indeed postulate that the fibrinolytic system balances the effects of the clotting system. An imbalance leads to intravascular coagulation on the one hand and afibrinogenaemia on the other (see p. 471).

Tests of importance in the bleeding diseases

Platelet count.

Bleeding time—the time taken for a small skin puncture to stop bleeding. It varies from 1 to 9 minutes, and is prolonged when there is a lack of platelets, which, as has been described, are essential for haemostasis.

Clotting time—the time taken for a specimen of whole blood to clot. At 37°C this should be from 5 to 15 minutes. The clotting time is prolonged if there is a deficiency of any of the factors concerned in the *intrinsic clotting system* or in the *common pathway* (Fig. 30.10). The test is insensitive, and a normal result can be obtained even in the presence of a very low level of some clotting factors. The test is not affected by the level of Factor VII (extrinsic system), but is prolonged when a circulating anticoagulant such as heparin is present in excess. The clotting time is widely used to control heparin therapy. Thrombocytopenia does not increase the clotting time, because only a trace of the platelet lipid factor is necessary for the formation of prothrombinase.

Prothrombin consumption test. The clotting time can be normal even though small amounts of prothrombinase are produced (see above). However, much unused prothrombin will remain, and this can be measured in the prothrombin consumption test. The test measures only those factors required for prothrombin production *via* the intrinsic system and is more sensitive than the clotting time (Fig. 30.10).

Partial thromboplastin time (PTT). This is the time taken for plasma to clot under the following three conditions:

1. The test is carried out in a glass tube—the surface activates Factor XII
2. A fraction of brain extract called 'cephalin' is added. This provides excess phospholipid and makes the test independent of the platelet count
3. Calcium chloride is added.

The PTT is a sensitive measure of the factors concerned in the *intrinsic* and *common pathways*.

Prothrombin time. In this test equal amounts of brain extract (containing tissue factor), calcium chloride solution, and test plasma are incubated and the time taken for clotting to occur is recorded. A control must be put up at the same time, and this should clot in 10 to 16 seconds. The prothrombin time is a measure of the factors concerned in the *extrinsic system* and in the *common pathway*. The intrinsic system is by-passed.

Capillary fragility test. This is performed by inflating the cuff of a blood-pressure manometer to a pressure between the diastolic and systolic for five minutes. If positive, the arm and forearm below the cuff show a petechial eruption. This occurs in platelet deficiency, because normally the platelets seal off any defects caused by a sudden rise in blood pressure. The test is also positive if the vessels themselves are abnormal, e.g. in scurvy.

The four tests which can most easily be carried out as an initial investigation of a patient with a bleeding disease are: the *platelet count*, the *bleeding time*, the *partial thromboplastin time (PTT)* and the *prothrombin time (PT)*. If both PTT and PT are normal, the defect is probably in the vessels or the platelets. If either PTT or PT is prolonged, there is probably a defect in the clotting system. If both PTT and PT are abnormal, the defect is most likely in the common pathway. If the PTT is prolonged and the PT is normal, it is the intrinsic system which is most likely at fault. A prolonged PT and a normal PTT is rare, and indicates a deficiency of Factor VII.

In practice, complex defects in haemostasis are best investigated in specialized centres where the activity of each individual factor can be assessed.

THE HAEMORRHAGIC DISEASES

These manifest themselves as petechial haemorrhages into the skin, mucous membranes, and viscera (a condition called *purpura*), larger extravasations into muscles, joints, and serous cavities, and by a tendency to prolonged bleeding after injury and operations. There are three factors to be considered in a bleeding disease:

1. The blood vessels
2. The platelets
3. The clotting factors.

It must be understood that most bleeding is due to a local vascular lesion or injury. Postoperative bleeding is usually due to a badly-ligated vessel or infection, and epistaxis (nosebleed) is usually due to a vascular disturbance in the nose. Purpura itself may be the result of local factors, e.g. *senile purpura* is due to a loss of connective-tissue support of the smaller vessels, and *orthostatic purpura* may appear on the skin of the legs of people who stand for long periods of time. Generalized purpura is usually a manifestation of a bleeding disease, due either to systemic vascular disease or to thrombocytopenia. It is not usually found in association with defects in the clotting factors. Postoperative bleeding (including that following dental extraction) is due either to thrombocytopenia or a defect in the clotting factors. It is never due to vascular disease acting alone.

Haemorrhagic diseases due to vascular disease

This takes the form of purpura, which may manifest itself internally as haematuria and haematemesis. Bleeding is seldom serious enough to endanger life. Important examples are:

Anaphylactoid (Henoch-Schönlein) purpura is a vasculitis in which small vessels are damaged by immune complexes. It occurs mostly in the young, and is accompanied by skin eruptions, haematemesis, and haematuria.

Scurvy. See page 283.

Infections, such as scarlet fever, haemorrhagic smallpox, and typhus, and also following the administration of *drugs* and *chemical agents* like aspirin and quinine, all of which damage the vascular endothelium by direct action or by the local deposition of immune complexes.

In these conditions there are no specific haematological abnormalities. The capillary fragility test is usually positive.

Haemorrhagic diseases due to platelet abnomalities

Thrombocytopenia

This is manifested by purpura which may be very marked, severe haematemesis and haematuria, and fatal bleeding into internal viscera, especially the brain. Prolonged postoperative bleeding is another danger, but serious bleeding after relatively minor trauma, such as dental extraction, is uncommon. The bleeding time is prolonged, but the clotting time and PTT are normal. The capillary fragility test is strongly positive and clot retraction is impaired.

Thrombocytopenia may be due to three factors: (1) increased platelet destruction, (2) increased platelet consumption, and (3) a failure of production.

Increased platelet destruction. The most important condition in this group is *idiopathic thrombocytopenic purpura*. This occurs as an acute self-limiting disease in young children, and as a more chronic condition in older children and young adults. One interesting variant of acute thrombocytopenia is *onyalai*, which affects young adult Black males in Africa and is associated with haemorrhagic bullae in the mouth and on other mucous surfaces.

Idiopathic thrombocytopenic purpura is due to an autoantibody of IgG class against platelets. The spleen sequesters the sensitized platelets and then destroys them. Splenectomy is therefore of value, as also is the administration of glucocorticoids.

Other causes of immunological platelet destruction are systemic lupus erythematosus and some drug-induced purpuras, for instance, those induced by quinidine, the thiazides, and the notorious hypnotic Sedormid which was once widely used. A different mechanism of platelet destruction is seen in splenic overactivity (see p. 462).

Increased platelet consumption. This occurs in disseminated intravascular coagulation, which is described later.

Failure of platelet production. This causes thrombocytopenia, as seen in bone marrow aplasia, acute leukaemia, and conditions where the bone marrow is extensively replaced by tumour.

Thrombocytopathia

In thrombocytopathia there is defective platelet function but a normal platelet count. There are a number of rare inherited conditions in which the platelets are abnormal, either showing an inability to aggregate with ADP or exhibiting a defective release reaction. In addition, there are a number of acquired conditions in which the platelet function is abnormal. Thus the drugs aspirin and indomethacin impair the release reaction and inhibit the production of prostaglandins by platelets. Another important example is uraemia. In all these conditions purpura develops in the face of a normal platelet count but with a prolonged bleeding time.

Haemorrhagic diseases due to defects in the clotting mechanism

Defects in the clotting mechanism are accompanied by massive bleeding into the tissues and from the body's orifices. Purpura is unusual, but intractable postoperative haemorrhage is characteristic; serious, even fatal, bleeding can occur after dental extraction. The partial thromboplastin time is prolonged, and if the defect is severe, so also is the less sensitive clotting time.

The clotting disorders may be inherited or acquired.

Inherited defects

Haemophilia A. This disease is due to a deficiency of Factor VIII. It is the most common inherited defect in clotting and affects males only, since it is inherited as a sex-linked recessive trait (p. 45). The bleeding is very severe, and a special feature is *haemarthrosis*, which is usually recurrent. The organization of the haematoma leads to obliteration of the joint by fibrous adhesions and bony ankylosis. When frozen plasma is warmed to 4°C, a precipitate forms which is rich in Factor VIII. *Cryoprecipitates* prepared in this way are now widely used in the treatment of haemophilia.

Haemophilia B (Christmas disease). This disease is due to a deficiency of

Factor IX. Its mode of inheritance and clinical manifestations are indistinguishable from those of haemophilia. Only by specialized tests can they be separated.

Although the bleeding time is normal in both haemophilia A and Christmas disease, the haemostatic plug which is formed in injured vessels is not stabilized by fibrin, and continued oozing and rebleeding is characteristic. Any fibrin which is formed tends to be removed by the activation of plasmin, and inhibiting this fibrinolytic enzyme might be expected to be of therapeutic value. Epsilon-aminocaproic acid is a plasmin inhibitor, and its administration parenterally before and after dental extraction has been reported to be of value. It can be used in addition to the injection of antihaemophilic globulin.

von Willibrand's disease. This is probably the second most common of the hereditary clotting disorders, and bears a close relationship to the haemophilias. The clotting disorder is complex and is not completely understood. The disease has features of a combined platelet and clotting-factor defect. Thus mucosal bleeding from the nose and gastrointestinal tract is considerably more common than in haemophilia, but cutaneous petechiae are rare. In severe cases haemarthroses and intramuscular haematomata occur. Post-traumatic and postoperative bleeding is an important feature.

Other bleeding diseases. There are a considerable number of rare inherited bleeding disorders which may manifest as postoperative bleeding. The treatment of all these conditions is basically similar. The deficient factor is replaced by either fresh plasma or some suitable concentrate.

Acquired clotting disorders

Hypoprothrombinaemia. In this condition there is not only a deficiency of prothrombin, but also of Factor VII, and sometimes of Factors V and X also.

The usual causes are *liver failure* or a *deficiency of vitamin K*. This vitamin is used by the liver for the synthesis of prothrombin and Factors VII and X. Vitamin K is fat-soluble, and is obtained partly from the diet and partly as a result of bacterial synthesis in the intestine. Its absorption is aided by the presence of bile salts, and it is therefore poorly absorbed in *obstructive jaundice*. Vitamin-K deficiency also occurs in the newborn due to an inability of the infant to synthetize it in the bowel. If the mother's intake is also deficient, a serious bleeding state may occur—*haemorrhagic disease of the newborn*. Another cause of hypoprothrombinaemia is the *administration of coumarin anticoagulants*. These inhibit the synthesis of the clotting factors.

Hypofibrinogenaemia. A deficiency of fibrinogen is usually acquired as the result of the entry of clotting factors into the circulation. This material sets up intravascular clotting, so that the residual blood becomes incoagulable. In addition there is usually an activation of plasminogen, and fibrinolysis and fibrinogen destruction occur together with the clotting. The condition is called *disseminated intravascular coagulation*, or the *defibrination syndrome*, and is characterized by dramatic bleeding. It is met with most commonly as a complication of pregnancy, when amniotic fluid enters the circulation and sets up both clotting and general fibrinolysis. It is also described after *severe trauma*, *lung operations*, *incompatible blood transfusions*, in the generalized *Schwartzman reaction*, and rarely in *widespread cancer*.

BLOOD GROUPS AND BLOOD TRANSFUSION

The red cells contain many antigens, but for practical purposes those concerned with the ABO and Rhesus blood groups are the most important.

The ABO system. The antigens concerned are glycoproteins. The basic antigen is called the H substance. Under the influence of the *A* and *B* genes, it is converted into A and B substances, depending on the presence of either or both genes. At birth there are no corresponding antibodies in the plasma, but within 3 to 6 months the antibodies corresponding to the antigen *not present* make their appearance. These are called *alloantibodies*, and are capable of agglutinating the red cells of normal people who are of a different blood group, but not those of the same blood group as that of the individual.

The following table describes the distribution of ABO antigens and antibodies:

Blood group	*Antibody normally present in plasma*
A	anti-B
B	anti-A
AB	none
O	anti-A and anti-B

Why these antibodies develop is not certain. It is known that many Gram-negative intestinal bacilli have high concentrations of blood-group specific substances, and it is possible that the infant forms antibodies against those to which it is not immunologically tolerant.

To perform a blood grouping it is necessary to treat a suspension of red cells with 'anti-A' and 'anti-B' serum (derived from a donor with a high titre of these antibodies). If 'anti-A' serum causes agglutination of the cells, they are group A; if 'anti-B' does it, they are group B. If they are agglutinated by both, they are group AB, and if by neither, they are group O. Although group-O cells contain H substance, anti-H is rarely present in the plasma of group-A and group-B subjects in sufficient strength to cause a significant reaction in the body. It will be noted that the naturally-occurring ABO antibodies are of the IgM class and 'complete', i.e. they agglutinate red cells in saline suspension (p. 453).

The Rhesus system. About 85 per cent of the White population of the world have a red-cell antigen which was first noted in Rhesus-monkey red cells. It is called the *Rh antigen*, and cells that contain it are described as Rh-positive. Rh-negative individuals do not normally have Rh antibodies in their plasma (c.f. the ABO system), but if they are immunized by Rh-positive red cells, they form antibodies very easily. Such immunization may follow a mismatched blood transfusion, or occur after the pregnancy of a Rh-negative woman bearing a Rh-positive fetus (p. 454).

Rh-grouping is done by suspending the red cells in serum obtained from a pregnant woman with a high titre of complete Rh antibody. Rh-positive cells undergo agglutination.

Blood transfusion

Indications. Blood transfusion is an essential procedure in clinical practice.

Not only is it mandatory for restoring the blood volume after *severe haemorrhage*, but it is also used extensively in *major operative procedures*. The administration of packed red cells plays a part in the treatment of *severe anaemia* of whatever cause, but if possible this should be treated with the specific agent, e.g. iron, vitamin B_{12}, etc., unless the patient's life is in danger. Various blood components are available from transfusion centres, and these are useful in *restoring deficient clotting factors*, such as Factor VIII, prothrombin, and fibrinogen. Blood transfusion plays no part in the therapy of agranulocytosis and severe infection, unless there is concomitant anaemia. Platelet and granulocyte transfusions are used in specialized centres only.

Storage of blood. Blood is collected aseptically from a healthy donor into a plastic bag in which there is an anticoagulant. The one most used is ACD, a mixture of citric *a*cid, trisodium *c*itrate, and *d*extrose. Blood is stored at 4°C, and must not be allowed to freeze or to exceed 10°C. It can be stored for periods up to 3 weeks. Up to this time most of the red cells survive in the recipient as well as do fresh cells.

Cross-matching. The important elements are the donor's red cells and the recipient's plasma. With rare exceptions the donor's plasma is not important, because the antibodies it contains are so diluted by the recipient's plasma that they are not likely to react with the recipient's cells. It is always preferable to use blood of exactly the same ABO and Rhesus groups as those of the recipient, but group-O blood can be used if necessary, provided it is properly cross-matched. Group O is called the 'universal donor', because it is not normally agglutinated by any serum. In extreme emergencies, where delay might lead to death from exsanguination, it is permissible to use uncross-matched group-O Rh-negative blood, but otherwise cross-matching is essential, because (1) there may be an error in sample identification, and (2) the recipient's serum may contain antibodies other than anti-A, anti-B, and anti-Rhesus.

Technique of cross-matching. (1) Mix a 2 per cent suspension of donor cells and recipient serum at room temperature for 1 hour. Absence of agglutination rules out a 'complete' antibody. (2) Mix the cells and serum at 37°C for 1 hour. Then centrifuge the cells, wash them three times in saline, and suspend them in an antiglobulin serum (Coombs test). Absence of agglutination rules out an 'incomplete' antibody.

Hazards of blood transfusion

Haemolytic transfusion reactions. These are usually due to the rapid destruction of the donor red cells by antibodies in the recipient's plasma, and are generally the result of transfusion of ABO incompatible blood, for example group A red cells into a group O recipient. *These mishaps are almost always due to an error in the identification of the patient, a specimen, or the unit of blood, rather than a technical failure to detect incompatibility.* The antigen-antibody reaction leads to the release of vasoconstrictor substances from the red cells, which cause widespread vascular phenomena. There is initial pain along the vein, and this is followed by facial flushing, headache, a sensation of constriction around the chest, and backache. A danger is severe renal arterial spasm with ischaemia of the kidneys. Free haemoglobin in the plasma causes mild renal vasoconstriction, and the presence of vasoconstrictor substances (as well as the original condition that necessitated transfusion) accentuates this markedly. ABO incompatibility leads to much more severe renal effects than does Rh incompatibility, and death from uraemia may occur.

Bacterial contamination of the blood due to the adventitious introduction of coliform organisms leads to fatal septicaemia.

Diseases introduced from the donor, the most important of which are malaria, syphilis, and viral hepatitis (see p. 260).

Febrile reactions are usually due to the presence of white-cell antibodies formed by the recipient as a result of previous transfusions or pregnancy. Another cause is pyrogens present in the bottles, tubing, or anticoagulant fluid. The fever is sharp, but usually lasts only a few hours.

Allergic reactions, usually urticarial are not uncommon, and are due to some antigen in the donor's plasma to which the recipient is hypersensitive. Life-threatening acute anaphylaxis is rare. Allergic reactions may also be due to the presence of IgE in the plasma of the donor.

Overloading of the circulation, leading to heart failure.

Air embolism is very rare with modern equipment.

Thrombophlebitis following the local irritation of the vein by the needle.

Transfusional haemosiderosis. This occurs when repeated transfusions are given frequently over a long period of time. There is a gradual accumulation of iron pigment which is not used in erythropoiesis, and it is deposited in the tissues, where it may set up fibrosis.

Sensitization. The transfusion of blood carrying antigens not present in the recipient's cells may stimulate the production of alloantibodies directed against the foreign antigen. These alloantibodies to red-cell, white-cell, platelet, or plasma-protein antigens may complicate future transfusions or pregnancies.

In modern centres blood transfusion is a lifesaving procedure. However, the possible complications are numerous, and except under emergency conditions, transfusion should never be attempted without expert supervision.

GENERAL READING

Hardisty R M, Weatherall D J (eds) 1974 Blood and its Disorders, 1540 pp Blackwell, Oxford
Wintrobe M M, Lee G R, Boggs D R, Bithell T C, Athens J W, Foerster J 1974 Clinical Hematology, 7th edn, 1896 pp Lea & Febiger, Philadelphia

READING FOR BLOOD TRANSFUSION

Boorman K E, Dodd B E, Lincoln P J 1977 Blood Grouping Serology, 5th ed, 495 pp Churchill Livingstone, Edinburgh
Giblett E R 1969 Genetic Markers in Human Blood, 629 pp Blackwell, Oxford
Mollison P L 1979 Blood Transfusion in Clinical Medicine, 6th edn, 884 pp Blackwell, Oxford
Race R R, Sanger R 1975 Blood Groups in Man, 6th edn 659 pp Blackwell, Oxford
Wallace J 1977 Blood Transfusion for Clinicians, 392 pp Churchill Livingstone, Edinburgh

PART TWO

Diseases of individual systems and organs

31

Disorders of the circulation

THE BLOOD PRESSURE

The function of the circulatory system is the maintenance of adequate perfusion of blood to all the tissues of the body. Each ventricular contraction ejects a quantity of blood into the arterial system, and in the systemic system the expansion of the elastic arteries prevents an undue rise in pressure. Nevertheless, the arterial pressure rises to a maximum (normally 120 to 150 mm Hg), and during the subsequent diastole it falls steadily as blood flows away through the arterioles to the various vascular beds. The lowest pressure (diastolic pressure) reached is generally 60 to 90 mm Hg. The major resistance encountered by the blood is in the arterioles, so that by the time the capillaries are reached, the pressure is only about 30 mm Hg. The blood flow in the major arteries is pulsatile. The elasticity of the major vessels and the high resistance provided by the arterioles reduce this pulsation, so that in the capillaries and veins the blood flow is constant. It follows that whereas blood escapes from capillaries and veins in a constant ooze, it spurts out when an artery is cut.

The physiological mechanisms involved in maintaining the blood pressure will not be described in detail. In the main they involve the regulation of arteriolar tone by the autonomic division of the nervous system in response to stimuli from the aortic and carotid baroreceptors. Low blood pressure (hypotension) is characteristic of shock and Addison's disease. Hypertension will now be considered.

Systemic hypertension

A considerable rise in blood pressure is normal in response to emotion, physical exercise, and sexual intercourse. A persistent or recurrent elevation of the blood pressure at rest is abnormal, and is termed *hypertension*. Two types are recognized.

Primary, or essential, hypertension. This is the common form of high blood pressure, and its cause is unknown. It is a condition that is more common in women than in men, and is especially prevalent in North American Blacks. Primary renal or adrenal abnormalities have been postulated but never proven.

Secondary hypertension. Hypertension is characteristic of phaeochromocytoma, where it is due to the effects of adrenaline and noradrenaline produced by the tumour (p. 625). Hypertension is also seen in some adrenal cortical tumours, and is an accompaniment of both Conn's and Cushing's syndromes (p. 626). The most common cause of secondary hypertension is renal disease.

The classical experiments of Goldblatt proved that in the dog an obstruction to the renal arterial blood flow could produce hypertension. This is due to the release from the kidney of the proteolytic enzyme *renin*, which acts on a plasma globulin, *angiotensinogen*, converting it into *angiotensin I*. Another plasma enzyme converts this into *angiotensin II*, an octapeptide which induces vasospasm and produces hypertension.

In the human hypertension sometimes, but not always, occurs in acute and chronic glomerulonephritis, pyelonephritis, and other renal diseases. It is not certain whether the mechanism of its production is similar to that of the Goldblatt experiments; present evidence is against such a pathogenesis. Hypertension in unilateral renal lesions is sometimes relieved by nephrectomy, but unfortunately this is not always so.

Effects and complications of hypertension

Haemorrhage. Weakened blood vessels tend to rupture more commonly in the hypertensive subject than in the normal; dissecting aneurysm of the aorta, ruptured berry aneurysms of the circle of Willis, and cerebral haemorrhage are all more common in the hypertensive subject.

Arteriolosclerosis. The small arteries and arterioles of many organs show thickening of their walls, particularly the tunica intima, with hyaline material. This thickening is most marked in the afferent arterioles of the renal glomeruli; gradually as these vessels close down the glomeruli and tubules that they supply become atrophic and replaced by fibrous tissue. The kidneys become small and their surface granular. The condition is called *benign nephrosclerosis.*

The arterioles of the retina share in this generalized process. The thickening of their walls together with the ischaemic changes in the retina constitute *hypertensive retinopathy.*

Arteriolosclerosis also affects the central nervous system and is responsible for such vague symptoms as headache, lightheadedness, and giddiness. Personality changes and memory defects are also common. More severe lesions resulting from vascular occlusion or haemorrhage produce more definite effects, such as a hemiplegia.

Heart failure. Systemic hypertension causes left ventricular hypertrophy and ultimately left ventricular failure. It is a common cause of paroxysmal nocturnal dyspnoea.

Malignant hypertension. Hypertension, whether primary or secondary, may occasionally evolve into a malignant phase. The blood pressure becomes very high, causing necrosis of the arteriolar walls (*malignant arteriolosclerosis*). The kidneys and the brain are the two organs most severely affected. In the kidney glomerular destruction causes haemorrhage and culminates in uraemia (*malignant nephrosclerosis*). In the brain the changes cause haemorrhage and oedema. Swelling of the optic discs (*papilloedema*) is a useful sign of raised intracranial pressure; symptoms include mental confusion and seizures. The syndrome of malignant hypertension usually progresses rapidly over a period of weeks, and unless treated expeditiously results in death from uraemia, heart failure, or an intracranial vascular accident.

THROMBOSIS

In the vascular system it is the platelets and the clotting mechanism which guard against the danger of haemorrhage. The deposition of platelets and fibrin effectively patches any minor defect, and even severed vessels are soon sealed off. The control of platelet deposition and fibrin formation is an excellent example of a homeostatic mechanism designed to steer the body between the two hazards of haemorrhage and thrombosis. Under abnormal conditions an excessive deposit of platelets and fibrin may be formed, and this endangers the circulation by causing obstruction. This is *thrombosis.*

The coagulation mechanism. Coagulation, or clotting, may be defined as the conversion of fibrinogen to a solid mass of fibrin. The mechanism is described in Chapter 30 and here it will suffice to note that clotting can be initiated by clotting factors derived from either the blood (intrinsic) or tissues (extrinsic). The activation of the intrinsic system has two components:

1. Platelets which have become adherent to a surface liberate a lipid factor, and
2. an abnormal surface activates Factor XII (Hageman factor).

Minor degrees of injury are constantly being sustained by blood vessels, and a layer of platelets is soon laid down to prevent haemorrhage. Endothelial cells cover this platelet deposit so that the smooth lining of the vessel is restored, further deposition ceases, and the process is brought to an end. The presence of naturally occurring anticoagulant substances, like heparin and antithrombin III,[1] and the constant bathing by the stream of blood, tend to prevent clotting. Nevertheless, small quantities of fibrin are probably formed even under normal conditions, and there exists a *fibrinolytic mechanism* for its removal (p 467). The active agent *plasmin* is formed on the fibrin threads and leads to their dissolution. Thus, three mechanisms normally prevent the intravascular accumulation of fibrin:

1. Endothelialization of both platelet deposits and areas of damage
2. The fibrinolytic system
3. Factors that limit the deposition of platelets (see below).

Under abnormal circumstances these mechanisms are inadequate, and intravascular coagulation becomes excessive.

Platelet aggregation and adhesion are described on page 463.

Pathogenesis of thrombus formation[2,3]

Thrombosis may be defined as the formation of a solid mass in the circulation from the constituents of the streaming blood. The mass itself is called a *thrombus.* Thrombosis involves two distinct processes:

1. *The deposition of platelets on a vascular surface.* This occurs under three circumstances:

    a. When the endothelial lining is damaged or removed.

b. With vascular stasis, when the platelets fall out of the axial stream and impinge on the wall
c. In association with eddy currents, which deflect the platelets to an area on the wall.

Whenever any of these three factors operates to an excessive extent, an abnormal mass of platelets is formed. This is a *pale*, or *platelet, thrombus.*

Platelets do not adhere to a normal intact endothelial surface; although this may be due to the active blood flow sweeping them along, there is also a possibility that a chemical mechanism is involved. This involves the formation of thromboxane A_2 and prostacyclin, and is described below together with the role of the prostaglandins in thrombosis.

2. *The formation of a clot of fibrin in which the blood cells are trapped.*

If the platelet thrombus is not speedily endothelialized, or if there is stasis, blood clot is formed, and in its meshes are trapped the red and white cells. Thrombin is potent in causing platelets to adhere to each other, and its liberation during the process of coagulation readily leads to a further deposition of platelets. In this way a large mass is built up. When blood clot is the major component, it is called a *red,* or *coagulation, thrombus.* Frequently the thrombosis is made up of both red clot and pale platelet components, and is then called a *mixed thrombus.*

The crucial feature of thrombosis is the deposition of platelets on a vascular surface. This can occur only in the presence of a flowing stream, and is therefore produced spontaneously only in the living animal. The clotting is a secondary phenomenon. It follows that the terms 'clot' and 'thrombus' are quite distinct; a thrombus contains a variable amount of clot, but the important feature is a platelet scaffold which is lacking in a clot; it can be formed only *in vivo.** Clotting, on the other hand, may occur as part of thrombosis, and is also seen in a column of static blood *in vivo* or *in vitro.*

Since the cardinal process in thrombosis is the deposition of platelets on an intimal surface, it is evident that the integrity of the vascular system is all-important in preventing it. The two factors are:

1. The smooth endothelial lining which diminishes frictional resistance between the wall and the circulating blood, and
2. the streamline of blood along the complex circulatory pathways, which results in the formed elements moving in a central axial stream (p. 72).

The speed of flow prevents local stasis, and the absence of irregularities in the walls does not allow the development of eddy currents. The streamline of blood can be threatened in a variety of ways, which are illustrated in Fig. 31.1. These lesions all lead to local stasis as well as to the formation of eddy currents, and the platelets that cover them are actually performing a remedial function. They serve to smooth out the contours of the wall and restore the streamline of blood in the vessel. The small amount of clotting factors that they generate is dissipated in the flowing blood, and they themselves are rapidly endothelialized. It is when this process is retarded that the platelet mass grows, clotting factors accumulate,

* Highly artificial experimental procedures can, of course, provide an exception to this rule.

much fibrin is produced, and thrombosis proceeds even to the extent of obliterating the vessel lumen.

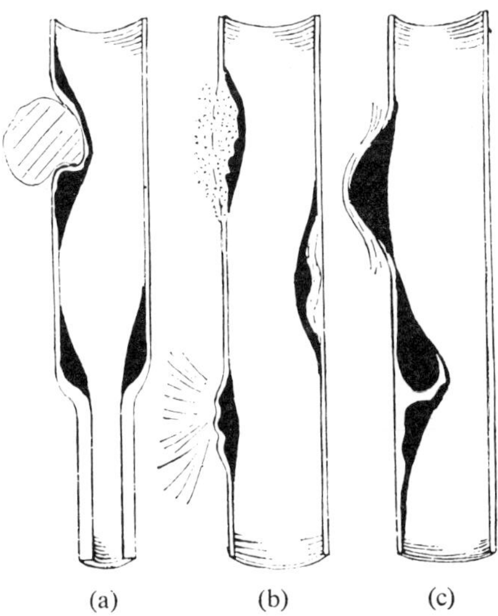

Fig. 31.1 This diagram shows seven different causes of a disruption of the normal streamlining of the blood flow, and the manner whereby platelets (shown in black) are laid down to restore the architecture.
(a) Bulging due to external pressure and spasm.
(b) Endothelial swelling and roughening due to inflammation, a plaque of thickening, e.g. atheroma, and corrugation due to adjacent cicatrization.
(c) Aneurysm, and a hard sclerotic valve.
(*From Hadfield G 1950 Annals of the Royal College of Surgeons of England 6: 219.*)

Role of the Prostaglandins in Thrombosis[4]

The prostaglandins are potent agents derived from 20-carbon polyunsaturated fatty acids that are present in the phospholipids of all cell membranes. They have been named by letter (approximately in order of discovery) and by figures one to three according to the number of double bonds in the molecule. The group containing two double bonds has attracted most attention. They are synthetized from *arachidonic acid* which is released from cell-membrane phospholipid by the action of phospholipase A_2. The enzyme cyclo-oxydase converts arachidonic acid into the two unstable *prostaglandin endoperoxides*, PGG_2 and PGH_2*. In platelets these endoperoxides are converted into *thromboxane* A_2 (TXA_2), which is a powerful agent that causes vasoconstriction and platelet aggregation.

When platelets adhere to a vessel wall TXA_2 is formed, platelet aggregation is encouraged, and a platelet thrombus is formed. However, the endoperoxides formed by the platelets can also be used by cells of the vessel walls; these cells convert the endoperoxides into *prostacyclin* (PGI_2, formerly called prostaglandin X), which is a vasodilator and can inhibit platelet aggregation. A balance between

* These endoperoxides can also be converted into PGE_2 and $PGF_{2\alpha}$. Together with PGE_1 these are thought to be important mediators of acute inflammation (p 86).

the formation of thrombaxane A_2 by the platelets and prostacyclin by the vessel wall may well be an important factor in determining the extent of thrombus formation. Damage to a vessel wall may impede prostacyclin formation and thereby encourage thrombus formation.

The vessel wall synthetizes prostacyclin from its own precursors, as well as from endoperoxides released by platelets. Thus the continuous formation of prostacyclin may be an important homeostatic mechanism whereby platelets which are forced on to the vascular endothelium (or on areas of minimal damage) are prevented from building up an abnormal platelet thrombus. Prostacyclin in the circulation, partially derived from the lungs, appears to be an additional protective mechanism. When it is remembered that platelet deposition on arterial walls is thought to be a major factor in the pathogenisis of atherosclerosis, it will be readily understood why research into the formation and properties of the prostaglandins is currently so active.

Causes of thrombosis

Three factors (*Virchow's triad*) must be considered in regard to the mechanism of thrombosis:

The vessel wall. The various types of anatomical changes in the vessel wall which may lead to platelet deposition have already been depicted (Fig. 31.1). In general these abnormalities play an important part in thrombosis involving the heart and arteries. In the veins they are of less importance.

The flow of blood. The importance of *eddy currents* has already been noted. These lead to platelet deposition, and the resulting thrombus is pale. This occurs in fast moving streams, e.g. over the heart valves and in arteries. *Stasis* is the most important cause of extensive thrombosis involving veins. It is also a factor in inducing thrombosis in the sac of an aneurysm.

The constituents of the blood. An increase in the platelet count, an increased tendency to platelet adhesion and aggregation, a decrease in the clotting time, and decreased antithrombin activity all contribute to thrombosis. The interaction of these factors is complex, but changes in them help to explain the thrombosis that occurs after parturition, splenectomy, trauma, and severe haemorrhage, and also the thromboses that complicate hyperlipidaemia and the administration of certain drugs, e.g. the birth-control pill.

It should be noted that usually more than one factor is implicated in causing thrombosis. For instance, there is regional stasis and a high platelet count after an operation, and atheromatous plaques act both by causing a loss of the endothelium and inducing eddy currents.

Venous thrombosis

Although disease of the vessel walls is uncommon, stasis is particularly evident in the veins, especially in those of the legs. Thrombosis with a large element of clotting is therefore common. Two distinct entities should be recognized: phlebothrombosis and thrombophlebitis.

Phlebothrombosis

In this important condition there is extensive thrombosis and clot formation in the veins of the calf. It is due mainly to stasis, and is seen whenever the circulation in the legs is impaired. This occurs whenever the cardiac output is reduced, e.g. in heart failure, shock, and when the metabolic rate is reduced as when a patient is put to rest in bed. The venous return from the legs is greatly facilitated by the squeezing action of the surrounding muscles, and this important mechanism is in abeyance in the bedridden patient. The arms are much less likely to be affected, since they are in constant use in all conscious patients. Following trauma the increased platelet count, increased platelet adhesiveness, and decreased clotting time are further factors favouring thrombosis. Direct damage to the veins, e.g. by a fractured bone, or even the pressure of a pillow on the calf muscles, may be additional precipitating factors. It follows therefore that phlebothrombosis is common in the leg veins whenever a patient is put to bed, especially in the elderly,

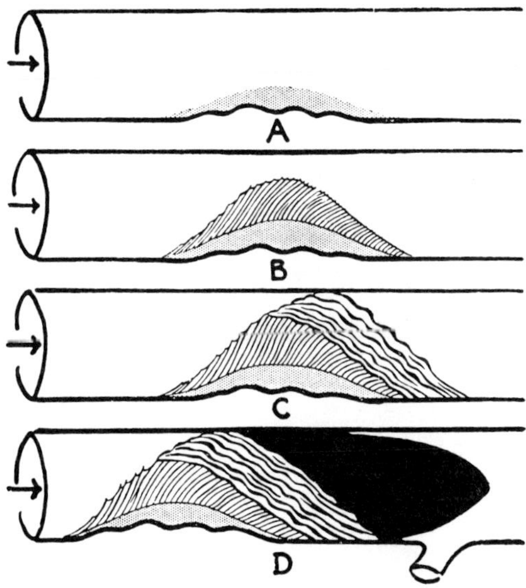

Fig. 31.2 The pathogenesis of phlebothrombosis.
A. Primary platelet thrombus.
B. Coralline thrombus.
C. Occluding thrombus.
D. Consecutive clot to the next venous tributary.
(*From Hadfield G 1950 Annals of the Royal College of Surgeons of England 6: 219.*)

if the heart is failing, or if there is shock or severe trauma, such as after a major operation or a severe haemorrhage. Indeed, it occurs in about 35 per cent of patients after major surgery, and is even more frequent in cases of recent myocardial infarction.[5]

Pathogenesis of phlebothrombosis. Five stages can be recognized (Fig. 31.2).

Primary platelet thrombus. Following some trivial intimal damage, platelets adhere to the vein walls and form a mass of palc thrombus. This has been likened to the formation of a snow-drift during a snow-storm. Under normal circumstances this would produce no ill-effect, but if stasis is superadded, fibrin formation ensues and a large coralline thrombus is produced.

Coralline thrombus. As fibrin formation occurs and further platelets accumulate, the latter take the form of upstanding laminae growing across the stream. Between the laminae there is complete stasis, and fibrin is deposited; in it numerous red and white cells are trapped. This is an example of a mixed thrombus, and on section the alternating layers are seen (Fig. 31.3). The retraction of the fibrin layers leads to the characteristic ribbed or rippled appearance seen when the surface of the thrombus is examined. The elevated platelet ridges are called the *lines of Zahn*, and are a characteristic feature of a thrombus formed in a fairly rapid

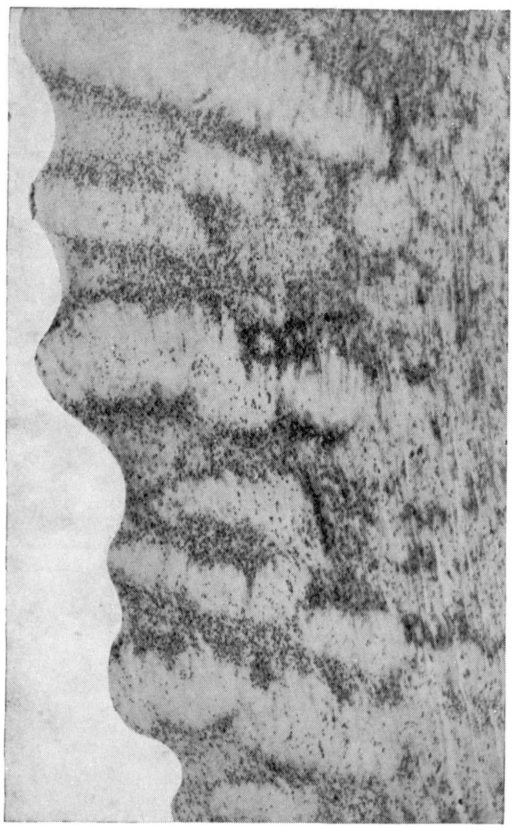

Fig. 31.3 Coralline thrombus. Photomicrograph of vertical section including free surface of a coralline thrombus adjacent to the wall of a large artery. Pale platelet laminae are seen projecting from the surface. Coagulated plasma containing leucocytes lies between them. Many leucocytes are adherent to the platelet laminae. (*From Hadfield G 1950 Annals of the Royal College of Surgeons of England 6: 219.*)

stream of blood. Their presence is a useful indication that a structure found in a vessel is a thrombus formed during life and not a post-mortem clot (p. 492).

Occluding thrombus. The growth of the coralline thrombus progressively occludes the lumen of the vein, and the ensuing stasis rapidly leads to the formation of an occluding thrombus.

Consecutive clot. Once the vein is occluded, blood flow stops and with it stops the thrombosis. The stationary column of blood beyond the thrombus extending to the next entering tributary undergoes coagulation. This is called the consecutive clot (Fig. 31.4), and its free end, or tail, points like a dagger towards the heart.

Propagated clot. When stasis is marked, the clotting process extends up a considerable length of the vein past the entering tributaries to produce a long propagated clot (Fig. 31.4). As this retracts, it lies free in the lumen, and is attached only at the point of original thrombosis. This long, loose structure can easily become detached and carried to the right side of the heart as an embolus.

Clinical features. Clinically phlebothrombosis is remarkably silent. There is little pain in the limb, but direct squeezing pressure on the calf muscles may elicit tenderness. Careful measurement may detect slight oedema. Frequently the first indication of phlebothrombosis is the occurrence of pulmonary embolism.

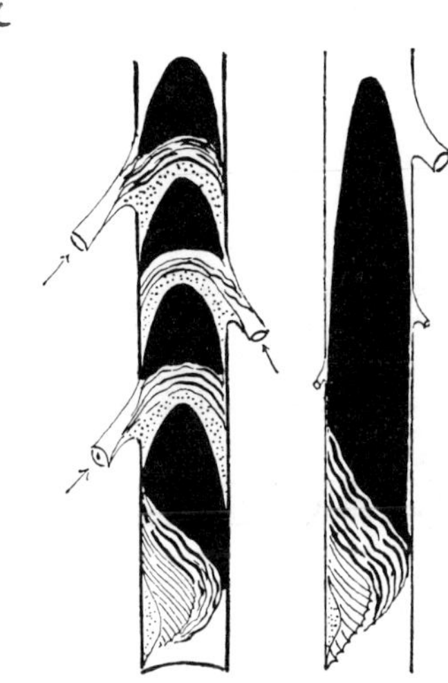

Fig. 31.4 Methods of propagation in phlebothrombosis.
(a) With thrombus formation at each entering tributary.
(b) Clotting *en masse* in an extensive length of vein.
(*From Hadfield G 1950 Annals of the Royal College of Surgeons of England 6: 219.*)

Several methods are available for the detection of phlebothrombosis:

1. *Phlebography.* Contrast medium is injected into a foot vein, and the venous circulation of the leg and thigh are studied radiographically.

2. *Radio-active iodine-labelled fibrinogen test.* In this test ^{125}I-labelled human fibrinogen is administered intravenously (after giving suitable doses of potassium iodide to block any uptake of the radio-active iodine by the thyroid gland). The labelled fibrinogen is incorporated into the thrombi, and the concentration of the isotope in the local area is detected and measured by an external counter.

3. *Doppler ultrasound method.* Using a special apparatus one can detect the flow of blood through a vessel by placing a sensor on the overlying skin. Complete absence of flow denotes thrombosis.[6]

The prevention of postoperative deep vein thrombosis involves leg exercises whilst the patient is in bed, early ambulation, avoidance of pressure on the calf and the administration of heparin.[7]

Complications. Small emboli lodge in the lungs, and may produce infarction. A more serious complication is massive pulmonary embolism which can produce sudden death. This usually occurs from 7 to 10 days after injury or operation.

Varicose veins. A common cause of phlebothrombosis is varicose veins, but the circumstances are so different from those of deep vein thrombosis of the leg veins that this topic will be considered separately.

Elongation and irregular dilatation of veins is known as *varicosity*. It is generally assumed that persistent increase in pressure is a cause of this; oesophageal varices can certainly be explained in this manner (see Ch. 34). Nevertheless, the common condition of varicose veins of the legs is not well understood. An inherited defect of the venous walls or valves has been postulated. There also seems to be a familial factor in the incidence of this common disease. Other suggested causes are the standing for long periods over many years that is required in some occupations and the lack of support for the walls of the veins that is seen in fat people. Because pregnancy seems to initiate varicose-vein formation, the disease is more common at an earlier age in women. Once varicose veins have formed, their valves become incompetent, so that on standing the full hydrostatic pressure of blood is applied to the vessel wall and further dilatation ensues. The extremely sluggish blood flow through the veins can predispose to thrombus formation, but *embolism from this is extremely rare*. The major effect of varicose veins is to produce venous stasis. The increased hydrostatic pressure leads to oedema, and the skin exhibits *stasis dermatitis*. Trivial injuries lead to persistent ulcerations that characteristically overlie the medial malleoli. Even though these ulcers can enlarge, they are not painful. In this respect they contrast with the ulceration caused by arterial disease (ischaemic ulcers).

Thrombophlebitis

Inflammation of a vessel wall may follow the injection of irritant chemicals, e.g. anaesthetic agents, or be a complication of an adjacent area of infection, e.g. a staphylococcal abscess. In either event thrombosis occurs in the area of damage, but as stasis is not present, extensive propagation of the clot does not occur. The thrombosis is therefore relatively localized and firmly adherent. The condition is characterized by pain and swelling in the region of the vein, and is therefore clinically very obvious.

Embolism is most uncommon except in thrombophlebitis due to pyogenic infection, when the organisms invade the thrombus and cause its softening, so that small infected emboli are released into the circulation. The condition is called *pyaemia*, and the numerous infected emboli become impacted in distant organs, e.g. the lung, where they produce metastatic, or pyaemic, abscesses. If thrombophlebitis affects the portal vein, the *pyaemic abscesses* are found primarily in the liver. This is an occasional complication of suppurative appendicitis.

Two particular types of thrombophlebitis are worthy of special note:

Thrombophlebitis migrans. Migratory thrombophlebitis is characterized by thrombosis affecting many veins at different times. It is a well-recognized complication of malignant disease, especially carcinoma of the pancreas.

Painful white leg (phlegmasia alba dolens). The painful white leg that is seen in pregnant women in the third trimester—or more often immediately following delivery—is due to iliofemoral venous thrombosis. It is thought that inflammation also involves the lymphatics and that this contributes to the formation of such massive oedema.

Thrombosis in the atria of the heart

Atrial thrombosis is generally due to stasis, and the condition is analogous to phlebothrombosis. The thrombi commonly occur in the atrial appendages, and are seen whenever there is stasis, e.g. in heart failure, especially if accompanied by atrial fibrillation. The thrombi may become detached as emboli either in the pulmonary or the systemic circulation depending upon which atrium is involved.

Thrombosis in arteries

In the high-velocity arterial system the most important cause of thrombosis is disease or spasm of the arterial wall itself. This acts in three ways.

1. Eddy current formation leads to the deposition of platelets.
2. There is ulceration of the endothelial lining
3. Disease of the arterial wall may so weaken it that aneurysmal dilatation occurs. This leads to local stasis.

The causes of arterial thrombosis are thus those of arterial damage, and it is appropriate to describe the common types of arterial disease at this point.

DISEASES OF ARTERIES

Arterial disease and its complications are responsible for about 40 per cent of all deaths. Arteritis forms a distinct group, but the degenerative diseases (arteriosclerosis) are by far the most important.

Arteritis. Causes of inflammation of the arterial wall include:

Trauma, as when an artery adjacent to a fracture is injured.

Infective. Arteritis may occur in pyogenic infections, and if the vessel wall undergoes necrosis, severe haemorrhage can result. A good example of this is the fatal haemorrhage from the lingual artery that sometimes ends the life of a patient with an ulcerating carcinoma of the tongue. Neoplastic invasion plays its part, but the major weakening effect is the result of infection. Similarly, destruction of an artery at the base of a gastric ulcer is a common cause of bleeding. Fortunately, in many chronic inflammatory lesions the artery responds by proliferation of its intimal lining so that the lumen becomes steadily occluded (*endarteritis obliterans*) and bleeding is restricted.

Idiopathic inflammatory conditions. There are a number of diseases in which inflammation of the arterial wall leads to thrombosis. *Thromboangiitis obliterans* (*Buerger's disease*) is the best known. It is seen predominantly in young men. It affects the veins and arteries of the legs, and causes ischaemia which leads to intermittent claudication (pain in the calf muscles on exercise) and ultimately gangrene commencing in the toes. *Giant-cell arteritis* is a disease of elderly people; the affected artery shows thrombosis and a chronic inflammatory granulomatous reaction with many giant cells formed around disrupted elastic fibres. The disease can affect any artery, but commonly it is the temporal one and pain in the temple is a marked feature. The ophthalmic artery is sometimes involved and blindness may result. Rarely the lingual artery is occluded, when ischaemia and pain can affect the oral structures, e.g. the tongue. *Polyarteritis* and other forms of vasculitis can also cause thrombosis.

Neoplastic infiltration. (p. 334).

Arteriosclerosis. This term embraces what is loosely called degenerative arterial disease, and is extremely important. It includes the following:

Mönckeberg's medial sclerosis. This affects the large muscular arteries especially those of the lower limbs. The tunica media shows hyaline change and *calcification.* It produces dramatic radiological appearances but does not cause any ill-effects, and is therefore unimportant.

Diffuse hyperplastic sclerosis. In this condition the small muscular arteries and arterioles become progressively thickened. The lesions are most marked in hypertension and have already been described.

Atheroma (or atherosclerosis). This is the most important type of arteriosclerosis.

Atherosclerosis

Atheroma is the commonest killing disease in all highly advanced civilized communities, and its lesions are present to some degree in almost every adult member. The disease characteristically affects the large elastic arteries like the aorta and its main branches. Of the medium-sized vessels the coronary and cerebral arteries are most commonly involved. This is extremely unfortunate in view of the vital nature of the organs they supply, and it accounts for the lethal effects of atheroma. Atheroma may be considered as consisting of two types of condition.

Basic lesions of atherosclerosis

Type I: Superficial yellow plaques in the intima. Lipid-containing cells (probably muscle cells) accumulate in the subendothelial layer of the vessel and later break down to release their fatty content into the tunica intima. In this way are produced the yellow streaks that are a common necropsy finding in the aorta. When the fatty deposits occur in small arteries, they do not produce appreciable narrowing of the lumen. These early yellow plaques are sometimes referred to as *atheroma.*

Type II: Accumulation of fatty material in the intima with additional fibrosis. This is the common type of lesion seen in middle age and old age. The lesions consist of intimal plaques and contain a central mass of fatty, yellow, porridge-like material (from the Greek *athere* meaning porridge) consisting predominantly of cholesterol and its esters. This material is covered by dense fibrous tissue, which gives the plaque a white, pearly appearance. This type of lesion is generally designated atherosclerosis.

Advanced and complicated lesions of atherosclerosis

Four further changes may be seen in the plaques as they progress:

Haemorrhage. Proliferation of vessels from the vasa vasorum produces increased vascularity in the connective tissue surrounding the atheromatous plaque. Rupture of one of these vessels leads to bleeding into the plaque. In a small vessel like the coronary artery this bleeding can produce acute obstruction.

Thrombosis. Eddy currents around the plaque can lead to superadded thrombosis.

Ulceration. Sometimes the fibrous covering of the plaque becomes detached so that ulceration is combined with thrombosis.

Calcification. The fatty material in the atheromatous plaque undergoes dystrophic calcification.

Aetiology and pathogenesis[8,9]

The cause of atherosclerosis is not yet known, but genetic factors seem to play a part, since the disease sometimes appears in many members of a family. In some instances there are clues to the pathogenesis. Thus, atherosclerosis is more common in persons having diabetes mellitus, which is itself a familial disease. Likewise, there are some inherited conditions of abnormal lipid metabolism in which high blood lipid levels are associated with the early development of atheroma.

It is not known whether the lesions of type I atheroma progress to those of type II, or whether the two types are independent diseases. Experimentally, lesions resembling the human fatty streaks can be produced in animals by feeding them with an abnormal diet—usually one containing a high content of cholesterol. It is believed that certain types of diet predispose human beings to develop atheroma. Much of the cholesterol in the body is produced endogenously, but the level of plasma cholesterol is related to the types of lipid that are eaten. A diet high in saturated animal fats appears to predispose a person to atheroma.

Lesions resembling type II atherosclerosis can occur after the arterial wall has been injured. A thrombus forms and its subsequent degeneration and partial organization produce an atheromatous plaque. Either lipid deposition or thrombosis could be involved in the pathogenesis of human atheroma, and there is currently much controversy as to the relative importance of these two mechanisms. Furthermore, they are not mutually exclusive. Initial lipid lesions produced by dietary imbalance could progress by additional thrombosis. Injury and superadded thrombosis release chemicals (e.g. histamine and 5-hydroxytryptamine) that could alter the endothelial permeability and allow plasma lipoproteins to enter the intima. Degradation of the lipoprotein together with failure to remove the lipid component is believed to be the mechanism of lipid accumulation in atheroma.

Recent investigations have laid stress on the role of the smooth muscle cells of the intima. It has been found that platelets release a factor that causes these cells to proliferate. Thus injury to the vessel wall (e.g. by hypertension, local trauma, abnormal lipoproteins, or hyperlipidaemia) could lead to the formation of a platelet thrombus. Smooth muscle cells of the intima could proliferate, and as lipoproteins enter the vessel wall they could be taken up by the cells and the lipid component retained. In this way could be produced the early fatty streaks (type I) lesions. It is evident that the pathogenesis of atherosclerosis is very complex indeed. The increase in the incidence of the disease has now reached pandemic proportions and this is a reflection of our ignorance.

Effects of atherosclerosis

Gradual obstruction. Atherosclerosis of small vessels such as the coronary or cerebral arteries produces intimal thickening and progressive occlusion of the lumen. This leads to ischaemia of the area supplied.

Thrombosis. This leads to sudden complete obstruction and often to infarction.

Dilatation and aneurysm formation. The presence of an atherosclerotic plaque causes atrophy of the adjacent media. The wall consequently weakens, and the artery involved may show either a diffuse enlargement, called *ectasia*, or a localized dilatation, called an *aneurysm*. These effects are seen most often in the aorta, in which the atherosclerosis is most severe. The lesions of atherosclerosis tend to be more advanced toward the more distal regions of the aorta, and it is therefore in the abdominal portion that aneurysm formation is most common. The aneurysm is generally below the origin of the renal arteries, and rupture of such a lesion leads to exsanguination and death.

Embolism. It is not uncommon for atheromatous material, or overlying thrombus, to become detached and embolize distally. Usually such emboli are small and are inapparent clinically. Nevertheless, the steady occlusion of many small vessels is probably a factor in the peripheral ischaemic disease of the lower leg as well as the progressive ischaemic renal disease that often accompanies atherosclerosis.

Aneurysms

An aneurysm is a local dilatation of an artery or a chamber of the heart due to a weakening of its walls. It may be localized and saccular or diffuse and fusiform.

Causes. The weakening of the wall may be due to:

1. Congenital deficiency, e.g. berry aneurysms of the circle of Willis (p. 608).
2. Trauma. Sometimes an injury can damage not only an artery but also an adjacent vein, thereby establishing a connexion. This formation is called an *arteriovenous aneurysm*, or *fistula*. It is important, because so much blood can be diverted from the peripheral tissue that heart failure ensues.
3. Inflammation, e.g. syphilitic aortitis may cause an aneurysm of the thoracic aorta. The condition is now rare.
4. Degeneration, e.g. atheromatous. This is by far the most common type of aortic aneurysm.

Effects. Aneurysms produce harmful effects in a number of ways:

Pressure. An aneurysm of the thoracic aorta may press on the oesophagus and cause difficulty in swallowing, or on the recurrent laryngeal nerve and lead to changes in the voice.

Haemorrhage. Rupture of an aneurysm leads to bleeding; for a while this can be quite trivial because of the plugging effect of the thrombus lining the sac. Nevertheless, when an aneurysm, such as one of the abdominal aorta, has begun to bleed, it is not long before massive haemorrhage follows and the patient dies of exsanguination.

Thrombosis. The sac of an aneurysm soon becomes filled by laminated thrombus (Fig. 31.5). This is due in part to the damage to the endothelial lining and in part to the local stasis.

Ischaemia. This is due to blockage of the branches of the artery at the site of the aneurysm, an effect produced either by local pressure or by thrombotic occlusion.

Dissecting aneurysm of aorta

The basic defect is degeneration in the media of the aorta (*medionecrosis*), the aetiology of which is unknown. If there is rupture of one of the small vessels

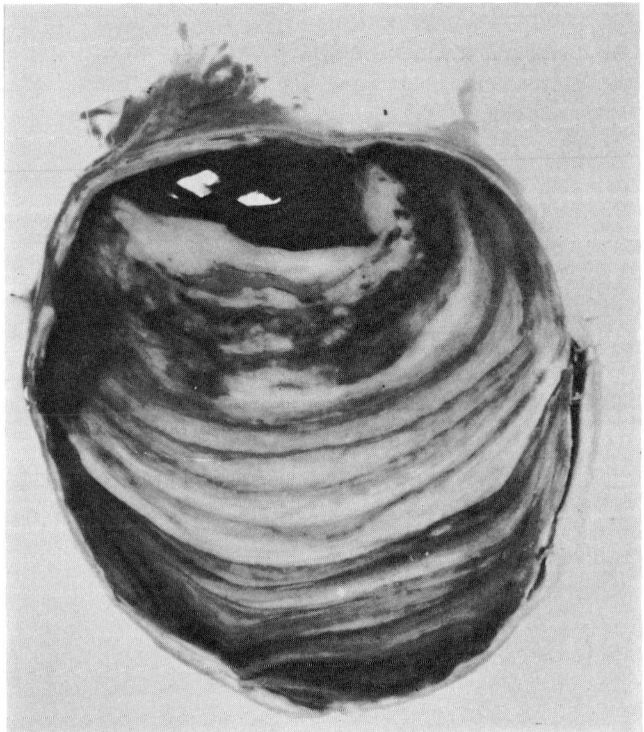

Fig. 31.5 Laminated thrombus in an aneurysmal sac. In this cross-section the sac is seen to be almost completely occluded with laminated thrombus. (C31b.4. *Reproduced by permission of the President and Council of the Royal College of Surgeons of England.*)

supplying the wall of the aorta (vasa vasorum), bleeding occurs into the media. This steadily splits the arterial wall into two layers, and eventually a tear extends into the main lumen. This usually occurs in the ascending aorta. Blood is then forced in considerable quantity through this tear, and it produces an extensive stripping of the arterial wall, even down into the abdominal aorta. The disease is quite common, and is usually heralded by the sudden onset of severe chest pain. The effects are serious because the dissection causes blockage of the ostia of important branches of the aorta.

The consequences vary considerably from case to case.[10] Thus, the coronary arteries may be occluded and myocardial infarction results. There is a varying degree of obstruction to the arteries supplying the upper limbs so that the pulses at the wrist are often either weak or unequal. Blockage of the renal arteries leads to infarction and anuria. The outer coat of the aneurysm usually ruptures, causing fatal haemorrhage into the pericardium, the mediastinum, the retroperitoneal space, or the peritoneal cavity.

Thrombosis in the heart

Thrombosis in the atrium. This has been described on page 487.

Thrombosis in the ventricles. Thrombosis is usually seen in the left ventricle overlying an area of infarction or in an aneurysmal sac.

Coiled thrombi are found in the pulmonary trunk and right ventricle in massive pulmonary embolism. These should not be confused with *post-mortem* clots. The latter are formed after death, and their shape conforms to that of the cavity in

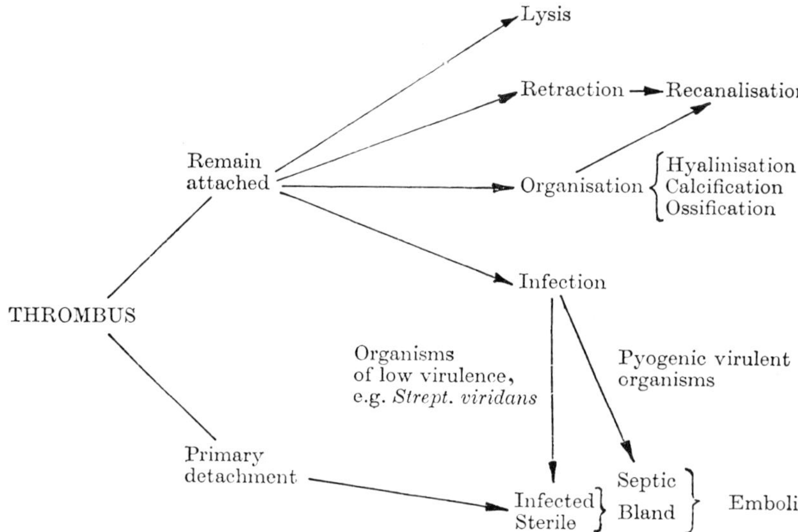

Fig. 31.6 The possible fate of a thrombus.

which they are formed. They are shiny and elastic, and never exhibit the lines of Zahn which are characteristic of thrombi. Furthermore, in conditions accompanied by a high ESR the blood may separate before it clots, so that there is an upper portion consisting largely of coagulated plasma. This is pale yellow, and is usually called the 'chicken-fat clot', while the clot underneath contains sedimented red cells. This is the so-called 'red-currant-jelly clot'.

Thrombosis on the valves. Thrombi on heart valves are called vegetations and are described on pages 513–516.

Fate of thrombi

Fig. 31.6 summarizes the possible fate of a thrombus.

1. Many thrombi undergo lysis, and leave no trace of their previous existence. The fibrinolytic mechanism is of importance (p. 467).

2. If an occluding thrombus in an artery or vein contains much clot, it retracts sufficiently for blood to pass by. In this way a new channel is formed. Endothelium quickly lines this passage, and recanalization occurs. In the pulmonary arteries a thin web of connective tissue may be all that remains of a previous life-threatening thrombo-embolism.
3. A thrombus which is not removed may become organized. In veins the granulation tissue invades it from the mural aspect, and endothelium grows over the thrombus from the adjacent intima. In large, elastic arteries the vasa vasorum from the adventitia do not penetrate as far as the intima, and organization is therefore impaired. Some occurs from the adjacent endothelium, but it is possible that thrombi in arteries undergo degeneration, and are converted into atheromatous plaques.
4. Organized thrombi may become hyalinized and calcified. This is common in the pelvic veins, and the *phleboliths* so produced may be seen on radiographic examination.
5. Thrombi may become detached to form emboli.

EMBOLISM

An *embolus* is an abnormal mass of undissolved material which is transported from one part of the circulation to another. The most satisfactory classification is based upon its composition.

Types. Five categories may be recognized.

Thrombi and clot. This may be bland or infected
Gas—air and nitrogen
Fat
Tumour
Miscellaneous.

1. Emboli composed of thrombus or clot[11]

Pulmonary embolism. The source of the thrombo-emboli is generally one of the veins, most often in the legs. Small emboli block branches of the pulmonary arteries and produce either no effects or else infarction (p. 502). Large quantities of thrombus and propagated clot, however, produce the syndrome of massive pulmonary embolism. In this the main pulmonary artery and its branches are plugged by a mass of coiled thrombus (Fig. 31.7). The clinical effects are dramatic. The patient experiences sudden dyspnoea and chest pain. The obstruction of the right ventricular outflow results in a dramatic fall in left ventricular output; hypotension occurs and consciousness is lost. Death frequently follows. The prevention of massive pulmonary embolism is the prevention of phlebothrombosis. Patients confined to bed must be given leg exercises to increase the venous circulation. Postoperative physiotherapy and early ambulation have done much to reduce this complication of trauma and surgery.

Systemic embolism. The emboli usually arise in the heart, commonly from the left atrium in mitral stenosis or heart failure. Systemic embolism is also a

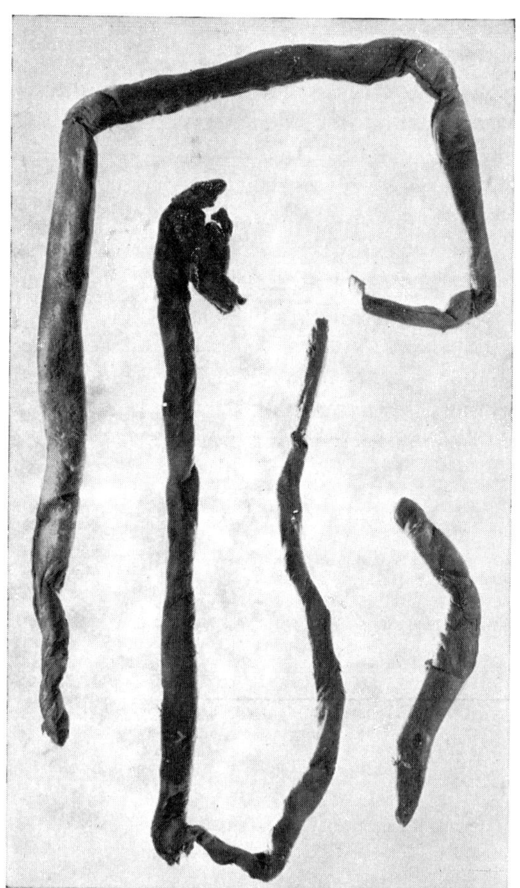

Fig. 31.7 Massive pulmonary embolism. These thrombi were removed from the pulmonary arteries of a man who died suddenly a week after an abdominal operation. There was extensive phlebothrombosis in both calves. Note that the calibre of the thrombi corresponds with the lumina of the leg veins. (C40.5. *Reproduced by permission of the President and Council of the Royal College of Surgeons of England.*)

feature of infective endocarditis, and it may arise from the mural thrombus formed over a myocardial infarct.

2. Gaseous emboli

Air.[12] Air may inadvertently be introduced into a systemic vein, e.g. during a mismanaged blood transfusion. If in considerable quantity, it travels to the heart where it produces foaming in the right ventricle. The right ventricle compresses this foam but cannot expel it. Death therefore occurs rapidly.

During pleural aspirations air may inadvertently be introduced into the pulmonary venous circulation and reach the left side of the heart. From here it may travel to the coronary and cerebral vessels and occlude them. The blockage often has a fatal result.

Nitrogen: the decompression syndrome.[13, 14] Bubbles of nitrogen appear in the circulation in those who, having been exposed to a high atmospheric pressure, are suddenly decompressed. This occurs in divers, tunnellers, and pilots. Nitrogen, being soluble in lipids, also appears as bubbles in the central nervous system. This effect may result in considerable damage to the spinal cord. Severe pain is produced ('the bends'), and permanent damage or death may ensue.

3. Fat emboli[15]

Globules of fatty marrow may enter the small veins after a fracture of a long bone; with multiple injuries this embolization may be quite extensive. Usually the emboli are trapped in the lungs and have no harmful effects because of the enormous capacity of the vascular bed. Occasionally, however, emboli pass through the pulmonary capillaries and enter the systemic circulation, where they produce the syndrome of *systemic fat embolism.* Multiple emboli lodge in the kidneys causing haematuria, the brain, where they lead to severe neurological changes, and the skin, where they cause small petechial haemorrhages.

4. Tumour emboli

It is probable that all malignant tumours invade the local blood vessels at an early stage of the disease, and that isolated malignant cells are of frequent occurrence in the circulation. The majority of these emboli are destroyed; only a small percentage develop into metastatic deposits. Occasionally, for instance in carcinoma of the lung, a large mass of tumour becomes detached, and a massive embolus blocks a major artery, e.g. the femoral.

5. Miscellaneous emboli

Foreign bodies.[16] A large number of foreign bodies have been reported to undergo embolism, e.g. a polyethylene tube may become detached in a vein and travel to the right side of the heart.

Parasites. Various parasites and their ova are carried in the blood stream.

Red cells. The blockage of small vessels by sludged aggregates of red cells is commonly seen in infections and following trauma (p. 409).

Amniotic fluid. An occasional complication of pregnancy is the sudden introduction of amniotic fluid into the veins of the uterus. This produces a syndrome characterized by shock and a generalized bleeding tendency. This is not attributable to the phenomenon of embolism, but to the initiation of diffuse intravascular clotting and fibrinolysis.

HYPOXIA

Hypoxia is a state of impaired oxygenation of the tissues.

Types. Four are commonly described:

Hypoxic, due to a low oxygen tension (Po_2) in the arterial blood. This is a feature of central cyanosis (p. 504).

Anaemic, due to an inadequate level of haemoglobin, which carries the oxygen in the blood.

Stagnant, or *ischaemic,* due to an inadequate supply of blood to the tissues. This, as will be seen, is due either to heart failure or some local vascular obstruction, and is a feature of peripheral cyanosis.

Histotoxic, due to cellular intoxication which prevents the uptake of oxygen, e.g. cyanide poisoning.

ISCHAEMIA

Ischaemia is defined as a condition of inadequate blood supply to an area of tissue. It produces harmful effects in three ways:

Hypoxia. Oxygen deprivation is undoubtedly the most important factor producing damage in ischaemic tissue, especially in respect of very active cells, e.g. muscle. On the other hand, it plays no part in the lesions produced by pulmonary arterial obstruction, because the alveolar walls derive their oxygen supply directly from the alveolar air.

Malnutrition. This is probably of little importance, because the blood contains much more glucose and amino acids than could be metabolized by the amount of oxygen which it contains.

Failure to remove waste products. The accumulation of metabolites is the most probable explanation of pain in ischaemic muscles. The presence of waste products or the failure to maintain important electrolyte or other balances is probably a factor in pulmonary infarction.

Causes of ischaemia

General

Ischaemia may be caused by an inadequate cardiac output; not all tissues are equally affected because of the redistribution of the available blood. The extremities (e.g. finger-tips) tend to be most severely affected, but the ischaemia is rarely sufficiently severe to cause structural damage. Not so, however, with the ischaemia that follows the sudden cessation of the heart's action. Sudden cardiac arrest may occur during the induction of anaesthesia or as a result of coronary thrombosis. The blood supply to the whole body is stopped, but manifestations are in fact confined to a single organ, the brain, which is particularly sensitive to hypoxia. If the arrest continues for 15 seconds, consciousness is lost, and if the condition lasts for more than three minutes, irreparable damage is done.[17] The neurons degenerate and are replaced by glial tissue. If cardiac arrest lasts for more than about eight minutes, death is inevitable. It follows that *all who deal with patients should be capable of diagnosing cardiac arrest* (*absent heart sounds*) *and dealing with it by the manoeuvre of external cardiac massage.*

Local

By far the most important cause of ischaemia is obstruction to the arterial flow. It should not, however, be forgotten that extensive venous and capillary damage can also produce ischaemia.

Arterial obstruction. Most of the causes of obstruction have already been described. They will therefore be summarized:

Thrombosis.

Embolism. The effects of an embolus are potentiated by the reflex spasm of the arterial wall, and completed by the rapid development of thrombus over the embolus.

Spasm (see below).

Atherosclerosis. This produces partial obstruction in medium-sized vessels, e.g. cerebral, coronary, and renal arteries.

Occlusive pressure from without, e.g. tourniquets and ill-fitting plasters.

Venous disease. Extensive venous obstruction leads to engorgement of the areas drained by the affected veins. This may reach such an intensity that blood flow is impeded and ischaemia results. Mesenteric vein thrombosis is a good example of this; it leads to intestinal infarction. Venous stasis secondary to varicose veins of the legs leads to ischaemic changes of the skin (stasis dermatitis). Ultimately chronic ulceration occurs, often precipitated by local injury.

Diseases of small vessels. In consideration of vascular disease the capillaries and arterioles are usually forgotten. There are, nevertheless, many conditions in which so many vessels in an area are occluded that ischaemia results. Because an additional effect is bleeding, petechial haemorrhages are a common feature of small-vessel disease even though the extent of the occlusion is insufficient to lead to ischaemia of the total area involved. Some causes of these diseases are briefly described below:

Frostbite.[18] The harmful effects of cold on exposed parts are due in large measure to small vessel damage. In mild cases there is an inflammatory reaction causing large blisters to form; if the damage is severe, the vessels become completely occluded by thrombus and gangrene occurs.

Occlusion of capillaries by red cells. This response occurs in severe sludging, and is a component of shock.

Occlusion by fibrin. This occurs in disseminated intravascular coagulation. The kidney is the organ most affected.

Occlusion by precipitated cryoglobulins. In cryoglobulinaemia exposure of the extremities to cold leads to vascular occlusion and petechial haemorrhages.

Fat embolism.

Decompression syndrome.

External pressure. The best example of this is a bedsore. Continual pressure on one area produces such ischaemia that necrosis of the skin and underlying tissues occurs. *It is a major duty of nurses to move non-ambulatory patients often enough that no pressure sores develop.*

Occlusion by antigen-antibody interaction. This is a feature of such immune complex phenomena as the Arthus reaction.

Vasculitis. The term vasculitis is used to describe an inflammatory reaction in the wall of small vessels. Typical lesions occur in the Arthus reaction; the immune complex deposition in the vessel wall causes damage associated with a marked polymorph infiltration and thrombosis (Fig. 13.1). This type of type III hypersensitivity is thought to occur in many drug reactions as well as in some infections. The petechial haemorrhages seen in the skin in septicaemia and in infective endocarditis are explained on this basis. Internal organs are affected; the kidney appears to be the most vulnerable. In some examples of vasculitis no cause can be found. The disease then appears to be a component of polyarteritis nodosa.

Vascular spasm

Although vascular occlusion is generally caused by an organic lesion, there are a number of conditions in which spasm of the vessel wall plays a most important part. Spasm may occur in either veins or arteries; it is debatable whether the capillaries are capable of independent contraction in humans.

Venous spasm. Trauma applied directly to a vessel wall can cause marked spasm. This is sometimes a source of great difficulty during an inexpert venepuncture. Venous spasm has not been incriminated as a cause of tissue ischaemia.

Arterial spasm. Trauma to arteries frequently produces local spasm, a function which may be of life-saving importance. Cases of avulsion of a limb are on record in which, due to spasm of the main artery, the patient did not die of massive haemorrhage.

This ability of arteries to contract can be utilized by the surgeon who is faced with severe bleeding during the course of an operation. It is a wise policy to pack the wound and await the onset of spasm rather than make heroic though blind efforts with a pair of haemostats. Although this response of the arterial wall to trauma may be of benefit, its effects are sometimes detrimental. Trauma to an artery, e.g. by the close proximity of a bullet path, the pressure of a plaster, or the application of a tourniquet, may at times produce such persistent and widespread spasm that the area involved becomes ischaemic and infarcted. *Absence of the pulse of a limb beyond an area of trauma must be regarded seriously, and efforts should be made to relieve the spasm, lest permanent damage be caused.*

Spasm of small arteries is a feature of ergot poisoning and Raynaud's phenomenon.* It may lead to gangrene of the extremities. Widespread arteriolar spasm is a feature of shock (p. 408), and has also been incriminated in primary hypertension (p. 477).

The effects of arterial and capillary obstruction

The effects depend largely upon the degree of ischaemia produced, and may range from sudden death to virtually no damage at all. The following are the possibilities:

No effects occur if the affected area is well supplied by blood vessels which form collateral anastomoses.

Functional disturbances. Sufficient blood may reach the area to supply its needs under resting conditions but not under those of activity. This is the cause of the pain in the chest (*angina pectoris*) in patients with coronary artery disease, and the *intermittent claudication* in those with peripheral vascular disease (p. 499).

Cellular degeneration may affect the parenchyma of an organ and terminate in necrosis. This may be a patchy affair leading to atrophy; it is generally accompanied by replacement fibrosis or, in the central nervous system, gliosis. This type of lesion is seen under two conditions:

1. Sudden complete arterial obstruction of short duration
2. Partial arterial obstruction of gradual onset.

* *Raynaud's disease* is an idiopathic condition in which the digital arteries are unduly sensitive to cold. When cooled, the hands or feet become pale and later cyanosed due to spasm of the digital arteries. In Raynaud's phenomenon, or syndrome, similar attacks occur, but the condition appears to be a complication of some other disease, e.g. cryoglobulinaemia, scleroderma, or lupus erythematosus.

Infarction. See below.

Sudden death. This occurs in massive pulmonary embolism and coronary occlusion.

Factors determining the extent of ischaemia in arterial obstruction

There are three crucial factors:

Speed of onset. If it is sudden the effects are more severe than if it is gradual, because there is less time for an effective collateral circulation to develop.

Degree of obstruction. A complete obstruction is obviously much more serious than a partial one.

Anatomy of the collateral circulation. Some arteries have no anastomotic channels; these are called *end arteries.* The central artery of the retina is a classical example; if obstructed there is complete ischaemia of the area supplied. With most arteries there is sufficient anastomosis to ensure that the blood reaches the affected area even when a main branch is occluded. If the anastomotic vessels are well developed, ischaemia is an uncommon phenomenon. The stomach illustrates this well, for it is supplied by three separate arteries which anastomose freely.

Subsidiary factors. There are four subsidiary factors modifying the effects of arterial blockage.

The pathology of the collateral circulation. It stands to reason that if the collateral vessels are severely affected with spasm or atheroma they are not likely to assist in maintaining a good alternative blood supply.

The oxygenation of the arterial blood.

The efficiency of the heart.

The nature of the affected tissue. Brain and heart are much more vulnerable to ischaemia than are any other organs. The effects on these organs are described elsewhere. Connective tissue survives much better than does the parenchyma of an organ. The causes and effects of ischaemia on the limbs are described below.

PERIPHERAL VASCULAR DISEASE

'Peripheral vascular disease' is an inclusive term that is used to describe all those conditions in which the blood supply to the limbs is impaired. Usually it is the legs that suffer. The following diseases all play their part:

Atherosclerosis. This tends to affect the large vessels such as the iliac and femoral arteries.

Buerger's disease. This is an occasional cause (p. 487).

Thrombosis. This may be secondary to atherosclerosis.

Embolism. Emboli may be large thromboemboli or small clumps of atheromatous material.

Small-vessel disease. Arteriolosclerosis associated with hypertension and diabetic microangiopathy (see p. 275) are the most important.

Effects of peripheral vascular disease. The effects are serious and disabling. The ischaemia of the leg leads to atrophy of many structures, including the bones (osteoporosis) and the skin. Trivial injury can lead to chronic, persistent, extremely painful ulceration. Ischaemia of the muscle leads to pain on walking (intermittent claudication) and, ultimately, to pain at rest. Dry gangrene leading to a loss of the limb is an all-too-frequent end-result.

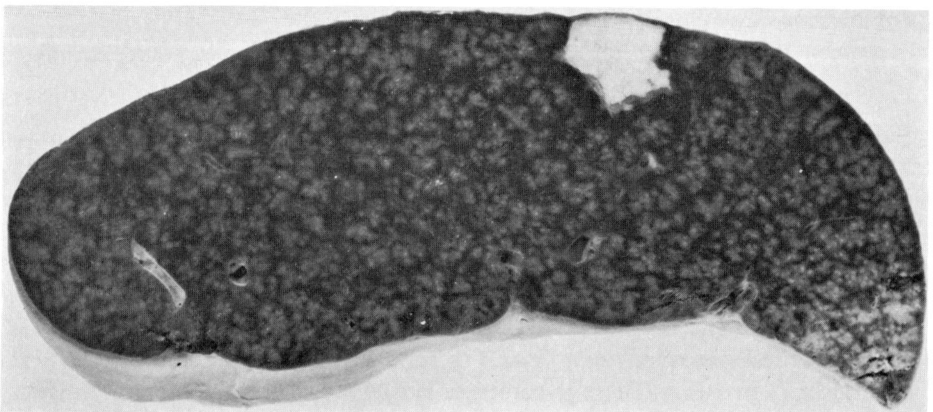

Fig. 31.8 Infarct of spleen. Note the pale, wedge-shaped infarct under the capsule. The lymphoid follicles are unduly prominent. The patient had *Strept. viridans* endocarditis. (H26.1. *Reproduced by permission of the President and Council of the Royal College of Surgeons of England.*)

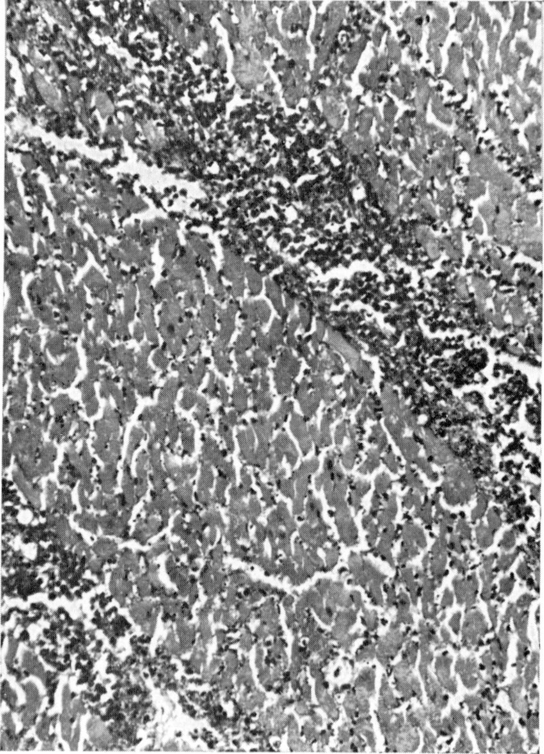

Fig. 31.9 Myocardial infarction. The muscle fibres are necrotic, but their structure is easily recognisable. There is a profuse cellular infiltration, including many polymorphs, around the necrotic tissue $\times 150$.

INFARCTION

Infarction may be defined as the circumscribed necrosis of tissue due to deprivation of blood supply. It usually leads to a circumscribed area of coagulative necrosis, which is subsequently organized into scar tissue. The process is as follows:

1. There is death of the cells in the area deprived of its blood supply. Blood, either from anastomotic vessels or by venous reflux, continues to seep into the devitalized area for a short time. Thus most infarcts contain a great deal of blood in the early stages, and are swollen and red in colour. The red cells entering the affected area escape from the damaged capillaries and lie free in the dead tissue. Infarcts of lax tissue, e.g. lung and intestine, are much more engorged than are those of compact organs, e.g. kidney and heart.

2. The dead tissue undergoes necrosis. In solid organs the associated swelling of the cells may squeeze the blood out of the infarct. In this way it becomes paler. Infarcts of the spleen and kidneys are characteristically pale, and present a wedge-shaped area of coagulative necrosis, the apex of which is the blocked supplying artery, and the base the capsule of the organ (Fig. 31.8). Infarcts of the heart are also pale, but their shape is more irregular due to the arrangement of the vascular supply.

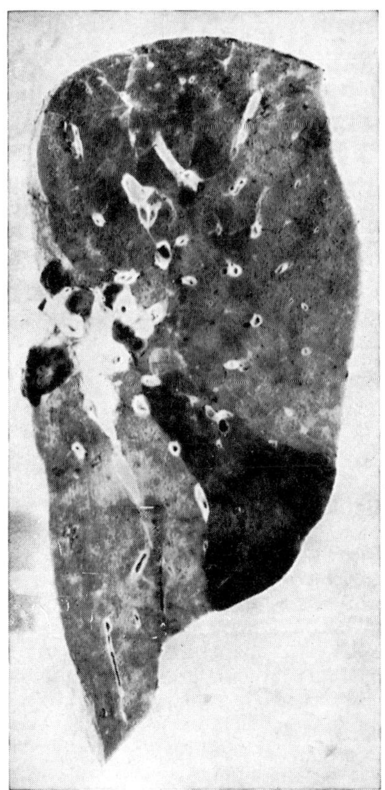

Fig. 31.10 Infarct of lung. Note the dark wedge-shaped infarct in this left upper lobe. It is stuffed with blood. (R27.3. *Reproduced by permission of the President and Council of the Royal College of Surgeons of England.*)

3. There is progressive autolysis of the necrotic tissue and haemolysis of the red cells. Microscopically an infarct shows a characteristic structured necrosis with the outlines of the cells being recognizable as ghosts without nuclei. This petrified-forest appearance may persist for many months. (Fig. 31.9).

4. At the same time the surrounding normal tissue undergoes an acute inflammatory reaction. The polymorph infiltration may be so intense as to simulate a pyogenic infection for a while. This is rapidly followed by macrophage activity.

5. The infarct gradually shrinks and becomes replaced by granulation tissue. Its central portion may, however, take many months to organize, and not infrequently shows dystrophic calcification.

Infarcts in particular organs present certain additional features. In the *lung* the infarct is so filled with blood that it remains red and generally organizes in this stage (Fig. 31.10). In the *intestine* the necrotic bowel wall is soon invaded by putrefactive organisms and becomes gangrenous. In the *limbs* sudden obstruction leads to infarction and wet gangrene, while slow obstruction produces the so-called dry gangrene (p. 66).

In the *central nervous system* the process is somewhat different, because the necrotic tissue undergoes rapid colliquative necrosis. The end-result is either a glial scar or else, if the infarct is large, a cyst surrounded by a layer of glial tissue.

Infarction of the lung does not occur in healthy people even if a major pulmonary artery is occluded. This is because the bronchial arteries supply well-oxygenated blood. If the bronchial arterial supply is itself impaired, as in heart failure, obstruction to a branch of the pulmonary artery may then lead to infarction. The usual cause of this is an embolus arising from one of the systemic veins. It will be recalled that phlebothrombosis is itself often associated with heart failure.

GENERAL READING

Hudson R E B (1965) Cardiovascular Pathology. Arnold, London. This book now in three volumes is useful for reference

REFERENCES

1. Leading Article 1976 Antithrombin. Lancet 1: 1333
2. Stehbens W E, Biscoe T J 1967 The ultrastructure of early platelet aggregation *in vivo*. American Journal of Pathology 50: 219
3. Mustard J F 1975 Function of blood platelets and their role in thrombosis. Transactions of the American Clinical and Climatological Association 87: 104
4. Moncada S, Vane J R 1979 Arachidonic acid metabolites and the interactions between platelets and blood-vessel walls. New England Journal of Medicine 300: 1142.
5. Leading Article 1971 Prophylaxis of venous thrombosis. British Medical Journal 1: 305
6. Meadway J, Nicolaides A N, Walker C J, O'Connell J D 1975 Value of Doppler ultrasound in diagnosis of clinically suspected deep vein thrombosis. British Medical Journal 4: 552
7. Leading Article 1975 Prevention of postoperative thromboembolism. Lancet 2: 63
8. Ross R, Glomset J A 1976 The pathogenesis of atherosclerosis. New England Journal of Medicine 295: 369 and 420
9. Leading Article 1977 Monoclonal theory of atheroma. British Medical Journal 1: 1371
10. Leading Article 1976 Diagnosis of dissecting aneurysm of the aorta. Lancet 2: 299
11. Sasahara A A, Stein M Eds 1965 Pulmonary Embolic Disease 312 pp Grune and Stratton, New York

12. Ward M K, Shadforth M, Hill A V L, Kerr D N S 1971 Air embolism during haemodialysis. British Medical Journal 3 : 74
13. Dewey A W 1962 Decompression sickness, an emergency recreational hazard. New England Journal of Medicine 267 : 759 and 812
14. Collins J J 1962 An unusual case of air embolism precipitated by decompression. New England Journal of Medicine 266 : 595
15. Leading Article 1972 Fat embolism. Lancet 1 : 672
16. Dimmick J E, Bove K E, McAdams A J, Benzing G 1975 Fiber embolisation—a hazard of cardiac surgery and catheterisation. New England Journal of Medicine 292 : 685
17. Dickinson C J, Pentecost B L 1974 In Clinical Physiology, ed Campbell E J M, Dickinson C J, Slater J D H, 4th edn, p 69, Blackwell, Oxford
18. Washburn B 1962 Frostbite. New England Journal of Medicine 266 : 974.

32

Diseases of the heart

Before commencing dental treatment it is particularly important to ascertain that the heart is normal, because unless precautions are taken, dental treatment may precipitate serious mischief in a patient with heart disease. Congenital lesions and valvular abnormalities predispose to infective endocarditis, and myocardial disease may lead to sudden death during anaesthesia.

The types and causes of heart disease are many and various; the effects, however, are few in number and stereotyped in nature. Since the heart is a pump, it follows that the diseased and failing heart often pumps inefficiently. The consequences of this are circulatory disturbances which together constitute the syndrome of heart failure. The main features of this will be described after individual diseases of the heart have been considered.

Two types of heart disease may be recognized. There is the group of malformations which are due to faulty development and are therefore congenital (*congenital heart disease*), and there are those disorders occurring in a normally developed heart.

CONGENITAL HEART DISEASE

Congenital heart disease is a subject of importance to the dentist because the abnormality can predispose to infective endocarditis. Developmental anomalies range from those that are so severe as to be incompatible with continued fetal life (these lead to abortion), to others that are mild and symptomless. Between these two extremes there are cases in which signs or symptoms become evident during infancy or childhood.

The incidence of congenital heart disease in newborn babies is at least 7 per 1000. Two-thirds of the affected infants die before their first birthday, so that only 2 or 3 of every 1000 school children have a cardiac malformation.

Signs and symptoms of congenital heart disease

Factors that alert the clinician to the possibility of congenital heart disease include the following:

Murmurs. These are often loud and may be heard over the precordium. Indeed, they may be felt (*thrills*) by the palm of the hand placed over the chest.

Evidence of heart failure—either left or right.

Evidence of a right-to-left shunt, central cyanosis. Central cyanosis occurs whenever the defect allows deoxygenated blood to by-pass the lungs and enter the circulation. Central cyanosis affects all the tissues, and can be differentiated from peripheral cyanosis, which is due to stagnation and occurs in the skin when the temperature is reduced and there is vasoconstriction, but not in the mucous membranes which have a good blood supply. In 'blue babies' cyanosis is present in infancy, and often Fallot's tetralogy is responsible. Central cyanosis can occur in severe lung disease as well as a result of pulmonary arterio-venous shunts.

Polycythaemia. This is due to the effects of hypoxia on the bone marrow.

Clubbing of the fingers and toes. This is generally present when the cyanosis has been present for a long period. The pathogenesis is obscure. Clubbing is also found as an idiopathic congenital anomaly of little consequence; furthermore, it is a feature of chronic suppurative lung disease (e.g. bronchiectasis and lung abscess), lung cancer, and *Streptococcus viridans* endocarditis.

Squatting. Patients with cyanotic heart disease typically assume a squatting posture after exertion to obtain relief from their dyspnoea.

Hypoxic spells. The degree of hypoxia may suddenly progress to the extent that the patient loses consciousness, has convulsions, and may even die. Such alarming episodes are most common in young children.

Underdevelopment. Unless the congenital heart defect is corrected, the child may show poor development. Respiratory infections are common, and death may occur from them or from heart failure.

Aetiology of congenital heart disease

Some types of congenital heart disease are familial and there is an evident genetic influence. The association with Down's syndrome is well established.

The heart develops during the third to eighth week, and external agents acting during this period can cause congenital heart disease. If the mother contracts rubella there is a high incidence of congenital heart disease. Measles and mumps have also been suggested as likely aetiological agents. The thalidomide babies (see p. 376) also exhibited cardiovascular anomalies.

Individual lesions of congenital heart disease

Patent ductus arteriosus (Fig. 32.1)

Before birth the pressure in the aorta is slightly below that of the pulmonary artery and the ductus transmits blood from the artery to the aorta. After birth the baby starts to breathe, and as the lungs inflate, so the pressure in the pulmonary artery falls and that in the aorta rises. Normally the ductus becomes obliterated, but should it fail to close, blood flows from the aorta to the pulmonary artery thereby increasing the volume of blood passing through the lungs and returning to the left atrium and ventricle. The heart can cope with this situation for a while, but pulmonary hypertension develops and eventually there is a reversal of flow so that cyanosis ensues. If the shunt is large, it may cause cardiac failure in infancy, but more often the effects are less severe. There is a tendency for the child to tire easily, and there is growth retardation. Death generally occurs before the age of 40 due either to heart failure or the effects of infection (bacterial endarteritis).

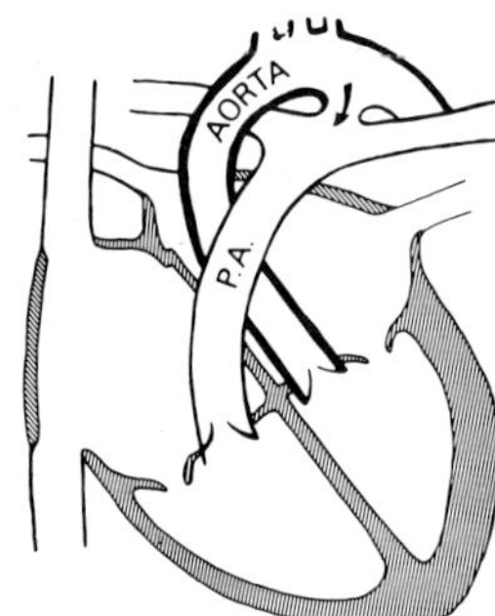

Fig. 32.1 Patent ductus arteriosus

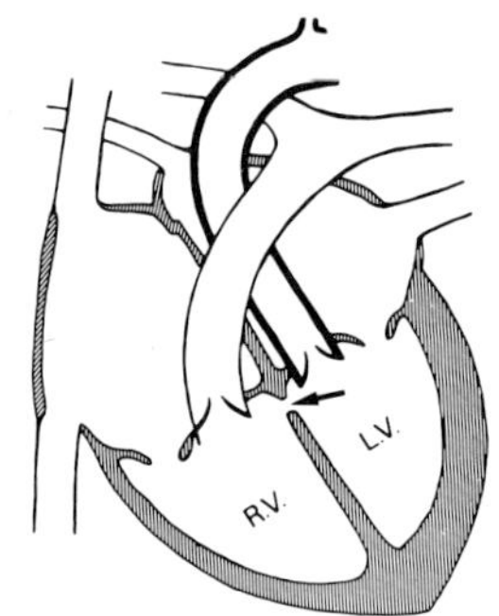

Fig. 32.2 Ventricular septal defect

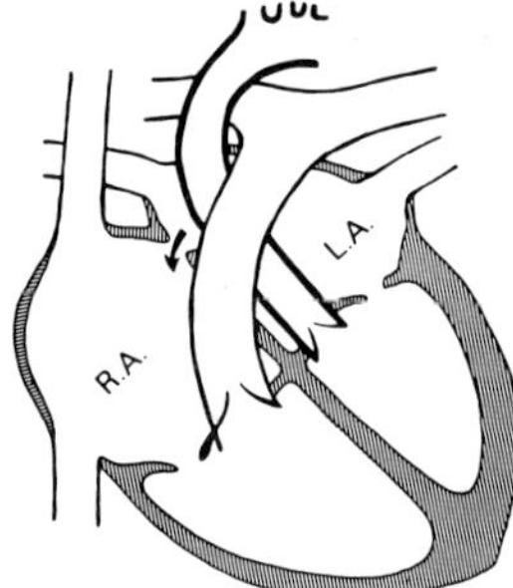

Fig. 32.3 Atrial septal defect

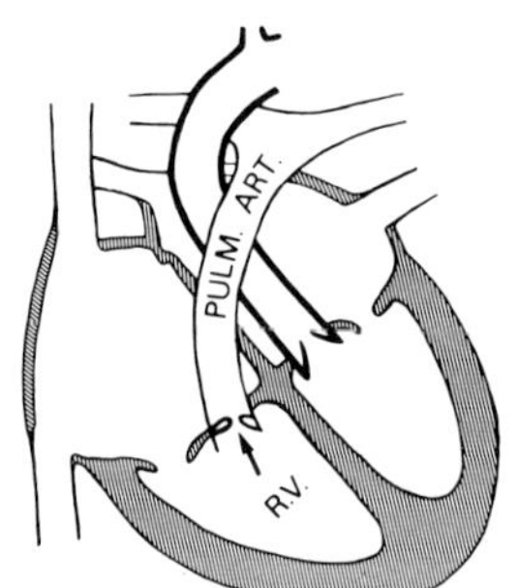

Fig. 32.4 Pulmonary stenosis

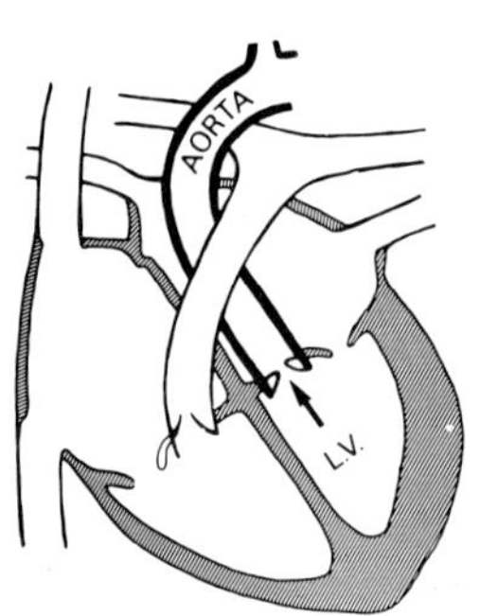

Fig. 32.5 Aortic stenosis

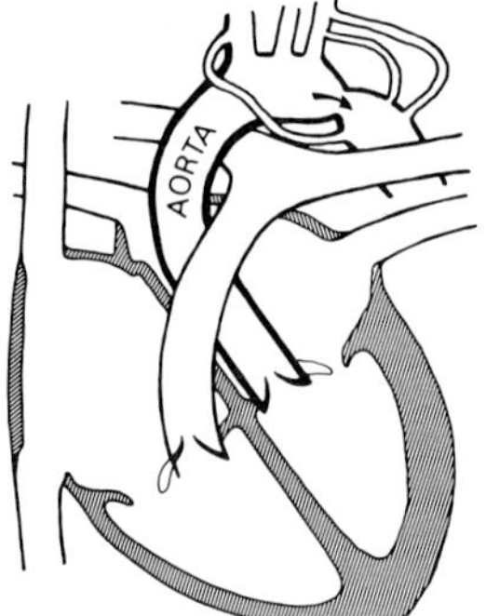

Fig. 32.6 Coarctation of aorta

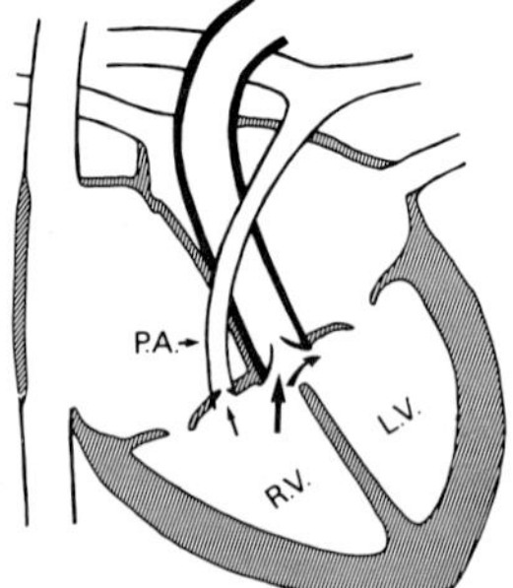

Fig. 32.7 Fallot's tetralogy

Figs. 32.1 to 32.7 Congenital heart lesions. See the text for descriptions of the individual lesions. (*Illustrations by the Photographic Section of the Oral Pathology Department of the Birmingham Dental School.*)

The treatment is division or ligation of the ductus, but it is essential to ensure that no other anomalies are present. With complex heart disease the ductus may indeed provide the only lifeline communication between the left and the right sides of the circulation.

Ventricular septal defects (Fig. 32.2)

In ventricular septal defects the shunt of oxygenated blood from left to right through the defect causes the same changes in the heart and pulmonary blood flow as those of patent ductus arteriosus. Eventually pulmonary hypertension may lead to right-sided heart failure.

If the ventricular septal defect is large, early surgical intervention is required to save the child's life. With small defects there may be no symptoms and the condition may remain undiagnosed. In intermediate cases there is cardiac enlargement, diminished exercise tolerance, and a tendency to respiratory infections which ultimately lead to heart failure. Ventricular septal defects may close spontaneously during the first few years of life, and such patients have a normal life expectancy. The treatment of ventricular septal defects is open-heart surgery and closure of the defect either by stitches or the insertion of a prosthetic patch.

Atrial septal defects (Fig. 32.3)

An atrial septal defect is the most common congenital anomaly found in adults. A left-to-right shunt results in overfilling of the right atrium and therefore an increased output of the right ventricle. Children with this lesion tire easily and suffer from frequent respiratory infections. Cardiac failure may develop between the ages of 20 and 40 years, and most untreated cases are dead by the age of 45. The treatment is operative closure of the defect, generally best performed between the ages of 5 and 10 years.

Pulmonary stenosis (Fig. 32.4)

Pulmonary stenosis is relatively common and the obstruction may be supravalvular, valvular, or subvalvular. It usually occurs as a result of unequal division of the truncus arteriosus during development. Right ventricular hypertrophy results in all but the mildest cases; the limits of hypertrophy are eventually reached and cardiac failure occurs.

Aortic stenosis (Fig. 32.5)

Aortic stenosis is an uncommon form of congenital heart disease, but congenital abnormalities of the aortic valve are not uncommon. Usually the valve is bicuspid. This may cause symptoms during childhood, but frequently it remains asymptomatic until old age. The valves then become rigid, and this is thought to be a major aetiological factor in calcific (calcareous) aortic stenosis (see p. 517).

Coarctation of the aorta (Fig. 32.6)

In this condition the aorta is narrowed either at the level of the entrance of the ductus arteriosus or immediately before or immediately after this. Blood then reaches the lower half of the body *via* collateral vessels. The importance of this condition is two-fold. Firstly the area of stenosis may become infected (infective endarteritis), and secondly there is systemic hypertension confined to the upper part of the body. This leads to left ventricular hypertrophy and failure, and an increased liability to cerebral haemorrhage. Unless treated, life is seldom prolonged over the age of 40 years. Coarctation is associated with Turner's syndrome.

Transposition of the great vessels

Owing to a failure of rotation, the aorta arises from the right ventricle and the pulmonary artery from the left ventricle. If this were the only anomaly life would not be possible, and a compensatory defect must also be present. The patient's survival after birth depends upon there being some communication, e.g. a septal defect, between the two sides of the heart. Transposition of the great vessels is one of the common fatal anomalies in children under 1 year of age.

Dextrocardia

Occasionally the heart develops as a mirror image of the normal. If this mirror image involves all the organs of the body, the condition is called *complete situs inversus* and the patient lives a normal life. If, however, only the heart is affected the results are serious, because other defects are also present.

Multiple defects

Developmental anomalies are often multiple. Not only may they be found in other organs, but several lesions may be present in the heart itself. A common combination is that found in the *tetralogy of Fallot* (Fig. 32.7). This comprises:

1. Pulmonary stenosis
2. Ventricular septal defect
3. Over-riding of the septum by the aorta, so that the blood from the right and left ventricles enters the aorta
4. Hypertrophy of the right ventricle—this is compensatory.

In Fallot's tetralogy there is usually cyanosis at birth, but initially it may only be apparent during crying or feeding. Dyspnoea usually occurs early. The child exhibits the squatting phenomenon before the age of 3 years, and clubbing of fingers and toes is common. If untreated, survival past 21 years of age is uncommon.

ACQUIRED HEART DISEASE

Arteriosclerotic heart disease

The myocardium is supplied by blood through the two coronary arteries. These vessels are particularly liable to be affected by atherosclerosis, which causes a narrowing of their lumina and subsequent myocardial ischaemia.

Gradual coronary occlusion

At first myocardial ischaemia is symptomless. However, in some patients although there is no effect on the resting heart, with exercise the ischaemia of the muscle causes pain (*angina pectoris*). Characteristically this is felt in the precordium, and spreads into the neck and down the left arm. The pain comes on with exercise, particularly in cold weather and after a heavy meal. It is relieved by rest and by placing a tablet of nitroglycerin under the tongue. This drug is readily absorbed from the buccal mucosa, and acts by causing peripheral vasodilatation which lowers the systolic blood pressure and lessens the load on the left ventricle.

The structural effects of myocardial ischaemia are patchy necrosis and subsequent replacement by fibrous tissue. The result is *myocardial fibrosis*. The left ventricular muscle is invariably affected and ultimately this leads to left ventricular failure.

Sudden coronary occlusion

Myocardial infarction or an *acute fatal dysrhythmia* is the common effect. These conditions are described below.

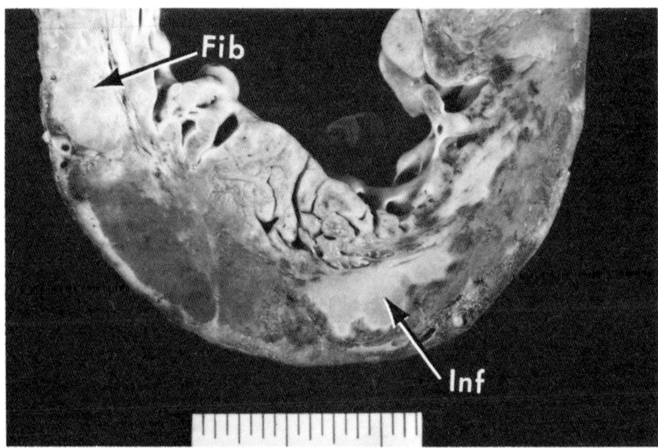

Fig. 32.8 Recent myocardial infarction. The specimen shows part of the wall of the left ventricle. The recent infarct (Inf) is pale and has a haemorrhagic border. The lesion is about ten days old. Fibrosis in other areas (Fib) is the result of a previous myocardial infarction.

Effects of Acute Myocardial Ischaemia

Acute functional derangements

The left ventricle fibrillates in some cases, whereas in others ischaemia of the conducting system causes heart block. Sudden death is most common during the first 24 hours after the onset of ischaemia, and the value of acute coronary care units is that immediate external cardiac massage or defibrillation can save the life of a number of these patients.

Myocardial infarction

If the patient survives, the ischaemic muscle undergoes necrosis. The infarct appears as a firm, yellow area of coagulative necrosis with some surrounding haemorrhage and later inflammation (Fig. 32.8). Necrotic muscle releases its enzymes into the blood stream, and a rise in the level of SGOT, LDH, CPK, and HBD is a useful indication of myocardial infarction (see p. 64). Likewise an increase in the white-cell count and slight fever are manifestations of the inflammation. Electrocardiographic changes are important manifestations in myocardial infarction, and are often diagnostic (Fig. 32.14D).

Extensive myocardial necrosis is seen under the following circumstances:

1. *Following coronary artery thrombosis*, which is itself secondary to atherosclerosis. In the past it has often been assumed that nearly all myocardial infarcts were due to coronary thrombosis: the two terms (myocardial infarction and coronary thrombosis) are thus commonly used almost interchangeably. It is now realized that thrombosis is not always present, and it may even occur in the coronary artery *after* infarction has already taken place.

2. *With coronary artery stenosis only.* When no thrombus can be found in the stenosed coronary vessels, it is assumed that some additional factor is concerned. Additional strain on the left ventricle may occur if the blood pressure rises suddenly or if there is an increased heart rate (tachycardia). Sudden lowering of the blood pressure, as is seen in shock, is sometimes a factor, since although it diminishes the load of the left ventricle, the blood flow through the coronary arteries is diminished even more so. Infarction associated with widespread coronary-artery stenosis without thrombus is often widespread, and involves the subendocardial myocardium rather than producing a more localized infarct that involves the entire thickness of the muscle wall (transmural infarction). (See Fig. 32.9).

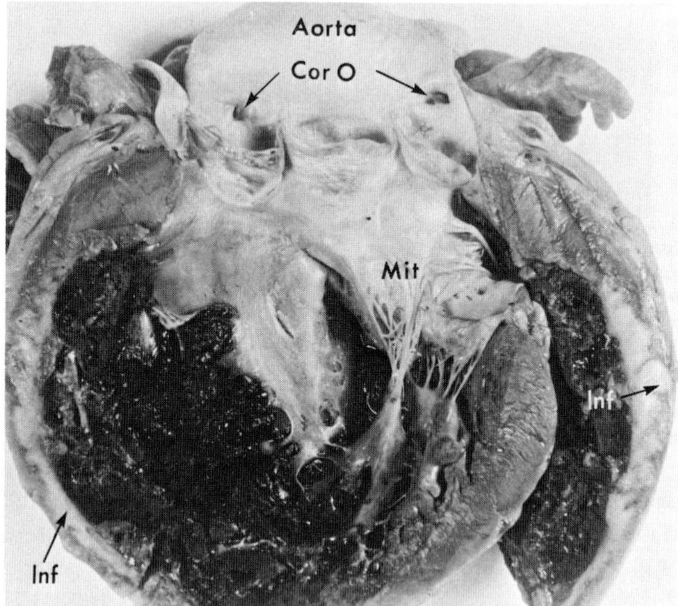

Fig. 32.9 Myocardial infarction with extensive mural thrombosis. The dilated left ventricle has been opened, and part of its lateral wall has been swung over to the left. The anterior cusp of the mitral valve (Mit) is clearly shown. Part of the aorta is included in the specimen, and the orifices of the two coronary arteries (Cor O) can be seen immediately above the three cusps of the aortic valve. There is extensive infarction (Inf) of the left ventricular wall immediately adjacent to the endocardium. Attached to the infarcted muscle there is dark mural thrombus. Both coronary arteries were markedly stenosed by atheroma, but no occluding thrombus was present. It is not uncommon to find this pattern of myocardial infarction in the absence of a thrombosed coronary artery.

3. *With neither coronary artery stenosis nor coronary artery thrombosis.* Severe hypotension, as occurs in shock, may be present in some cases, but in others no explanation can be found. Multiple small emboli or thrombi have been postulated, and their early dissipation might explain why they are not found at necropsy. Experimentally it can be shown that this is possible, for ADP infused into the coronary artery of a pig leads to the formation of platelet emboli and to infarction. Whatever the mechanism, there is little doubt that myocardial infarction can occur in humans without large occlusive arterial thrombosis.

Clinical features of myocardial infarction. The sudden onset of severe pain in the centre of the chest is characteristic of myocardial infarction. The pain is relieved neither by rest nor nitroglycerin. It is frequently accompanied by sweating. Although the typical heart attack is accompanied by severe pain, it is not uncommon for the pain to be relatively mild and atypical. Indeed, there may be no pain at all, and the presence of extensive infarction comes as a surprise at the necropsy of a patient who has died of heart failure for unknown reasons.

Four early complications of myocardial infarction should be noted:

Heart failure. Acute heart failure, due directly to myocardial damage or to dysrhythmia, can produce a low cardiac output and a state of shock (*cardiogenic shock*). Persistent hypotension is serious, and can lead to renal ischaemic tubular necrosis and renal failure.

Pericarditis. This occurs if the infarct involves the pericardial surface.

Mural thrombosis. This complication is seen if the infarct involves the endocardium (Fig. 32.9). Portions of thrombus may break off and embolize to systemic organs like the brain and kidney, producing serious and sometimes fatal results.

Rupture. Occasionally the necrotic muscle ruptures, and this causes haemopericardium and sudden death. Both this complication and systemic embolism are likely to occur at the end of the first week.

About 70 per cent of patients with myocardial infarction survive the first attack. The infarct is organized and replaced by a fibrous scar which may later bulge. The aneurysm of the left ventricle so formed impedes the function of the chamber for with each systole it expands, and thereby diminishes the output of the ventricle. Rarely the aneurysm may rupture. Usually the patient is left with some degree of heart damage, and may have further episodes of infarction.

Hypertensive heart disease

In systemic hypertension the left ventricle is subjected to a continuous strain. It responds by hypertrophy of its muscle fibres, and for a time bears the strain well, but eventually the enormously thick ventricular wall fails. Often there is associated coronary atherosclerosis. The chronic left ventricular failure is followed by congestive heart failure. In addition, some patients develop sudden nocturnal attacks of pulmonary oedema. The victim is seized by an ominous sense of suffocation; the condition is called paroxysmal (nocturnal) dyspnoea (p. 538).

Rheumatic heart disease

Acute rheumatic fever is a disease of childhood and affects those between 5 and 15 years of age. It typically occurs 2 to 3 weeks after a streptococcal sore throat, and is currently believed to be due to an immune-complex reaction between large amounts of streptococcal antigen and antibody present in the patient's plasma. The soluble antigen-antibody complexes appear to localize in the small blood vessels of the heart and joints, and by activating complement lead to tissue damage. The reason for the localization of the lesions in rheumatic fever is not known.

The disease is characterized by fever, flitting pain and swelling of the joints, subcutaneous nodules particularly over bony prominences, and most important of all, involvement of the heart. The pericardium is inflamed, and lesions are found in the myocardium. These take the form of *Aschoff nodes*. They consist of a central area of necrotic collagen surrounded by a zone of inflammatory cells—polymorphs, macrophages, and giant cells. These have up to four vesicular nuclei (with prominent nucleoli) and a basophilic cytoplasm, and are called Aschoff giant cells. Fibroblasts are also present, and the Aschoff node ultimately undergoes

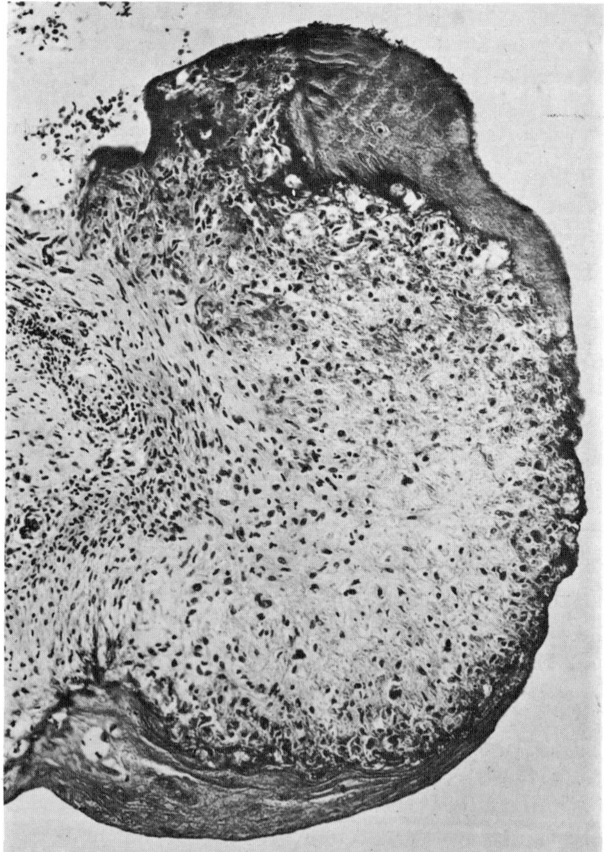

Fig. 32.10 Organizing rheumatic vegetation. The base of the thrombus has been invaded by granulation tissue, while a layer of fibrin (in which there are doubtless aggregations of platelets) still remains on the surface. × 110.

fibrosis. Occasionally death from myocardial failure occurs during the acute stage of rheumatic fever, but the microscopic Aschoff nodes seem quite inadequate as an explanation. Dilatation of the valve ring leads to *mitral regurgitation* and this contributes to the heart failure.

The most important lesion of acute rheumatic fever is that which involves the valves. Inflammation (valvulitis) leads to swelling and deposition of small thrombi (called *vegetations*) on the cusps, especially along the line of their closure (Fig. 32.10). While most other lesions of acute rheumatic fever undergo resolution, those of the valves do not. They tend to progress to a state of chronic inflammation, and the cusps become thickened, fibrosed, and contracted. Adjacent cusps adhere

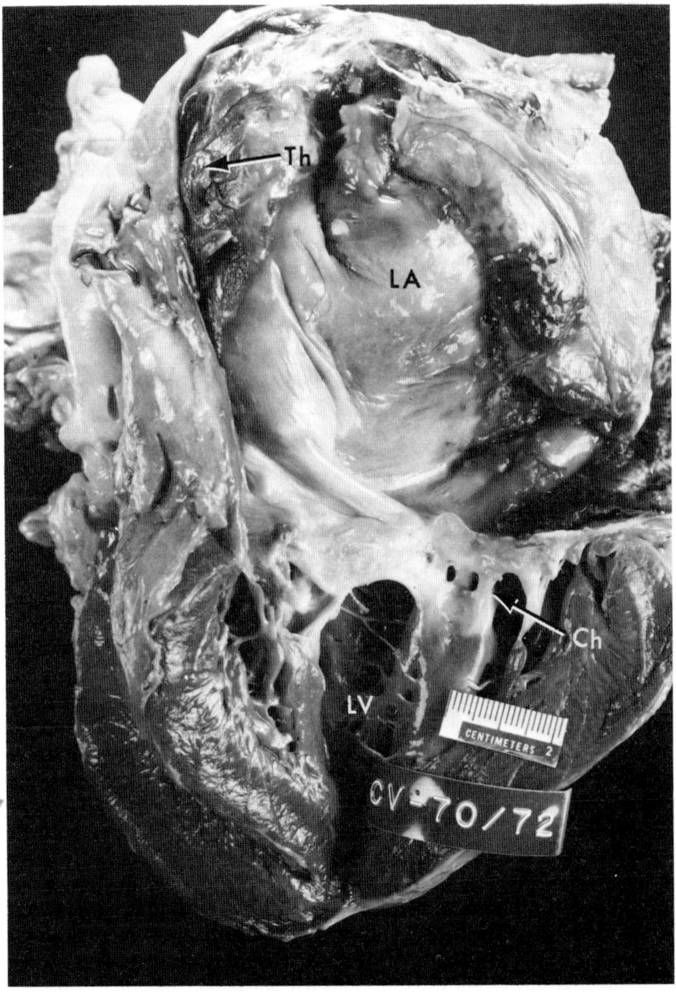

Fig. 32.11 Mitral stenosis due to chronic rheumatic disease. The heart has been opened by an incision passing from the left atrium (LA) to the left ventricle (LV). The left atrium is enormously dilated, and thrombus (Th) is adherent to its walls. The mitral valve is markedly fibrosed, and its chordae tendineae (Ch) are greatly thickened and shortened. The left ventricle shows no abnormality, thereby indicating that the major functional effect of the valvular lesion was that of stenosis. (*Photograph by courtesy of Dr M D Silver.*)

to each other rendering the orifice *stenotic*, while the rigid leaflets and thickened, contracted chordae tendineae lead to *regurgitation*. If the aortic valve is affected, it is usually rendered both stenosed and incompetent.

Not all patients who suffer from an attack of acute rheumatic fever have persistent heart-valve damage. Nevertheless, the disease has a tendency to recur, and with each attack valvular damage increases. Since the disease is precipitated by streptococcal infection, long-term antibiotic therapy is often instituted as a prophylactic measure.

In those patients unfortunate enough to progress to chronic rheumatic heart disease, mitral stenosis is the commonest valvular lesion found (Fig. 32.11). This causes hypertrophy and great dilatation of the left atrium. Stasis may lead to the formation of thrombus on the wall of the atrium, particularly if there is atrial fibrillation. Systemic embolization may follow. In mitral stenosis the left atrial pressure rises, and there is pulmonary venous congestion. The effect of this is to make the lungs more rigid so that breathing is more difficult and requires more effort: this causes dyspnoea. Intra-alveolar bleeding leads to haemoptysis, and gradually to brown induration of the lungs. In mitral stenosis the left ventricle is under no strain, and is therefore small. Should, however, there be an additional factor of regurgitation, or an aortic valvular lesion, the left ventricle becomes enlarged and might subsequently fail. The back-pressure effect on the lungs eventually leads to pulmonary hypertension and right ventricular failure.

In chronic rheumatic heart disease the valves of the left side of the heart are affected much more frequently and severely than those of the right side.

Endocarditis

Non-bacterial thrombotic endocarditis

Small warty or friable vegetations along the line of closure of the mitral or aortic valves are not uncommon as a *post-mortem* finding. The vegetations are sterile and may be formed on normal or deformed valves. They are of importance in two respects. Occasionally they become detached and embolize to the brain. About 10 per cent of cerebral embolism has been attributed to this mechanism. Secondly the vegetations may form a nidus for the development of infective endocarditis. Usually however, the vegetations of non-bacterial thrombotic endocarditis are of no significance and are removed, probably by lysis.

Infective endocarditis

In this condition the valve cusps are invaded by organisms which are usually bacteria, hence the usual name 'bacterial endocarditis'. But nowadays fungal infections of the valves are seen, and also rickettsial infection in Q-fever, and the condition is better called 'infective endocarditis'.

Acute infective endocarditis. During the course of septicaemia, organisms may invade the heart valve and produce an endocarditis which is characterized by the deposition of large friable thrombi (vegetations) on the valve surfaces. The valves themselves may undergo ulceration and rupture. Unless treated, the condition is terminal and leads to *pyaemia*, as fragments of infected thrombus become detached and enter the arterial circulation—usually the systemic. The common infecting organisms are *Staph. aureus* and pneumococci.

Subacute infective endocarditis (and endarteritis). The adjective 'subacute', hallowed by tradition, is meaningless; the course of the disease is chronic. It is much more helpful to describe the condition in terms of the causative organism than its course. The usual organism is *Strept. viridans*, but sometimes other bacteria, e.g. *Staph. albus, Strept. faecalis*, anaerobic streptococci, *H. influenzae*, and coliform organisms, are responsible. A special type may occur in Q-fever, and fungal cases due to *Candida albicans* are also well known (Fig. 32.12). The organism involved is one of relatively low virulence.

The disease occurs typically on a vascular wall which has been previously abnormal, usually as the result of rheumatic fever. Sometimes a congenital lesion, e.g. a bicuspid aortic valve, coarctation of the aorta, or patent ductus arteriosus,

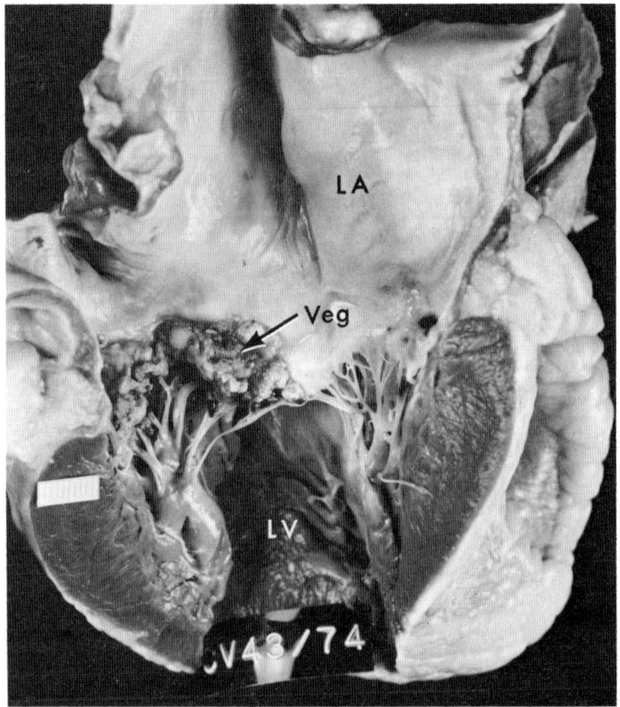

Fig. 32.12 Candida albicans endocarditis. The heart has been opened to show the mitral valve, the left atrium (LA), and the left ventricle (LV). Friable vegetations (Veg) are present of the anterior cusp of the mitral valve. Candida albicans was identified in the vegetations both by culture and in histological sections.

is the seat of trouble, indicating that the condition need not always be an endocarditis. The disease is being encountered more frequently in the elderly than it was previously, and usually there is no obvious preceding valvular disease to account for its localization. Perhaps minor degenerative lesions are present in the affected valve. The mitral and aortic valves are most commonly affected. The attachment area of ball-valve prostheses (usually aortic) is also liable to infection.

Prevention. The organisms reach the heart by the blood stream. *Strept. viridans* is a commensal organism in the mouth. A transient bacteraemia is a frequent event during dental extraction, and may even occur with vigorous mastication. In a healthy individual this is rarely of any consequence, but in a patient with an organic valvular lesion there is a distinct danger that the organisms will localize in damaged areas of the heart and set up endocarditis. Possibly the coincidental formation of non-bacterial thrombotic vegetations causes the organisms to become trapped and set up the infection.

As a prophylactic measure any patient known to have a valvular or congenital heart lesion should be given adequate antibiotic cover before being subjected to dental extraction. It should be given half an hour before the extraction—if given too early, there will be the possibility of the development of more resistant organisms. Long-term chemotherapy is likewise contra-indicated, because it merely results in the development of drug-resistant organisms, and, should endocarditis then occur, the infection might be with organisms that are resistant.

In patients who have recovered from infective endocarditis, a recurrence of infection can occur either with the same organism or with a different one. *Strept. viridans* infection can recur even in edentulous patients, and the extraction of sound teeth is not recommended for the prophylaxis of subacute infective endocarditis.

Clinical features. The disease runs a chronic course, and unless early, prolonged, and efficient treatment is instituted, the patient dies within one year—usually of heart failure due to valvular destruction or cicatrization, or of a progressive glomerulonephritis, probably of immune-complex allergic aetiology. *Pyrexia* of an irregular type, loss of weight, and *anaemia* are constant features, and the last is in part responsible for the *café-au-lait colour of the skin.* The chronic bacteraemia is responsible for RE hyperplasia which accounts for the *splenomegaly. Clubbing of the fingers* is often present, and multiple *embolic phenomena* are characteristic. Large emboli may cause infarction of the brain, intestine, kidney, or spleen; smaller ones have been presumed to be responsible for the *haematuria*, the *splinter haemorrhages* under the nails, and the *petechial haemorrhages of the skin.* However, it seems more likely that these small lesions are due to antigen-antibody complexes causing local vascular damage. *It is important to note that the emboli behave as if they were sterile.* The organisms which they contain are exposed to the bactericidal action of the blood when once they break off from the valves. It is known that the patient's blood contains a high content of antibodies against the causative organisms.

Pathological features. The vegetations are large, red, and friable, and are liable to break off and embolize. Histologically they consist of thrombus containing numerous bacterial colonies which are well protected from the blood stream. The vegetations are attached to the valve by means of granulation tissue, but this is neither profuse nor does it penetrate far into the vegetation. The organisms are once more beyond the reach of the blood. The poor vascularity of the valve cusps is probably the explanation of this inadequate organisation. It is a good example of frustrated repair, and as such is typical of chronic inflammation.

One of the curious features of this disease is that organisms of relatively low virulence are able to survive in the presence of a high degree of immunity. Their inaccessibility in the thrombus appears to be the explanation.

Diagnosis. A definite diagnosis hinges on obtaining a *positive blood culture.* But the disease is so serious that if the clinical picture suggests endocarditis, treatment should be instituted without waiting for pathological confirmation.

Prior to the days of antibiotics the disease was invariably fatal. With modern treatment cure is possible, but the healed valves are often grossly distorted and show calcification. Surgical replacement with a prosthesis is then required.

Calcific (calcareous) aortic stenosis

This condition, probably arising in a congenitally abnormal valve, usually affects elderly men. The aortic ring and later the valve cusps become calcified, and fuse together producing a tight stenosis. The left ventricle is hypertrophied, but in spite of the overaction of this chamber an inadequate amount of blood is pumped into the aorta. In particular the blood supply to the coronary vessels is impaired, and these patients are in constant danger of sudden death. Surgical replacement of diseased valves by a homograft or a plastic prosthesis is therefore indicated.

Valvular disease of the heart

It is convenient at this stage to summarize the valvular defects. Details of these will be found elsewhere in the book.

Mitral valve disease

Mitral stenosis. This defect is a common valvular disease of the heart and is nearly always due to chronic rheumatic disease.

Mitral regurgitation. Some degree of mitral insufficiency is common in chronic rheumatic mitral stenosis. It is also seen in heart failure when dilatation of the mitral ring leads to valve dysfunction. Occasionally mitral regurgitation results from infarction of the papillary muscles holding the valve cusps: the insufficiency can be due to dysfunction or to actual rupture of the muscle. Ulcerative bacterial endocarditis is a rare cause of mitral regurgitation. Mucoid change of the valve cusps is an occasional cause of mitral regurgitation.

Aortic valve disease

Aortic stenosis. Stenosis is usually combined with regurgitation in chronic rheumatic disease of the aortic valve. Congenital stenosis can affect the valve itself or, when the stenosis is produced by muscular hypertrophy (*congenital subaortic muscular stenosis*), the region below the valve. Calcific aortic stenosis occurs in later life. Occasionally it is the end-result of healed endocarditis; usually it develops on the basis of a congenitally abnormal valve which may be bicuspid.

Aortic regurgitation. There are a number of conditions in which the elastic tissue of the aorta and the aortic ring is so weakened that the ring becomes dilated. The valve cusps fail to meet, causing severe regurgitation to result. Syphilitic aortitis, the aortitis of ankylosing spondylitis, and medionecrosis of the aorta fall into this group. Sufficient dilatation to cause regurgitation is also occasionally seen in systemic hypertension.

Tricuspid valve disease. Tricuspid stenosis is generally of rheumatic origin, but it is rare. Triscuspid regurgitation, which is more common than stenosis, is generally due to dilatation of the valve ring in right-sided heart failure.

Pulmonary valve disease. Pulmonary stenosis is nearly always congenital in origin. Sufficient rheumatic endocarditis to cause deformity is rare.

Cardiac dysrhythmias

The term 'dysrhythmia' is used to describe any condition in which the heart is beating either too quickly, too slowly, or irregularly. The impulse that initiates cardiac contraction commences in the sinoatrial (S-A) node in the right atrium, spreads throughout the atria to the atrioventricular (A-V) node, and then travels down the conducting bundle of His to reach the two ventricles *via* the two major branches of the bundle of His. This regular spread of electrical impulse can be interrupted in many ways by various pathological conditions. Only some of the most common disorders will be described here (Figs. 32.13 and 32.14).

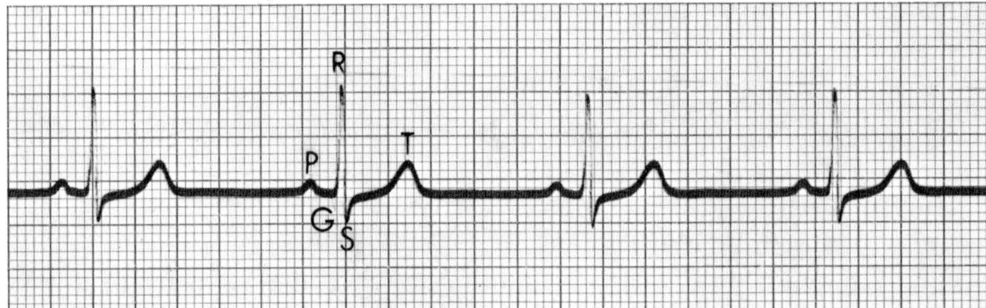

Fig. 32.13 The normal electrocardiogram (ECG). The electrocardiograph is a metre that amplifies and records the differences in electrical potential between two points (bipolar leads) on the surface of the body. Originally three standard leads were used (lead 1, left arm—right arm, lead II, left leg—right arm, and lead III, left leg—left arm), but the 'unipolar' or V leads are now commonly used. An exploratory electrode is placed on various parts of the chest wall; for example, VI lead is placed on the fourth right intercostal space near the sternum, and the second electrode is kept at zero potential.

The electrocardiogram is representative of the electrical activity in the heart, and this triggers muscular activity. P, the first wave, represents passage of activity through the atria (depolarization), and triggers atrial contraction. The QRS complex represents ventricular excitation corresponding to ventricular systole. The T waves represent ventricular recovery, or repolarization. The Q wave is a small negative deflection and is often absent. With the graph paper used for the standard electrocardiogram, each small square of the abscissa is 1 millimetre and represents 40 msec. The heart rate can be estimated by counting the number of millimetres between two consecutive R waves (or other portions of the complex) and dividing 1500 by this number. In the record shown above, the distance between each R wave is 29 or 30 millimetres, and this corresponds to a heart rate of just over 50 beats per minute. (*Photograph by courtesy of Dr R S Baigrie.*)

Ectopic beats. An ectopic beat arises prematurely from a site other than the S-A node. It may be in the atria, in the A-V node, or in the ventricle. Distinction between these types can be made only by study of the electrocardiogram. Following the ectopic beat there is a compensatory pause before the next normal heart beat. This sometimes produces the feeling of the heart 'turning over,' but apart from this, ectopic beats produce no symptoms. They are common in normal people, but they can also be an indication of myocardial disease. This association with myocardial disease applies particularly to the ventricular ectopic beats, which are seen in patients with myocardial ischaemia and in those who have taken too much digitalis (Fig. 32.14 c).

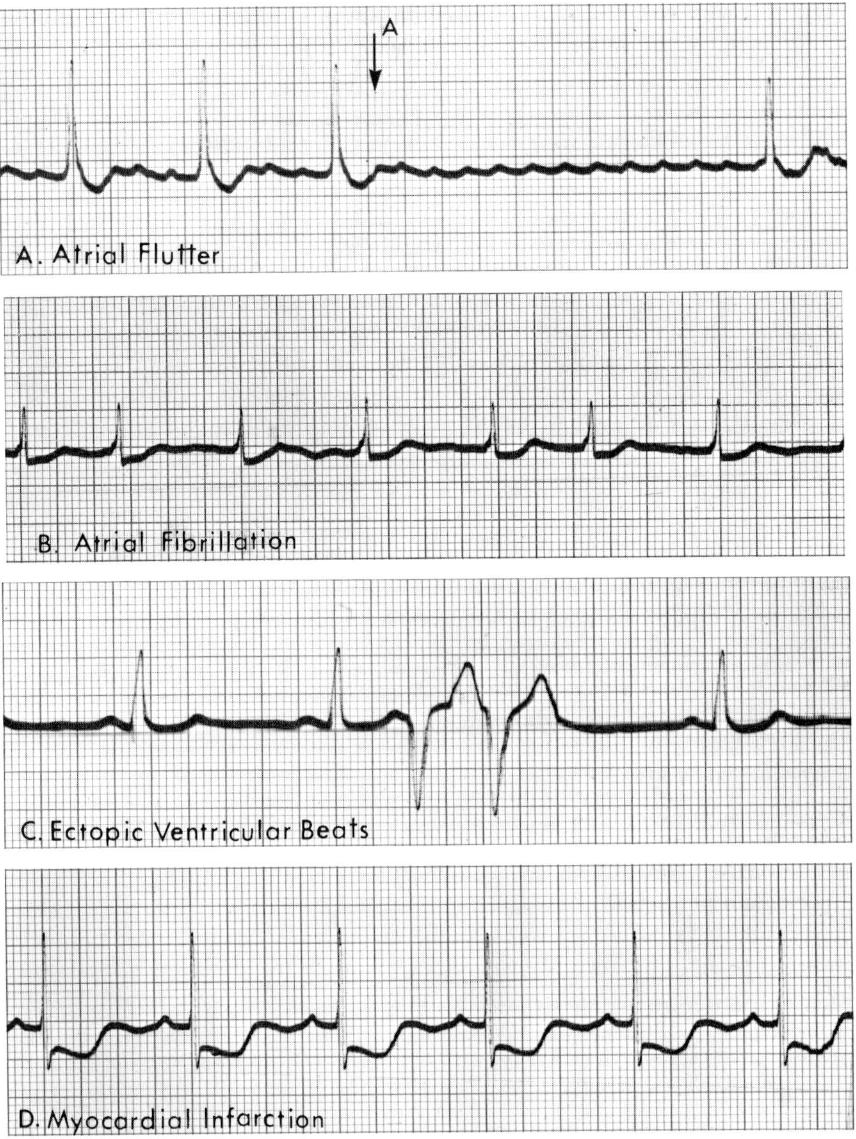

Fig. 32.14 Abnormal electrocardiogram. A, *Atrial flutter.* Normal P waves are absent and are replaced by a flutter wave occurring at approximately 300 per minute. Some impulses reach the ventricles and lead to ventricular complexes. At point A, pressure was applied to the carotid sinus, and this produced reflex vagal activity. The effect of this was to produce a temporary heart block, and for a period there was ventricular standstill. *B, Atrial fibrillation.* In this electrocardiogram no P waves can be seen, and the irregular atrial fibrillation indicates chaotic atrial activity. The ventricles respond in an erratic manner, so that the heart rate in addition to being fast (95 beats per minute) is irregular. *C, Ectopic ventricular beats.* Two ectopic beats are shown in which the QRS complex is abnormal. This abnormality is a reflection of the beats arising within the ventricles themselves, and not being a response to normal stimulation from the atria. *D, Myocardial infarction.* The outstanding feature of this electrocardiograph is depression of the ST segment. This change was seen shortly after an acute myocardial infarction. In other leads there was ST segment elevation, and analysis of the changes in the standard leads can give a good indication of the site of the infarct. (*Photograph by courtesy of Dr R S Baigrie.*)

Paroxysmal tachycardia. In this condition there are attacks of rapid heart action resulting from a regular succession of ectopic beats that last for a few seconds or as long as several days. *Paroxysmal atrial tachycardia* is the most common type and is generally not associated with heart disease. The *ventricular type* is more usually seen in patients with ischaemic disease; like ventricular ectopic beats, this condition may precede ventricular fibrillation in patients with myocardial infarction.

Atrial fibrillation. This is a common and important disorder. It appears to be due to multiple ectopic foci discharging at variable rates in the atria. Rapid fibrillary waves take place rather than normal atrial contraction, and the multiple impulses that reach the A-V node (up to 600 per minute) cannot all be conducted to the ventricles. Approximately 100 to 160 reach the ventricles at a completely irregular rhythm. Because not all ventricular contractions are powerful enough to open the aortic and pulmonary valves, the pulse rate as felt at the wrist is less than that heard at the apex of the heart. Rheumatic heart disease, particularly mitral stenosis, is the most common cause of atrial fibrillation, but in older patients ischaemic heart disease, systemic hypertension, and thyrotoxicosis are other important causes (Fig. 32.14 b).

Atrial fibrillation is generally treated by the administration of digitalis, which acts by impairing conduction in the bundle of His. Fewer impulses reach the ventricles, causing them to be slowed, so that each contraction is more effective. The atrial fibrillation itself is not terminated. Indeed, to try to stop the fibrillation itself may precipitate detachment of a mural thrombus from the atrium.

Atrial flutter. This form of dysrhythmia is less common than atrial fibrillation. The atria contract at a rate of about 300 beats per minute, being stimulated by a rapidly firing ectopic pacemaker. Atrioventricular block results in a slower ventricular rate (Fig. 32.14A).

Ventricular fibrillation. This is a most serious condition, and it is generally the immediate precursor of death in myocardial infarction. Immediate external electrical defibrillation is the most effective treatment if equipment is available.

Heart block. The term 'heart block' is used to describe depression of conduction between the atria and the ventricles. In the early stages, the time required for the impulse to reach the ventricles is merely prolonged, but as the condition progresses, occasional impulses fail to reach the ventricles and a beat is dropped. When conduction is completely blocked, there is *complete heart block*; no impulses from the atria reach the ventricles, which then beat at their own intrinsic rate of about 40 beats per minute. The chief causes of heart block are ischaemic heart disease and an overdose of digitalis. When complete heart block occurs suddenly, the ventricles may not start to beat for several minutes, and the patient rapidly loses consciousness and develops convulsions. These episodes are known as *Stokes-Adams attacks.*

Effects of cardiac dysrhythmias.

Irregular or rapid cardiac contraction may lead to a sensation in the chest that is described as *palpitation.* If the heart rate is either very rapid (e.g. over 160 beats per minute, as in paroxysmal tachycardia and atrial fibrillation) or very low (e.g. below 40 beats per minute, as in complete heart block), the cardiac output is diminished, particularly on exercise. If the heart is otherwise normal, this change in rate may be of no immediate consequence, but if it is superadded to some other heart disease, the results can be serious. Tachycardia increases the heart's requirement for oxygen, and the energy expended is wastefully used by ineffective contractions. Furthermore, during tachycardia the coronary blood flow is decreased. Most of the coronary blood flow takes place during diastole, so that with tachycardia diastole is shortened and the blood flow is diminished. The heart muscle therefore has an increased need for oxygen at the same time that its supply is reduced. The ischaemia that results further impairs myocardial activity and can lead to necrosis, either patchy or massive.

HEART FAILURE

The most important chambers of the heart are the two ventricles. These fill during diastole from the low-pressured venous reservoirs, an effect aided by atrial contraction. Normally the heart is able to expel all the blood which flows into it. If the venous return is increased in volume, the increased filling of the heart stretches its muscle fibres and the force of the next contraction is increased. This is *Starling's Law of the Heart.* The cardiac output is thus gauged to the venous return, and the heart can satisfy the needs of the body under all normal circumstances.

Under resting conditions the ventricles do not empty completely with each systole, but with exercise their contraction results in more complete emptying. This is mediated by an increase in sympathetic tone,* and acting with the greater filling due to the increased venous return, it results in a larger volume (the stroke volume) of blood being ejected with each heart beat. In addition, the heart rate increases. Therefore the heart has a considerable *functional reserve*, and can increase its output from the resting level of 5 litres per min to 25 to 30 litres per min.

Prolonged overwork of any chamber causes hypertrophy of the muscle of its walls. This is an additional cardiac reserve, but it should be remembered that the hypertrophied myocardium usually fails unless the strain on it is removed. A large heart is a diseased heart.

When, in the presence of an adequate venous return, the heart fails to supply blood to meet the needs of the body the condition is known as *heart failure.* At first the effects of this are to be seen on exercise, but as the failure increases so the effects are apparent even at rest. Either the left or the right ventricle may fail separately. More usually the heart fails as a whole, and the condition is called *congestive heart failure.*

Effects of right ventricular failure

Rise in central venous pressure.† A failure of the right ventricle to eject all the blood which it receives leads to distension of the right atrium by a back-

* A change in the force of contraction of the heart without a corresponding change in the initial length of the muscle is called an *inotropic effect.* The alkaloids of digitalis are used in heart failure because they have an inotropic effect.

† This is the pressure in the right atrium minus the negative intrathoracic pressure.

pressure effect. The pressure in the great veins rises, and the *jugular veins are seen to be distended with blood* when the patient sits up in bed. To some extent this *aids* heart function, because the raised pressure causes increased filling of the heart. This by stretching the myocardium *increases* the force of contraction. However, a point can be reached beyond which increased stretching causes a *decrease* in cardiac contraction. Exercise, by increasing the venous return, further reduces the cardiac output; the patient is therefore bedridden. Once past this critical point, therapeutic bleeding increases the cardiac output by reducing the venous pressure. This is the basis for the time-honoured practice of bleeding as a treatment for heart failure. In right-sided heart failure all the organs of the body are congested. This is particularly well seen in the liver, where the centres of the lobules are deeply congested and red (see nutmeg liver, p. 523). Congestion is evident in the skin, especially of the face.

Cyanosis. The sluggish circulation allows a more complete deoxygenation of the blood as it passes through the tissues. In the skin this may be detected by the bluish coloration known as *cyanosis.* Cyanosis is evident when the capillary blood contains more than 5 g reduced haemoglobin per dl. It should be noted that cyanosis due to stasis (*peripheral cyanosis*) is not necessarily due to heart disease. It is seen whenever the circulation is sluggish, e.g. in polycythaemia (where the blood is very viscous), in an area affected by venous obstruction, and in shock. Some people are so sensitive to cold that their ears, nose, and finger-tips become cyanosed even on exposure to a cool atmosphere.

Polycythaemia. An increased red-cell count occurs as a result of bone marrow hypoxia.

Oedema. Oedema of the dependent parts is a prominent sign of heart failure. It accumulates around the legs and genitalia, and, during recumbency, the sacral region. The pathogenesis of the odema is complex. In part it is due to the chronic passive venous congestion of the tissues, but a more important factor is the reduced cardiac output. The reduced output of the right ventricle leads to a corresponding fall in that of the left ventricle, for the quantity of blood entering this chamber is the same as the right ventricular output. This reduced cardiac output acts on the kidneys and causes salt and water retention (see congestive heart failure).

Effects of left ventricular failure

Rise in pulmonary venous pressure. The venous distension affects the lungs which become congested and tense. The effort of breathing is increased, and this causes distress (*dyspnoea*). *Pulmonary oedema* is an ever-present danger, and may come on with dramatic suddenness. Rupture of capillaries leads to *haemoptysis*, and the blood which remains in the lungs is converted into haemosiderin. This produces a brown pigmentation of the lungs and stimulates fine fibrosis, a condition called *brown induration of the lung*. It is the result of longstanding chronic venous congestion.

It should be noted that in primary left ventricular failure the output of the two ventricles is the same, but the left is functioning with the aid of an increased venous filling pressure. The right ventricle, on the other hand, is working normally. This leads to a redistribution of blood, more being retained in the pulmonary circuit than is normal. In addition to producing pulmonary congestion and oedema, the rise in pulmonary pressure (*pulmonary hypertension*) ultimately causes the right ventricle to fail, and *congestive heart failure* ensues.

Effects of congestive heart failure

The inadequate cardiac output causes ischaemia of many organs. Selective vasoconstriction, e.g. of the skin vessels, causes sufficient redistribution of blood so that the important organs do not suffer damage in the initial stages. Cutaneous arteriolar constriction is an important factor in the pathogenesis of *peripheral cyanosis*. The two organs in which the effect of ischaemia is most marked are the liver and the kidneys.

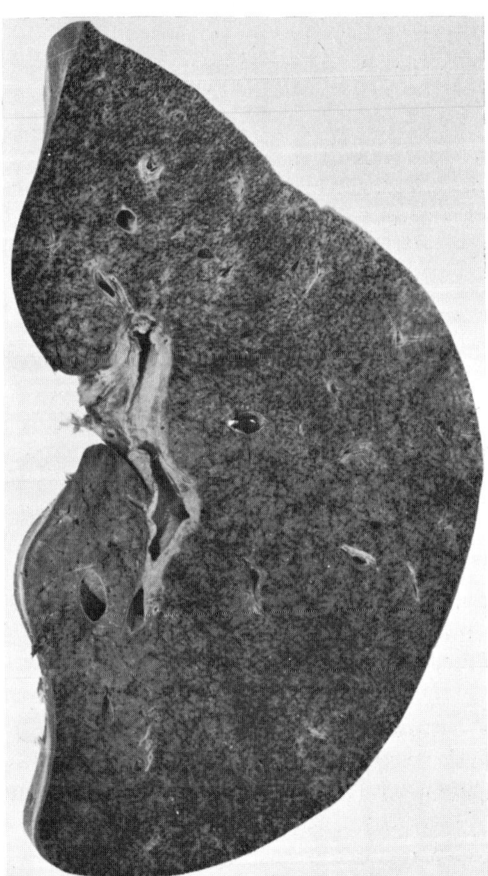

Fig. 32.15 Nutmeg liver. The pattern of alternating dark congestion and pale fatty change is apparent. (A 95.2. *Reproduced by permission of the President and Council of the Royal College of Surgeons of England.*)

In the liver the ischaemia leads to necrosis of the cells in the centres of the lobules, while the less severely affected peripheral cells show fatty change. The result is the characteristic *nutmeg liver* of congestive heart failure—the centres of the lobules are red and the peripheries yellow (Fig. 32.15 and 32.16).

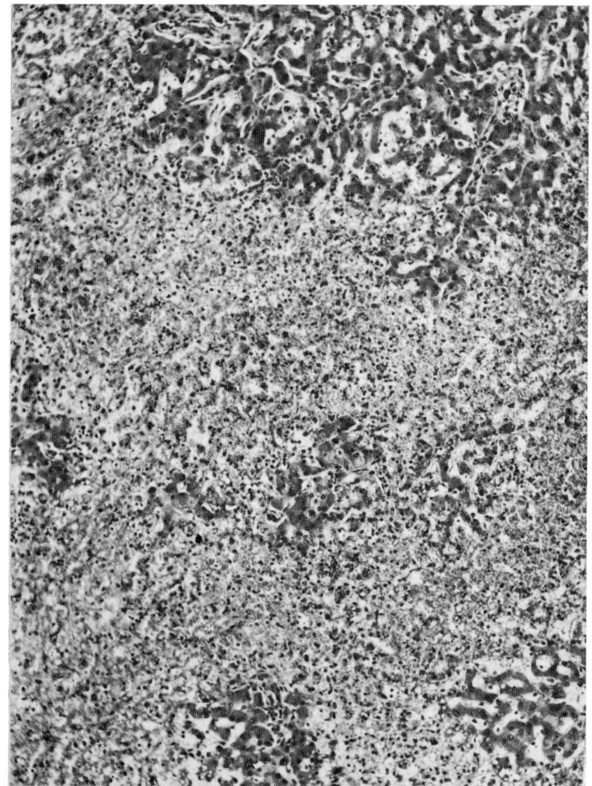

Fig. 32.16 Chronic venous congestion of the liver. There is a virtual disappearance of the liver cells in the central zones of the lobules, and their replacement with engorged, dilated sinusoids. The peripheral cells show fatty change. × 90.

In the kidneys no morphological changes other than congestion are evident, but the impaired renal blood flow leads to *salt and water retention.* This is a very important factor in the causation of cardiac oedema. Venous distension plays its part in determining the location of the oedema rather than in causing its formation.

In the terminal stages of left-sided heart failure *the brain* receives an inadequate blood supply, and this causes an impairment of consciousness and sometimes dementia.

The causes of heart failure

As previously described, the heart can easily increase its output during exercise. It cannot, however, maintain the high output for long, nor can it continue to function in the face of a high-output pressure. Any condition which imposes a sustained burden on the heart will eventually lead to its failure. It may also fail because of myocardial damage. The causes of heart failure may be considered under three headings:

Overburdening due to a sustained increase in ventricular pressure

This occurs in systemic and pulmonary *hypertension* and also in *aortic and pulmonary valvular disease*. If the semilunar cusps fuse together to produce a narrowing, or *stenosis*, of the valve orifice, the chamber behind the diseased valve, the ventricle, has to generate a high pressure to force blood through the stenosed valve. Hypertrophy of the ventricle occurs, but in time failure ensues. It should be noted that when the mitral valve is diseased, the over-distension of the left atrium causes pulmonary hypertension such that *right ventricular failure soon follows*.

Myocardial disease

Myocardial disease is by far the most important cause of heart failure. It is generally due to ischaemia secondary to atherosclerosis of the coronary arteries (p. 508). Other causes of myocardial failure are myocarditis (e.g. rheumatic and diphtheritic), amyloidosis, and myxoedema. Sometimes a large heart in a normotensive individual fails without obvious myocardial, coronary, or valvular damage. In a few cases this has been attributed to alcoholism, beriberi, or the excessive ingestion of beer to which cobalt salts have been added during its manufacture. In the remainder no cause is found and the cases are placed in a group called the *cardiomyopathies*. The diagnosis is one of exclusion of known causes.

Overburdening due to a sustained increase in cardiac output

Valvular defects. When the aortic valve becomes rigid and *incompetent*, blood flows back into the left ventricle during diastole. An increased volume of blood must therefore be ejected in systole. The actual output of the ventricle is increased, but the effective output is unaltered. A similar result is seen in *mitral regurgitation*, but here the wasted ventricular output is diverted to the left atrium. In both aortic regurgitation and mitral regurgitation left ventricular failure ensues. Pulmonary and tricuspid disease produce comparable effects on the right side.

High-output failure. There are a number of conditions in which there is a sustained increase in the true cardiac output; the most easily understood is thyrotoxicosis, where the increased metabolic rate demands an increased output from the heart. Anaemia and a large arteriovenous shunt have a similar effect. There are a number of diseases, e.g. chronic lung disease and advanced cirrhosis of the liver, in which the cardiac output even at rest is high for no very obvious reason. Whenever the resting cardiac output is increased, the heart copes with the load for a while, but ultimately fails. Even in failure the output may be above the normal, but is still inadequate to meet the demands of the body because these demands are themselves greater than normal. This condition is called *high-output failure* in contrast to the more common type of heart failure, called *low-output failure*, in which the cardiac output is less than that of a normal person of similar stature.

Additional factors causing heart failure

Anxiety raises the heart rate and blood pressure, thereby adding an additional burden on the left ventricle. Thus anxiety may precipitate an attack of paroxysmal nocturnal dyspnoea (p. 538). By raising the metabolic rate *pyrexia* causes an increase in the cardiac output. *Pregnancy* has a similar effect as a result of an increased blood volume and the necessity of supplying blood to the fetus. The effects of *dysrhythmias* have been considered earlier in this chapter.

GENERAL READING

Abelmann W H 1971 The cardiomyopathies. Hospital Practice, 6: 101

Braunwald E 1974 In Harrison's Principles of Internal Medicine, ed. by Wintrobe M M et al., 7th edn. ch 233 (Heart Failure). McGraw-Hill, New York

Braunwald E, Sobel B E 1974 In Harrison's Principles of Internal Medicine ch 234 (Cardiac Dysrhythmias)

Briller S A 1974 In Harrison's Principles of Internal Medicine, ch 229 (Electrocardiography)

Brod J 1972 Pathogenesis of cardiac oedema. British Medical Journal 1: 222

Campbell E J M, Dickinson C J, Slater J D H 1974 Clinical Physiology, 4th edn. ch 2 (The Heart and Circulation). Blackwell, Oxford

Davis J O 1970 The mechanisms of salt and water retention in cardiac failure. Hospital Practice 5: 63

Harris P, Heath D 1977 The Human Pulmonary Circulation, 2nd edn. Churchill Livingstone, Edinburgh

Hudson R E B 1965 and 1970 Cardiovascular Pathology, 3 Volumes. Arnold, London

Perloff J K 1970 The clinical manifestations of cardiac failure in adults. Hospital Practice 5: 43

Wood P 1968 Diseases of the Heart and Circulation, 3rd edn. Eyre and Spottiswoode, London

33

Diseases of the respiratory system

Normal function[1]

The function of the respiratory system is to enable gaseous exchange to take place between the blood and the atmosphere. Air is inhaled, and as it passes through the nose, nasopharynx, larynx, and trachea it is filtered and humidified. It eventually reaches the small air sacs, or alveoli, of the lung where it comes into close contact with blood in the capillaries. Conditions for gaseous exchange are ideal: oxygen is added to the blood and the carbon dioxide which is removed is exhaled. The gas in the alveoli is maintained at a fairly constant composition by the act of breathing. This has two components—ventilation and distribution.

Ventilation. This is the bellows-like action of the chest, by which fresh air is drawn in and stale air expired. The volume is approximately 7.5 litres per minute in the adult at rest.

Distribution. The inspired air is so distributed in relation to the volume of blood perfusing the lung that the composition of the alveolar gas is maintained at a constant level. Since the arterial blood, as it leaves the lung, is in equilibrium with the alveolar gas, it follows that the gaseous tensions of oxygen and carbon dioxide in the arterial blood are also maintained at this same constant level.

Respiratory failure

If through the dysfunction of the lungs there is oxygen lack or CO_2 retention, the condition is called *respiratory failure*. In the arterial blood under normal conditions the partial pressure of oxygen, usually written Po_2, is about 100 mm Hg (or 13.3 kilopascals, abbreviated to kPa) and the partial pressure of carbon dioxide (Pco_2) about 40 mm Hg (or 5.3 kPa). In respiratory failure the Po_2 is under 60 mm Hg and the Pco_2 over 49 mm Hg.

Lack of Oxygen (hypoxia). The arterial blood is normally saturated with oxygen, but in respiratory failure both the tension and quantity of oxygen in the blood are reduced. As the blood passes through the tissues it becomes increasingly desaturated, and cyanosis of the exposed parts occurs. The hypoxia stimulates red-cell production in the bone marrow, and leads to polycythaemia. This increases the viscosity of the blood, and by causing stagnation in the tissues contributes to the cyanosis. In addition there is a further strain on the heart, and *heart failure* may occur. Usually the right ventricle is affected, because in most lung diseases causing respiratory failure there is considerable destruction of lung tissue and obliteration of pulmonary vasculature. This causes pulmonary hypertension and strain on the right ventricle.

Retention of carbon dioxide. An increased tension of CO_2 in the arterial blood (hypercapnia) produces vasodilatation of the vessels of the skin and brain. The skin is hot and flushed, and the brain becomes hyperaemic and oedematous. Clinically the latter is manifest as confusion, drowsiness, tremor, and finally coma and death.

Dyspnoea

In a healthy person the rate and depth of respiration are so regulated that the individual is unaware of the movements involved in breathing. *Tachypnoea* is an increased rate of respiration, and is seen when pain restricts respiratory movement, as in pleurisy, or when the lungs become increasingly rigid, as in congestion or fibrosis. Tachypnoea is sometimes accompanied by an increase in depth of breathing, and the term *hyperpnoea* embraces both conditions. *Dyspnoea* is a condition in which the act of breathing causes distress. It occurs under two main circumstances: (1) *when tachypnoea or hyperpnoea are of marked degree;* (2) *when the ventilatory effect produced on inspiration is small in comparison with the muscular effort needed to produce it.* This occurs in any disease interfering with the respiratory excursions of the lung, for instance, fibrosis or congestion. Obstruction to the major air passages, whether due to pulmonary disease like chronic bronchitis or to strangulation, has a similar effect, and produces intense dyspnoea. Psychological factors also play a part. Thus the sudden blockage of a tube through which a person is breathing occasions intense dyspnoea. However, if the subject is asked to block the tube, the manoeuvre causes no immediate discomfort.

Bronchial obstruction

Causes

The common causes of bronchial obstruction are:

1. Tenacious mucus which is not expelled from the respiratory passages, e.g. in asthma
2. Chronic bronchitis
3. Inhaled foreign bodies, e.g. roots of teeth, peas, etc.
4. Tumours, usually carcinoma.

Effects

The effects of obstruction depend on whether the obstruction is partial or complete.

Partial obstruction. The partial obstruction of a bronchus impedes the ventilation of the lung distal to the obstruction. It follows therefore that the blood perfusing that part of the lung is inadequately oxygenated, and that in effect a quantity of venous blood is shunted directly into the pulmonary veins and thence to the left side of the heart. Since the blood leaving the lungs is normally fully saturated with oxygen, it follows that no amount of over-ventilation of the unaffected lung can compensate for this shunt effect. The arterial Po_2 is therefore lowered. A very important example of partial obstruction of the bronchi occurs in chronic bronchitis, especially after surgical operation (p. 539).

Infection. Infection commonly follows bronchial obstruction. Organisms that are inhaled into the affected lung segment become trapped in the mucus, their expulsion is impaired, and bronchopneumonia follows. The infection also involves the bronchial wall, and if long-continued will produce destruction of the muscle and cartilaginous component, so that the bronchus is weakened and tends to dilate (*bronchiectasis*). This is frequently seen distal to the obstruction caused by a carcinoma or a foreign body. Quite often bronchiectasis occurs in several parts of the lung as an idiopathic condition, and is thought to be the result of obstruction by mucus during some previous infection, such as measles or whooping-cough during childhood.

Complete obstruction. Where there is complete obstruction of a large bronchus, the lung distal shows a progressive absorption of its gas content until it becomes completely airless or *collapsed.*

PNEUMONIA

Pneumonia is defined as an inflammation in the alveolar parenchyma of the lung. Exudate usually fills the alveoli which are thereby rendered airless and solid. This is called *consolidation.* Sometimes, however, the inflammatory exudate is restricted to the alveolar wall. This is often called *interstitial pneumonia*, but the term *pneumonitis* is also used.

Two main types of pneumonia are recognized, depending upon the gross appearance of the lesions which result.

Lobar pneumonia

This is a disease that can affect healthy young adults, but an underlying debilitating disease, particularly chronic alcoholism, can predispose to it. The organism concerned is a pneumococcus of high virulence, and is acquired by inhalation from another victim or a convalescent carrier. The disease has a sudden onset with rigors, fever, and pain in the chest. The organisms which reach the lung produce a rapidly spreading inflammatory oedema which soon implicates a whole lobe, and sometimes several lobes (Fig. 33.1).

Pathogenesis

The fact that infection spreads so rapidly in a gigantic wave of oedematous exudate suggests that allergy is involved in the process. Perhaps the patient has already had a minor pneumococcal infection sufficient to produce an immune response. When now attacked a second time, the reaction of hypersensitivity accompanies the inflammatory response and renders it more intense. An alternative explanation is that lobar pneumonia is a primary infection. When the organisms reach the lungs, they gain entry rapidly into the blood stream, where they proliferate in the RE system, and then escape into the blood to produce a septicaemia. When they reach the lungs again, an allergic response occurs due to

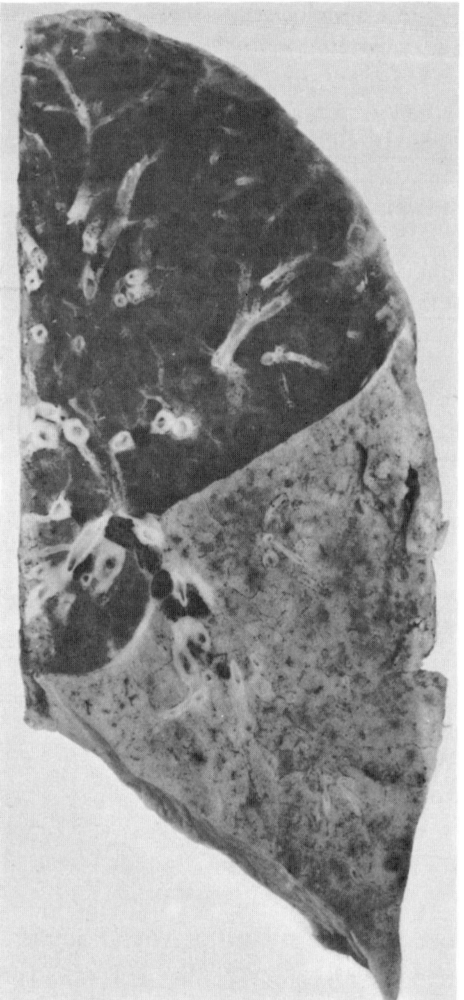

Fig. 33.1 Lobar pneumonia. The left lower lobe is consolidated in the stage of grey hepatization, while the upper lobe is unaffected. (R30.2. *Reproduced by permission of the President and Council of the Royal College of Surgeons of England.*)

their reaction with recently formed local antibodies. This mechanism would be analogous to that described in typhoid fever and syphilis.

Stages

Whatever the mechanism, there is no doubt that during the acute stage of the disease there is a septicaemia, and sometimes the pneumococci may localize themselves not only in the lungs but also in the meninges, peritoneum, joints, etc. During the first few days of illness the patient is desperately ill and may die; the lobe of lung affected is *congested* and shows *inflammatory oedema.* It is teeming with pneumococci.

The second stage of the disease is called *red hepatization*, because the congested, consolidated lung has the appearance of liver. Microscopically the alveolar capillaries are dilated, and the alveoli are filled with inflammatory exudate containing oedema fluid, fibrin, and many polymorphs (Fig. 33.2). A number of red cells are present also. Gradually the hyperaemia of the lung diminishes, the capillaries shut down, and the lung assumes a grey colour. This is the classical stage of *grey hepatization*. The alveoli are still filled with inflammatory exudate, but the polymorphs show disintegration and fibrin threads appear clumped

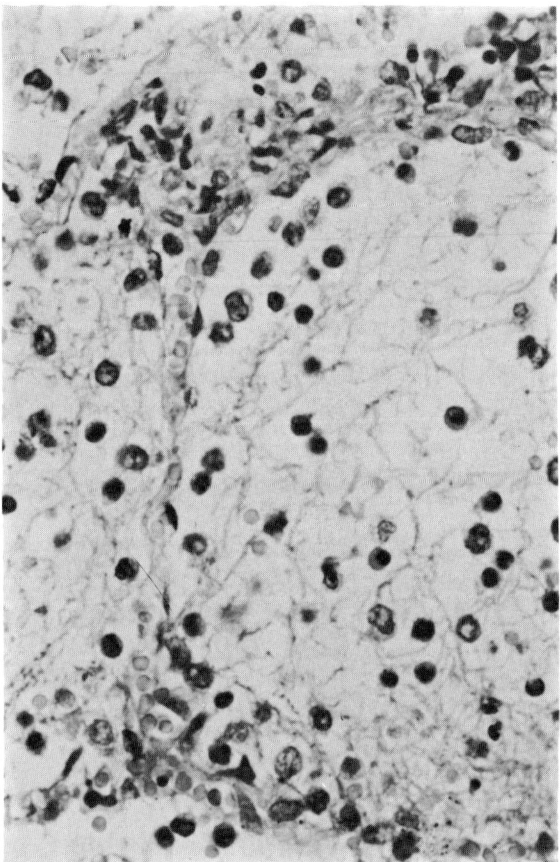

Fig. 33.2 Lobar pneumonia. The two adjacent alveoli are filled with a loose fibrinous exudate containing pus cells and macrophages. The alveolar capillaries are dilated and contain many red cells. This corresponds to the stage of red hepatization. × 200.

(Fig. 33.3). The fourth and final stage is that of *resolution*, in which demolition is accomplished by macrophages. The fibrin is removed with great rapidity, and all the debris is cleared away. Fluid exudate and macrophages leave the alveoli mainly by way of the lymphatics. With the removal of all the inflammatory exudate the lung returns to normal, and this is therefore an excellent example of complete resolution. Rarely the exudate in the alveoli is not demolished but persists and is organized into fibrous tissue.

During the acute stage of lobar pneumonia the overlying pleura shows acute inflammation, and is covered with a fibrinous exudate. This is responsible for the creaking pleural rub which may be heard clinically, and for the pain which occurs on inspiration.

Clinical course

Following the acute onset, the patient remains seriously ill for 7 to 10 days with high fever. Death may occur during this stage. As suddenly as the disease started,

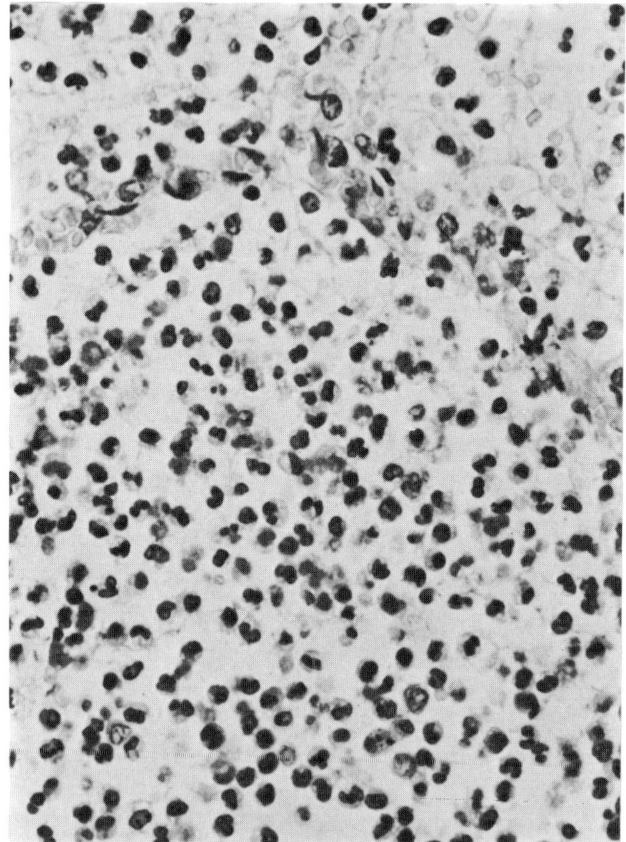

Fig. 33.3 Lobar pneumonia. The alveoli are crowded with pus cells, and the fibrinous exudate has condensed into thick strands. The alveolar capillaries are inconspicuous, and appear to have shut down. This corresponds to the stage of grey hepatization. × 200.

so it terminates. Sweating occurs, the temperature drops, and there is a sense of well-being. This is termed the crisis. In practice these stages are rarely seen today, since antibiotics rapidly terminate the course of the disease.

Complications. Lung abscess, pulmonary fibrosis, and empyema may occur but are uncommon, even in the untreated patient.

BRONCHOPNEUMONIA

In bronchopneumonia, unlike lobar pneumonia, there are discrete foci of inflammation round terminal bronchioles (Fig. 33.4). Patches of consolidation are scattered throughout several lobes of the lung, and the condition is usually bilateral (Fig. 33.5). The wildfire spread seen in lobar pneumonia is not present.

There are many varieties of bronchopneumonia. They are best considered under two headings:

1. *Endogenous bronchopneumonia*
2. *Exogenous bronchopneumonia.*

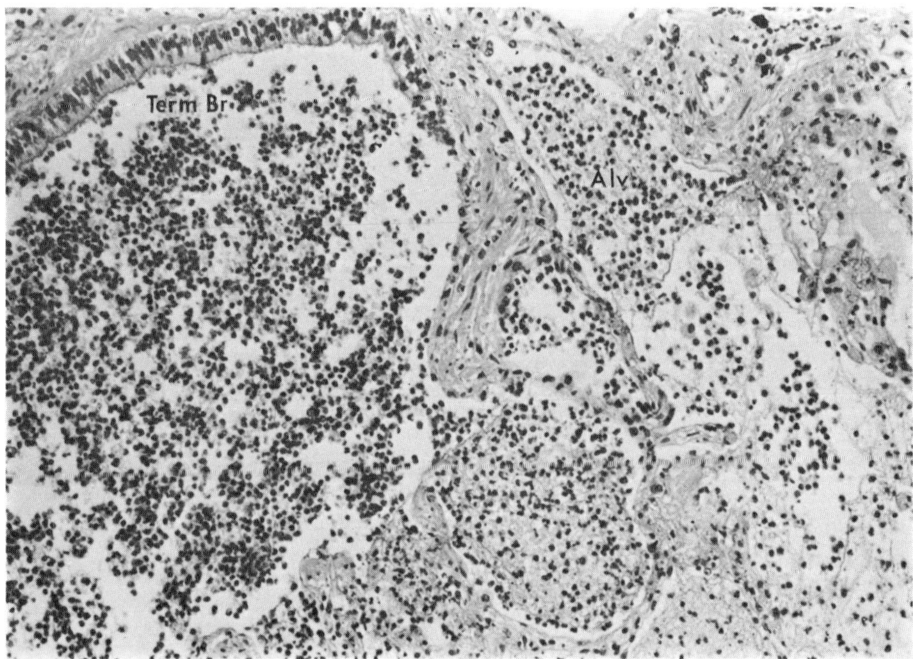

Fig. 33.4 Bronchopneumonia. Part of a terminal bronchiole (Term Br) is shown with its lining of ciliated columnar epithelium. The bronchiole is crowded with inflammatory cells, the majority of which are polymorphs. Alveoli (Alv) adjacent to the bronchiole also contain inflammatory exudate with polymorphs and fibrin. An alveolus further away from the bronchiole merely contains oedema fluid. × 100.

Endogenous bronchopneumonia

This type of bronchopneumonia is due to infection with commensal organisms normally resident in the upper respiratory passages. Of these the commensal pneumococci of low-grade virulence are by far the most important. They cause infection whenever the defence mechanisms of the host are impaired. The antagonists are therefore a weakly virulent endogenous organism and an enfeebled host. This contrasts with lobar pneumonia in which the contending parties are a highly virulent organism and a relatively healthy host.

Causes

The conditions leading to endogenous bronchopneumonia may be considered under two headings:

General factors. *Extremes of age.* Bronchopneumonia is commonest in infancy and old age.

General debilitating illness. The disease is a common terminal event in cancer, cerebrovascular accidents, and uraemia.

Impaired immune response. It may occur in agammaglobulinaemia, agranulocytosis, and as a complication of glucocorticoid therapy.

Local factors. Any local condition interfering with ciliary action and the upward movement of mucus is liable to be followed by bronchopneumonia. The causes may be listed.

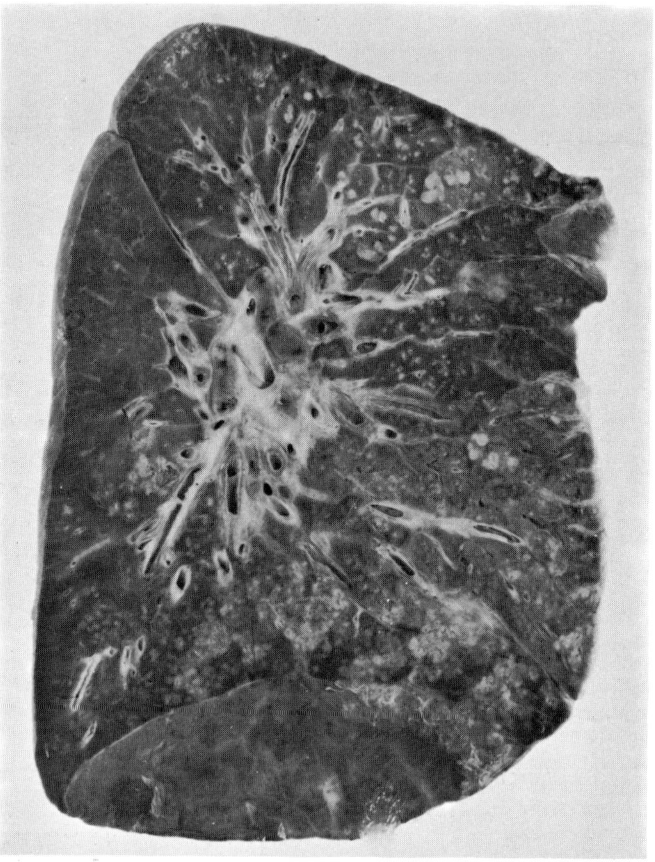

Fig. 33.5 Staphylococcal bronchopneumonia. There are discrete foci of consolidation scattered throughout the lung, and some have formed tiny abscesses. (R29.3. *Reproduction by permission of the President and Council of the Royal College of Surgeons of England.*)

Pre-existing acute respiratory disease. Bronchopneumonia often complicates influenza, measles, and whooping-cough. In these infections the ciliated bronchial epithelium is shed, and organisms which gain access to the lung cannot be removed.

Local obstruction. The trapped secretions form an admirable medium for bacterial growth, and bronchopneumonia is localized to the segment distal to the obstruction. Foreign bodies and tumours of the bronchi are well-known examples.

Chronic bronchitis and bronchiectasis. These are important predisposing causes of bronchopneumonia. Two factors are involved. In the first place the ciliated epithelium may be replaced by goblet cells or squamous cells, and this impedes the upward flow of mucus. Secondly the mucus itself is often of viscid consistency, and cannot easily be removed. An excessive amount of mucus appears in the *chronic venous congestion* of heart failure due to the additional fluid contributed by transudation.

Pulmonary oedema. In oedematous lung tissue it seems likely that the macrophages are unable to perform their normal function. Infection is therefore quite a common sequel to oedema from whatever cause. The basal oedema which occurs in debilitated, bedridden patients, in those who are unconscious, and following operations often progresses to pneumonia, and is called *hypostatic pneumonia.*

Bronchopneumonia is of much longer duration than lobar pneumonia. If the primary condition is incurable, the pneumonia is merely a welcome terminal event, and there will obviously be little attempt at healing. Even in the childhood bronchopneumonias that follow measles and whooping-cough, a prolonged course is the rule, and is often punctuated by relapses and remissions depending upon whether the organism or the host is gaining the upper hand. Both the onset and the end of the disease are gradual.

Lesions of bronchopneumonia

The disease is usually basal and posterior in distribution and is bilateral. If an area of bronchopneumonia is examined microscopically, it is found to consist of acutely inflamed bronchioles full of pus. Some of the surrounding alveoli contain oedema fluid in which there are macrophages and polymorphs, while others are filled with a dense fibrinous exudate in which there are innumerable polymorphs. Some are collapsed as the result of the absorption of air distal to the blocked bronchioles, whereas neighbouring alveoli are empty and distended due to compensatory dilatation (Fig. 33.4). In contrast to lobar pneumonia, where all alveoli in a lobe are at about the same stage of the inflammatory process, in bronchopneumonia there is a very varied picture.

Sequelae of bronchopneumonia

Resolution. This is much less frequent than in lobar pneumonia.

Progressive fibrosis of the lung. This is correspondingly more frequent. It is due to organization of the inflammatory exudate in the alveoli. In addition there is often a continuance of the inflammatory process, so that more and more lung tissue is destroyed and converted into fibrous tissue. This is, of course, the condition of chronic inflammation, and bronchopneumonia often becomes chronic. In due course the infection spreads, and the muscle and elastic tissue of the adjacent bronchi are destroyed and replaced by granulation tissue. In consequence the lumina widen, and eventually the dilatation becomes so extensive that secretion accumulates forming the nidus of further infection and inflammatory destruction. This is the pathogenesis of *bronchiectasis*, which is both a sequel of bronchopneumonia and a predisposing cause of further attacks (Fig. 33.6)

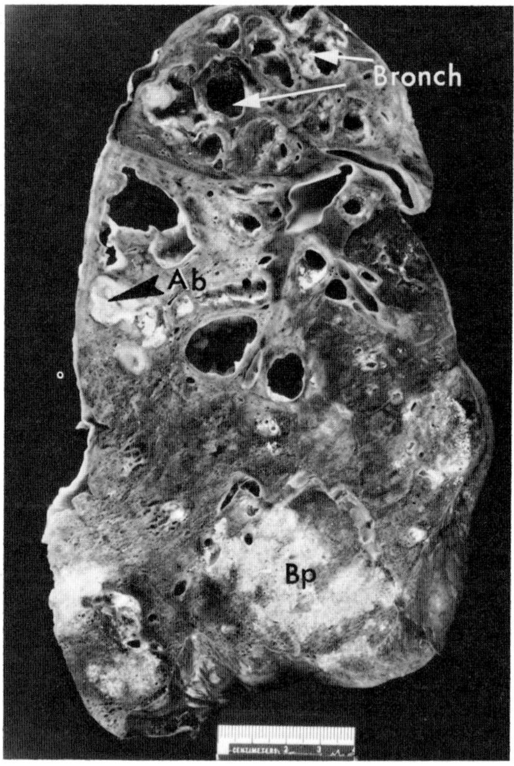

Fig. 33.6 Bronchiectasis with chronic lung infection. Since the age of 7 years this patient had had repeated attacks of pneumonia. When he was 24 years of age a diagnosis of cystic fibrosis was made (see p. 290). He was treated with vitamins and pancreatic enzymes by mouth, but continued to be plagued by repeated lung infections. The terminal event was an overwhelming infection with *Pseudomonas aeruginosa*, and he died at the age of 32 years. This specimen shows the effects of repeated bronchopneumonia. Towards the base of the lung there are several areas of bronchopneumonia (Bp), and the discrete areas of consolidation have fused together to become confluent. Nevertheless, the appearances are not those of lobar pneumonia. In another area the pneumonia has progressed to abscess formation (Ab). Towards the upper part of the lung there is great dilatation of bronchi, and the upper lobe shows the typical appearances of advanced bronchiectasis (Bronch). Much of the intervening lung has been destroyed.

Suppuration. Abscess formation is not uncommon, particularly when the host's resistance is exceptionally poor and the causal organism is *Staph. aureus.*

Exogenous bronchopneumonia

A variety of virulent organisms when inhaled may lead to severe bronchopneumonia. The host may be a healthy adult, or else be enfeebled as a result of a previous disease. Examples of virulent organisms causing exogenous bronchopneumonia are:

Staph. aureus, as a result of hospital cross-infection.

Strept. pyogenes. This was particularly common in the 1918 influenza pandemic.

Yersinia pestis—pneumonic plague.

Mycobacterium tuberculosis and the deep-seated fungal diseases. This type of disease is quite distinct, as the lesions produced are characteristically chronic. They are described in Chapter 15.

Mycoplasma pneumoniae is discussed on page 242.

Pneumonia may be due to a variety of *viruses.* Coxsackie viruses, ECHO viruses, and paramyxoviruses have commonly been incriminated in acute pneumonia especially in children. *Respiratory syncytial virus* is a common offender.

The microscopic features of this group of pneumonias are poorly defined, since death from the uncomplicated disease is rare. There is usually a lymphocytic and macrophage infiltrate in the alveolar walls so that the lesion may be described as an *interstitial pneumonia.* There is a variable amount of exudate in the alveoli themselves, and the fibrin component often becomes compressed against the alveolar walls as an eosinophilic lining, or *hyaline membrane.*

OEDEMA OF THE LUNGS[2]

The systolic pressure in the pulmonary artery is 15 to 25 mm Hg, and being much lower than that in the systemic vessels, it follows that there is less tendency to oedema formation. The osmotic effect of the plasma proteins is relatively unopposed. Nevertheless, when oedema does occur, two factors tend to ensure that it persists and even spreads.

1. The loose nature of the lung prevents any appreciable rise in tissue tension, a factor which in other tissues limits the extent of oedema formation.
2. When once the lungs become oedematous, ventilation ceases, the vessels become hypoxic, and they tend to leak. It follows that in all examples of pulmonary oedema the fluid has a high protein content. It is not possible to distinguish between transudates and exudates as in other tissues.

Causes of pulmonary oedema

Acute inflammation. Oedema occurs in the early stages of pneumonia. It is particularly marked in acute lobar pneumonia, and was seen in the broncho-pneumonia which complicated influenza in the 1918 pandemic. The lungs were described as showing acute haemorrhagic oedema rather than bronchopneumonia of the classical type. Such a picture is also seen in poisoning with certain gases, e.g. phosgene, chlorine, and nitrogen peroxide. Acute pulmonary oedema also follows the inhalation of gastric juice such as may occur if a patient vomits during the inexpert administration of a general anaesthetic.

Heart failure. Acute pulmonary oedema is a frequent complication of left ventricular failure and is also common in mitral stenosis. Although increased pulmonary venous pressure is the usual explanation offered for this complication, it is unlikely that this is the major cause of pulmonary oedema in heart failure. More important is the effect of a *redistribution of the blood volume*: attacks of acute pulmonary oedema occur quite suddenly, sometimes at night, and they are probably initiated by peripheral vasoconstriction. The amount of blood in the peripheral circulation is thus diminished, and the excess volume is displaced into the pulmonary circulation where it appears as oedema fluid. Support for this contention is the fact that acute pulmonary oedema is a well-known hazard of adrenaline administration. This drug causes peripheral vasoconstriction. It must never be given to patients with acute pulmonary oedema of cardiac origin. In bronchial asthma this drug is beneficial, but in cardiac asthma it can be lethal.

The terms *cardiac asthma* and *paroxysmal nocturnal dyspnoea* are often applied to these attacks of acute pulmonary oedema. The patient wakes up breathless with a sense of oppression in the chest and sits up, but the dyspnoea increases. Mounting restlessness drives the patient out of bed to seek the fresh air at the window. The sense of suffocation becomes intense, and with it there is profound distress. The skin has an ashen cyanosis, and there is profuse sweating. Blood-stained sputum may be coughed up, and in severe cases a rapidly spreading pulmonary oedema results in death.

Overloading the circulation. If an excessive volume of fluid is administered intravenously, some of the excess is accommodated in the great veins, but the remainder is diverted to the pulmonary circulation and leads to oedema formation. It is obvious that patients already in heart failure are particularly liable to this complication. Transfusion must be carried out very slowly, and packed red cells should be used instead of whole blood if anaemia is to be corrected.

Cerebral damage. Acute pulmonary oedema is sometimes seen following damage to the brain, e.g. after trauma or cerebral haemorrhage. The most likely explanation is that there occurs considerable sympathetic activity, which by leading to peripheral vasoconstriction causes diversion of the circulating fluid to the lungs, as described above.

THE PNEUMOCONIOSES[3]

This group of diseases, produced by the *inhalation of dust*, are mostly occupational in origin. The most important is *silicosis*, which is seen in miners and those who work with finely divided silica. Following the inhalation of this dust there results a chronic inflammatory condition which eventually leads to extensive fibrosis (p. 146). *Asbestosis* produces a similar effect, but, unlike silicosis, is also important in predisposing to cancer of the lung and mesothelioma of the pleura.[4]

Anthracosis, which is due to the inhalation of carbon, is the most common of the dust diseases, because to some extent it affects all city dwellers. The condition is particularly severe in coal miners, but since carbon induces little inflammatory reaction or fibrosis, the miners experience no ill-effects unless there is co-existent silicosis.

CHRONIC BRONCHITIS, EMPHYSEMA, AND BRONCHIAL ASTHMA

In the past, chronic bronchitis, pulmonary emphysema, and bronchial asthma have often been grouped together as *chronic nonspecific lung disease* or *chronic obstructive pulmonary disease*, since they are frequently diagnosed together and have many clinical and pathological features in common. Nevertheless, these conditions are often found separately. Since the origin of these diseases is poorly understood, it is advisable to consider each of them as a separate entity rather than to try to group them under one heading.

Chronic bronchitis[5]

Definition and lesions. This is best defined as a condition in which there is a chronic or recurrent increase in the volume of bronchial mucus, sufficient to cause expectoration, and which is not due to localized bronchopulmonary disease. It is much commoner in tobacco-smokers than in non-smokers, and is very prevalent in England but less so in North America. The bronchial mucosa is thickened by hyperplasia of the mucous glands, and there is an increase in the number of goblet cells in the lining epithelium. True chronic inflammation is not a feature, and Laennec's 'bronchial catarrh' would be a better name.

Recurrent inflammation is a common complication, and may be due to infection or the effects of irritant chemicals—smog is particularly dangerous in this respect.

Effect. The effect of chronic bronchitis is impairment of ventilation due to bronchial narrowing. The mucosa is thickened and there is excess mucus in, and spasm of, the bronchi. Dyspnoea is a prominent symptom, and as the disease progresses respiratory failure develops. The arterial blood is unsaturated and cyanosis occurs. Hypercapnia and right ventricular failure are also common.

The administration of anaesthetics to chronic bronchitics and patients with bronchial asthma is particularly hazardous, since any further increase in mucous production or spasm of the bronchi is liable to precipitate respiratory failure.

Pulmonary emphysema[6,7]

Definition. The word, introduced by Laennec, is derived from the Greek, meaning an inflation. It is defined as a condition in which there is an increase beyond the normal in size of the terminal air passages. Two distinct types occur.

Dilatatory emphysema. Emphysema due to dilatation of the air passages occurs as a compensatory phenomenon following the removal, collapse, or destruction of the adjacent lung. It is of no importance as a cause of respiratory failure.

Destructive emphysema. This is of great importance, and the unqualified term 'emphysema' is generally taken to mean this condition. There is destruction of the alveoli in the walls of the terminal air passages, which are therefore widened. Sometimes large air-filled sacs, or *bullae*, are formed and little lung parenchyma remains. The effect of this lung destruction is to impair gaseous exchange. CO_2 can escape rather more easily than oxygen can be taken up. A common effect is therefore arterial desaturation and cyanosis. Dyspnoea is often marked.

Bronchial asthma[8]

Asthma may be defined as a condition of widespread narrowing of the bronchial airways, which *changes its severity over short periods of time* either spontaneously or under treatment, and is not due to cardiovascular disease. It is characterized by *paroxysms of wheezing dyspnoea.* The bronchial obstruction is caused partly by spasm of the bronchial muscle and partly by the presence of viscid mucus. The disease often has an hereditary basis, and is one of the manifestations of atopy (p. 184). Its pathogenesis is complex; attacks may be the result of hypersensitivity to some inhaled antigen, but psychological and other factors are undoubtedly involved.

TUMOURS OF THE LUNG

The vast majority are epithelial in origin.

Bronchial 'adenoma'

This term, which now serves no useful purpose and should be dropped, has been applied to a group of bronchial tumours that form about 1 per cent of pulmonary neoplasms. The most common type is the carcinoid tumour which arises from neurosecretory cells. The tumour arises in the wall of a large bronchus and causes partial, and finally complete, obstruction. Distal *bronchopneumonia* and *bronchiectasis* are frequent. The tumours are of intermediate type; they invade locally but do not commonly metastasize. Hence lobectomy or pneumonectomy is usually curative.

Other uncommon types of bronchial tumour included under this heading are the mucous-gland adenoma, the adenoid cystic carcinoma, and the mucoepidermoid carcinoma (see p. 253).

Carcinoma[9, 10]

Cancer of the lung now ranks as the commonest lethal cancer in males, and is also frequent in females. Cigarette smoking and atmospheric pollution are major factors in its aetiology. Asbestosis is a predisposing cause, and it was also common in the Schneeberg miners who inhaled radioactive substances.

Gross Appearance. Two common types of tumour may be recognized:

Peripheral lung cancers. These tumours presumably arise in one of the small bronchi or bronchioles, and appear as fairly discrete tumour masses situated in the lung parenchyma. Symptoms are often absent until the pleura and chest wall are invaded, or distant metastases appear.

Central lung cancers. These arise in one of the major bronchi, and therefore cause early obstruction with resulting collapse, bronchopneumonia, and bronchiectasis (Fig. 33.7). Frequently the patient presents with fever and symptoms of pneumonia. Haemoptysis is common, the bleeding being either from the tumour itself, or, more often, from the inflamed dilated bronchi beyond.

Spread. Lung cancer spreads by all the classical routes:

Local spread to involve lung parenchyma, pleura, bronchi, arteries, and veins.

Lymphatic spread to the hilar and mediastinal nodes. This usually occurs early, and is most marked with the oat-cell tumours.

Blood-borne metastases. Secondary tumours are common in the *liver, bones, adrenals,* and *brain.* Even the spleen and bowel, organs not commonly the site of metastases from other tumours, may be involved. It is the frequency of distant spread which makes the prognosis so poor.

Diagnosis. Haemoptysis, recurrent or 'unresolved' pneumonia, or a persistent shadow on the radiograph should always lead to thorough investigation, particularly if the patient is a smoker. Sputum examination may reveal malignant cells. The tumour may be seen and biopsied at the time of bronchoscopy. Even if the tumour is beyond the range of the bronchoscope, mucus or pus may be aspirated from individual bronchi. The finding of malignant cells in a specimen will then localize the tumour. Mediastinoscopy is a useful procedure in which the mediastinum is examined with an instrument that is inserted through a small

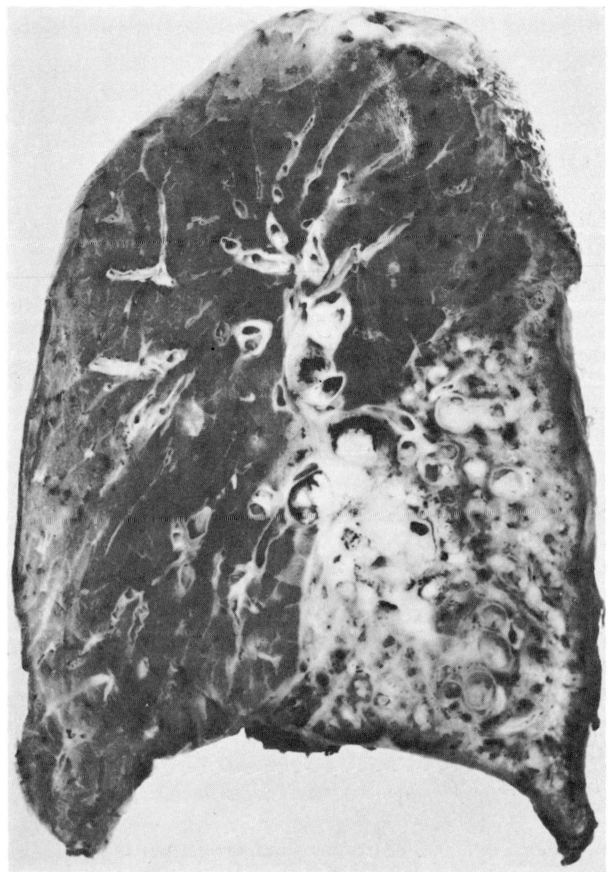

Fig. 33.7 Carcinoma of the lung. This has arisen from the left lower lobe main bronchus and has infiltrated into the lower lobe, which has also undergone fibrosis secondary to collapse, bronchiectasis, and bronchopneumonia. The local hilar lymph nodes are involved. The tumour proved to be a squamous-cell carcinoma. (R45.1. *Reproduced by permission of the President and Council of the Royal College of Surgeons of England.*)

incision in the neck. Enlarged lymph nodes may be detected and biopsied. This investigation also gives the surgeon an indication of whether the tumour is operable. If these investigations are negative, thoracotomy and direct biopsy may be necessary, since a policy of 'wait and see' is rarely justifiable. Carcinoma of the lung should also be borne in mind as a cause of the carcinomatous syndromes described on page 333.

Histological Types. Although arising from a mucus-secreting epithelium, cancers of the lung are remarkable for their histological variations.

Squamous-cell carcinoma. Microscopically this resembles squamous-cell carcinoma arising elsewhere, except that well-differentiated examples are not common. The tumours arise either in areas of squamous metaplasia or by tumour metaplasia in an adenocarcinoma—the latter explanation is the more likely. These tumours may be either central or peripheral, and have the most favourable prognosis.

Adenocarcinoma. These tumours are almost always peripheral, and tend to be more frequent in women. Areas of squamous metaplasia are common.

Anaplastic carcinoma. These tumours show little or no differentiation; two variants are recognized:

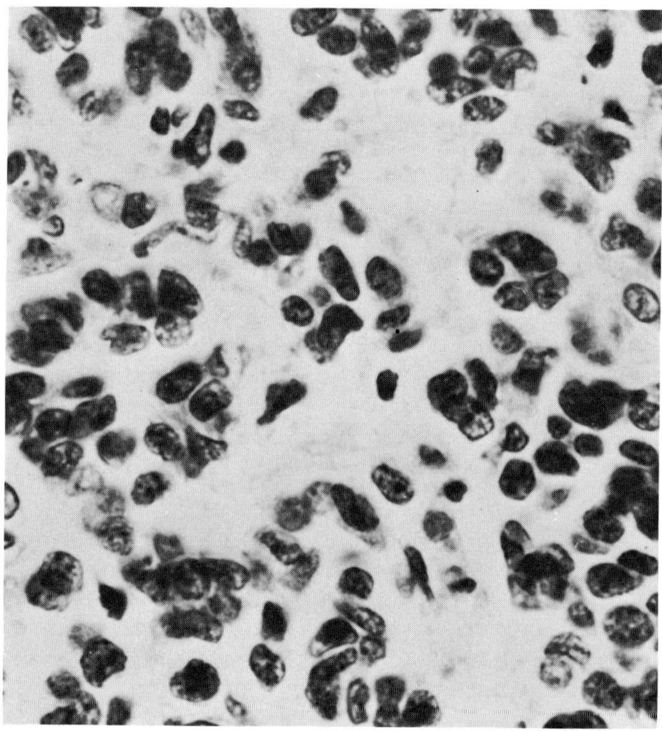

Fig. 33.8 Oat-cell carcinoma of lung. The tumour is composed of sheets of uniform, small, darkly-staining cells, nearly all the substance of which is nuclear. Many have a fusiform shape which gives rise to the descriptive term 'oat cell'. × 320.

Large-cell tumours, which are most probably tumours at the anaplastic end of the scale of squamous-cell carcinoma or adenocarcinoma.

Small-cell, or oat-cell, carcinoma. Oat-cell carcinoma of the lung is a distinct tumour, being derived from neurosecretory cells of the bronchial mucosa akin to the argentaffin cells of the intestine. In this respect it shares a common origin with the carcinoid tumour. The tumour is composed of small, darkly-staining cells, may form small rosettes, and may be round or oat-shaped (Fig 33.8). The tumours are frequently large, and their origin is difficult to determine. They metastasize early and widely. An enormous mediastinal mass may be produced, which impedes the heart's action by directly invading the pericardium and myocardium, and by compressing the great vessels. The tumours are very radiosensitive, but the prognosis is extremely bad.

THE PLEURA

The pleural cavities are normally potential spaces situated between the visceral and parietal pleurae, each lined by flattened mesothelial cells. An accumulation of fluid in the pleural space is called a *hydrothorax*, or *pleural effusion*. There are two types:

A transudate. The fluid has a low protein content and few cells. The most common causes are congestive heart failure and the nephrotic syndrome.

An exudate. An exudate is formed as a result of inflammation or neoplasia involving the pleura. The protein content approximates that of the plasma; inflammatory or neoplastic cells are present in the fluid.

Pleurisy

Inflammation of the pleura (pleurisy or pleuritis) is usually secondary to underlying inflammatory or neoplastic lung disease. This may be apparent, as in lobar pneumonia or in a large area of infarction, or it may be inapparent, as in the pleurisy that accompanies a small tuberculous lesion. Occasionally the cause of the pleurisy is to be found below the diaphragm, e.g. a subphrenic abscess.

Fibrinous pleurisy. 'Dry pleurisy' is associated with a audible friction rub, and can be extremely painful, particularly on deep inspiration. Organization of the exudate leads to the formation of fibrous pleural adhesions.

Serous or serofibrinous pleurisy. 'Pleurisy with effusion' can lead to the accumulation of so much fluid that the affected lung is collapsed. Persistent pleural effusion should always be adequately investigated. Fluid can be withdrawn through a needle and sent for bacteriological and cytological examination. Tuberculosis and carcinoma (primary or metastatic) are two causes that must be considered.

Empyema thoracis

The presence of pus in the pleural cavity is called an 'empyema'. It is generally formed as an extension of infection from a contiguous structure, e.g. bronchopneumonia, a lung abscess, or a subphrenic abscess.

Pneumothorax

The presence of air in the pleural cavity is called a 'pneumothorax'. It may arise suddenly in an apparently healthy person (*spontaneous pneumothorax*), and it is usually due to the rupture of a small subpleural emphysematous bulla. The onset is sudden with severe pain in one side of the chest. Collapse of the lung causes dyspnoea and cyanosis; their severity depends on the amount of air that escapes into the pleural cavity. The condition tends to recur.

Pleural tumours

The most common primary malignant tumour of the pleura is the mesothelioma. This tumour, which is related to asbestosis, forms an encasing mass around the lung. Metastatic tumours, particularly from carcinoma of the breast and lung, are frequent in the pleural cavity.

GENERAL READING

Comroe J H, Forster R E, Dubois A B, Briscoe W A & Carlsen E 1962 The Lung: Clinical Physiology and Pulmonary Function Tests, 2nd edn. 390 pp. Year book medical publishers, Inc. Chicago

Spencer H 1977 Pathology of the Lung, 3rd edn. vols 1–2, 1099 pp. Pergamon Press, Oxford

REFERENCES

1. Campbell E J M & Cade J F 1974 In Clinical Physiology (ed) Campbell E J M, Dickinson C J & Slater J H, 4th edn. Blackwell, Oxford, p 100
2. Staub N C 1970 The pathophysiology of pulmonary edema. Human Pathology 1: 419
3. Wyatt J P 1971 Occupational lung diseases and inferential relationships to general population hazards. American Journal of Pathology 64: 197
4. Leading article 1968 Cancer and asbestos. British Medical Journal 3:448
5. Heard B E 1969 Pathology of Chronic Bronchitis and Emphysema 136 pp. Churchill, London
6. Reid L 1967 The Pathology of Emphysema. Lloyd-Luke, London
7. Leading article 1974 Pathogenesis of emphysema. British Medical Journal 1: 527
8. Pepys J 1972 Asthma. British Journal of Hospital Medicine 7: 709
9. Ashley D J B and Davies H D 1967 Cancer of the lung. Histology and biological behavior. Cancer 20: 165
10. Kreyberg L, Liebow A A & Uehlinger E A 1967 Histological typing of lung tumours, International histological classification of tumours No. 1. World Health Organisation, Geneva.

34

Diseases of the alimentary tract

Although the alimentary tract is usually regarded as being within the body, it is in fact a long tube exposed at each end to the exterior. Its contents, ranging from food in the mouth to faeces in the rectum, are never within the body proper. This is an ideal arrangement, for within the lumen the chemical changes necessary for digestion can occur under conditions which could not be tolerated inside the body itself. One effect of this arrangement is that many litres of digestive fluids are poured into the alimentary tract each day. Normally nearly all of this is reabsorbed, but it can readily be appreciated that if much escaped to the exterior the volume of fluid lost could reach alarming proportions. Vomiting and diarrhoea are potent causes of water and electrolyte depletion, and this is described in Chapter 28. In the present chapter the digestive aspects of the alimentary tract are considered as well as some of its common afflictions.

The mouth, pharynx, and oesophagus[1]

In the mouth food is masticated and mixed with saliva, which, by virtue of its mucus content, performs a lubricating action in addition to commencing carbohydrate digestion by the enzyme ptyalin.

Swallowing (*deglutition*) is triggered off by the voluntary contraction of the pharyngeal and buccal muscles. This, by raising the larynx and tongue, throws the bolus of food against the posterior pharyngeal wall. Thereafter a wave of peristalsis sweeps the bolus down the muscular oesophagus into the stomach.

Difficulty in swallowing (dysphagia). This is caused by a great variety of lesions, a few of which will be mentioned.

1. *Painful conditions* inhibit the voluntary initiation of the act of swallowing, e.g. aphthous ulceration and acute tonsillitis.

2. *Mechanical interference with deglutition* is seen when the pharynx or tongue is infiltrated with scirrhous carcinoma or amyloid.

3. *Mechanical obstruction.* This usually occurs in the oesophagus, and is caused by *carcinoma* (Fig. 34.1), either squamous-cell, which is usually in the middle third of the oesophagus, or adenocarcinoma arising from the lower portion or the stomach. Less common are *benign strictures*, secondary either to chronic peptic ulcer at the lower end or to the destruction and scarring caused by swallowing corrosive acids and alkalis. The dysphagia of the *Plummer-Vinson syndrome* is associated with obstruction at the upper end of the oesophagus (p. 450); a web is

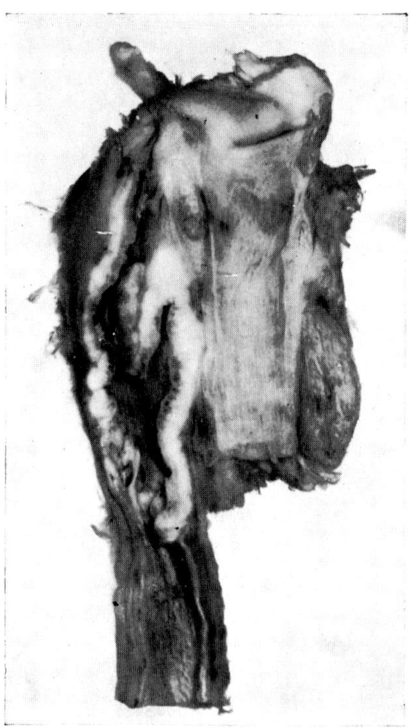

Fig. 34.1 Postcricoid carcinoma of oesophagus. This is a vertical section through the larynx and adjacent oesophagus. The upper part of the oesophagus is surrounded by an infiltrating tumour which has almost completely occluded the lumen. Carcinoma of the oesophagus tends to invade locally and metastasize late, but by the time a diagnosis has been made resection is often difficult or impossible, so that the prognosis is poor.

often present in the anterior aspect of the cricopharyngeal area, but whether or not this causes a mechanical obstruction has been debated for years and is still undecided.

4. *Paralysis of the muscles of deglutition*, e.g. in poliomyelitis affecting the brain-stem and in pseudobulbar palsy (p. 609).

5. *Neuromuscular incoordination.* In elderly people incoordination of the peristaltic waves and muscular spasm may produce a sensation of obstruction and severe pain. In *achalasia of the cardia* there is a degeneration of the ganglion cells of the lower oesophagus, which results in disturbed peristalsis and a failure of relaxation of the cardiac sphincter. As a result the oesophagus becomes greatly dilated.

6. *Psychiatric.* Difficulty in swallowing and a sensation of a foreign body in the throat are familiar accompaniments of fear and anxiety.

For clinical purposes dysphagia may be divided into two groups:

Oropharyngeal dysphagia, in which attempted swallowing may lead to the inhalation of food or its regurgitation through the nose.

Oesophageal dysphagia, in which the common symptom is a sense of obstruction in the chest during swallowing. Carcinoma is the lesion most to be feared, especially if the symptoms are progressive and difficulty in swallowing first affects solids and finally liquids.

Acute streptococcal sore throat. This is an acute infection of the tonsils and adjacent pharynx by *Streptococcus pyogenes.* The onset is sudden, and the sore throat is accompanied by fever, leucocytosis, and malaise. The tonsils and adjacent pharynx are swollen and red, and a white inflammatory exudate is seen on the surface. If the strain of streptococcus produces abundant erythrogenic exotoxin, and if the patient has no immunity to this toxin, the sore throat is shortly followed by an erythematous skin rash. At that stage the disease is called *scarlet fever.*

Streptococcal sore throat is an important disease, because in a number of patients it is followed by acute glomerulonephritis or acute rheumatic fever—conditions that are considered elsewhere.

It should not be assumed that every sore throat, even if accompanied by tonsillar exudate, is due to the streptococcus. Viral infections, for instance those caused by adenovirus and the causative agent of infectious mononucleosis, can have a very similar clinical appearance, although the onset is generally more insidious. In the past it was essential to consider diphtheria in the differential diagnosis; now, however, the disease is extremely uncommon in the Western world. The diagnosis of diphtheria rests on obtaining a positive culture from a throat swab.

The stomach

In the stomach the masticated food is softened, moistened, lubricated, and partly digested by the gastric juice. It is kneaded by strong muscular contraction into a semiliquid mass called *chyme*, which is passed steadily into the *duodenum.*

The gastric juice has four major components:

Mucus, which has a lubricating action
Intrinsic factor, without which vitamin B_{12} cannot be absorbed
Pepsin, which commences protein digestion
Hydrochloric acid. This has an important bactericidal action, and also provides the correct pH for the action of pepsin. Its presence is important in the pathogenesis of one of the common disabling afflictions of human beings—*peptic ulceration.*

Wherever acid gastric juice comes into contact with a non-acid-secreting mucosa, peptic ulceration is liable to occur. It is therefore seen at the pylorus, along the lesser curve of the stomach, in the first part of the duodenum, at the lower end of the oesophagus, and at the site of anastomosis between the stomach and small intestine following gastro-enterostomy.

Acute ulceration

Acute erosions.[2] Acute shallow ulcers, commonly called erosions, are often seen in the stomach. They are usually multiple, and appear to be caused by dietary indiscretions, alcohol, and the action of irritant drugs, e.g. aspirin. They are shallow and involve little more than the covering epithelium. Healing is rapid and complete. Slight bleeding is common, and may occasionally be severe.

Acute ulceration of the stomach or duodenum is also seen as a complication of burns and any severe injury, e.g. major surgery, and may be related to vagal overactivity. There are usually multiple ulcers and they usually heal rapidly with minimal scarring, but may occasionally erode a large vessel or perforate into the peritoneal cavity, giving rise to severe haemorrhage or peritonitis. Sometimes, after trauma, there is a generalized oozing of blood from the congested gastric mucosa. In this way much blood is lost without an obvious localized bleeding point.

Chronic peptic ulcer

Chronic ulcers are usually solitary, and present a characteristic appearance. The destructive process penetrates beneath the mucosa to the underlying muscle layers, and this produces a deep, round or oval, punched-out ulcer with straight edges. For reasons which are not known regeneration of the epithelium is inhibited, and chronic inflammation ensues. Healing of the destroyed stomach or duodenal wall is by granulation tissue, and the base of the ulcer consists of inflamed vascular granulation tissue covered by necrotic tissue which forms a slough. Bleeding is therefore common. Deeper in the base of the ulcer the granulation tissue matures to form scar tissue.

Clinical features. Pain in the epigastrium is common and is related to the gastric acidity and spasm of the muscle. It is usually relieved by meals and especially by the administration of alkalis.

Complications. *Haemorrhage.* Repeated bleeding is a common cause of iron-deficiency anaemia (p. 449). Sometimes the ulcer becomes attached to an adjacent structure, e.g. the pancreas, and a large artery is eroded. This leads to a massive haematemesis and melaena.

Perforation. When the ulcer penetrates to the peritoneal surface it produces a localized fibrinous inflammation which may cause adjacent structures to become adherent to it. If this does not occur the ulcer may perforate, and the gastric or dudodenal contents are poured into the peritoneal cavity. The patient immediately experiences excruciating pain, and generalized peritonitis soon develops.

Cicatrization. As an ulcer heals, the scar tissue is apt to contract and cause stenosis. Pyloric ulcers are particularly liable to this complication, and the resulting pyloric stenosis causes severe vomiting. This leads to dehydration and metabolic alkalosis.

Aetiology. Remarkably little is known about the cause of peptic ulceration. Without the acid content of the gastric juice peptic ulceration cannot occur, but hypersecretion of acid is not constantly related to ulcer formation. Hyperchlorhydria is usually associated with duodenal ulcers but not with gastric ulcers. Other factors that may play a part in the formation of ulcers are a demanding occupation, overwork, smoking, and emotional stress. Genetic factors have also been incriminated; thus, duodenal ulceration is more common in patients who are of blood group O. All of these factors, however, appear to be contributory—the precise pathogenesis of the ulceration is not known.

Cancer of the stomach

This tumour is not uncommon in Northern European communities, but its incidence is now lower than that of colonic cancer. It is very common in the Japanese. The tumour is either of the fungating, cauliflower type, or else it appears as a typical malignant ulceration. Occasionally the tumour cells invade the stomach wall so diffusely that no definite mass exists. Instead the whole wall is thickened by dense scirrhous tumour (*diffuse infiltrating carcinoma of the stomach* or *linitis plastica*). Histologically the cancer is usually a poorly-differentiated adenocarcinoma. Even with early excision the prognosis is extremely bad because there is usually early spread to the regional lymph nodes and the liver.

The small intestine

The small intestine consists of the duodenum, the jejunum, and the ileum and, in all, is about 20 feet long. The chyme that leaves the stomach is acted upon by bile, the pancreatic enzymes, and the intestinal secretion (*succus entericus*). The last contains few enzymes; the most important of these is *enterokinase*, which converts trypsinogen to trypsin—a conversion that is an essential step in the activation of pancreatic enzymes. The function of the small intestine is therefore the final breakdown of fat, carbohydrate, and protein, as well as the absorption of the products formed. The complex structure of the mucosa with its numerous villi is well adapted to this function. Likewise, the microvilli of each luminal cell are designed for absorption of the products of digestion. The glycocalyx (Fig. 2.5) is thought to contain enzymes, including the important disaccharidases. These are responsible for splitting disaccharides (e.g. sucrose and lactose) into monosaccharides (e.g. fructose and glucose); in this form these sugars can be absorbed.

From this brief account of the functions of the small intestine it is evident that any derangement caused by disease can easily by accompanied either by malabsorption or by the loss of large quantities of fluid and electrolytes.

Acute inflammations of the small intestine

Food poisoning. Acute enteritis is often accompanied by inflammation of the stomach. Such an acute *gastroenteritis* produces vomiting, diarrhoea, and abdominal pain; it may be severe, but it is rarely fatal. Many causes of gastroenteritis can be recognized:

1. *Chemicals.* Poisoning may be deliberate (e.g. by ingestion of arsenic) or accidental (e.g. by ingestion of poisonous mushrooms or spoiled potatoes).
2. *Bacterial toxins.* If *Staphylococcus aureus* or *Clostridium welchii* are allowed to grow in food, such as in a meat pie, they produce toxin that causes acute gastroenteritis when ingested.
3. *Bacterial infection.*[3] Many strains of *Salmonella* are recognized that produce an acute, but fleeting, infection of the small intestine. Enteropathic strains of *Escherichia coli* cause some cases of infantile diarrhoea as well as some examples of traveller's diarrhoea (variously known as 'Delhi belly,' 'Gyppy tummy,' 'Montezuma's revenge,' etc).
4. *Viral infection.* The important causative agent is the rotavirus. Other viruses, e.g. enteroviruses and adenoviruses have been identified in the faeces, but their significance is unknown.
5. *Idiopathic.* No agent can be incriminated in many cases.

Typhoid fever. Typhoid fever is a specific type of enteritis and is described in Chapter 7.

Cholera. Cholera has often been described as an acute enteritis, when in fact its pathogenesis is quite different from that of a simple inflammation. The disease, which is caused by a vibrio, has been responsible in the past for several pandemics that have originated in the Bengal basin. The disease is characterized by the sudden onset of intense vomiting and diarrhoea, which rapidly lead to dehydration and hypovolaemic shock, to be followed by death within 2 or 3 days in about one third of the cases. With efficient treatment by fluid and electrolyte administration, the mortality can be reduced to under 1 per cent.

Cholera is acquired by ingesting water or food contaminated with the organism. The bacteria are not killed by the acid in the stomach, and thus pass into the small intestine where they multiply and elaborate enterotoxin that acts on the plasma membrane of the intestinal epithelial cells. Cyclic AMP is formed and induces a tremendous outpouring of water and electrolytes into the intestinal lumen. A large quantity of fluid flows into the colon, which is unable to absorb the load. The result is a severe diarrhoea with watery stools ('rice-water stools').

Crohn's disease (regional enteritis)[4]

Crohn's disease is a chronic inflammatory disease that can affect any part of the alimentary tract, even the mouth, but it is usually most obvious in the lower small

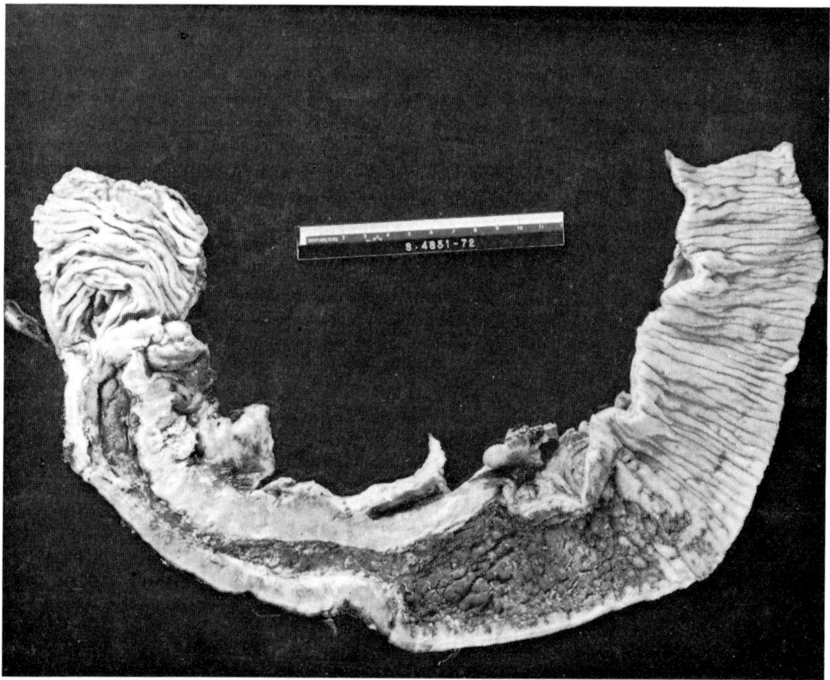

Fig. 34.2 Crohn's disease of ileum. Resected specimen of the terminal ileum, ileocaecal junction, caecum, and a small portion of the ascending colon from a man aged 22 years. The terminal ileum shows great thickening and rigidity of its wall; the lumen is reduced in size and the mucosa has a characteristic cobblestone appearance. The disease stops sharply at the ileo-caecal valve. Microscopically, the affected bowel showed transmural oedema, fibrosis, and the presence of non-caseating tuberculoid granulomata. (*Photograph by courtesy of Dr J. B. Cullen*).

intestine. The bowel shows a chronic inflammatory response that involves the entire wall. The lumen becomes narrowed, leading to the development of intestinal obstruction (Fig 34.2); constipation alternates with diarrhoea. An outstanding feature of the disease is the formation of small abscesses on the mucosal surface of the bowel; these penetrate the muscularis to the serous coat. The inflammatory reaction leads to a localized peritonitis with adhesions between the abdominal organs. Sinuses and fistulae develop, so that communications are established between adjacent loops of intestine, the colon, the bladder, and the skin surface. The cause of the disease, which tends to affect young adults, is unknown. Treatment by resection of the affected bowel is sometimes successful, but recurrence in other areas is quite common. The course is therefore protracted, and the condition presents great problems both to patient and attendants.

The malabsorption syndrome

This is described in Chapter 18.

THE LARGE INTESTINE

The colon has two main functions: the absorption of water and electrolytes and the formation of a convenient receptacle for faeces, so that they may be discharged at the individual's own convenience. Acute inflammation of the colon results in a derangement of its functions, and the diarrhoea that results causes great inconvenience as well as a considerable loss of water and electrolytes. Two severe infections are recognized:

Bacillary dysentery[3]

This is an acute infection of the colon caused by organisms of the genus *Shigella*. The incubation period is short (24 to 48 hours), and the disease is characterized by fever, abdominal pain, and diarrhoea which can lead to severe dehydration and death. The faeces are fluid and contain blood, mucus, and pus.

Amoebic dysentery

This is caused by a protozoon, *Entamoeba histolytica*, which invades the colonic mucosa and produces shallow ulceration. The disease may be acute with severe bloody diarrhoea, but more usually it is chronic, and the patient has several foul-smelling, sometimes blood-stained stools each day. Occasionally the amoebae invade the blood stream and cause *amoebic hepatitis*; a liver abscess may ensue.

Both types of dysentery are most common in the tropics and in those who live under crowded, unhygienic conditions.

Idiopathic ulcerative colitis[4]

Now the commonest cause of serious bowel disease in Britain and North America, idiopathic ulcerative colitis affects all age groups and often starts in young adult life.

The diseases generally commences with an acute attack of colicky abdominal pain accompanied by diarrhoea and the passage of blood, mucus, and pus in the faeces. Fever and malaise are also present. The acute attack generally subsides and is followed by chronic ulcerative colitis with recurrent exacerbation of symptoms. Pain, diarrhoea, and the passage of blood, mucus, and pus are intermittent.

The disease generally affects the rectum and distal colon most severely, and in the acute phase it is characterized by intense hyperaemia of the mucosa. On proctoscopy the mucosa bleeds at the slightest touch. In due course mucosal ulcers

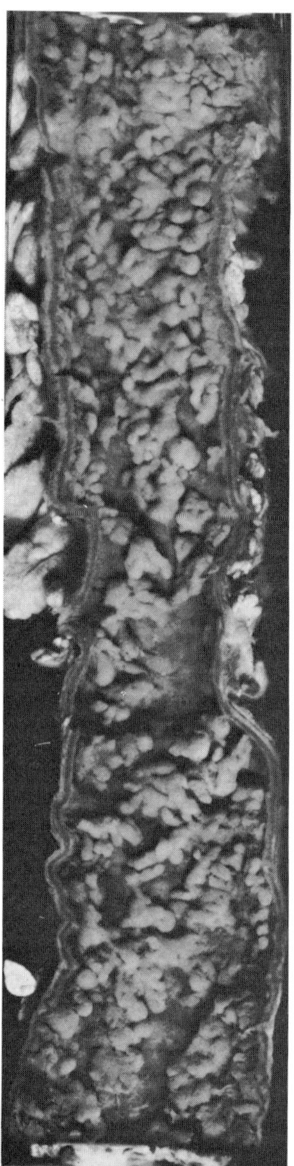

Fig. 34.3 Chronic ulcerative colitis with pseudopolyposis. The apperance of these multiple foci of polypoid overgrowth of epithelium is to be distinguished from true polyposis coli. In pseudopolyposis the bowel itself is chronically inflamed, and in this specimen the wall is considerably contracted. Furthermore, the intervening mucosa is roughened and inflamed. In polyposis coli there is no evidence of inflammation. (EA 70.1, *Reproduced by permission of the President and Council of the Royal College of Surgeons of England*)

develop, these tending to undermine the mucous membrane so that tags, or pseudopolyps, are formed (Fig. 34.3). The ulcers are covered by a slough. Deep to this is an inflammatory reaction from which the blood and pus are derived.

In chronic ulcerative colitis the disease tends to remain confined to the mucosa.

Because the muscle coat itself and the peritoneal surface of the colon are not generally affected, adhesions do not form between adjacent viscera and there is usually no perforation or fistula formation. In this respect the disease differs markedly from Crohn's disease, which can also affect the colon.

Ulcerative colitis generally pursues a chronic intermittent course, producing misery to the patient and leading to anaemia, general debility, and loss of weight. A further complication is the development of carcinoma. It has been estimated that about one third of the patients who suffer from the disease for more than 12 years develop cancer. For this reason and because of the symptoms of the disease, total colectomy is sometimes performed, and the patient is left with a permanent ileostomy. The ileum is brought to the surface of the anterior abdominal wall, a permanent opening is created, and a suitable container is attached.

Ulcerative colitis is occasionally very acute, either at its inception or at some stage in its development. The colon becomes acutely congested, its muscle becomes atonic, and the bowel dilates enormously. This type of disease follows a fulminating course; generally, the transverse colon is involved, and the patient becomes extremely ill. Multiple perforations develop, and the patient dies of toxemia associated with peritonitis. This variant of ulcerative colitis is called *acute toxic megacolon.*

Diverticular disease of the colon

The current Western diet, which contains inadequate cellulose (roughage), is believed by some authorities to be responsible for the high frequency of colonic diverticula. This disease is most frequent in the distal part of the colon—particularly the sigmoid area. Apart from the presence of numerous diverticula, the most striking change is muscular hypertrophy and shortening of the colon—presumably due to the muscular overactivity that is necessary to propel the small, hard faeces. The diverticula themselves consist of outpouches of the mucosa that penetrate weak points in the muscular coat. Often they are covered merely by a thin layer of peritoneum. Sometimes the orifices of the diverticula become obstructed by faecal material, and inflammation ensues. Overlying peritonitis with the formation of adhesions, pericolic abscesses, and fistulae develops. The condition is then called *diverticulitis.* Sometimes a mass of chronic inflammatory tissue forming in the bowel wall is sufficient to cause obstruction and to simulate carcinoma. Occasionally diverticular disease can cause massive bleeding, which is life-threatening.

Carcinoma of the large intestine

The large bowel ranks with lung and breast as the most common site of fatal malignant disease in Europeans. The rectum and sigmoid colon are most frequently involved (Fig. 34.4). The tumour is usually a well-differentiated adenocarcinoma, and it breaks down to produce a typical carcinomatous ulcer. This tends to encircle the gut and produce obstruction. The passage of blood and mucus in the stools with constipation alternating with diarrhoea are the usual clinical features. The tumour invades locally, metastasizes to the regional lymph nodes, and finally invades the blood stream to give metastases in the liver and elsewhere. Growth is often relatively slow, so that the prognosis following resection is well correlated with the stage of the tumour (see p. 337).

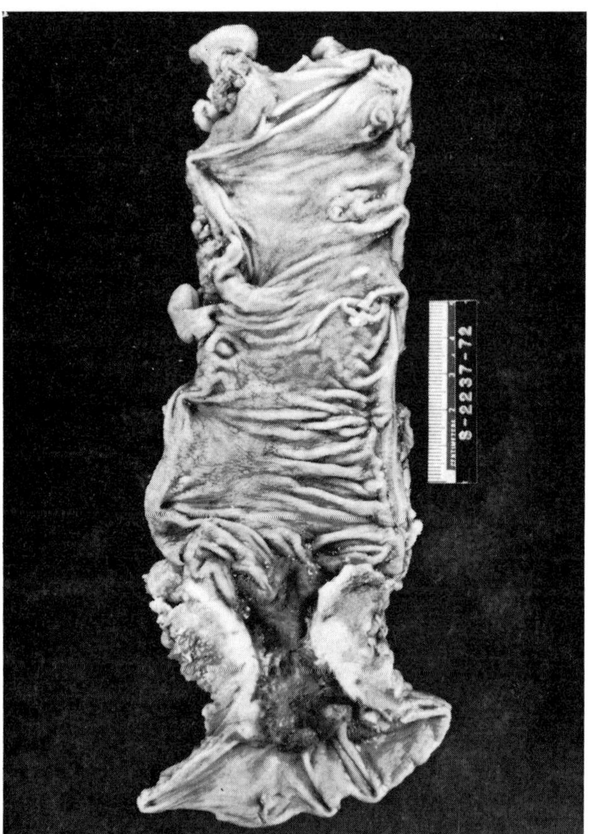

Fig. 34.4 Carcinoma of colon. This resection specimen from a man aged 66 years shows an adenocarcinoma at the recto-sigmoid junction. The tumour involves the whole circumference of the gut, and has produced stenosis. The pericolic fat has been invaded, and several regional lymph nodes contained metastatic carcinoma. (*Photograph by courtesy of Dr J. B. Cullen*)

Carcinoid tumours of the intestine

These are not common but are of great interest. They occur in the appendix, ileum, colon, and occasionally in the stomach and pancreas. They are derived from the argentaffin cells, and are of intermediate malignancy. Tumours of the appendix tend to remain localized, but the ileal ones sometimes produce metastases in the liver. These lead to the *carcinoid syndrome*—diarrhoea, valvular lesions of the right side of the heart, asthmatic attacks, and periodic flushing of the face. The pathogenesis of this syndrome is not clear, but the release of 5-hydroxytryptamine by the tumour, the activation of the plasma kinins, and the deposition of platelets on the heart valves are all involved.

REFERENCES

1. Morson B C, Dawson I M P 1972 Gastrointestinal Pathology, A reference book in 676 pages, Blackwell, Oxford
2. Leading article 1974 Erosive gastritis. British Medical Journal 3: 211
3. Christie A B 1974 Infectious Diseases: Epidemiology and Clinical Practice, 2nd edn. Churchill Livingstone, Edinburgh. See, in particular, Chapter 2, 'Food Poisoning: Salmonellosis'; Chapter 4, 'Bacillary Dysentery'; and Chapter 5, 'Infantile Gastroentiritis'
4. Colcock B P 1972 Benign ulcerative and granulomatous lesions of the bowel. Surgery Annual 4: 285

35

Diseases of the liver

The liver is the largest organ in the body and its functions are manifold. Both anatomically and functionally it occupies a key position in relation to the digestive system, for nearly all the venous blood from the gastrointestinal tract reaches it *via* the portal vein. It is therefore not surprising that the liver performs many functions connected with fat, carbohydrate, and protein metabolism. Another activity of the liver is the secretion of bile, which, in addition to having a digestive role, also contains the end-products of haemoglobin metabolism.

Degenerative conditions

The liver cells, or *hepatocytes*, are very susceptible to the effects of many poisons. Poisonous mushrooms (*Amanita phalloides*), carbon tetrachloride, chloroform, and many drugs (important among which is the anaesthetic agent halothane) can all cause severe liver damage, either by direct action or by some type of hypersensitivity response. Infections, in particular with the viruses of hepatitis, can also produce liver damage (see Ch. 16).

The effects of hepatotoxic agents can vary from mild cloudy swelling and fatty change to extensive necrosis.

Hepatic necrosis

Types. If the liver cells are severely affected, they die and undergo necrosis. This usually has a *zonal distribution*, which means that the cells of a particular zone in every lobule undergo necrosis—*centrilobular necrosis* is the most common (Fig. 35.1 (*b*)). Sometimes the foci of necrosis are erratically distributed; this is termed *focal necrosis*, or spotty necrosis. It is typical of viral hepatitis.

Occasionally the necrosis is more extensive and involves wide tracts of liver. Whole lobules are destroyed, and the name *massive necrosis* is appropriate.

Results. The outcome of necrosis depends upon the severity of the lesions:

Zonal and focal necrosis. The patient may have no symptoms, or suffer from an acute febrile illness with jaundice and gastrointestinal symptoms and then recover. The necrotic liver cells autolyse and are removed. The sinusoidal structure and reticulin framework of the liver lobules remain intact, and as the surviving liver cells divide, the destroyed ones are replaced, and there is complete restoration of the liver to normal (Fig. 35.1 (*a*)).

Massive necrosis. The patient may die of liver failure in the acute phase—this is seen after acute poisoning and occasionally in viral hepatitis, but quite often no cause can be found. If the patient survives, the lobular structure of the necrotic liver collapses, and the destroyed areas are replaced by scar tissue. Isolated groups of liver cells show regeneration, but since there is no normal scaffold on which they may disperse, they form irregular nodules called *regeneration nodules*. The final result is a form of *cirrhosis of the liver* (Fig. 35.1 (*c* and *d*)).

Hepatocellular degeneration and fatty change

The changes are described in detail in Chapter 4. Cloudy swelling, hydropic

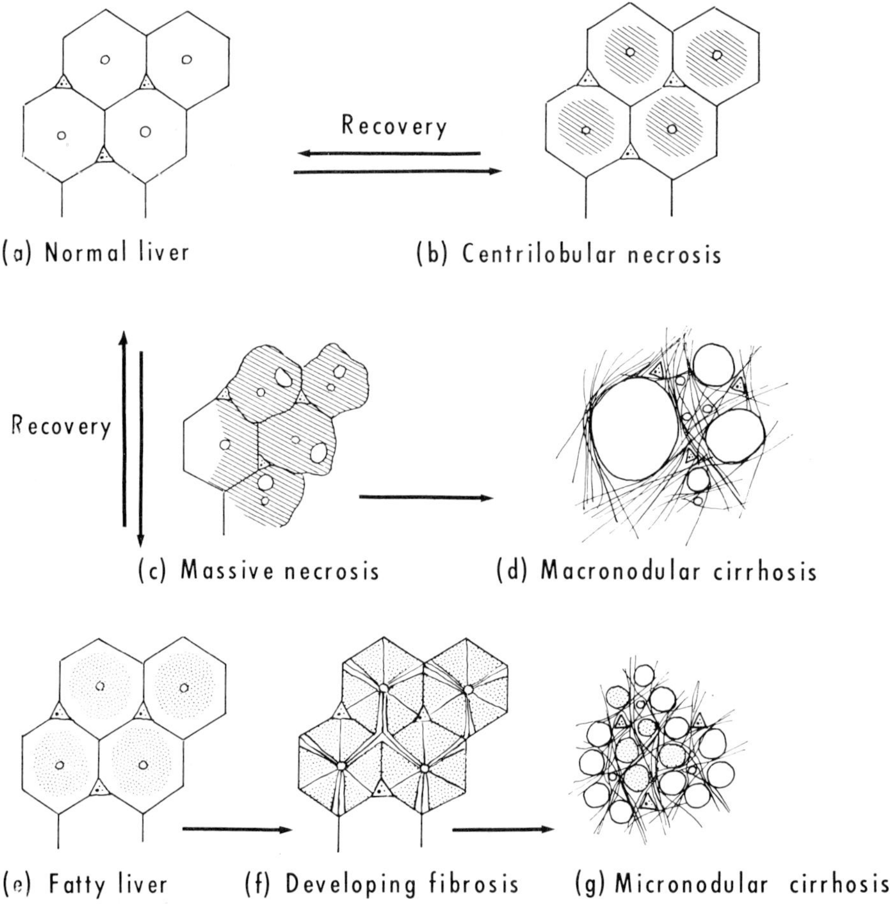

Fig. 35.1 The pathogenesis of cirrhosis. (a) Depicts four normal liver lobules as hexagonal structures each with a central hepatic vein. Between the lobules are the portal triads, each containing branches of the hepatic artery, bile duct, and portal vein. In (b) there is centrilobular necrosis, and when liver cell regeneration occurs there is complete return to normal. (c) Shows massive necrosis with collapse of the affected lobules. When regeneration occurs, a coarsely nodular cirrhotic liver is produced as depicted in (d); in some areas normal lobules will be found. A fatty liver (e) may return to normal. However, if it persists over a long period, fibrous septa form and these divide up the lobules (f). Some liver cells degenerate, and as regeneration occurs a finely nodular cirrhotic liver develops (g). No normal lobules remain. (*Drawn by Margot Mackay, Department of Art as Applied to Medicine, University of Toronto.*)

degeneration, and fatty change may all result from the effects of poisons, hypoxia, or infection. Fatty change is the most important lesion, and is often caused by an inadequate diet. It is also common in *chronic alcoholism.*

If the cause of the fatty liver is removed, complete recovery is usual—not so if the condition is allowed to persist indefinitely, particularly if it is due to alcoholism. Gradually fibrous tissue forms, and hepatic cells become isolated as the lobules are split up (Fig. 35.1 (*f*)). Some cells undergo necrosis, others regenerate, and there results a finely nodular cirrhotic liver not fundamentally different from that seen after massive necrosis (Fig. 35.1 (*g*)). The fatty liver of kwashiorkor does not predispose to cirrhosis.

Alcohol and the liver

There can be little doubt that alcohol abuse can adversely affect the liver; whether this is due to a direct toxic action of alcohol on the liver cells or to an effect of the imbalanced diet of the addict has yet to be decided. The liver of the chronic alcoholic often shows fatty change, and in some subjects this progresses to cirrhosis. Acute episodes of alcohol intake result in patchy liver cell necrosis. The cells contain alcoholic hyaline, and foci of necrosis are accompanied by a polymorph infiltration. This condition, which is called *alcoholic hepatitis*, is a phase in the evolution of alcoholic cirrhosis.

Hepatitis

Acute viral hepatitis

Two distinct epidemiological types of acute viral hepatitis are known. In *infective hepatitis* due to virus A, the disease commonly occurs in institutions like schools and military camps. It is contracted by the ingestion of contaminated food, and has an incubation period of about 1 month. In *serum hepatitis*, caused by virus B, the disease is usually contracted by an injection of contaminated serum. The nature of the infective agents is described in Chapter 16.

Symptoms of viral hepatitis. The onset is usually insidious with mild fatigue, lassitude, and sometimes fever. Nausea, vomiting, and diarrhoea are not uncommon, and an aversion to both food and cigarette smoking is a curious symptom. Such an influenza-like illness may be the only manifestation of hepatitis, but in other patients the disease progresses and jaundice appears, at first evident in the conjunctivae and later in the skin. Some tenderness over the liver may be noticed, and enlargement of the organ may be detected. Recovery is the usual end-result, but it may take 3 or 4 months, or even longer. The two forms of hepatitis have similar clinical features, although serum hepatitis tends to be more severe, and in an appreciable number of cases the disease progresses either to massive hepatic necrosis ending in death or to a chronic form of liver disease culminating in cirrhosis.

Chronic hepatitis

The term *chronic hepatitis* encompasses a number of different conditions that have three features in common:

1. Infiltration of liver by inflammatory cells, usually lymphocytes and plasma cells. The infiltrate is concentrated in the portal triads
2. Necrosis of liver cells
3. Fibrosis of the liver that may terminate in cirrhosis.

The diagnosis of chronic hepatitis is generally made on the liver biopsy. The following types can be recognized:

Chronic active hepatitis. This disease is characterized by recurrent attacks of hepatitis, ultimately developing into cirrhosis, usually of the macronodular type, which is fatal within 10 years. The disease was first described as affecting young people, 75 per cent of the patients being women. Hypergammaglobulinaemia is a characteristic feature, and both antinuclear factor and rheumatoid factors are usually present. Although the disease was originally called *lupoid hepatitis*, there is no evidence that the condition is related to lupus erythematosus itself. Nevertheless, over half the patients also have arthritis. Antibodies that react with smooth muscle are present in most cases, and the disease therefore has a strong autoimmune component.

The syndrome of chronic active hepatitis has now been extended to include other groups of patients. Some are middle-aged women, and others are men who usually have HBsAg in their blood. Autoantibodies are usually present, but this autoimmune component is less striking than in the original lupoid hepatitis.

Other types of chronic hepatitis. There are other types of chronic hepatitis that do not fit into the entity designated chronic active hepatitis. Some are cases of patients who have recovered from an acute attack of viral hepatitis, and yet have evidence of continuing liver damage. Others are asymptomatic and yet are chronic carriers of the hepatitis antigen. Still others have neither HBsAg nor demonstrable autoantibodies in their plasma. Viral infection, resolving alcoholic hepatitis, and drug-induced liver damage are suggested as possible causes in the heterogeneous group of conditions labelled chronic hepatitis.

Cirrhosis of the liver

The term 'cirrhosis' (from Greek *kirrhos*, orange yellow + *nosos*, disease) was introduced by Laennec, who was impressed by the tawny colour of the liver in this condition, but this is due merely to fatty change of the liver cells. The important structural features of cirrhosis are the *destruction of the liver parenchyma* and its *replacement by fibrous tissue*, thereby disrupting the normal lobular architecture. There is also active regeneration of the liver cells occurring at the same time as this fibrous reparative process. The *formation of regenerative nodules* is the third essential component of cirrhosis (Fig. 35.2).

Cirrhosis is best regarded as an *end-stage condition*, as it can be the end-result of liver damage due to many causes—poisons, alcohol, inadequate diet, infection, genetic error, etc. Classifications are very unsatisfactory since in many cases the cause is unknown (cryptogenic cirrhosis). A descriptive classification is the most useful and is based on the liver's nodularity. If the nodules are small and of uniform size (Fig. 35.3) the term *micronodular cirrhosis* is applied. This contrasts with *macronodular cirrhosis* (Fig 35.1 d), in which the nodules are of varying size and many of them are large. Micronodular cirrhosis may be idiopathic, but is often found in alcoholics with fatty liver; the macronodular type follows massive necrosis. It must be emphasized that there is no sharp line of division between these two types of cirrhosis.

Symptoms and complications of cirrhosis. Cirrhosis is commonly asymptomatic until some complication makes the condition obvious. The appearance of jaundice, oedema of the ankles, or progressive abdominal enlargement may bring the disease to the attention of the patient. Increasing

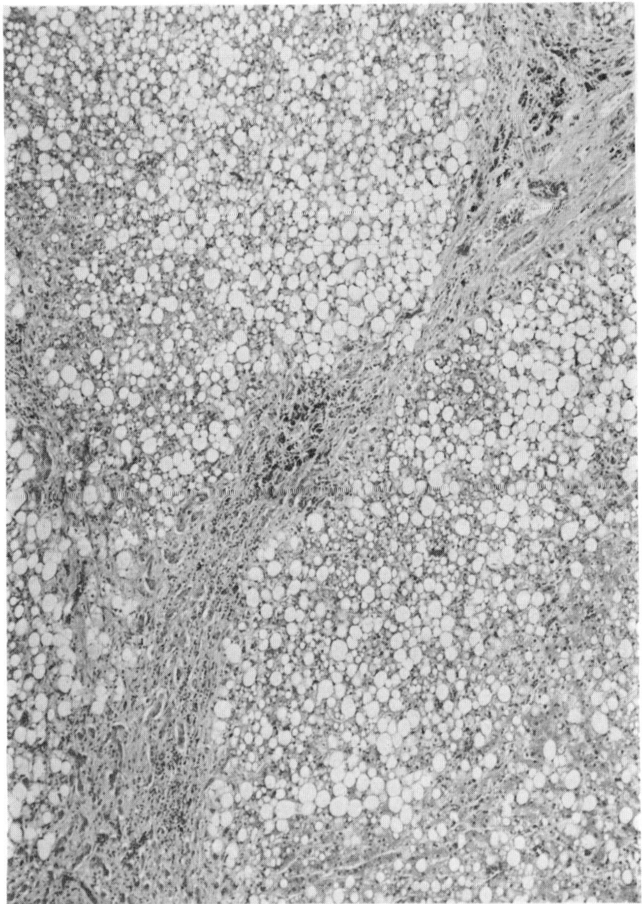

Fig. 35.2 Micronodular cirrhosis. A thick strand of cellular fibrous tissue intersects two nodules, the cells of which show severe fatty change. × 40.

weakness, loss of weight, loss of body hair, and testicular atrophy are all features that may appear. Commonly the first symptom is massive haematemesis and the rapid development of hepatocellular failure with coma and death.

During the development of cirrhosis many branches of the portal and hepatic veins are obliterated. The pressure in the portal radicles rises (*portal hypertension*), and blood from the portal vein is shunted into the systemic veins following the development of anastomoses. This *portal-systemic shunting* of blood has two serious effects:

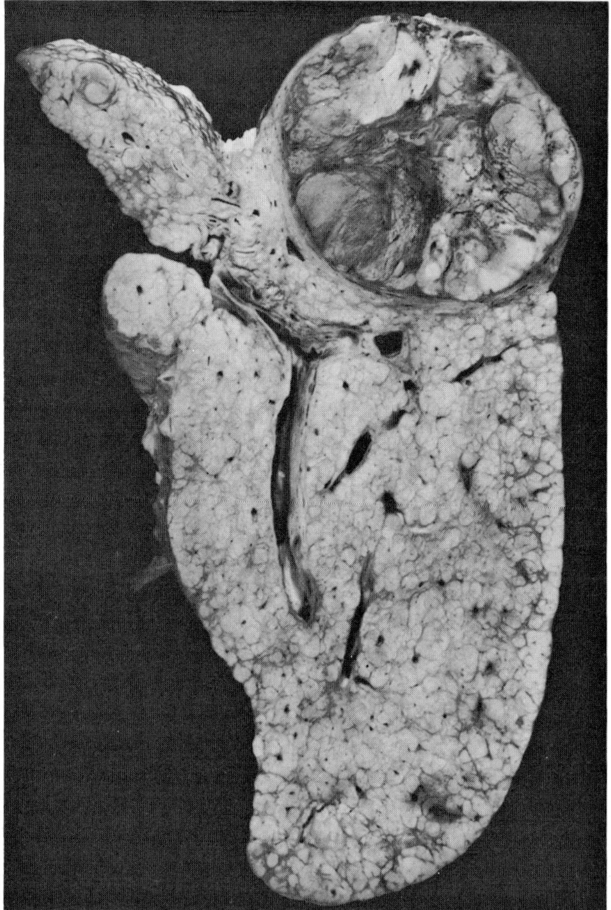

Fig. 35.3 Cirrhosis of the liver. A section through the liver shows the regular pattern of small, uniform nodules typical of micronodular cirrhosis. At the top of the specimen there is a large rounded tumour which, in the fresh state, was white in colour and partly bile stained. Histologically it was a well-differentiated adenocarcinoma. The patient was an elderly man who had no history of liver disease, but died with a haemoperitoneum consequent on rupture of the hepatoma. (A108.1, *Reproduced by permission of the President and Council of the Royal College of Surgeons of England.*)

Haemorrhage. An important group of anastomoses develops at the lower end of the oesophagus. The veins are thin-walled and tend to bleed. Sudden, massive, and often fatal haemorrhage is the result. The blood is usually vomited up (*haematemesis*).

Intoxication. Products from the intestine by-pass the liver and reach the remainder of the body. This leads to a *faecal odour* of the breath, and is thought to be the cause of the confused mental state and *coma* which patients dying of cirrhosis often develop.

Ascites. Fluid in the peritoneal cavity is common in cirrhosis, and is in part due to the portal hypertension. Hypoalbuminaemia and hyperaldosteronism are other factors in the pathogenesis of ascites and the generalized oedema which sometimes develops.

The main cause, however, appears to be obstruction of the flow of blood through the liver. This obstruction is postsinusoidal, and results in an increased rate of formation of lymph in the liver. Normally the lymph is drained away by lymphatics into the thoracic duct, but in cirrhosis the vast excess of lymph produced oozes, or weeps, from the liver, and drips into the peritoneal cavity. The ascites of cirrhosis of the liver is therefore a type of lymphoedema. If this ascites is relieved by draining the fluid, much albumin is also removed, and this adds to the patient's problems. Furthermore, the sudden removal of a large quantity of fluid can lead to hypovolaemia and shock.

Hepatocellular failure. The other symptoms of terminal cirrhosis—including neuro-psychiatric features, coma, and haemorrhagic tendency—are described under hepatocellular failure.

Biliary cirrhosis

Obstruction to the bile duct, particularly if combined with infection (cholangitis), can sometimes lead to such severe liver-cell damage that cirrhosis develops. There is, in addition, a *primary form of biliary cirrhosis.* This is most frequently encountered in middle-aged women. Itching is usually the first symptom, and this is followed by the development of obstructive jaundice. The disease has an autoimmune component, for the blood contains IgM antibodies active against bile-duct components as well as IgG antimitochondrial antibodies. The detection of the latter is a useful diagnostic feature of primary biliary cirrhosis.

Bile formation and jaundice

Of all the symptoms of liver disease, *jaundice*, or *icterus*, is the most immediately apparent. Nearly all the tissues in the body are coloured a bright yellow. In addition to the skin, the conjunctivae and oral mucous membrane are discoloured, and in the early stages jaundice is sometimes most apparent in these sites, especially in dark-skinned individuals. Jaundice is due to an excessive amount of bilirubin in the plasma and tissues. Its development can be understood only in relation to bilirubin metabolism (Fig. 35.4).

Bilirubin metabolism. When red cells are broken down, the porphyrin moiety of the haemoglobin is converted into *bilirubin* in the cells of the reticulo-endothelial system. Bilirubin is insoluble in water, and following its release from the RE cells it is carried in the blood stream attached to albumin. The liver has three important functions in regard to bilirubin:

1. It *extracts* it from the blood
2. It *conjugates* it with glucuronic acid to form bilirubin diglucuronide
3. It *excretes* the conjugated bilirubin into the bile.

Under normal conditions 15 to 20 per cent of the bilirubin excreted is derived from sources other than red-cell destruction. Some of this originates from the bone marrow during the formation of haemoglobin (*ineffective erythropoiesis*); the remainder is derived from the metabolism of porphyrins present in enzymes and elsewhere. The amount formed by ineffective erythropoiesis may be increased in disease, for example pernicious anaemia, and contribute to the jaundice.

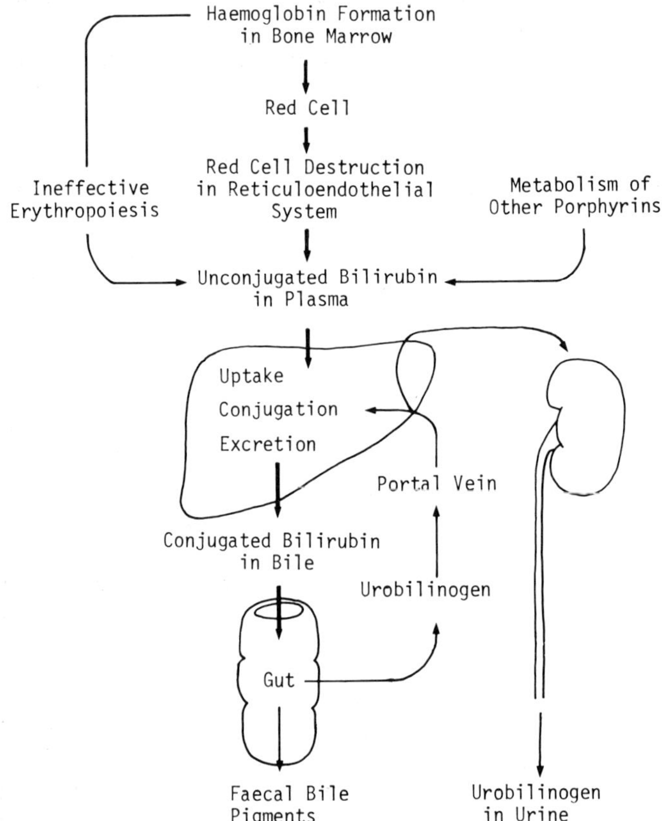

Fig. 35.4 Metabolic pathways in the formation and excretion of bilirubin.

Bilirubin is estimated in the plasma by means of the diazo reagent. Bilirubin diglucuronide reacts directly with this reagent to form diazobilirubin, a red dye that can be measured colorimetrically. This is called the *direct van den Bergh reaction;* the amount of conjugated bilirubin is increased in the plasma in cases of obstructive jaundice (see below). Unconjugated bilirubin, on the other hand, since it is insoluble in water, does not react with the diazo reagent until it is brought into solution by the addition of alcohol. This is called the *indirect van den Bergh reaction;* it measures the total bilirubin content of the plasma, since after the addition of alcohol both conjugated and unconjugated bilirubin are measured. The normal plasma bilirubin level is 5 to 17 μmol per litre (0.3 to 1.0 mg per dl).

Types of jaundice

Obstructive jaundice. This occurs when there is an obstruction to the passage of conjugated bilirubin from the liver cells to the intestine. The bilirubin diglucuronide is absorbed back into the blood, and if the obstruction is complete the patient rapidly becomes deeply jaundiced. The conjugated bilirubin is soluble in water, and is easily excreted by the kidneys. Therefore the *urine is dark*. This contrasts with the faeces, which are clay coloured due to the lack of bile pigments. Little stercobilinogen is formed in the intestine, little is returned to the liver, and virtually none escapes into the urine. Two major types of obstructive jaundice may be recognized. In one (*extrahepatic cholestasis*) the bile duct is blocked, for instance by a gallstone in its lumen or by a carcinoma of the head of the pancreas. In the second type the obstruction is assumed to be in the liver itself (*intrahepatic cholestasis*). One important cause of this is the administration of certain drugs, for example chlorpromazine (Largactil) and other phenothiazine derivatives. Intrahepatic cholestatic jaundice is an occasional complication of pregnancy; it is also seen in the acute fatty alcoholic liver and sometimes during the early stages of acute viral hepatitis.

Three other characteristic features of obstructive jaundice should be noted:

1. *Pruritus.* Often severe, the condition is probably due to retention of *bile salts*
2. *Malabsorption.* Due to the lack of bile in the intestine, this is a feature of chronic biliary obstruction
3. *Hypercholesterolaemia.* This condition is due to increased synthesis by the liver rather than to biliary obstruction. Lipid-laden macrophages accumulate in various organs, and may form tumour-like masses called *xanthomata.* These lesions tend to be bright yellow because of their content of carotene; they are most obvious in the skin.

Haemolytic jaundice. This is the second type of jaundice to be considered. The excessive destruction of red cells causes an increased rate of bilirubin formation, and the liver is unable to deal with the increased load. The bilirubin in the blood is unconjugated, and is therefore insoluble in water and not excreted in the urine. This type of jaundice is said to be *acholuric.* The faeces contain an excess of stercobilin, and the amount of urobilinogen returned to the liver is increased. Haemolytic jaundice rarely reaches the intensity of the obstructive variety. An exception to this is that seen in haemolytic disease of the newborn. Because unconjugated bilirubin is relatively soluble in lipids, bile pigments pass into the brain tissue and can cause severe damage to the developing central nervous system in severe cases of haemolytic jaundice of infancy. This is called *kernicterus.*

Hepatocellular jaundice. This is considered below.

Hepatocellular failure

It is convenient to complete this survey of liver disease by summarizing the important features of liver-cell failure. It is often called *cholaemia*, and may occur as a terminal event in many forms of liver disease. Thus it is seen in necrosis, cirrhosis, and occasionally when the organ is extensively involved by tumour.

Manifestations of liver-cell damage

Jaundice. This is due partly to a failure of the liver to take up bilirubin from the blood, and partly to its failure to excrete conjugated bilirubin. This hepatocellular variety of jaundice is therefore of mixed type. Normally the liver converts most of the stercobilinogen absorbed from the intestine into bilirubin, and excretes it in the bile. In liver-cell damage this function is impaired, and an excess of stercobilinogen reaches the kidney and is excreted as urobilinogen (Fig. 35.4).

Neuropsychiatric manifestations (hepatic encephalopathy). These pathological conditions assume many forms. Patients with chronic liver disease often exhibit steady deterioration in their intellect: forgetfulness and confusion can progress to stupor and finally to coma. Ataxia and a characteristic 'flapping' tremor of the outstretched hands are noteworthy accompaniments. The neuropsychiatric manifestations may be chronic, with the patient exhibiting personality changes, mental deterioration, and other neurological symptoms. On the other hand, the syndrome may be acute and terminate in coma with convulsions.

Animals with a portacaval, or Eck shunt,* can be maintained in a reasonable state of health if given a low-protein diet. If given a large protein meal, they develop coma and die rapidly ('meat intoxication'). It is believed that these manifestations are caused by nitrogenous substances; their precise nature is not known. Hepatic encephalopathy is seen in patients who have undergone a similar portacaval anastomosis in the treatment of cirrhosis of the liver.

The liver is the principal site of deamination of amino acids and is probably the only organ that can convert the ammonia so produced into urea. The other site of ammonia formation is the intestine, where it is formed by bacterial decomposition of protein. Shunting of this ammonia from the portal blood into the systemic circulation is a possible cause of cerebral dysfunction.

Acute encephalopathy is sometimes precipitated by bleeding oesophageal varices; the explanation is that the large quantity of protein-containing blood passes into the intestine and amounts to a heavy protein meal. Since bacterial action in the intestine appears to lead to the formation of damaging nitrogenous products, the administration of the antibiotic neomycin is currently recommended.

Haemorrhagic tendency. The liver manufactures all the plasma clotting factors, with the exception of Factor VIII. In liver disease a haemorrhagic tendency is not uncommon. Surgery, even dental extraction, should be attempted with caution.

Hypoalbuminaemia. The liver also manufactures albumin, and it is not surprising that the plasma level falls in many chronic liver diseases. Hypoalbuminaemia contributes to the formation of ascites and generalized oedema.

Failure of detoxification. Many drugs, e.g. morphine and barbiturates, are detoxified or excreted by the liver. In patients with liver failure a normal dose of such a drug may precipitate coma and death.

A failure in the metabolism of oestrogen is the suggested cause of the testicular atrophy and gynaecomastia (enlargement of the male breast) that are associated with hepatic cirrhosis. Likewise, a failure to metabolize aldosterone may be the explanation of the hyperaldosteronism.

Fever. Pyrexia is not uncommon, but its cause is not known.

In the terminal stages severe electrolyte imbalance occurs. The patient sinks

* This is an artificial shunt made surgically between the portal vein and the inferior vena cava. Portal blood tends to flow directly into the vena cava rather than through the liver.

into a state of cholaemic coma with deepening jaundice, and the end is precipitated by renal, cardiac, or peripheral circulatory failure.

Tumours of the liver

Benign tumours are rare and unimportant. *Primary carcinoma* is an occasional complication of cirrhosis, and is therefore quite common in those countries where this disease is rife. Metastatic deposits of tumour are extremely common in the liver in cases of disseminated malignant disease. The common sites for the primary carcinoma are the breast, lung, and gastrointestinal tract.

A raised level of *alkaline phosphatase* in the plasma is characteristic of metastatic tumour and is a useful clinical test. Each nodule of tumour obstructs a number of small bile ducts, and the test is positive before there is significant retention of bilirubin. Jaundice is not common in tumours of the liver unless it is associated with cirrhosis or it occurs as a terminal event. This emphasizes the tremendous reserve capacity of the liver and its ability to regenerate (see also p. 129).

GENERAL READING

Sherlock S 1975 Diseases of the Liver and Biliary System, 5th edn, 821 pp, Blackwell, Oxford

Scheuer P J 1974 Liver Biopsy Interpretation, 3rd edn, 171 pp, Baillière, Tindall and Cassell, London

Schiff, L (ed) 1975 Diseases of the Liver, 4th edn, 1461 pp, Lippincott, Philadelphia and Toronto

36

Diseases of the kidney

The function of the kidneys

The kidneys are essential for life because of the part they play in the excretion of waste products and in the regulation of the extracellular fluid. They control the concentration of its various electrolytes, contribute to acid-base balance, and are intimately concerned in the regulation of water balance. These functions depend on the secretion of urine, which entails two distinct processes:

1. The passive filtration of plasma through the glomeruli, so that the escaping fluid is similar to plasma except that it is virtually free of protein
2. The passage of this filtrate through a complex system of tubules, where its content of solutes is altered and its pH is modified. The resulting fluid is urine.

The glomerulus and its tubule together constitute the *nephron*, and this opens into a large collecting tubule which empties into a calyx of the renal pelvis. From here the urine passes down the ureter to the bladder, where it is held until it can be voided by micturition.

Many alterations take place in the composition of the glomerular filtrate as it passes through the tubules:

There is reabsorption of all the glucose, about 80 per cent of the water, and many electrolytes from the *proximal convoluted tubule.*

There is an active secretion of hydrogen and potassium ions by the *distal convoluted tubule*, and this is balanced by a reabsorption of sodium, chloride, and bicarbonate ions.

There is reabsorption of more water in the *distal convoluted tubules and the collecting tubules*—this function is under the control of the pituitary antidiuretic hormone, which makes the tubular cells more permeable to water exchange, while sodium reabsorption from the *distal tubule* is controlled by aldosterone.

Renal failure: Uraemia

Renal failure is a state in which the body's metabolism is deranged as the result of dysfunction of the kidneys. Renal insufficiency usually first manifests itself in a disturbance of urine formation and this is followed by various systemic effects which culminate in a clinical syndrome described as *uraemia.* The most conspicuous biochemical feature of uraemia is the retention of nitrogenous substances in the blood. An indication of the extent of dysfunction may be obtained by measuring the plasma urea level . . . normally 2.5 to 6 mmol per litre or 15 to 35 mg per dl . . . or if expressed as blood urea nitrogen (BUN) it is 2.9 to 8.9 mmol per litre or 8 to 25 mg. pr dl. The plasma creatinine level rises similarly.

Clinical features of uraemia

Since the diagnosis of uraemia is largely clinical, it is convenient to describe its main features at this stage:

1. Cerebral symptons, e.g. drowsiness, headache, convulsions, and coma. These are possibly due to disturbances of fluid balance and the retention of ill-defined waste products.
2. Deep, sighing respirations, which are due to metabolic acidosis.
3. Muscular twitchings, and occasionally muscular spasms, due probably to hypocalcaemia.
4. Nausea, vomiting, and diarrhoea. These are possibly due to the excretion of urea into the stomach and intestine, where it is converted into ammonia by the urease secreted by local organisms.
5. Hiccup, gastrointestinal bleeding, pruritus (itching of the skin), purpura, and acute fibrinous pericarditis.
6. Infection, particularly bronchopneumonia, is common, and may be the terminal event.

Although many of the features of uraemia are unexplained at the present time, it seems certain that electrolyte imbalance and failure in acid-base regulation are more important than is the retention of nitrogenous substances.

Renal insufficiency may either appear acutely, or else develop gradually as a terminal feature of chronic destructive renal disease. These two types will be considered separately.

Acute renal failure. This manifests itself by a sudden diminution in the urinary output (*oliguria*), and this may be followed by complete cessation (*anuria*). This must not be confused with sudden failure to pass urine due to an obstruction, an event which commonly affects men with prostatic enlargement and is called *retention of urine.*

Acute renal failure is a common clinical emergency, and is usually due to *sudden renal ischaemia due to vasoconstriction.* This occurs:

1. Whenever there is a sudden decrease in blood volume such as may follow severe haemorrhage, burns, and persistent vomiting or diarrhoea
2. Following the escape of free haemoglobin or myoglobin into the circulation, as after incompatible blood transfusions and crushing injuries to the muscles of the limbs
3. Following certain complications of pregnancy.

If the cause is remedied in time, the change may be reversed without any structural damage to the nephron, but if it persists, necrosis of parts of the tubules follows (*acute tubular necrosis*). This may lead to death, and even if the patient survives it may take many months for renal function to be completely restored.

Acute tubular necrosis and acute renal failure may also be caused by certain poisons, e.g. carbon tetrachloride (used in fire extinguishers) and diethyl glycol (used in antifreeze).

Other causes of acute renal failure include: acute bilateral renal artery obstruction such as is caused by dissecting aneurysm of the aorta, acute renal disease such as acute glomerulonephritis and pyelonephritis particularly when associated with papillary necrosis, and certain infections, e.g. leptospirosis.

The manifestations of acute renal failure are severe oliguria—complete anuria occurs in the worst cases—associated with the retention of nitrogenous substances, potassium, phosphate, and other anions in the blood. The pH of the blood falls due to the failure of tubular secretion of hydrogen ions (*metabolic acidosis*), and there is an increase in the volume of extracellular water. The patient may die of overhydration, potassium intoxication, infection, or the retention of unclassified toxic metabolic products.

If the patient survives, there follows a period when large quantities of urine are passed (*polyuria*), because the kidneys cannot conserve electrolytes and water. Life is then in jeopardy because of dehydration and electrolyte loss. Regeneration of tubular epithelium occurs quite rapidly, but a perfect functional recovery is unusual.

Chronic renal failure. This too is common in clinical practice, and is usually due to *chronic destructive renal diseases* like chronic pyelonephritis, glomerulonephritis, and bilateral renal tuberculosis. *Vascular disease*, e.g. malignant hypertension, is another cause, and so is *obstruction to the outflow of urine*, as follows prostatic enlargement, urethral stricture, and cancer of the pelvic organs. *Hypercalcaemia* (p. 300) and *diabetes mellitus* (p. 275) also lead to kidney damage and chronic renal failure.

The manifestations of chronic renal failure are complex and diverse. There is usually moderate dehydration, as the diseased kidneys cannot conserve water and sodium properly. Potassium is usually retained, and a metabolic acidosis develops. Phosphate retention is a prominent feature, and it may, if longstanding, lead to a reciprocal lowering of the plasma calcium level and secondary hyperparathyroidism.

Many chronic renal diseases are complicated by *hypertension*. A fall in afferent arteriolar pressure stimulates renin formation (p. 478), but it is uncertain whether this is the means whereby hypertension occurs in renal disease.

Another feature of chronic renal failure is intractable *anaemia*. The kidneys secrete erythropoietin (p. 448), and it may be that the production of this hormone is impaired in chronic renal disease. Both acute and chronic renal failure, if unrelieved, culminate in *uraemia* which is the harbinger of death.

The protein-losing kidney

Normally only a trace of protein escapes into the glomerular filtrate, and this is reabsorbed by the proximal tubule. There are a number of conditions in which the permeability of the glomerulus is increased, so that large amounts of protein escape into the filtrate and are voided with the urine. Albumin, the smallest of the plasma proteins, is affected the most severely, and hypoalbuminaemia results. The occurrence of proteinuria, hypoalbuminaemia, and oedema is called the *nephrotic syndrome*, and it may be a complication of such chronic diseases as glomerulonephritis, diabetes mellitus, renal amyloidosis, and systemic lupus erythematosus. It may also occur in *nephrosis* as a primary lesion of the glomerulus. Several entities are recognized. In some types, particularly the nephrosis of children, the glomeruli appear normal by light microscopy but abnormalities can be detected electron-microscopically. In other types, the basement-membrane zone is seen by light microscopy to be thickened, a change which is described as 'membranous'. The disease is alternatively known as idiopathic membranous glomerulonephritis.

The main features of the nephrotic syndrome are:

1. Severe proteinuria
2. Hypoproteinaemia, especially affecting the albumin level of the plasma
3. Generalized oedema due in part to the hypoproteinaemia and perhaps also to hyperaldosteronism
4. Susceptibility to infection, due possibly to a loss of immunoglobulins in the urine
5. A raised level of lipids in the blood. The plasma cholesterol (normally 6.5 mml per litre or about 250 mg per dl.) may exceed 26 mml pr litre or 1000 mg pr dl. The cause of this is unknown.

In the early stages renal function is well maintained and the blood pressure is normal, but later renal failure and uraemia may occur.

Glomerulonephritis

Glomerulonephritis is a term applied to a group of diseases that are not obviously of infective nature, and in which the glomeruli are primarily affected. Although many classifications have been proposed, none has been found to be satisfactory. The types at present recognized have been delineated on the basis of three parameters:

1. Clinical features. The clinical features of glomerulonephritis vary enormously. The onset may be acute with haematuria and oliguria (*acute glomerulonephritis*), or the onset may be insidious with signs of renal failure developing over a period of many months (*chronic glomerulonephritis*). Proteinuria is invariable, and if severe leads to the nephrotic syndrome. One important type of glomerulonephritis is associated with infection by *Streptococcus pyogenes*. This post-streptococcal glomerulonephritis may be either acute or chronic.

2. Immunological findings. Glomerulonephritis is a feature of immune-complex disease, and it is thought that renal damage follows the deposition of immune complexes in the glomeruli. The kidneys are therefore damaged as 'innocent bystanders'.The immune complexes can contain antigen derived from organisms (e.g. streptococci and malaria parasites), tumour antigen (the nephrotic syndrome can complicate malignancy), or endogenous antigen (e.g. DNA-anti DNA complexes in lupus erythematosus).

Occasionally deposits of immunoglobulin are found in the kidney that are directed against kidney antigens, usually glomerular basement membrane material. The detection of antigens and immune complexes in kidney disease is performed by immunofluorescent techniques.

3. Histopathological findings. Light microscopy, aided by electron microscopy, reveals several types of changes. For example there may be proliferation of mesangial cells and deposits of material (mostly immunoglobulin) in the glomerular basement membrane zone (*proliferative glomerulonephritis*, see Figs. 36.1 and 36.2). Widening of the basement membrane zone may be sufficiently

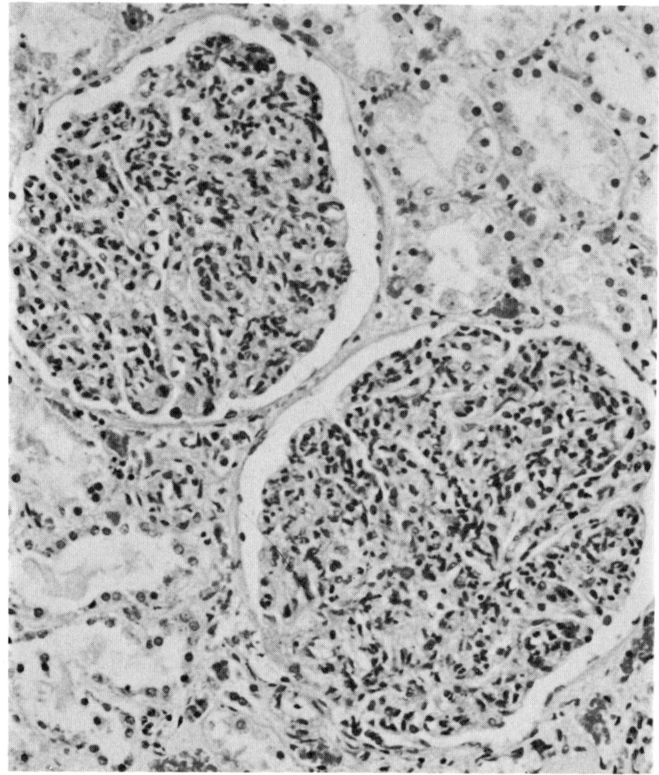

Fig. 36.1 Acute glomerulonephritis. The two glomeruli included in the section are considerably enlarged. They are hypercellular due to an infiltration of polymorphs and a proliferation of mesangial cells. The vascular lumina have been occluded, with the result that few red cells are present in the tuft. × 200.

marked to be visible on light microscopy (*membranous glomerulonephritis*). Both these patterns may be combined (*membranoproliferative glomerulonephritis*). When the glomerular damage is severe, it often stimulates the parietal epithelial cells to proliferate and produce a *crescentic glomerulonephritis* (Fig. 36.3).

A characteristic electron microscopic finding in glomerulonephritis is fusion of the foot processes of the epithelial cells (podocytes) of the glomeruli (Fig. 36.4). This appears to be an effect of the increased permeability of glomerular vessels to protein and is therefore present whenever there is proteinuria.

The technique of needle biopsy, by which a core of kidney substance can be

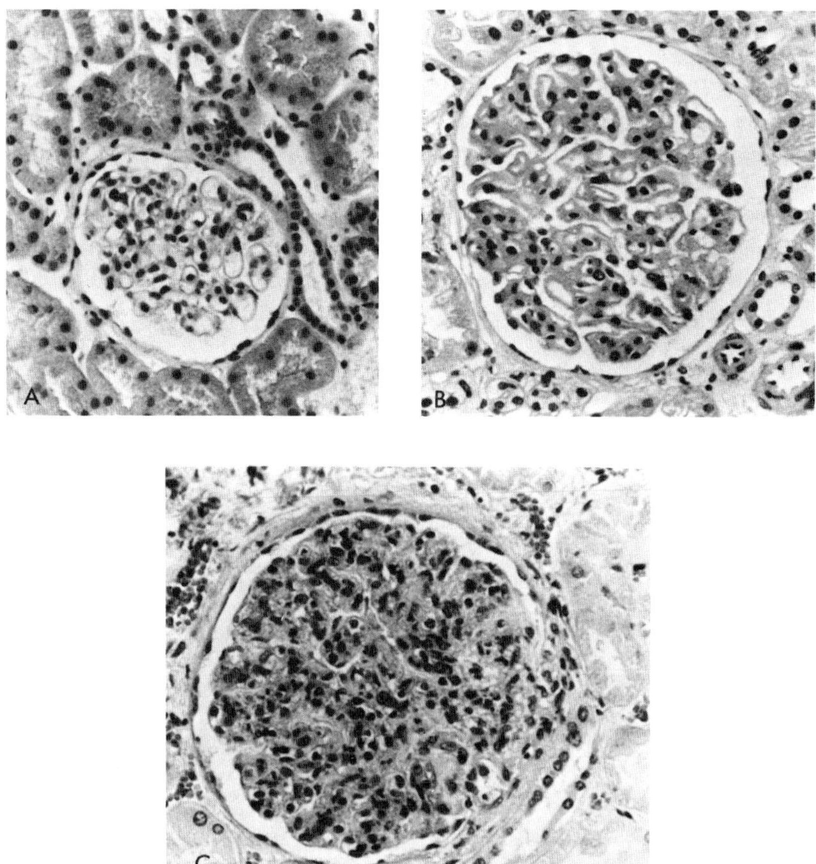

Fig. 36.2 Glomerulonephritis. *A*. Normal glomerulus. *B*. Membranous glomerulonephritis. Note the thickening of the basement membrane of the glomerular capillaries. *C*. Proliferative glomerulonephritis. The glomerulus is enlarged and shows increased cellularity that is due partly to mesangial proliferation and partly to a polymorph infiltration. × 450.

removed safely during life, has greatly aided the investigation of renal disease in patients. The material obtained is particularly suited for immunofluorescent studies and electron microscopy as well as for routine light-microscopic examination.

Types of glomerulonephritis

The diagnosis of glomerulonephritis is the task of the expert who has access to such sophisticated tools as electron microscopy and immunofluorescence: for a detailed account of the various types specialised texts should be consulted.

In one type of glomerulonephritis (*minimal-change glomerulonephritis*) the glomeruli appear normal under light microscopy, but under electron microscopy fusion of the foot processes of the epithelial cells is revealed. Most patients with this type of disease are children with a nephrotic syndrome. In *post-streptococcal glomerulonephritis* (Bright's disease) the changes during the acute phase are those of a proliferative glomerulonephritis. The illness occurs from 1 to 6 weeks after a streptococcal infection, and is characterized by oliguria and haematuria with oedema, particularly of the face. Infection with certain strains of *Streptococcus pyogenes* (nephritogenic strains e.g. type 12) are particularly liable to be followed by glomerulonephritis, and the organisms are thought to share an antigen with the human glomerulus. Cross-reacting antibodies are assumed to cause the renal damage. The majority of patients (about 80 per cent) recover completely, and death rarely occurs during the acute phase; this is generally due to heart failure associated with hypertension. A number of patients develop a rapidly-progressive disease which terminates in uraemia. These patients show severe glomerular

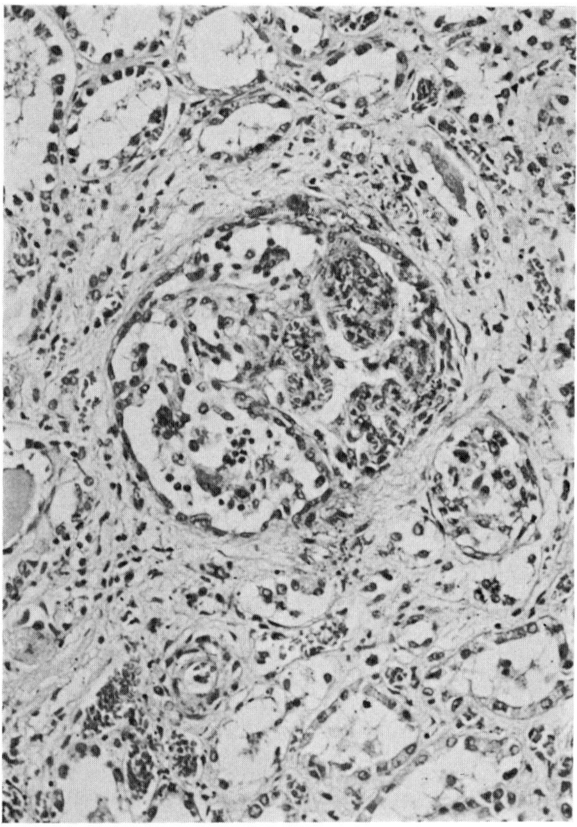

Fig. 36.3 Chronic glomerulonephritis. The glomerular tuft is severely deformed and shows a somewhat lobular appearance. There are adhesions between the tuft and the cells of the parietal layer of Bowman's capsule. In one segment these cells have proliferated sufficiently to form an early crescent. The proximal convoluted tubules are atrophic and there is some increase in the amount of interstitial tissue. × 200.

damage with crescent formation (Fig. 36.3). The remainder develop a slowly-progressive disease with the glomeruli ultimately being replaced by hyalinized collagenous tissue. The tubules undergo atrophy and there is fibrous replacement of the renal parenchyma (chronic glomerulonephritis). The disease may be silent for a long time apart from moderate proteinuria, but eventually the manifestations of chronic renal failure and uraemia develop. Hypertension and heart failure are common. Some cases develop a nephrotic syndrome.

At autopsy the kidneys are reduced in size and display a fine granular surface (Fig. 36.5). At this stage it is frequently impossible to be certain of the nature of the original disease. Such *end-stage kidneys* can result from many types of glomerulonephritis, nephrosclerosis, chronic pyelonephritis, interstitial nephritis, diabetic nephropathy, etc.

Other types of renal disease

Lupus nephritis. Glomerulonephritis of either a proliferative or a membranous type is common in systemic lupus erythematosus (Fig 36.4). It often causes a nephrotic syndrome and ultimately leads to renal failure.

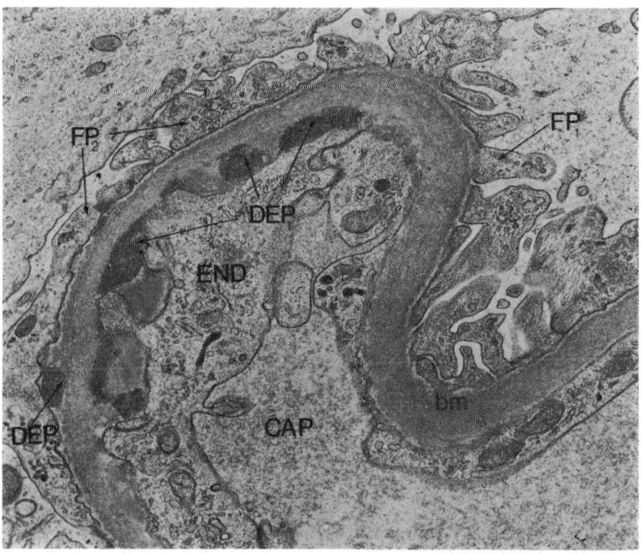

Fig. 36.4 Electron micrograph of glomerulus in systemic lupus erythematosus. In some areas the foot processes (FP_1) of the podocytes appear relatively normal, but elsewhere they are swollen and spread over the basement membrane (bm) of the capillary (FP_2). This change is commonly described as 'fusion of the foot processes'. Prominent subendothelial deposits are present (DEP_1). Subepithelial deposits are smaller and less obvious (DEP_2). In this patient the deposits were shown by immunofluorescence to contain IgG and components of complement. × 27 500. (*Photograph by courtesy of Dr Y. Bedard.*)

Nephrosclerosis. Nephrosclerosis is a term used to descibe the renal lesions of systemic hypertension (see Ch. 31). In the *benign type*, the arteriolosclerosis causes patchy ischaemia. The affected nephrons become atrophic and are ultimately replaced by scar tissue. Hence, the kidneys in benign nephrosclerosis show thinning of the cortex and a granularity of the surface. In malignant hypertension the arteriolar necrosis causes extensive patchy foci of necrosis (*malignant nephrosclerosis*). Renal failure is a common cause of death.

Interstitial nephritis. Interstitial nephritis is characterized by an inflammatory reaction in the interstitial tissues. This is associated with tubular damage, and the glomeruli are spared until late in the course of the disease. Acute interstitial nephritis can lead to death from acute renal failure; however, the disease is usually chronic. Some cases are caused by drug intake—particularly intake of the pencillin derivative methicillin. Another group is due to the prolonged intake of large doses of analgesic drugs, particularly aspirin-phenacetin mixtures (causing *analgesic nephropathy*). The condition generally arises from self-medication. Many cases of interstitial nephritis are idiopathic and are difficult to distinguish from chronic pyelonephritis, since the pathological findings of the two diseases are very similar.

Diabetic nephropathy. This condition is described in Chapter 17.

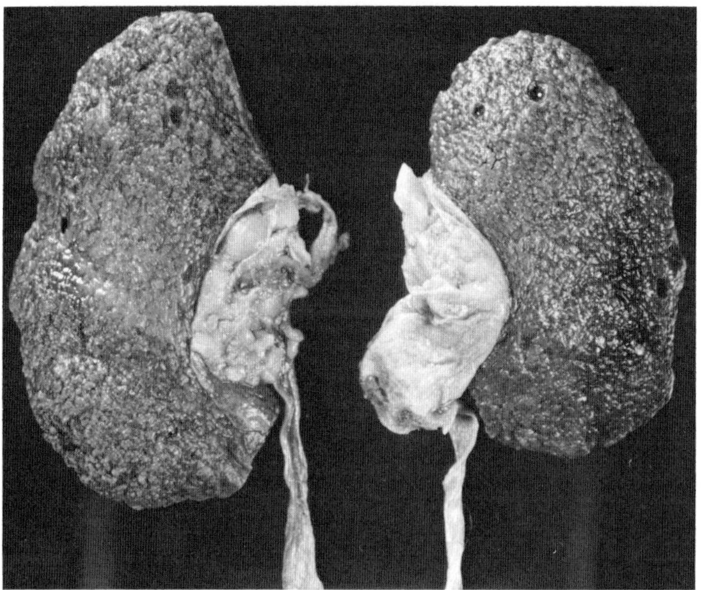

Fig. 36.5 Chronic glomerulonephritis. Both kidneys are reduced in size and display a fine granular surface. The patient had developed acute glomerulonephritis following a streptococcal sore throat. Renal failure and systemic hypertension slowly evolved over the next 15 years. Death was due to cerebral haemorrhage. These are typical end-stage kidneys, and it is not possible to distinguish between the various types of chronic renal disease by a gross examination of them.

Renal and urinary tract infection: pyelonephritis

Bacterial infection of the urinary tract is very common and constitutes a major medical problem. The infecting organisms are usually the Gram-negative intestinal bacilli, including *Escherichia coli*, *Pseudomonas aeruginosa*, and *Proteus* species. Two routes of infection have been described, but their relative importance has been long debated:

Haematogenous infection. It is believed that some infection is blood-borne from the colon. Normally organisms that avoid the reticuloendothelial cells of the liver pass into the systemic circulation; they escape into the glomerular filtrate and are expeditiously voided in the urine. If there is an obstruction to the outflow of urine, these organisms flourish and set up acute inflammation of the bladder (*cystitis*), of the renal pelvis (*pyelitis*), or of the kidney and renal pelvis (*pyelonephritis*).

Ascending infection. There is a rival hypothesis that infection ascends from the perineum and lower urinary tract. Acute cystitis is more common in women (particularly during pregnancy), and it is probable that this is due to the shortness of the urethra and the ease with which vulval organisms can ascend to the bladder. Likewise, urinary-tract infection often follows repeated catheterization. Direct introduction of urethral organisms into the bladder can therefore be implicated. Following acute cystitis 'ascending infection' due to reflux of urine up the ureters can occur.

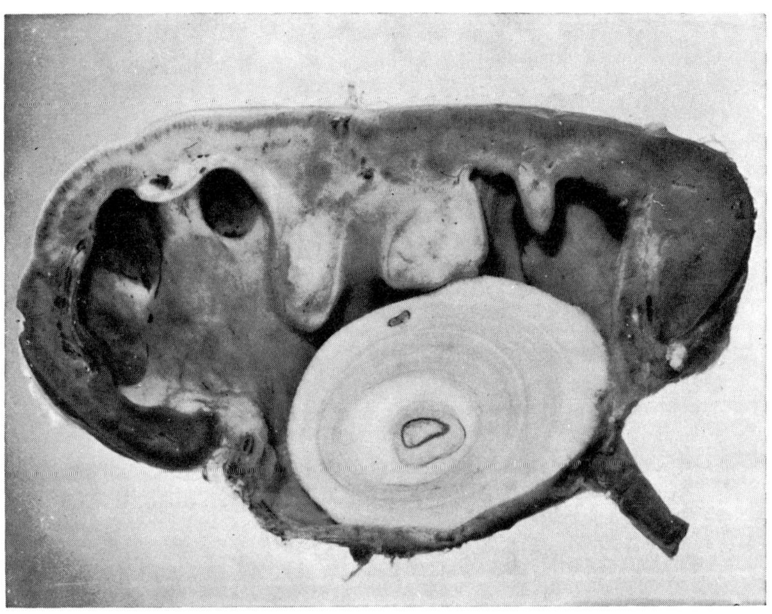

Fig. 36.6 Hydronephrotic kidney. The pelvis is greatly dilated, and it contains a large calcium phosphate calculus which has been sectioned to reveal its laminated structure. The kidney substance has been severely destroyed. (U25.3 *Reproduced by permission of the President and Council of the Royal College of Surgeons of England.*)

It is evident that obstruction to the urinary flow is the most important factor predisposing a person toward infection. Pyelonephritis can be unilateral if one ureter is obstructed, such as by a stone (Fig. 36.6). If there has been previous blockage, the hydronephrotic kidney becomes infected to produce a sac of pus known as *pyonephrosis*. Urethral obstruction, such as that due to prostatic enlargement, generally causes bilateral pyelonephritis.

The clinical features of acute urinary tract infection are those of an acute infection: rigors and a sudden rise in temperature. Pain is experienced in the loins in pyelonephritis. With cystitis and urethritis the inflammation leads to urgency of micturition together with pain and burning on passing urine. The acute attack generally subsides rapidly either under treatment or spontaneously.

The urine in acute cystitis and pyelonephritis contains numerous pus cells; organisms can usually be seen in a stained smear of an uncentrifuged specimen. Haematuria is common.

Chronic pyelonephritis. In many cases of acute urinary infection, there is recurrence or the development of chronicity. This is *chronic pyelonephritis*, the commonest cause of chronic renal failure. Its pathogenesis is uncertain, for there is often no obvious obstruction to or stasis in the urinary passages. It may be that intrinsic renal lesions, especially the scars of previous infections, are the predisposing factors for smouldering infection. There is a gradual destruction of the renal parenchyma, which is heavily infiltrated by lymphocytes, plasma cells, macrophages, and variable numbers of pus cells. The glomeruli are gradually converted into hyaline masses, the tubules undergo atrophy and obliteration, and

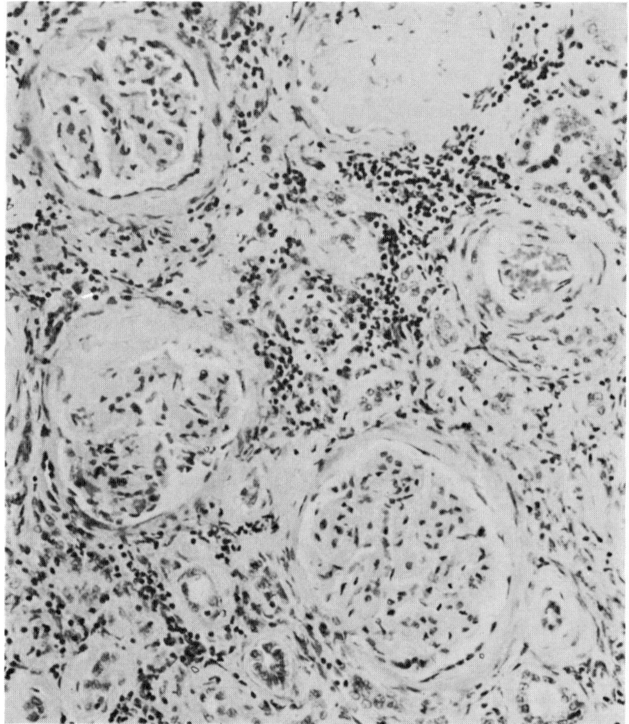

Fig. 36.7 Chronic pyelonephritis. Most of the renal parenchyma has been replaced by fibrous tissue heavily infiltrated by lymphocytes in some parts. The glomeruli are partly fibrosed, and there is well-marked periglomerular fibrosis. The tubules are atrophic. × 90.

the parenchyma is replaced by fibrous tissue (Fig. 36.7). At first, the process occurs in wedge-shaped subcapsular foci, but eventually it becomes diffuse. Surviving tubules undergo dilatation, and are often filled with eosinophilic protein material which gives them a thyroid-like appearance. Hypertensive vascular changes are often severe. Ultimately the kidney resembles that found in chronic glomerulonephritis. Indeed, the end stages of many renal diseases are barely distinguishable from one another.

The relationship between urinary-tract infection and urinary calculi (or stones) should be noted. Infection predisposes to the formation of *secondary stones* consisting of calcium salts. The presence of these stones predisposes to recurrent infection. Likewise primary calculi (these include stones composed of calcium oxalate, uric acid—sometimes associated with gout—and mixed calcium oxalate and phosphate—sometimes associated with hypercalcaemia and hypercalciuria as in hyperparathyroidism) may also cause urinary-tract obstruction and predispose to infection. Another noteworthy effect of calculi is the production of haematuria associated with severe pain (*renal colic*). This contrasts with the *painless haematuria* characteristic of carcinoma of the bladder or kidney

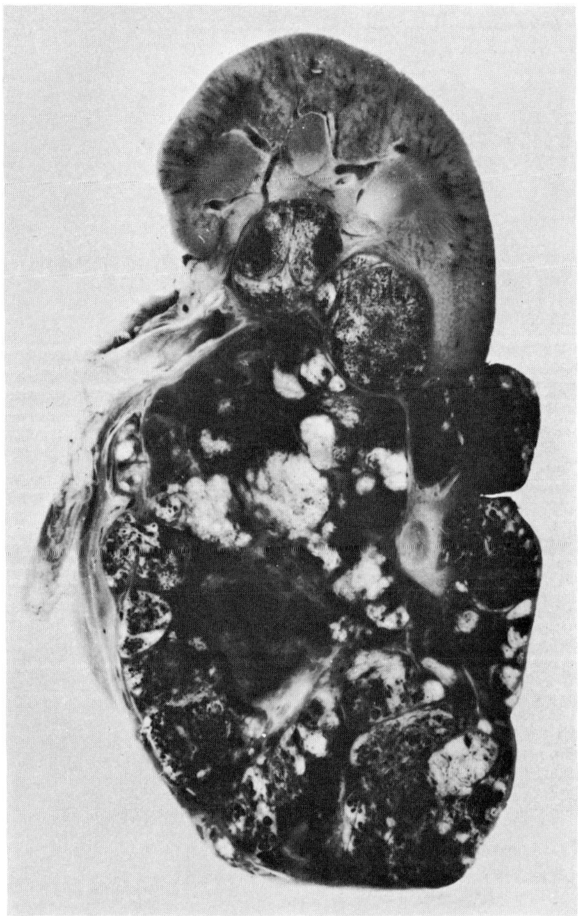

Fig 36.8 Carcinoma of the kidney. The lower pole has been replaced by a large encephaloid tumour which is infiltrating into the upper pole and compressing the ureter. Note the variegated appearance of the tumour. (EU30.1. *Reproduced by permission of the President and Council of the Royal College of Surgeons of England.*)

Tumours of the kidney

Adenoma. The common benign renal tumour is the *adenoma.* It usually appears as a pin's-head-sized, white or yellow nodule situated just beneath the capsule. Its cells are usually arranged in a papillary cystadenomatous pattern, and they sometimes have a clear cytoplasm, thereby closely resembling those of the carcinoma.

Carcinoma of the kidney. This is the malignant counterpart of the adenoma.

It presents at a pole of the kidney as a large encephaloid mass, which on section has a variegated appearance: areas of orange are interspersed amid white stroma and red foci of haemorrhage (Fig. 36.8). Microscopically it consists of large spheroidal cells with a clear cytoplasm (Fig 36.9). These cells resemble those of the adrenal cortex, and it was once believed that the tumour arose from ectopic adrenal rests situated on the surface of the kidney. This belief was the origin of the name *hypernephroma*, which is still sometimes used in connexion with the tumour.

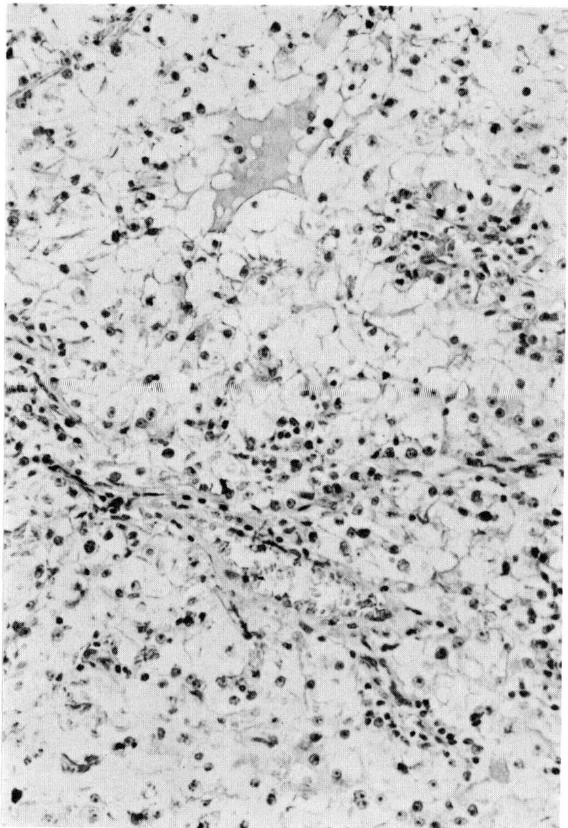

Fig. 36.9 Clear-cell carcinoma of the kidney. The tumour consists of sheets of large round and polygonal cells with a copious clear cytoplasm and darkly-staining nuclei. × 100.

It arises in fact from the renal tubular epithelium, and all grades of transition can be found between it and the tubular adenoma. The clear appearance of the cells is due to their high content of lipid and glycogen, both of which tend to be lost during histological processing. The carotenoids dissolved in the lipid give rise to the orange colour of the tumour. The correct name for this tumour is *clear-cell carcinoma of the kidney.*

Clinically carcinoma of the kidney is often silent for a long time. Haematuria and an abdominal mass are two common presenting features. Distant lymphatic and blood-borne metastases are common, the liver, lungs, and bones being especially vulnerable. Indeed, a skeletal metastasis is sometimes the first indication of the tumour.

Another interesting feature is the phenomenon of dormancy (p. 337)—bony deposits may suddenly erupt many years after the successful removal of the affected kidney.

The other important renal tumour is the *nephroblastoma,* or *Wilms's tumour*, an embryonic tumour of infancy discussed in Chapter 24.

GENERAL READING

Black D A K (1972) Renal Disease, 3rd edn, 871 pp. Blackwell, Oxford

De Wardener H E (1973) The Kidney, 4th edn. 432 pp. Churchill, London

Pitts R F (1968) Physiology of the Kidney and Body Fluids, 2nd edn. 266 pp. Year Book Medical Publishers, Chicago

37

Diseases of bone and joints

BONE

Introduction

In early embryonic life condensations of mesenchyme are laid down at the sites of future bone formation, and by the end of the second month ossification commences. In the development of some bones, notably the cranium and the clavicle, there is a direct conversion of the membranous sheet of mesenchyme to bone. Bones formed in this way are called *membrane bones.* The base of the skull and the long bones develop in a different way: in these the mesenchyme differentiates into cartilage which is subsequently *replaced* by bone. The cartilage cells swell up and die, and the intervening matrix then calcifies. This *calcified cartilage* is eroded by osteoclasts, and at the same time osteoblasts lay down lamellar bone (see below); the process continues at the epiphyseal ends of long bones until adult stature is reached. This type of bone formation is called *endochondral ossification.* Some bones, for example the mandible, are formed by a mixture of the two processes of ossification.

Structure of bone[1–5]

Bone is composed of calcified osteoid tissue; the latter consists of collagen fibres embedded in a mucoprotein matrix (osseomucin). The exact composition of the calcium salts is not known, but they are generally considered to have a hydroxyapatite structure.

Depending upon the arrangement of the collagen fibres, two histological types of bone may be recognized.

Woven, immature, fibrillary, or non-lamellar bone. This shows irregularity in the arrangement of the collagen bundles and in the distribution of the osteocytes. The osseomucin is usually basophilic, and is less abundant than in mature bone. It also contains less calcium.

Formation. Woven bone is formed wherever ossification occurs primarily in loose connective tissue. This occurs in three situations:

1. During the formation of membrane bones
2. When bone forms in the midst of the differentiating granulation tissue of a healing fracture
3. In certain bone disorders and in osteogenic tumours.

Lamellar or mature bone. In this type of bone the collagen bundles are arranged in parallel sheets either in the form of concentric Haversian systems or flat plates.

In the outer dense *cortex* of a long bone Haversian systems predominate, while flat plates are seen under the periosteum and endosteum. This type of bone is called *compact bone.*

The central portion of long bones is hollowed out to form the medullary cavity, which contains marrow. Only a few spicules of bone remain. These are constructed of flat bundles of collagen, although in the wider trabeculae Haversian systems may be found. The central trabeculated part of the bone is called *cancellous,* and it should be noted that, like 'compact' bone, this is a term related to the gross appearance.

Formation. Lamellar bone is formed when bone is laid down on a previously calcified structure. This may be:

1. calcified cartilage, as in normal endochondral ossification and in replacement of the cartilage which forms during the healing of a fracture
2. woven bone, as during the early growth of membrane bones
3. lamellar bone itself, as during the circumferential growth of all bones.

In the normal adult the entire skeleton is composed of lamellar bone.

Metabolic functions of bone

The relationship of bone to calcium metabolism and the functions of parathyroid hormone and calcitonin are described in Chapter 19. An important enzyme of osseous tissue is *alkaline phosphatase*; it is manufactured by osteoblasts, but its precise role in bone formation is not understood. Nevertheless, since some of the enzyme escapes into the blood, the plasma level is a good index of the over-all osteoblastic activity within the body. The measurement of the alkaline phosphatase level in the plasma is therefore a useful aid in the diagnosis of generalized bone disorders.* The level is normally 1.5 to 5 units (Bodansky), or 3 to 13 units (King-Armstrong), in adults and slightly higher in children.*

Although bone appears rigid and inert, it is as susceptible as the soft tissues to adverse circumstances and deleterious agents; indeed, the effects on bone are often more severe and permanent.

There is a continuous process of remodelling throughout life with bone resorption by *osteoclasts* and bone deposition by *osteoblasts,* each keeping pace with the other. If either predominates osteoporosis or osteosclerosis results. *Osteoporosis* is a condition in which osteoid matrix, although reduced in amount, is normally mineralized. The bony trabeculae are greatly thinned, and the bone as a whole is weakened and liable to fracture.

* Very high plasma levels of alkaline phosphatase are found in obstructive jaundice. Liver disease must therefore be considered. The total plasma alkaline phosphatase activity consists of the summation of the effect of five isoenzymes. These can be measured separately. Bone alkaline phosphatase is the most unstable and is the one referred to here. Another important alkaline phosphatase is derived from liver and its plasma level is raised in bile-duct obstruction.[6] The level is not only raised in obvious jaundice due to main bile-duct obstruction, but also with multiple bile-ductule obstruction when jaundice is absent. A raised level is therefore a useful indication of the presence of multiple secondary carcinoma.

Osteoporosis may be brought about by either excessive destruction of bone or defective formation, and may occur in a number of conditions in a localized or generalized form (pp. 588 and 585).

In *osteosclerosis* there is excessive formation of osteoid, which being calcified, makes the bones appear dense on a radiograph.

Classification of generalized bone disorders

There is no very satisfactory classification of generalized bone disorders, but they may be considered under three headings:

1. *Developmental abnormalities,* of genetic or unknown cause
2. *Abnormalities due to metabolic disorders.* These include endocrine disturbances and vitamin deficiencies or excesses, and are described in Chapters 39 and 18 respectively
3. *Abnormalities occurring in the adult,* generally of unknown cause.

Although this is a convenient classification, there is an overlap between the groups, and in some examples a localized form of the disease may occur.

DEVELOPMENTAL ABNORMALITIES

There are a few rare conditions of bone which are due to some failure during the developmental process.

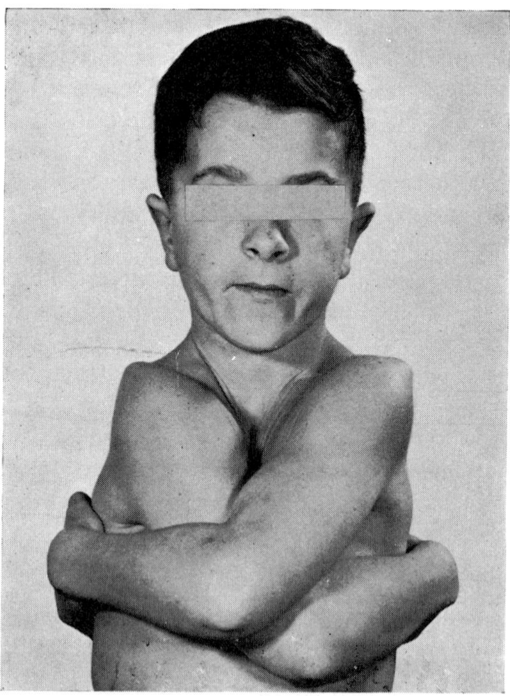

Fig. 37.1 Cleidocranial dysostosis. The two shoulders can be approximated across the chest because of the absence of intervening clavicles. (*Photograph by courtesy of Professor T D Foster.*)

Cleidocranial dysostosis[7]

This condition is sometimes inherited as a dominant trait, and is characterized by the complete agenesis of a bone or part of a bone. The clavicle is most often affected, but defects have also been reported in the pelvic girdle and long bones. When the clavicles are absent, the subject is able to approximate the shoulders across the chest (Fig. 37.1).

There may also be retardation or failure of closure of the fontanelles, and the two halves of the frontal bone may not fuse. There is also associated a general failure of eruption of the teeth.

Osteogenesis imperfecta (fragilitas ossium)[8]

This condition may be present at birth (*congenital type*) or may develop later (the *tarda form*).

In the congenital type, which is inherited as an autosomal recessive trait, multiple fractures occur *in utero* or during birth, and the prognosis is poor. In the tarda form, inherited as an autosomal dominant trait, the condition is less severe, for, if the child survives, the tendency to fracture decreases after puberty.

The bones in osteogenesis imperfecta are generally thin and brittle. The cortex is thin, and there is a decrease in the amount of cancellous bone. The fragility results in the frequent occurrence of fractures which occur either spontaneously or as a result of trivial injuries. Although there is rapid healing of the fractures, the bone is of abnormal consistency. The multiplicity of fractures generally leads to severe deformities.

The pathogenesis of the disease is obscure, but it is thought that there is a generalized hypoplasia of mesenchyme. This theory is supported by the fact that affected subjects are of short stature, and have lax ligaments which lead to hypermobility of the joints. In addition the sclera is sometimes thin and semi-

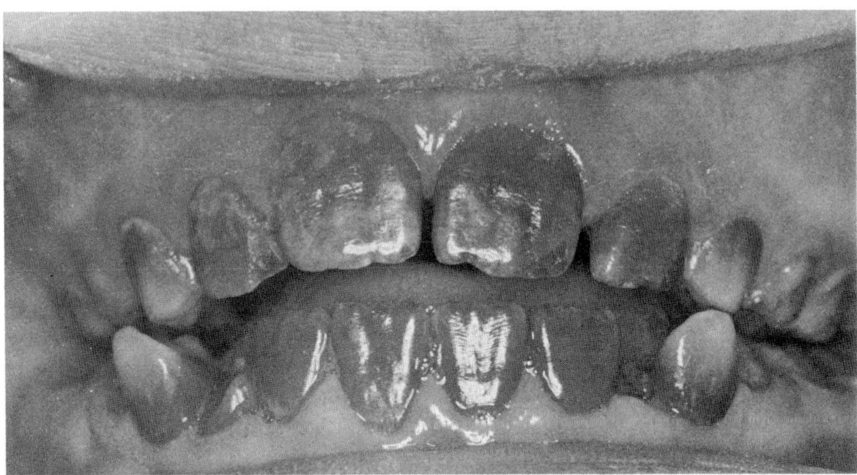

Fig. 37.2 Dentinogenesis imperfecta. The enamel, being translucent, allows the discoloured dentine to show through, producing the bluish brown appearance that gives rise to the descriptive term 'opalescent dentine'.

translucent, so that it appears blue due to the pigmentation of the underlying choroid.

Dentinogenesis imperfecta (hereditary opalescent dentine). This is a condition affecting that part of the tooth of mesenchymal origin (dentine), and may be seen in association with osteogenesis imperfecta or may occur without any bony involvement (Fig. 37.2).

Fibrous dysplasia

The aetiology of this condition is unknown. It is characterized by the appearance of areas of bone resorption and replacement by fibrous tissue in which there are thin trabeculae of woven bone in the shape of Chinese characters. The marrow space is also obliterated in the affected areas. Any bone may be affected, either in its entirety or only focally. Fibrous dysplasia includes a wide variety of conditions which may well be excluded from this group as our knowledge increases. Two main types are described:

Polyostotic fibrous dysplasia. This manifests itself early in life. There is an insidious onset, and a pathological fracture may be the presenting symptom. The condition usually affects one side of the body only. When the skull and facial bones are involved there is much disfigurement. The disease process usually ceases when growth has ended.

A more severe form of the condition is accompanied by pigmentation of the skin (café-au-lait spots), endocrine dysfunction resulting in sexual precocity in young girls, and disturbances of growth and development (*Albright's syndrome*). The reason for the pigmentation and endocrine disturbance is not known.

Monostotic fibrous dysplasia. Some authorities believe that this is a reparative reaction following trauma or infection. Despite the histological similarity to the polyostotic form it does not seem to progress to the latter. Monostotic fibrous dysplasia is much more common than the polyostotic form. It occurs in young people, and may affect any bone including the jaw in from 10 to 15 per cent of cases.[9,10]

Familial fibrous dysplasia ('cherubism')[11]

This disease, first described by Jones in 1933, resembles monostotic fibrous dysplasia but is inherited as an autosomal dominant trait with incomplete penetrance. The bone is replaced by loose, oedematous fibrous tissue in which there are scattered giant cells. Bony trabeculae like those of fibrous dysplasia are not present.

Characteristically there is enlargement of the jaws and there may be submaxillary lymphadenopathy. Involvement of the orbital floor with upward displacement of the eyes combines with the large jaws to give a cherubic appearance.

Bony expansion of the jaws occurs particularly in the mandibular molar region—it commences in the first 2 to 3 years of life, and gradually ceases as growth terminates. There may be a premature loss of primary teeth and some disturbances of the permanent dentition with an absence of teeth and failure of eruption of those present.

Radiographs of the jaws show extensive symmetrical areas of radiolucency which have a multilocular appearance. Involvement of bones other than those of the skull and mandible can occur, but it is rare.

There is some doubt as to the exact nature of the condition. Jones, who coined the named cherubism, considered that it was an anomaly of dental development. Others regard it as a fibrous dysplasia or a bone dysplasia. Others do not commit themselves, and consider the condition a familial osseous dysplasia or fibrous swelling of the jaws.[12]

Achondroplasia (chondrodystrophy fetalis)

This disease is transmitted as an autosomal dominant trait. The essential feature is defective endochondral bone formation, and the long bones of the limbs are therefore short. The trunk and head are of normal size, but the middle third of the face is depressed due to the premature cessation of cartilaginous growth and synostosis of the bones of the cranial base. There is relative or true protrusion of the lower jaw. This type of dwarf, who has normal intelligence, is very muscular and agile, and is frequently seen in the circus ring.

Osteopetrosis (Albers-Schönberg disease, marble-bone disease)[13]

There is increased deposition of bone in this condition, so that the bones are hard, heavy, and inelastic. The cortex is greatly thickened, and the marrow cavity is much reduced in size. This disease is inherited as an autosomal recessive trait.

Although the bones are thickened and hard, they are liable to fractures because of their inelasticity. Leuco-erythroblastic anaemia may occur as a result of the reduction of bone-marrow space. Later on blindness, deafness, and facial paralysis develop, because the cranial nerves are constricted as they pass through the bony foramina of the skull.

ABNORMALITIES OF BONE OCCURRING IN THE ADULT

Generalized osteoporosis[14, 15]

Osteoporosis is a condition of bone atrophy, and has aptly been defined as a lesion in which the volume of bone tissue per unit volume of anatomical bone is reduced.[15] There is a reduction in the amount of osteoid tissue, which, however, remains normally mineralized. It must be distinguished from *osteomalacia,* in which osteoid is present in abundance but is poorly calcified. The radiological appearance of osteoporosis is a reduction of bone density; it must, however, be remembered that this can be detected in routine films with certainty only when the content of calcium is reduced by at least a half. Refined techniques may be more sensitive.[16]

Causes of generalized osteoporosis. *Disuse osteoporosis.*[17] Prolonged recumbency produces considerable osteoporosis in most bones. It would seem that stress and strain are a necessary stimulus for the maintenance of bone structure. Immobilization leads initially to osteoclastic resorption of bone and the mobilization of excessive amounts of calcium, which results in hypercalciuria and sometimes renal-stone formation. This is then followed by a phase of quiescence in which the bone shows little osteoclastic or osteoblastic activity. If movement is resumed, the bones gradually return to normal. The blood levels of calcium, phosphate, and phosphatase are normal in disuse osteoporosis.

Idiopathic osteoporosis. Osteoporosis, especially of the pelvis, spine, and ribs, is not uncommon in old age (*senile osteoporosis*), and compression of the vertebral bodies causes backache as well as a considerable loss of height. The condition is also seen in women who have passed the menopause (*post-menopausal osteoporosis*), and this has been attributed to hormonal imbalance (Fig. 37.3). Occasionally osteoporosis occurs in a younger age-group for no very obvious reason.

Other types of osteoporosis. Osteoporosis is also seen when collagen formation is impaired as in:

1. Scurvy
2. Excessive glucocorticoid levels, e.g. Cushing's disease and with prolonged administration of adrenocortical hormones
3. Impaired supply of protein, e.g. starvation and the malabsorption syndrome.

Effects of generalized osteoporosis. Symptoms are generally referable to the spine and pelvis, which are the parts of the skeleton most severely affected in generalized osteoporosis. Chronic backache and kyphosis are common, and collapse of the vertebrae may produce episodes of acute pain. Diminution in height is characteristic, and may be as much as 8 inches before being noticed by the patient. Fractures may complicate osteoporosis; thus minimal trauma may cause the fracture of a limb bone, particularly the lower forearm bones and the femur.

Paget's disease of bone (osteitis deformans)

Described first by James Paget in 1876, this condition is considered by some to be an inflammatory disease. However, despite much study its aetiology and nature are unknown. It occurs in people over the age of 40 years, predominantly in the male sex. It is perhaps more common than was originally thought, as routine radiographs sometimes reveal solitary lesions in the spine and pelvis without clinical manifestations. The involved bones show much thickening of the cortex due to the dominance of osteoblastic activity.

Initially the bone is softened due to osteoclastic resorption, and the affected area shows increased vascularity. The bending of softened, weight-bearing bones results in deformities, and is adequate reason for the alternative name of osteitis deformans. Later there is irregular subperiosteal deposition, and the bones become hard and thickened (Fig. 37.4). Microscopically the irregular new-bone formation results in a characteristic mosaic appearance (Fig. 37.5). The plasma calcium and phosphate levels are within normal limits, but the alkaline phosphatase may be raised as much as fifty times above normal.

The skull is frequently affected, and later it may become obviously enlarged. When the jaws are affected the teeth show marked hypercementosis. Bone pain may be an early feature. Blindness, deafness, headaches, and facial paralysis are complications that may occur as a result of compression of the nerves due to the increased bone formation. Sarcoma of bone complicates the condition in about 1 per cent of patients. The reasons for this is not known; it appears that the excessive proliferative activity of the bone leads eventually to neoplastic growth.

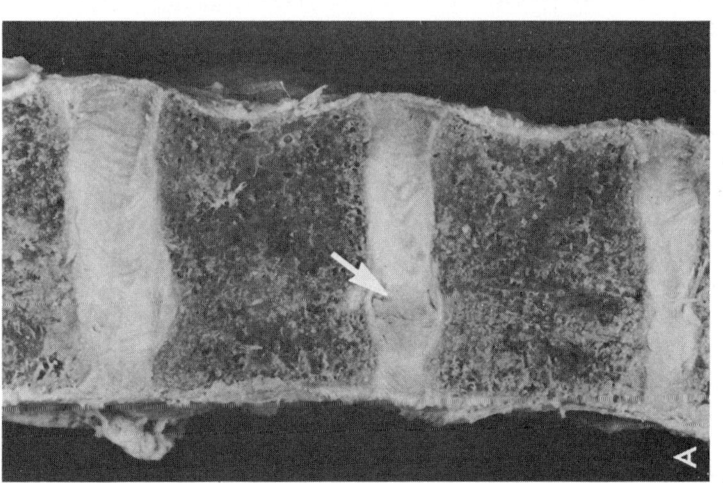

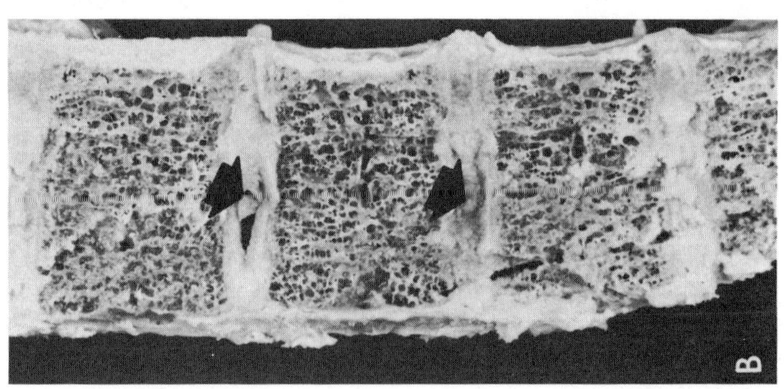

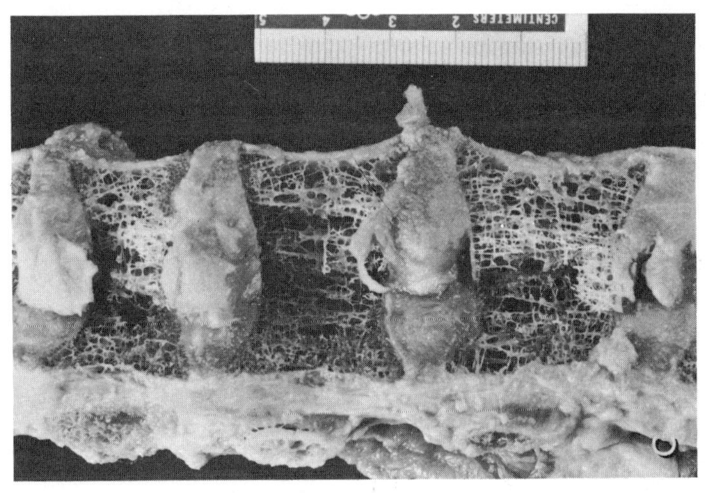

Fig. 37.3 Normal and osteoporotic vertebral bodies. *A*. Normal vertebral bodies. *B*. Moderate osteoporosis. *C*. Severe osteoporosis. The vertebral bodies have been sectioned to show their internal structure. Note the well-formed cancellous bone of the normal vertebral bodies in *A* as well as the structure of the intervertebral discs. One small focus of degeneration can be seen (white arrow). In *B* the specimen shows well-developed osteoporosis, but the over-all shape of the vertebrae is preserved. The discs show severe degenerative changes (black arrows). In *C* the specimen shows severe osteoporosis. The vertebrae have been compressed by the bulging discs.

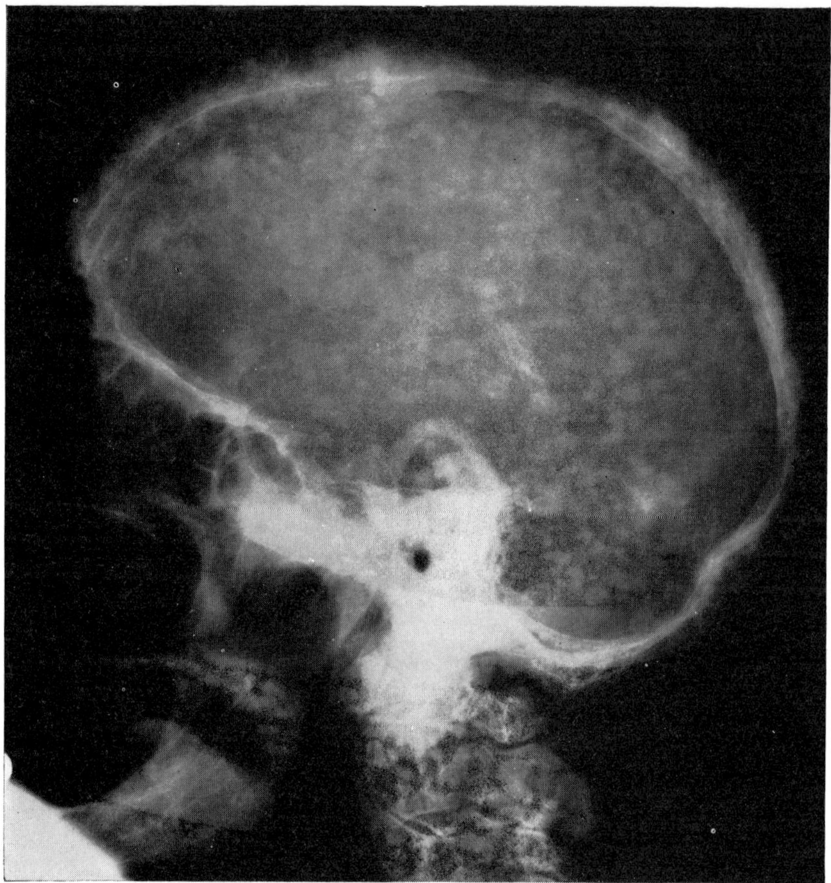

Fig. 37.4. Paget's disease affecting the skull. Note the uneven thickening of the outer table and the blurring of the demarcation between the inner and outer tables. (*Radiograph by courtesy of Professor H C Killey.*)

BONE DISORDERS CAUSED BY PHYSICAL DISTURBANCES

Localized osteoporosis

Due to immobilization. The local disuse of a bone causes osteoporosis in the same way as does total recumbency, and the immobilization of a joint leads to marked osteoporosis of the adjacent bones. This occurs after fractures and also in diseases of the joints themselves, e.g. tuberculous and rheumatoid arthritis. It is very pronounced in paralysed limbs; indeed, if paralysis occurs in childhood, as after poliomyelitis, the whole limb including the bones fails to attain adult size.

Sudeck's acute bone atrophy is probably an example of disuse atrophy. It follows quite trivial trauma to the hands, and more rarely the feet. Examples of this condition have also been noted in the mandible.[18] This condition is associated with marked pain and swelling, and there is radiological evidence of rapidly progressing osteoporosis. The pain is usually out of all proportions to the extent of the injury, and the most likely explanation of both the osteoporosis and the oedema is disuse consequent on the pain.

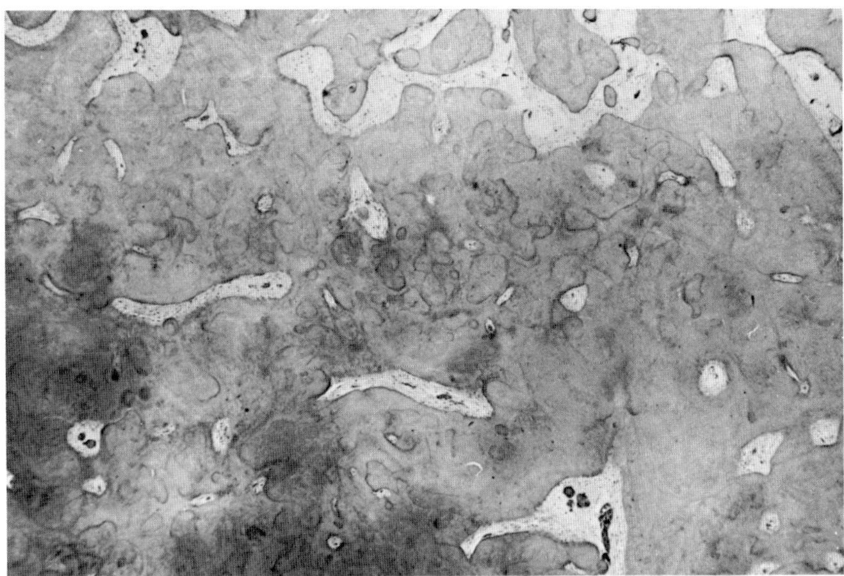

Fig. 37.5 Paget's disease of bone. There are massive, irregular trabeculae of bone that have been deposited haphazardly on one another during the process of new-bone formation that follows the initial osteoclastic resorption of bone. The disorientated blocks of bone are joined together by irregular cement lines which produce the mosaic pattern that is virtually specific to Paget's disease, and characteristic of its final, burnt-out phase (Photography by courtesy of Professor R. M. Browne.)

Pressure atrophy. Expanding lesions which exert pressure on the surrounding bone cause local ischaemia due to compression of the blood vessels, and atrophy results. Thus a benign tumour or cyst may produce a sharply-defined area of rarefaction. In an attempt to offset the weakness that ensues more bone is produced by the periosteum opposite the lesion, so that the mass appears to cause expansion of the bone. This is well seen in the giant-cell tumour and in the ameloblastoma. It should be noted that cartilage, being avascular, does not undergo pressure atrophy. Therefore an aneurysm of the descending aorta pressing on the vertebral column causes atrophy of the vertebrae but spares the intervertebral discs. For the same reason benign tumours and cysts do not destroy the epiphyseal cartilage of a long bone.

Fractures[2, 19, 20]

Exciting causes

Excessive mechanical force

Direct violence, e.g. depressed fracture of the skull.

Indirect violence, e.g. fractures of the condyles of the mandible following a blow on the chin (Fig. 37.6).

Muscular action. Sudden unexpected strains during violent exercise may cause fractures in normal bones (*spontaneous fractures*). Likewise the violent convulsive movements of tetanus and strychnine poisoning may result in the collapse of a vertebral body, causing wedging.

Abnormal bone. A fracture may occur in a diseased bone subjected to a normal strain (*pathological fracture*). Any lesion which causes weakness may be responsible, e.g. osteitis fibrosa cystica, osteogenesis imperfecta, simple bone cyst, and tumour. Secondary carcinoma must always be borne in mind, and indeed a pathological fracture may be the first indication of a malignant lesion, e.g. carcinoma of lung or breast.

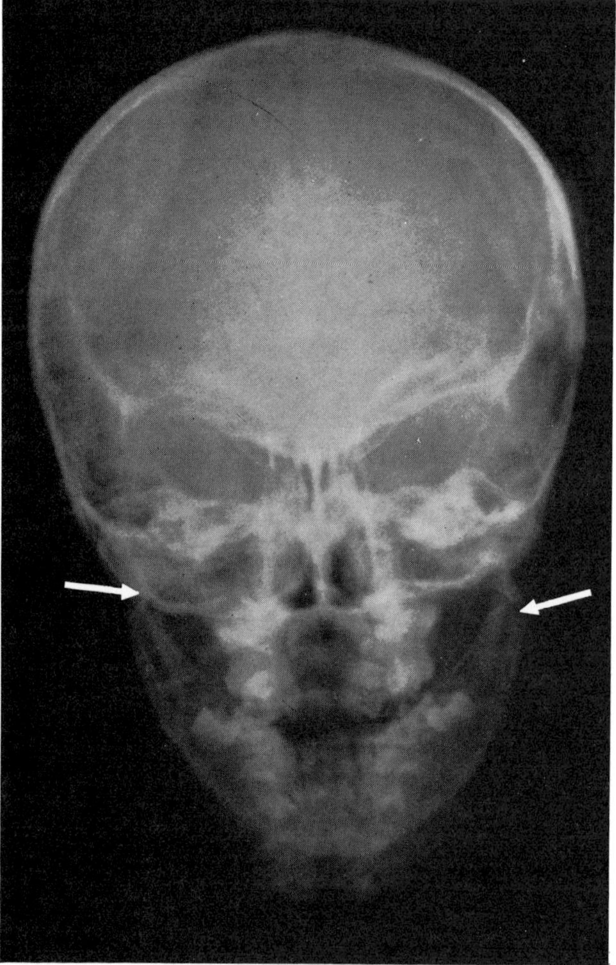

Fig. 37.6 Fractured condyles in a child aged 3 years following a fall on her chin.

Stages in fracture healing (bone regeneration)

The stages in healing of a fracture are illustrated diagrammatically in Fig. 37.7. It must be remembered that the entire area is not all at the same stage of healing at the same time; while the centre may be at an early stage, the changes adjacent to the bone ends are much more advanced. However, for descriptive purposes it is convenient to divide the healing process into separate stages.

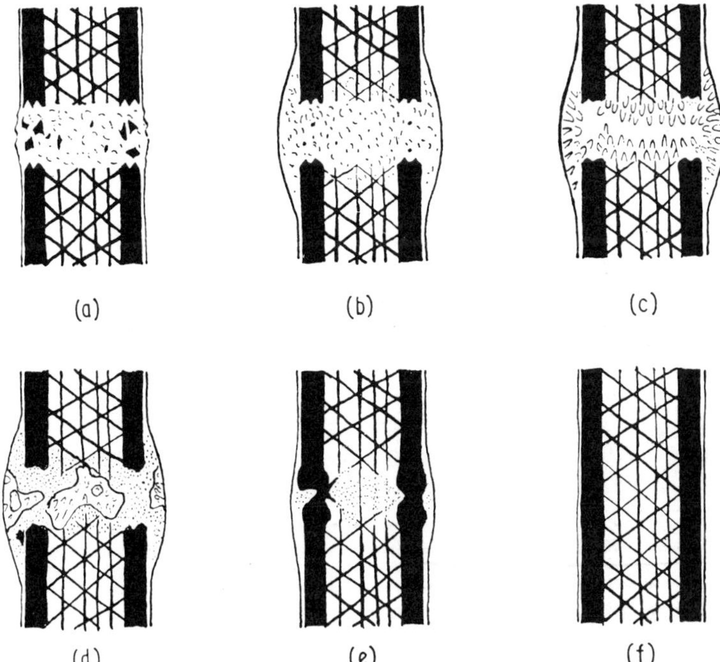

Fig. 37.7 Stages in the healing of a fracture.
(a) Haematoma formation.
(b) Stages 2 and 3. Acute inflammation followed by demolition. Loose fragments of bone are removed, and the bone ends show osteoporosis.
(c) Stage 4. Granulation tissue formation.
(d) Stage 5. The bone ends are now united by woven bone, cartilage, or a mixture of the two. The hard material is often called callus, and can be divided into three parts—internal, intermediate, and external. The intermediate callus is that part which lies in line with the cortex of the bone, while the external callus produces the fusiform swelling visible on the outside of the bone.
(e) Stage 6. Lamellar bone is laid down, and calcified cartilage and woven bone are progressively removed.
(f) Stage 7. Final remodelling.

Stage 1: haematoma formation. Immediately following the injury there is a variable amount of bleeding from torn vessels, and a haematoma is formed.

Stage 2: traumatic inflammation. The tissue damage excites an acute inflammatory response, with vasodilatation and a polymorphonuclear leucocytic infiltration. The hyperaemia has been held responsible for the decreased density of the adjacent bone ends often noted radiologically. This 'decalcification' is presumably a form of osteoporosis due to osteoclastic activity, but the pathogenesis is not clear. The connective-tissue changes that accompany the inflammatory reaction cause a loosening of the attachment of the periosteum to the bone. The haematoma therefore attains a fusiform shape.

Stage 3: demolition. Macrophages invade the clot and remove the fibrin, red cells, inflammatory exudate, and debris. Any fragments of bone which have become detached from their blood supply undergo necrosis, and are attacked by macrophages and osteoclasts.

Stage 4: formation of granulation tissue. Following the demolition there is an ingrowth of capillary loops and mesenchymal cells derived from the periosteum and endosteum. The importance of the periosteum in fracture union has been much disputed in the past. The cells of its deeper layer certainly have osteogenic potentiality, and together with its blood vessels contribute to the granulation tissue.

In fractures of the neck of the femur the head is dependent upon the periosteum for its blood supply. If this is damaged, there is ischaemic necrosis of the head. Hence in this situation the integrity of the periosteum is of great practical importance. In a rib following subperiosteal resection the periosteum alone is capable of effecting complete regeneration. Here it probably acts partly by forming a limiting membrane around the haematoma, and partly by providing cells and blood vessels for the granulation tissue.

In fractures of the long bones, however, it must not be forgotten that a very extensive area of cancellous bone is exposed. From this the endosteal osteoblasts and the medullary blood vessels grow out to form the granulation tissue. Under these circumstances the periosteum is of much less importance.

During these early phases the pH is low, and this is spoken of as the *acid tide*.

Stage 5: woven bone and cartilage formation. The mesenchymal 'osteoblasts' next differentiate to form either woven bone or cartilage. The term 'callus', derived from the Latin and meaning hard, is often used to describe the material uniting the fracture ends regardless of its consistency. When this is granulation tissue the 'callus' is soft, but as bone or cartilage formation occurs it becomes hard. The word is used loosely by surgeons, radiologists, and pathologists, but exact definition of its various stages is difficult and serves no useful function. If the term is used, it is probably best to apply it to the calcified hard tissue uniting the bone ends.

Formation of woven bone. The osteoblasts form both the collagen fibres and the osseomucin, in which they are embedded. The osteoid is in this way formed by the maturation of granulation tissue, and as in the repair of ordinary connective tissue progressive devascularization occurs. The collagen bundles are irregularly arranged with no attempt at lamellar structure.

After about 10 days the pH of the uniting fracture increases. During this *alkaline tide* the osteoid undergoes calcification, and thereby becomes woven bone. Osteoblasts produce an alkaline phosphatase which may play a part in the calcification, in that it may lead to a local supersaturation of phosphate due to its effect on hexose phosphates. Resorption of bony spicules may at the same time produce a local supersaturation of calcium ions.

The bone ends thus become united by woven bone. It forms a fusiform mass which is arbitrarily divided into internal, intermediate, and external callus (Fig. 37.7).

Woven-bone formation is found whenever the bone ends are adequately immobilized. It normally occurs in human fracture healing, and is a predominant feature in healing of tooth sockets. In experimentally-produced fractures in animals adequate immobilization is difficult to attain, and then the granulation tissue matures not to woven bone, but to hyaline cartilage as described below.

Formation of cartilage. The mesenchymal cells ('osteoblasts') behave as chondroblasts and form cartilage, i.e the cells actively lead to the formation of a specialized ground substance in which the collagen fibres are embedded. These cartilage cells swell and die, and the intervening matrix undergoes calcification. Cartilage formation is seen in fractures in which movement occurs, not only in experimental animal fractures, but also human fractures where complete immobilization is impractical, e.g. ribs.

In many fractures both cartilage and woven bone are formed. Both are capable of forming a calcified scaffold on which the final adult-type, lamellar bone can later be built. The two embryological methods of bone formation, endochondral and intramembranous ossification, are faithfully repeated in later life during the regeneration of bone.

Stage 6: formation of lamellar bone. The dead calcified cartilage or woven bone is next invaded by capillaries headed by osteoclasts. As the initial scaffolding ('provisional callus') is removed, osteoblasts lay down osteoid which calcifies to form bone. This time its collagen bundles are arranged in orderly lamellar fashion. For the most part they are disposed concentrically around the blood vessels, where they form Haversian systems. Adjacent to the periosteum and endosteum the lamellae are parallel to the surface as in the normal bone. This phase of deposition of definitive lamellar bone merges with the last stage.

Stage 7: remodelling. The final remodelling process, involving the continued osteoclastic removal and osteoblastic formation of bone, results in the formation of a bone which differs remarkably little from its previous state. The *external callus* is slowly removed, the *intermediate callus* becomes converted into compact bone containing Haversian systems, while the *internal callus* is hollowed out into a marrow cavity in which only a few spicules of cancellous bone remain.

The healing of a socket following the extraction of a tooth is similar to that of a fracture. After an extraction the socket fills with blood which forms a clot, which within a few days is replaced by granulation tissue. Woven bone is laid down in the socket and this is later replaced by lamellar bone. There is a covering of compact bone. As the alveolar bone is no longer required to support the tooth, remodelling takes place and results in a reduced ridge in that area. The extraction of a tooth produces an open wound, and the healing process also includes epithelialization over the granulation tissue.

A complication that sometimes occurs is the condition known as a 'dry socket'; this is a focal osteomyelitis and may occur if the blood clot disintegrates or is lost. The exposed bone becomes necrotic, and sequestration follows. The condition is extremely painful and healing is slow.

It is interesting to note that the healing of a fracture has some features in common with the process of axial regeneration in amphibia. Thus there is dedifferentiation of cells and the formation of a blastema in which the cells subsequently differentiate along several lines.

Abnormalities of fracture healing

Repair, or fibrous union. Although the cells of the granulation tissue are called osteoblasts, they are capable of differentiation along several lines. They can form bone, but if immobilization is not complete, cartilage may develop. When movement is even more free, the cells behave as fibroblasts, and the bone ends become united by ordinary scar tissue. Whether this can ever undergo ossification is debatable. It is claimed by some authorities that fibrous tissue can become replaced by bone, but that it is a very slow process. From a practical point of view fibrous union is an unsatisfactory end-result of healing, because in many cases it is permanent.

Occasionally with excessive movement the cells differentiate into synovial cells, and a false joint, or *pseudarthrosis,* results. This is a well-recognized sequel of fractures of the tibia.

Non-union. Complete lack of union between the fracture ends results from the interposition of soft parts. Muscle or fascia separating the bone ends may prevent the formation of a uniting haematoma. Under these conditions union of any sort is impossible. This phenomenon is utilized in the treatment of some disorders of the temporomandibular joint in order to create a new joint.

Delayed union. In the presence of a continuous haematoma any of the causes of delayed healing (p. 124) retard bone regeneration.

Causes of impaired healing. If the adverse conditions are severe, fibrous union may be the end result. In practice the following are the most important:

Movement. Movement of any sort is harmful, because it causes damage to the delicate granulation tissue, and thereby excites an inflammatory reaction. In surgical practice every attempt is made to reduce movement to a minimum. In the case of impacted fractures this is usually easy, but in other instances where the bone ends are mobile, recourse may have to be made to pins, plates, or other forms of internal splinting. The bone ends must not be over-distracted, for this leads to slow healing. Indeed, if on the contrary the bone ends are brought together under high compression, there is rigid immobilization and healing is accelerated.[21]

Infection. By prolonging the acute inflammatory phase, infection is an important cause of slow union or non-union. Since the tension engendered by the formation of exudate in a bone is liable to lead to extensive ischaemic necrosis with sequestrum formation, it is particularly important to avoid contaminating previously closed fractures during open reduction. Rigorous asepsis must be maintained by employing a no-touch technique.

Poor blood supply. While complete loss of blood supply results in necrosis of bone, poor blood supply leads to slow granulation tissue formation and therefore slow union. Certain sites are notorious for this complication, e.g. fractures of neck of femur, shaft of tibia, and the carpal scaphoid. In these situations the avoidance of other possible causes of delayed healing, e.g. movement, is particularly important. The slow healing of fractures in old age is probably due to ischaemia.

Traumatic myositis ossificans. If there is an extravasation of the fracture haematoma into the surrounding muscles, its subsequent organization and ossification results in the condition of *traumatic myositis ossificans.*

DISORDERS OF THE BONE MARROW

Disorders of the haematopoietic tissue of the marrow produce obvious effects in the circulating blood, and are considered in Chapter 30. There remain a number of disorders of uncertain nature which affect the reticulo-endothelial system as a whole, but since bone lesions are common it is convenient to consider them here.

Lipid-storage diseases[22]

The lipid-storage diseases are examples of inherited disturbances of lipid metabolism associated with a specific enzyme defect. Excess lipid accumulates in various organs, the RE cells being particularly affected in Gaucher's and Niemann-Pick disease. Several types of each of these diseases are known, and they are inherited as recessive traits.

Gaucher's disease. In this disease there is a massive accumulation of a glucocerebroside due to a deficiency of the enzyme glucocerebrosidase. Glucocerebroside is probably derived from effete white and red cells in the RE system and it is not surprising that here is found the main accumulation of lipid. The swollen RE cells are called Gaucher cells and their presence causes massive enlargement of the spleen and liver. Destructive lesions may occur in the bones, especially the femur, due to collections of Gaucher cells in the marrow eroding the cortex, which is thinned. The marrow replacement may cause a leuco-erythroblastic anaemia.

The adult form of the disease runs a protracted course. In the brain glucocerebroside is derived from gangliosides, which have a rapid turnover in infancy. It follows that central-nervous-system involvement with severe mental retardation and death is a feature of the infantile and juvenile neuropathic forms of Gaucher's disease.

Niemann-Pick disease. This rare and usually fatal disease occurs predominantly in Jewish children. It is familial, and is due to a defect in the metabolism of a phospholipid, sphingomyelin, which accumulates in the RE system as well as certain parenchymal cells. Not only are the spleen, lymph nodes, and bone marrow involved, but the kidney, lungs, brain, and adrenals may also be affected. There is physical and mental retardation. A generalized rarefaction with circumscribed foci of bone resorption may occur.

Histiocytosis X[23]

The three conditions in this category, Letterer-Siwe disease, Hand-Schüller-Christian disease, and eosinophilic granuloma of bone, although differing markedly in clinical behaviour, are nevertheless regarded as variants of the same disease process. Their differences are probable due to the age at which they occur—the younger the patient, the more severe is the form. Histologically there is a focal infiltration of large macrophages which may sometimes contain lipid. Interspersed among them there are polymorphs, eosinophils, and small round cells. The nature of the disease process is unknown.

Letterer-Siwe disease. This acute fatal condition occurs in young children. There is enlargement of spleen, liver, and lymph nodes. In fact there is a universal destructive proliferation of the RE cells, and few organs escape. Although classically a disease of the young, it can occur at any age.

Hand-Schüller-Christian disease. This disease runs a more chronic course, and affected children may survive into adult life. Characteristically there are focal areas of radiolucency in the skull. If the orbit is involved, exophthalmos (protrusion of the eyeballs) results, and if the sella turcica is implicated, diabetes insipidus may develop as a result of destruction of the posterior lobe of the pituitary. Loosening of the teeth is also quite a common feature if the jaw is affected. The destructive histiocytic lesions may eventually heal by fibrosis.

Eosinophilic granuloma of bone. A much older group is affected by this disease, which usually produces a solitary, localized area of bone destruction. Occasionally, however, multiple lesions are present, and when these are widely scattered the disease is not clearly delineated from Hand-Schüller-Christian disease. The affected areas are swollen and painful. The jaws are frequent sites of predeliction, and the lesions present diagnostic difficulties when they are closely related to the teeth.

TUMOURS[24]

Tumours of bone

The tumours of bone form a complex group of neoplasms, for in spite of the apparent simplicity of bone structure, the histogenesis of some of the tumours which arise from it is quite obscure. The occurrence of tumours in the adjacent marrow and the frequency of skeletal metastases add further to the confusion.

Quite often the initial diagnosis of bone tumour is made on radiological grounds, but it must be emphasized that histological confirmation by biopsy is essential before treatment is attempted. The 'characteristic' appearances of certain tumours, e.g. osteosarcoma, are often absent, and furthermore may be mimicked by other lesions.

Benign tumours

Osteoma, chondroma, fibroma, etc. are all recognized, but are rare, especially in the jaws. Many lesions described as tumours are in fact hamartomata, e.g. angioma, or variants of other non-neoplastic conditions, e.g. fibrous dysplasia, reaction to trauma, etc.

Intermediate tumours

Giant-cell tumour of bone (osteoclastoma). This tumour of uncertain histogenesis is usually found in patients between 20 and 40 years of age. It is composed of a mixture of spindle cells and giant cells resembling osteoclasts (Fig. 37.8). The tumour destroys bone locally by pressure atrophy and in some cases by actual invasion. This produces the characteristic soap-bubble appearance seen radiologically. About 15 per cent of giant-cell tumours metastasize to the lungs.

The tumour is usually seen in the long bones, and is very rare in the jaws. In the past it was commonly reported in the jaws, but this was probably due to the misdiagnosis of other non-neoplastic conditions. Some of these should be noted:

Central giant-cell reparative granuloma. This appears as a central, expanding lesion in the tooth-bearing portion of the jaw, usually the mandible. It occurs between the ages of 10 and 25 years, and closely resembles a giant-cell tumour histologically. Nevertheless, it is thought to be non-neoplastic; it never metastasizes, and is perhaps a reaction to haemorrhage.

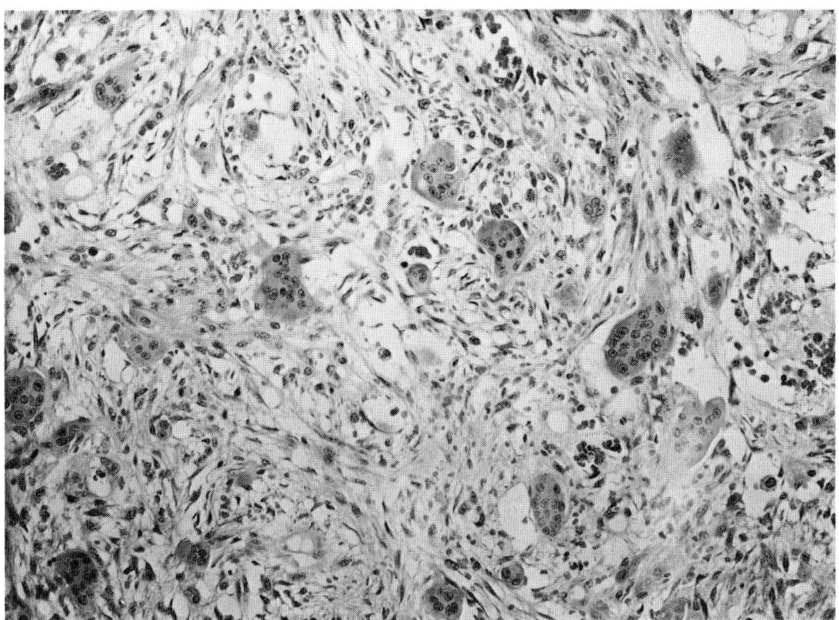

Fig. 37.8 Giant-cell tumour of bone. The tumour is composed of very large giant cells resembling osteoclasts and also a smaller spindle-shaped fibroblastic element. × 200.

Brown tumour. See p. 297.

Peripheral giant-cell reparative granuloma (giant-cell epulis). This should not be confused with a giant-cell tumour. It arises from the gingivae or periosteum as a result of chronic infection or irritation (see Fig. 21.1, p. 314).

Malignant tumours

Fibrosarcoma, angiosarcoma, etc. are described, but are rare.

Chondrosarcoma. This tumour is composed of atypical cartilage cells, but it is notoriously difficult to distinguish from a benign chondroma histologically. Local invasion and later metastasis to the lungs are the main features.

Osteosarcoma. Osteosarcoma is the most common and the most malignant of this rare group of primary bone tumours. It usually occurs in children and young adults, but is found in older persons as a complication of Paget's disease or as a result of the deposition of radioactive substances in the bone. The tumour is composed of malignant osteoblasts which are usually very pleomorphic; giant cells are often abundant. Well-differentiated tumours produce variable amounts of cartilage together with osteoid, which may or may not calcify to form bone (Fig. 37.9). The surrounding normal bone is destroyed, and radiologically a poorly-differentiated tumour appears *osteolytic,* as there is an irregular bony defect. The tumour lifts up the periosteum, and if neoplastic bone is formed, it tends to be laid down around the periosteal vessels as they penetrate the tumour mass. This leads to the characteristic sun-ray appearance of the *osteosclerotic* type

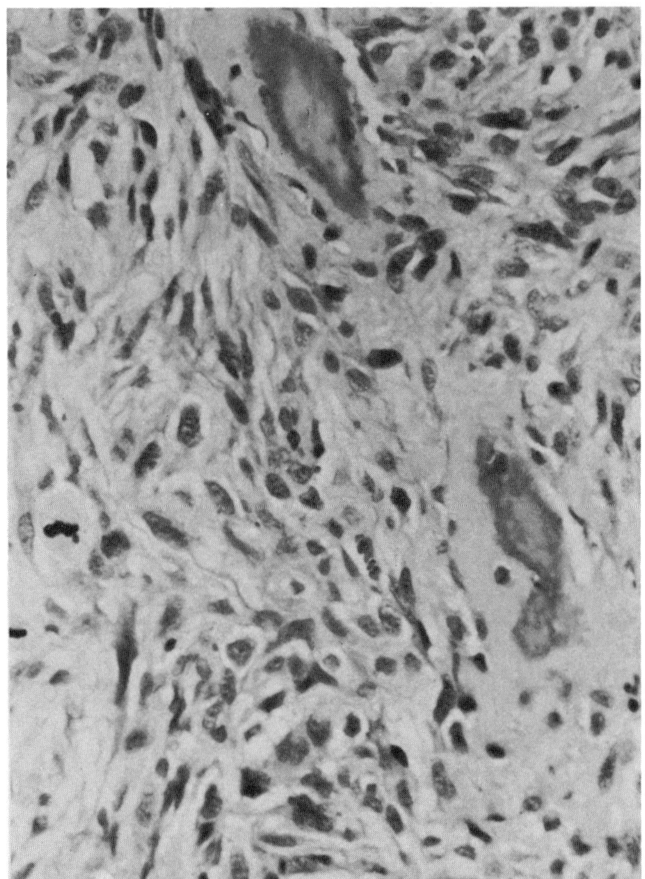

Fig. 37.9 Osteosarcoma. The tumour consists of sheets of spindle-shaped cells intimately connected with the intervening stroma. Two spicules of osteoid are included. Note the mitotic figure at the left edge of the section. × 350. (*Photograph by courtesy of Dr A D Thomson.*)

of tumour (Fig. 37.10). The outlook for a patient with osteosarcoma is extremely poor, for pulmonary metastases appear early.

Tumours of bone marrow (myelogenic tumours)

These rare tumours arise in the haematopoietic and reticulo-endothelial cells of the bone marrow. The three included in this group are *Ewing's tumour, reticulum-cell sarcoma,* and *multiple myeloma.*

Ewing's tumour. This tumour occurs in young children, and most often affects the shaft of a long bone. It is composed of sheets of small round cells, and is osteolytic. The raised periosteum may produce layers of new bone around the tumour, leading to an onion-like appearance radiologically. The nature of Ewing's tumour is obscure. It appears to be a distinct entity, but can be closely mimicked by reticulum-cell sarcoma and metastatic neuroblastoma. It is radiosensitive, but the prognosis is bad because it usually metastasizes to other bones and viscera.

Reticulum-cell sarcoma. This tumour occurs in an older age-group. It is

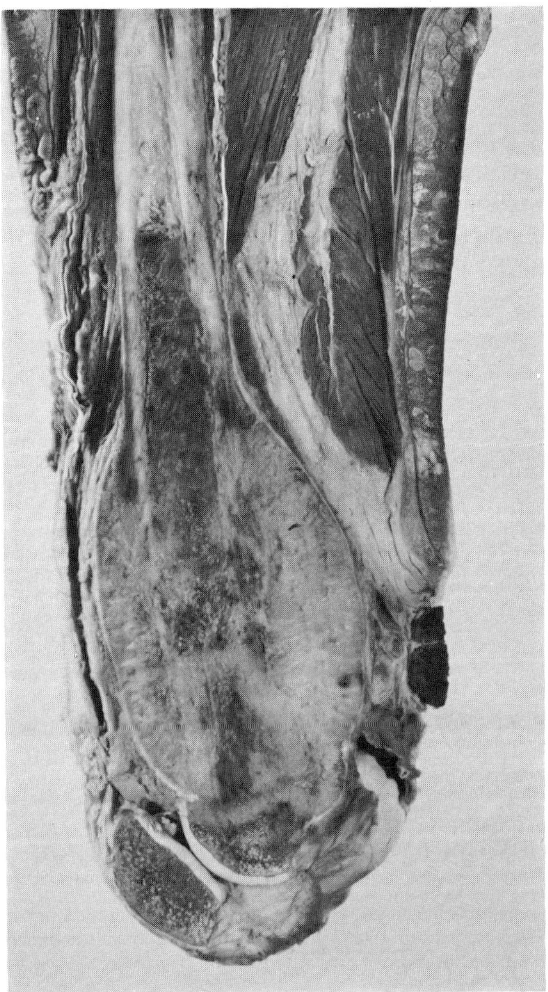

Fig. 37.10 Osteosarcoma. This has arisen from the lower end of the femur and has spread almost to the knee joint. The tumour has lifted up the periosteum, and has assumed a fusiform shape. There is a radiating ('sun-ray') disposition of newly-formed bony spicules in this spindle-shaped mass. (S72.5. *Reproduced by permission of the President and Council of the Royal College of Surgeons of England.*)

osteolytic, and nearly always appears as an isolated tumour. It is radiosensitive, and its prognosis is better than that of Ewing's tumour.

Myeloma. A tumour composed of neoplastic plasma cells is occasionally encountered as a *solitary myeloma* in the tonsil or nasopharynx. More commonly the tumours are multiple and are found in the bones, especially the vertebrae, ribs, sternum, and skull (*multiple myeloma*). The disease occurs in patients over the age of 40, and the osteolytic tumours produce characteristic punched-out areas on a radiograph (Fig. 37.11). The results of these tumours are serious. Not only do they lead to the destruction of the surrounding cortex and cause spontaneous fractures and collapse of the vertebral column, but they may also produce so much demineralization of the skeleton that hypercalcaemia and renal failure may follow. Pain is an early symptom.

The tumour cells form large amounts of a homogeneous immunoglobulin called *myeloma protein* (p. 434). Some tumours produce an excess of its component light chain, which has a molecular weight of about 22 000 daltons (*Bence-Jones protein*), and is small enough to pass through the glomeruli into the urine, where it can be recognized by its tendency to precipitate between the temperatures of 60°C and 80°C, and to redissolve on further heating. On cooling a similar phenomenon occurs between 80°C and 60°C. This protein may also precipitate in the tubules of the kidney, causing obstruction and renal failure.

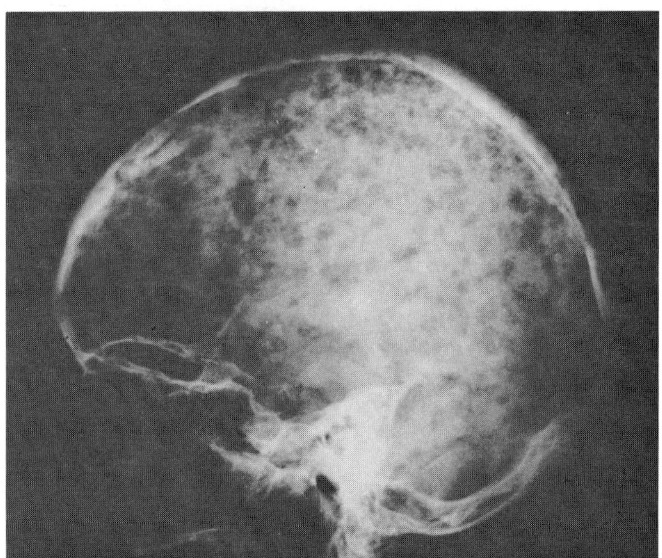

Fig. 37.11 Multiple myeloma. This radiograph of the skull shows numerous osteolytic tumour deposits that produce a typical moth-eaten appearance resulting from the punched-out areas where bone has been destroyed. An appearance similar to this can be produced by secondary carcinoma. (*Photograph by courtesy of Dr D E Sanders.*)

Metastatic tumours

Secondary tumours of bone are much more common than the primary ones. They develop from blood-borne metastases of carcinoma of the prostate, breast, bronchus, kidney, stomach, and thyroid. They are characteristically osteolytic, with the exception of carcinoma of the prostate which is osteoplastic. Pathological fractures and pain are the usual presenting symptoms.

The jaws are rarely affected, but when secondary deposits do occur it is usually in the mandibular molar area. A deposit in the jaws has been known to give rise to symptoms before the primary growth manifested itself.

DISEASES OF JOINTS

A joint consists of two or more opposing *cartilage-covered bone ends* united by a sleeve of connective tissue called the *capsule,* the innermost layer of which is modified into a secreting membrane called the *synovium.* This consists of one or more layers of flattened or cubical cells that secrete a clear, pale, viscid fluid (*synovial fluid*) which contains small quantities of albumin and globulin and also a significant amount of mucin. Not only does the synovial fluid lubricate the joint, but it is also the main, if not the only, source of nourishment of the hyaline cartilage covering the bone ends. The amount of synovial fluid in the joint is very small—there is only about 0.5 ml in the knee joint.

Arthritis

This is an inflammation of a joint. There is usually an increased amount of synovial fluid present due to a concomitant inflammation of the synovial membrane (*synovitis*). Arthritis may be traumatic, as after the twisting or the forcible hyperextension or hyperflexion of a joint. This may lead to a minor tear of the capsule, called a sprain, but if more severe the rupture of the capsule may cause a partial or complete displacement of the bone ends. A partial displacement is called a subluxation, and a complete one a dislocation. Simple sprains heal spontaneously, but the weakness of a ruptured capsule may predispose to a recurrent dislocation.

Another type of arthritis is *infective* in aetiology. This may follow a penetrating joint injury, when the infection is introduced from outside, or it may be blood-spread during the course of a systemic illness. The most important type of haematogenous arthritis is the suppurative arthritis that occasionally occurs in the course of such pyogenic diseases an gonorrhoea, lobar pneumonia, and staphylococcal septicaemia. Sometimes the infection may be of a more chronic type, e.g. tuberculosis and syphilis. Suppurative arthritis, unless energetically treated in the early stages with antibiotics, leads to the rapid destruction of the articular cartilages, and the whole cavity is filled with exudate which organizes and obliterates the space. In this way the joint is destroyed, and the bone ends are united by fibrous tissue. This is called an *ankylosis,* and it may undergo ossification later. A bony ankylosis is characteristic of a burnt-out suppurative process, whereas tuberculous arthritis usually terminates in a fibrous ankylosis.

By far the most important types of chronic arthritis are *rheumatoid arthritis* and *osteoarthritis.*

Rheumatoid arthritis

This common disease occurs most frequently in young adults, especially women. It is characteristically polyarticular (affecting many joints) and symmetrical. The small joints of the hands and feet are usually worst affected, but the knees also suffer badly. It is a systemic disease, and in the active phases there is mild pyrexia, weight loss, and sweating bouts. A moderate anaemia often develops.

The affected joints are swollen, tender, and painful. In the early stages the synovial membrane is acutely inflamed; it proliferates into villous folds in which there is a heavy infiltration of lymphocytes and plasma cells. Later on the lymphocytic infiltration becomes more copious and lymphoid follicles may also develop. There is a steady encroachment of granulation tissue from the articular margin on to the cartilage. This inflammatory tissue forms a *pannus* over the cartilage and destroys it. The joint space is gradually obliterated by fibrous adhesions, and eventually ankylosis occurs. In this late stage there is severe atrophy of the adjacent bones and muscles, and the overlying skin is smooth and shiny. The results of advanced rheumatoid arthritis are tragic to see. Progressive contractures lead to flexion deformities seen especially in the distorted hands with the characteristic ulnar deviation of the fingers, and the flexed, ankylosed larger joints which render the patient immobile. There may be limited movement in the temporo-mandibular joints, and occasionally ankylosis occurs.

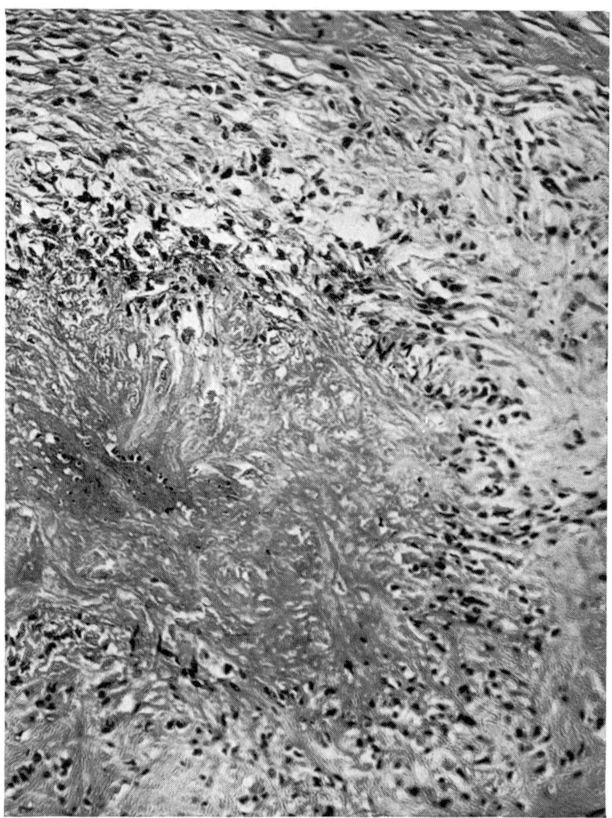

Fig. 37.12 Rheumatoid nodule. There is an extensive central area of necrotic connective tissue surrounded by a palisade layer of fibroblasts. In the periphery there is reparative fibrosis and a moderate small round cell infiltration. × 200 approx. (*From Bywaters E G L, Scott F E T 1960 Fig 6, Rheumatism and the connective tissue diseases. In: Dyke S C (ed) Recent advances in clinical pathology 3:301. Churchill, London.*)

The nature of rheumatoid arthritis is unknown, but the basic lesion seems to be a fibrinoid necrosis of collagen. It is therefore classed among the collagen diseases (Ch. 20). The systemic nature of the process is evidenced by *subcutaneous nodules* which develop over pressure points; these consist of a large area of necrosis surrounded by a palisade of fibroblastic cells and a diffuse zone of lymphocytes and plasma cells (Fig. 37.12). Inflammatory and fibrotic lesions are also encountered in the *heart and pericardium, lungs, arteries,* and *eyes.* Enlargement of the *spleen* and *lymph nodes* is also often present. *Amyloidosis* is an important complication; indeed, it is the only significant fatal lesion in rheumatoid arthritis, which may otherwise smoulder on for many years and produce complete crippling.

The sera of most patients with rheumatoid arthritis contain an autoantibody which reacts against human immunoglobulin. This antibody is called *rheumatoid factor,* but its significance in the pathogenesis of the disease is not known.

Ankylosing spondylitis. This condition resembles rheumatoid arthritis so much in its histological appearance and pathogenesis that some authorities used to regard it simply as a variant which attacked the spinal column primarily. But there are important differences: (1) young men are usually affected, (2) the vertebral joints and the large peripheral joints are affected, whereas the small distal joints are seldom involved, and (3) there is bony ankylosis of the spinal and peripheral joints, and the spinal ligaments and the margins of the intervertebral discs undergo ossification. In due course the spinal column is converted into a composite bony mass, the so-called bamboo spine. Subcutaneous nodules are not present, nor is the rheumatoid factor. There may be ocular and cardiovascular complications. There is a strong association between ankylosing spondylitis and transplantation antigen HLA-B27.

Osteoarthritis

Osteoarthritis, despite its name, is not an inflammatory disease of joints but rather a degenerative one; for this reason it is often called degenerative joint disease, or osteoarthrosis. It is one of humanity's commonest afflictions, for it is essentially an accentuation of the normal ageing process of articular cartilage. The nourishment of the hyaline cartilage is normally rather precarious, depending on the synovial fluid. The constant wear and tear on the joints after many years' activity leads to a gradual deterioration of the central parts of the articular cartilage; for this reason obesity predisposes to osteoarthritis of the weight-bearing joints. This process is greatly aggravated by concomitant trauma to a joint, for example that sustained during athletics. Osteoarthritis is a disease of later life, but it can affect a traumatized joint in a younger person. The spine and the large weight-bearing joints, especially the hips, are most severely affected, but the smaller joints do not escape. Osteoarthritis, unlike the rheumatoid variety, is not a systemic disease. The general health is not affected.

The condition commences with a softening and fraying of the articular cartilage. It becomes progressively thinner, and ultimately the underlying bone is exposed. This increases in density, and its surface becomes hard, worn, and polished, a change called *eburnation.* Meanwhile there is a proliferation of cartilage cells at the margin of the articular area. The new cartilage that is formed soon ossifies. The result is that the periphery of the articular cartilage is raised and bossed; this is called *lipping,* and is an important radiological finding. The peripheral new bone may become elongated into irregular *marginal osteophytes.* Not only do these interfere with the range of the joint's movement, but they may also become nipped off to form *loose bodies* (also called 'joint-mice'). These are a constant nuisance because they tend to be caught between the opposing bone ends during movement; the result is 'locking' of the joint, which may be excruciatingly painful if a fringe of synovium is included. A prominent site for osteophytes is the terminal interphalangeal joint of the fingers of elderly people. These produce the painless bony swellings called *Heberden's nodes.*

There is no primary synovial change, but later the membrane is thrown up into vascular villous folds. There is no inflammatory change except after locking, which produces a traumatic synovitis. These joints do not become ankylosed, but the destruction of articular cartilage and the osteophyte formation seriously limit movement, which may be very painful. Fortunately the operation of arthroplasty is now so successful that many people crippled with osteoarthritic hips have been restored to activity with artificial metallic or silastic joints.

Tumours of joints

The only significant one is the *synovioma,* and this arises much more often from the synovial membrane of a tendon sheath than from a joint. It is usually a benign tumour with cleft-like spaces and large giant cells.

There is a condition of generalized proliferation of the synovium, which is reddish brown in colour, found most often in the knee joint. Histologically there are giant cells, lipid-filled macrophages, and haemosiderin in the synovial villi, and the condition is called *pigmented villonodular synovitis.* The histological picture resembles that of a synovioma, and it is probable that this is a benign synoviomatous change in a joint. The blood pigment may be the end-result of repeated trauma.

The malignant synovioma resembles other sarcomata in its general behaviour.

REFERENCES

1. Bloom W, Fawcett D W 1975 In: A Textbook of Histology, 10th edn. Saunders, Philadelphia, p 244
2. Ham A W 1974 Histology, 7th edn. Lippincott, Philadelphia, p 378
3. McLean F C, Budy A M 1959 Connective and supporting tissues: Bone. Annual Review of Physiology, 21:69
4. Goldhaber P 1962 Some current concepts of bone physiology. New England Journal of Medicine, 266:870 and 924
5. Baker S L 1959 In: Shanks S C, Kerley P (eds) A Textbook of X-Ray Diagnosis, 3rd edn. Lewis, London, vol 4, p 55
6. Wieme R J, Demeulenaere L 1970 Journal of Clinical Pathology 24, Supplement (Association of Clinical Pathologists) 4:51
7. Forland M 1962 Cleidocranial dysostosis: A review of the syndrome and report of a sporadic case, with hereditary transmission. American Journal of Medicine 33:792
8. McKusick V A 1972 In: Heritable Disorders of Connective Tissue, 4th edn. (osteogenesis imperfecta). Mosby, St Louis, p 390
9. Houston W O 1965 Fibrous dysplasia of maxilla and mandible: clinicopathologic study and comparison of facial bone lesions with lesions affecting general skeleton. Journal of Oral Surgery 23:17
10. Zegarelli E V, Kutscher A H 1963 Fibrous dysplasia of the jaws. Dental Radiography and Photography 36:27
11. Jones W A 1965 Cherubism: a thumbnail sketch of its diagnosis and a conservative method of treatment. Oral Surgery, Oral Medicine and Oral Pathology 20:648
12. Lucas R B 1976 In: Pathology of Tumours of the Oral Tissues, 3rd edn. (cherubism). Churchill Livingstone, Edinburgh, p 405
13. Smith N H H 1966 Albers-Schönberg disease (osteopetrosis). Oral Surgery, Oral Medicine and Oral Pathology 22:699
14. Barzel U S 1970 Osteoporosis. Grune and Stratton, New York, pp 290
15. Leading Article 1971 Osteoporosis. British Medical Journal 1:566

16. Meema H E, Harris C K, Porrett R E 1964 A method for determination of bone-salt content of cortical bone. Radiology 82:986
17. Annotation 1963 Disuse osteoporosis. Lancet 1:150
18. Phillips R M, Bush O B, Hall H D 1972 Massive osteolysis (phantom bone, disappearing bone). Oral Surgery, Oral Medicine and Oral Pathology 34:886
19. Urist M R 1959 In: Patterson W B (ed) Wound Healing and Tissue Repair, The University of Chicago Press, Chicago, p 65
20. Pritchard J J 1963 In: The Scientific Basis of Medicine Annual Reviews, Athlone Press, London, p 286
21. Müller M E 1969 Compression as an aid in orthopaedic surgery. In: Apley A G (ed) Recent Advances in Orthopaedics, Churchill, London, p 79
22. Stanbury J B, Wyngaarden J B, Fredrickson D S (eds) 1972 The Metabolic Basis of Inherited Disease, 3rd edn. McGraw-Hill, New York, p 730 et seq.
23. Johnson R P, Mohnac A M 1967 Histiocytosis X: report of 7 cases. Journal of Oral Surgery 25:7
24. Lichtenstein L 1966 Bone Tumors, 3rd edn. Mosby, St Louis

38

Diseases of the central nervous system

The brain and spinal cord are of such complexity that only those features of neuropathology which are relevant to dental surgery will be described in this chapter.

Cellular components

The important component of the central nervous system is the nerve cell, or *neuron*. The highly specialized neurons with their long axonal processes are held in position and insulated from each other by a specialized connective tissue called *neuroglia*. This has three components:

The *astrocytes* are closely associated with the bodies of the nerve cells and the blood vessels.

The *oligodendroglia* encloses the axons and forms their myelin sheaths, an insulating function which is essential for the conduction of nerve impulses.

The *microglia*, as the name implies, are small cells, and are of mesodermal, reticulo-endothelial origin.

The extreme susceptibility of the neurons to hypoxia has been noted previously (p. 496). Permanent brain damage can easily occur if the brain is rendered ischaemic; this may occur during periods of hypotension in the course of a surgical operation. Inadequate ventilation of the lungs with oxygen is not uncommon during the inexpert administration of nitrous oxide as an anaesthetic, and is another important cause of cerebral hypoxia.

Meninges

The coverings, or *meninges*, of the central nervous system are three:

The *pia mater* closely envelops the brain and spinal cord.

The *dura mater* is closely adherent to the bony-ligamentous protective housing provided by the skull, vertebral column, and the connecting ligaments.

The thin, translucent *arachnoid* covering lies between the pia and the dura.

The space between the arachnoid and the pia is called the *subarachnoid space* and contains *cerebrospinal fluid* (*CSF*). This fluid originates in the choroid plexuses, perfuses the ventricles, and finally escapes through the foramina in the roof of the fourth ventricle to reach the subarachnoid space.

Effects of increased intracranial pressure

Although the rigid bony enclosure of the brain is a necessary protective shield, its presence has some attendant disadvantages. Any lesion which takes up space within the skull (*space occupying lesion*) tends to cause a rise in intracranial pressure, and this increases the pressure in the veins. Initially some CSF and venous blood are displaced, but soon, as venous obstruction is produced, there is a marked rise in CSF pressure, which has very serious effects. If of sudden onset, the blood supply to the brain is so reduced that the cerebral hypoxia causes rapid *loss of consciousness*. When the lesion develops gradually, severe *headaches* are common, and there is also progressive *mental impairment*. The traction on the cribriform plate, through which the optic nerve fibres leave the eye, causes compression on the nerves, thereby obstructing the normal flow of axoplasm. The result is swelling of the optic disc (*papilloedema*). Eventually *blindness* follows. *Haematoma*, *abscess* with inflammatory oedema, and *tumour* are examples of space occupying lesions.

Traumatic lesions of the central nervous system

An injury involving the jaws is sometimes accompanied by a much more important injury to the brain. Blows on the head produce damage to the region underlying the injury and to the brain at the opposite pole—this is the *contre-coup injury*. Minor injuries cause petechial haemorrhages and traumatic inflammatory oedema, while more severe ones may actually tear the brain (*laceration*), and haemorrhage may be of sufficient magnitude to cause death. Some degree of haemorrhage into the subarachnoid space is common in all head injuries, and can be detected by examining the cerebrospinal fluid obtained by lumbar puncture.

Subdural haemorrhage. It sometimes happens that a bridging vein is torn, and blood escapes into the loose subdural space to produce a subdural haematoma. If small, this is of little importance. If large, it organizes at the periphery and its centre remains fluid. The cyst which is formed imbibes fluid, and enlarges to form a *chronic subdural haematoma* which acts as a space occupying lesion. The injury which causes this type of lesion is often relatively mild, and in an elderly or alcoholic patient may be completely overlooked. Weeks later headaches and other signs and symptoms of raised intracranial pressure appear.

Extradural haemorrhage. This occurs when the *middle meningeal artery* is torn, usually in association with a fracture of the skull involving the temporal region. Unconsciousness may occur immediately after the injury, but the patient often recovers and feels well for a few hours. This *lucid interval* is deceptive, for presently, as the bleeding proceeds, increasing signs of raised intracranial pressure appear, and are followed by coma and death. It is evident that *all cases of head injury, except the most trivial, should be observed carefully for 24 hours.* This word of caution applies particularly to persons suspected of being drunk—a state which may be mimicked by the combination of medicinal brandy given by a well-wisher and an extradural haemorrhage.

Non-traumatic vascular lesions

Subarachnoid haemorrhage. This is not uncommon in the 20 to 50 year age-group. The haemorrhage stems from a ruptured aneurysm of one of the major cerebral arteries in the neighbourhood of the circle of Willis. The aneurysms lie in the subarachnoid space and are from 0.5 to 1.0 cm in diameter—because of this size they are often called *berry aneurysms.* They are thought to arise at the site of congenital defects in the elastic coat of the arteries. Sometimes they are multiple.

Cerebral haemorrhage and infarction. Atherosclerosis and hypertension both predispose to cerebral haemorrhage (sometimes called cerebral apoplexy). The common site is from the lenticulostriate artery, well named the artery of

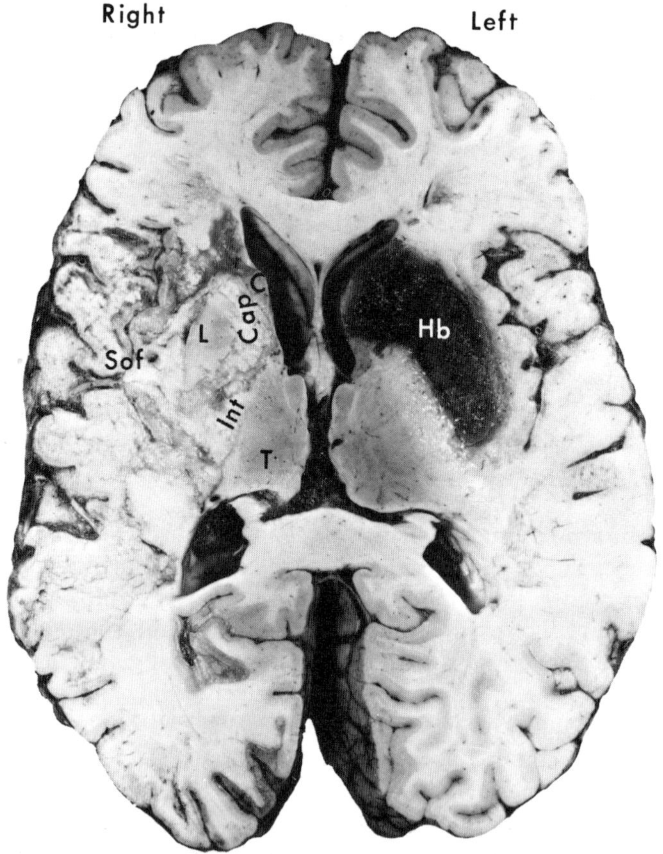

Fig. 38.1 Cerebral softening and haemorrhage. The brain has been sectioned horizontally, and is viewed here from below. There is severe damage. On the right-hand side there is extensive softening (Soft). Note the shrunken appearance of the affected area, which extends outwards to involve the grey matter of the cerebral cortex. The internal capsule (Int Cap) is severely affected. It lies between the lentiform nucleus and thalamus (T) posteriorly. Loss of the corticospinal fibres leads to an upper motor neuron lesion of the opposite side of the body. The patient had had a stroke three months before death. The attack, which had been attributed to a cerebral thrombosis, left the patient with left-sided hemiplegia. She subsequently had another stroke involving the opposite side. Note the extensive haemorrhage (Hb) that has occurred into the area of softening on the left side. (Photography by courtesy of Dr. N. B. Rewcastle).

cerebral haemorrhage, and the region of the brain affected is therefore the basal ganglia. The immediate effects of haemorrhage tend to be more severe than those produced by thrombosis. In both there is the clinical picture commonly called a 'stroke' (Fig. 38.1).

With haemorrhage there is usually sudden loss of consciousness, and as blood disrupts the substance of the brain, coma deepens and death ensues. This is not, however, inevitable, and the bleeding may stop.

Thrombosis often occurs during sleep, and although consciousness may be lost this is not invariable. Thrombosis causes *infarction*, which can itself lead to later haemorrhage in the damaged area.

The infarct is usually pale, and in those patients who survive the area softens (colliquative necrosis). The microglial cells enlarge, become phagocytic, and appear as large foamy macrophages. The damaged nerve fibres are not replaced to any extent, and the area heals by proliferation of astrocytes to produce a *glial scar*. The area of brain thus collapses, and sometimes a central cyst remains where once were the long tracts from the motor cortex to the spinal cord. It should be noted that any nerve cells destroyed are not replaced.

Cerebral embolism is another common cause of a stroke. The embolus generally originates from the heart, and the onset of the stroke is sudden.

In cerebral infarction the neurological picture is commonly that of *hemiplegia*—loss of voluntary movement on the side of the body opposite to that of the lesion.

Quite apart from acute episodes of thrombosis or embolism, cerebral athersclerosis can lead to multiple, bilateral, ischaemic lesions in the brain. The characteristic mental deterioration of old age is one effect, but if the lesions are extensive there may be severe bilateral damage to the corticospinal tracts. Bilaterally innervated muscles such as those of the tongue and pharynx are affected, and the condition is called *pseudobulbar palsy*.

Bacterial infections of the central nervous system

Pyogenic bacteria may produce a diffuse infection of the subarachnoid space, which is called *meningitis*, or a localized suppuration in the brain substance (*cerebral abscess*).

Meningitis

Mode of infection. Two routes of infection are common:

Blood-borne. H. influenzae and *N. meningitidis* (meningococcus) gain entry to the blood, presumably from an infection in the upper respiratory tract. The meninges are probably infected *via* the choroid plexuses, where the organisms are filtered out of the blood. The infection spreads through the ventricular system and reaches the subarachnoid space in the region of the basal cisterns. It is here that the most severe effects are encountered. The pia and arachnoid are acutely inflamed, and there is a massive polymorph and fibrinous exudate into the subarachnoid space. With modern chemotherapy the patients often survive, but even then the exudate may undergo organization, and the foramina in the roof of the fourth ventricle become blocked. Cerebrospinal fluid accumulates in the ventricular system which expands accordingly—this is one mechanism whereby *hydrocephalus* develops. In the young child the pressure exerted on the developing bones leads to a tremendous enlargement of the vault in the skull.

Tuberculous meningitis is mentioned on p. 218.

Local spread. Meningitis may follow the spread of infection from the middle ear or mastoid air cells—sites of infection that were once quite common in childhood. It is also a complication of a fractured skull when the wound is exposed to the exterior or the nasal cavity. Fracture of the cribriform plate of the ethmoid is followed by an escape of cerebrospinal fluid into the nose (*cerebrospinal rhinorrhoea*). Meningitis may follow.

Cerebral abscess

As with meningitis there are two modes of infection:

Blood-borne. Patients with chronic chest infections (empyema, lung abscess, and bronchiectasis) sometimes develop a cerebral abscess. The infection is presumably blood-borne; an alternative explanation is that spread occurs from an infected nasal air sinus—a common accompaniment of chronic chest suppuration.

Local spread. As with meningitis this occurs from an infected middle ear or nasal air sinus.

Viral infections

A large number of virus types cause infection of the central nervous system, e.g. the viruses of mumps, rabies, and the various forms of arbovirus encephalitis. Poliomyelitis is described on p. 256.

Diseases affecting the myelin sheath

The major nerve fibres both within the central nervous system and in the peripheral nervous system have a myelin sheath, which acts as an insulating covering, thereby aiding in transmission of impulses in the axon. Damage to the myelin sheath leads to impaired conduction, even though the axon itself may remain intact. Two groups of disorders are recognized:

1. The *demyelinating diseases*, of which multiple sclerosis is by far the most frequent
2. The *dysmyelinating diseases, or leukodystrophies*, in which myelin formation is impaired.

Multiple sclerosis

Multiple sclerosis, or disseminated sclerosis as it is also called, is a chronic disease characterized by exacerbations and remissions that often extend over many years. The brain and spinal cord show the development of well-circumscribed foci (plaques) of demyelination. During the acute phases there is an inflammatory reaction and severe impairment of nerve conduction. The nerve axons are generally preserved, and a considerable degree of functional recovery occurs after each phase. Depending on the site of damage, multiple sclerosis first manifests itself as sudden impairment of vision, inability to speak clearly (dysarthria), cerebellar dysfunction, or paralysis due to pyramidal tract damage. Alteration in emotional state and bladder dysfunction also occur. Each acute episode is followed by recovery; this occasionally is complete, but more frequently there is some residual damage, so that with the passage of years the patient ultimately becomes quite disabled.

Other demyelinating diseases

Several diseases are known that resemble multiple sclerosis but are more acute. Demyelination is also a feature of the encephalitis that occasionally follows certain viral infections, such as after vaccination for smallpox and rabies, as well as following certain naturally occurring viral diseases such as rubella.

The leukodystrophies

The leukodystrophies constitute a group of rare diseases in which there is a defect in the formation of myelin. Usually manifested during infancy or childhood, they are familial.

Toxic, deficiency, and metabolic disorders of the brain

The brain is a very active metabolic organ and although it represents about 2 per cent of the body weight, it is responsible for 20 per cent of the body's resting oxygen consumption. It is not surprising, therefore, that it can easily be affected adversely by many agents that interfere with metabolism. A few of these are listed below.

Poisons. Lead and arsenic are examples of agents that can cause permanent brain damage. Likewise, poisoning by carbon monoxide can cause necrosis of the basal ganglia and can lead to extrapyramidal syndromes, which are described later.

Deficiency of oxygen (hypoxia). The brain is extremely sensitive to oxygen deprivation. Even short periods of hypoxia can produce permanent damage. Hence care must be taken to avoid hypoxia when administering out-patient anaesthesia.

Vitamin deficiencies. *Vitamin B_1 (thiamine) deficiency.* In some patients vitamin B_1 deficiency causes focal areas of necrosis. Several syndromes can occur. For example, in *Wernicke's encephalopathy* there is paralysis of eye muscles and unsteadiness. It may be combined with loss of memory and confabulation (this is *Korsakoff's psychosis* that is associated with alcoholism combined with vitamin B_1 deficiency).

Pellagra encephalopathy. This condition is described in Chapter 18.

Subacute combined degeneration of the spinal cord. This condition is due to vitamin B_{12} deficiency and accompanies pernicious anaemia.

Metabolic encephalopathies. *Hepatic encephalopathy.* Degeneration of neurons is responsible for the mental deterioration encountered in chronic liver disease (see Ch. 35).

Chronic alcoholism. The pathetic state of some chronic alcoholics is a combined effect of alcohol, vitamin deficiency, and liver damage.

Hypoglycaemia. Poisoning with insulin causes hypoglycaemia, coma, convulsions, and death. Permanent neuronal loss can occur in those who survive; the changes resemble those of hypoxia. At one time, insulin convulsions were used as a treatment for certain psychiatric conditions, but this practice has now been abandoned.

Degenerative neurological diseases

There are many diseases of the nervous system in which neuronal degeneration occurs for no known reason. In some of these conditions there is a strong hereditary factor, whereas in others the degeneration is probably due to slow virus infection (e.g., in kuru and Creutzfeldt-Jakob disease; see Ch. 16). A few common examples of degenerative neurological diseases will be described.

Senile dementia. Cerebral atrophy with compensatory dilatation of the ventricles is a common event in old age.

Alzheimer's disease. This disease resembles senile dementia but occurs at an earlier age and is more severe.

Parkinson's disease. This common disease is due to selective degeneration of parts of the basal ganglia. The patient's muscles become rigid, the face is expressionless, and voluntary movement becomes difficult. A fine tremor completes the picture; 'pill rolling' movements of the fingers are characteristic. This *extrapyramidal syndrome* is also seen following encephalitis, vascular ischaemic episodes, and poisoning with carbon monoxide.

Huntington's chorea. Patients with this disease exhibit basal-ganglia degeneration as well as cortical neuronal loss. Bizarre grimacing and uncontrolled irregular jerking movement (chorea) are combined with progressive dementia in this disease, which is inherited as a mendelian dominant trait.

Motor neuron disease. Primary degeneration of the *Betz cells* in the motor areas of the cerebral cortex and their fibres in the pyramidal tracts, the *anterior horn cells*, and their *cranial equivalents* can occur either singly or in combination to produce a variety of syndromes.

Epilepsy

The term epilepsy comes from the Greek and means a seizure. It should be regarded as a syndrome rather than a disease entity because epilepsy is a symptom of an underlying brain disorder. It occurs in about 1 per cent of the population, and only about 5 per cent of the sufferers are mentally subnormal.

Epilepsy consists of a sudden, uncoordinated burst of impulses from a group of nerve cells. The seizure that results may be limited to a particular part of the brain and this constitutes *partial*, or *focal*, *epilepsy*. On the other hand, the seizure may cause loss of consciousness and may be accompanied by widespread brain dysfunction. This is *generalized epilepsy*.

Focal epilepsy

There are many areas of the brain in which epileptic discharges may originate and there are therefore many clinical variations of local fits. If the temporal lobe is affected, the patient experiences hallucinations which may be of smell, taste, hearing, or sight. Sometimes there is a feeling of great familiarity of the surroundings—this constitutes the 'déjà vu phenomenon'. In *Jacksonian epilepsy* the motor areas of the brain are affected, and the patient experiences muscular twitching confined to a particular area (e.g. a hand), and the twitching slowly extends to involve the whole limb or even the whole body. Sometimes after recovery from a Jacksonian fit the affected part remains paralyzed—this is called Todd's paralysis. In any type of partial epilepsy the focal discharging area may steadily extend its effect so that the initial local disturbances progress to involve a wide area and the condition then becomes an example of generalized epilepsy.

Generalized epilepsy

In generalized seizures there is loss of consciousness; two major types are described.

Grand mal seizures. There may be a *prodomal phase* lasting several hours or even days when the patient becomes aware that an attack is imminent. Often a change of mood is the forerunner of the attack itself. Grand mal seizures may commence with some sensory manifestation (a strange taste or feeling, or seeing flashes of light) or some motor activity (movement of one part of the body) which is described as the *aura*. This precedes loss of consciousness by a few seconds. Then follows the generalized convulsion. At first the muscles exhibit *tonic contraction*, and as the chest muscles contract the patient may emit a characteristic cry as air is forced past the glottis. The tonic phase is followed by a *clonic phase*, in which the muscles exhibit powerful jerking movements. Movement of the jaw and tongue causes saliva to froth at the mouth, and at this stage, which lasts about half a minute, the tongue may be bitten and the patient may sustain damage. The final phase is one of relaxation, and the patient passes from a comatose state into normal sleep. During the tonic and clonic phases the patient is often incontinent of urine and less frequently of faeces also.

Petit mal seizures. In petit mal seizures, sometimes described by the patient as 'dizzy spells' or 'fainting turns', there is a transient loss of consciousness. The patient develops a staring expression and there may be an upward rolling of the eyes. If the child is doing something, it will discontinue the activity for a few seconds, and then resume the action when the seizure is ended as though nothing had happened. The condition is most common in children, and attacks may cease at puberty.

Causes of seizures

Seizures can be induced in anyone provided a powerful enough stimulus (e.g. an electric current) is applied. There is indeed a *threshold level* for each individual, and any stimulus above this will result in an epileptic fit. In subjects with a 'normal' threshold there are many conditions (e.g. hypocalcaemia) which will induce seizures. Sometimes a local brain lesion will lower the threshold, and this results in epilepsy. When such lesions can be recognized the disease is labelled symptomatic epilepsy. When no cause can be identified resort must be made to the term idiopathic epilepsy.

Diseases causing symptomatic epilepsy. Amongst the numerous organic causes of epilepsy the following should be noted:

Cerebral tumours. This is the commonest type of symptomatic epilepsy, and in 10 per cent of the cases a seizure is the initial sign of the tumour. Glioma or metastatic carcinoma should always be considered as a likely cause of fits commencing in patients over the age of 40 years.

Cerebral trauma. Trauma may cause seizures immediately or after a period of time, in which event it is presumed that scarring of the brain is the cause.

Cerebrovascular disease. Fits may occur in cerebral haemorrhage and infarction.

Cerebral infections. Brain abscess and encephalitis may precipitate a seizure.

Metabolic diseases. Hypoglycaemia (insulin overdose), hypocalcaemia (tetany), uraemia, and hypoxia provide examples.

Sunstroke. See p. 415.

Drug intoxication. Certain drugs such as strychnine cause convulsions, but seizures may also follow the withdrawal of a drug (e.g. alcohol or barbiturates) in addicts.

Miscellaneous brain diseases. There are many diseases associated with seizures, for example, tuberous sclerosis and cerebral palsy.*

Convulsions are more common in infants due presumably to the fact that the nervous system is immature and more unstable. Many children have convulsions during the eruption of teeth, or with a sudden onset of fever. Hence, they are encountered with pneumonia, otitis media, and in the common viral infections. Such convulsions may be an isolated incident due presumably to some metabolic defect, or they may be the forerunner of more persistent seizures in later life. Seizures may occur following general anaesthesia, and patients prone to epilepsy require supervision for several hours postoperatively. Seizures may occur in the dental chair, and it is important to protect the patient from injury on equipment or biting the tongue.

Idiopathic epilepsy. When no morphological or biochemical cause of the seizures can be found the disease must be labelled idiopathic. Often when seizures begin in childhood no cause can be found, and it is possible that there is some specific genetic defect in cerebral metabolism. Patients with epilepsy may have their seizures precipitated by a variety of circumstances. Thus hyperventilation can cause a fit, as also may a flickering light or emotional disturbance. If such triggers can be recognized, then both idiopathic and symptomatic seizures may be averted.

In the treatment of epilepsy a variety of drugs are in use. One of the commonest is phenytoin (dilantin), and an important complication of the administration of this drug is gingival hyperplasia. Indeed this occurs in about 50 per cent of patients taking this medication. Good oral hygiene reduces the effect; if marked hyperplasia occurs, the advisability of using some other drug should be raised

* *Cerebral palsy* is a popular term for a condition in which there is a major disturbance of motor function that is generally non-progressive and has been present since infancy. Upper-motor-neuron damage with spasticity is the dominant feature. Cerebral palsy is not a distinct entity, but is the end-result of many processes—inherited defect, infection, birth trauma, etc. The term has been adopted by fund-raising societies (e.g. the Spastic Society), and is unlikely to disappear readily from medical terminology.

with the attending physician. Gingivectomy may be necessary if the hyperplasia is severe.

Tumours of the central nervous system

Primary tumours

The tumours are called *gliomata*; several types are described, the common one being derived from astrocytes. Well-differentiated astrocytomata invade slowly, but the poorly-differentiated tumours (Grades III and IV astrocytomata, or glioblastomata multiforme) are more malignant and kill rapidly. Although all gliomata are locally invasive and may metastasize within the central nervous system, one curious feature of these tumours is that *none of them ever produces distant metastases.* In spite of this, the prognosis is usually poor, because gliomata are difficult to remove surgically.

The *meningioma* is a benign tumour arising from the arachnoid granulations of the dura; it is therefore not a tumour of the brain itself. It is included here because the effects produced are very similar to those of a cerebral tumour. It produces pressure atrophy of the underlying brain; unless removed, a meningioma kills the subject by its local effects or because of an increased intracranial pressure.

Secondary tumours

These are as common as primary growths. Carcinoma of the lung in males and carcinoma of the breast in females are the common primary tumours in these cases.

GENERAL READING

Escourolle R, Poirier J 1973 Manual of Basic Neuropathology. Translated and adapted by Rubinstein L J. Saunders, Philadelphia

Foley J M 1974 In Pathologic Basis of Disease, ed. by Robbins S L, chapter 32, 'The nervous system'. Saunders, Philadelphia

Simpson J A, Mawdsley C 1974 In Davidson's Principles and Practice of Medicine, 11th edn., ed. by MacLeod J, pp 793–910, 'Diseases of the nervous system'. Churchill Livingstone, Edinburgh

39

Diseases of the endocrine glands

Introduction

While the nervous system exerts major control of the activity of higher animals, there is an additional mechanism whereby one group of cells can influence another. This is by their secretion into the blood stream of potent chemicals (hormones), which, being carried by the circulation, can exert influence on some distant part. Secreting cells which perform this endocrine function are being recognized in increasing numbers, for not only are they situated in the well-known endocrine glands, but are also found scattered in other tissues. For instance, when food enters the pylorus, the hormone called *gastrin* is secreted, and this stimulates the fundus of the stomach to produce hydrochloric acid. When acid enters the duodenum, *secretin* is formed, and this causes the pancreas to pour out its alkaline juice.

This chapter deals only with the common disorders of the major endocrine glands and the recently recognized APUD cells.

Mode of action of hormones

Hormones have an extremely potent and highly specific action on their target cells. This selective action is due to the binding of the hormone to specific cell receptors. The water-soluble hormones, such as adrenaline and glucagon, act on receptors situated in the cell membrane; cyclic AMP is formed, acting as a second messenger to stimulate or depress a characteristic biochemical activity (see Fig. 2.2, p. 8). In the case of insulin, cyclic GMP appears to be the second messenger. The lipid-soluble steroid hormones act on receptors in the cytoplasm, and the hormone-receptor complex, after modification, enters the nucleus and then acts by influencing the expression of the cell's genetic material.

THE HYPOTHALAMUS

Although the pituitary gland has been called the 'leader of the endocrine orchestra', it is now clear that it plays second fiddle to the hypothalamus, for many of the pituitary's activities are themselves controlled by hormones secreted in the hypothalamus (Fig. 39.1).

The hypothalamus consists of a complex collection of nerve cells and fibre tracts that participate in, and help regulate, many functions of the body. These include the autonomic nervous system, temperature, blood pressure, plasma osmolality,

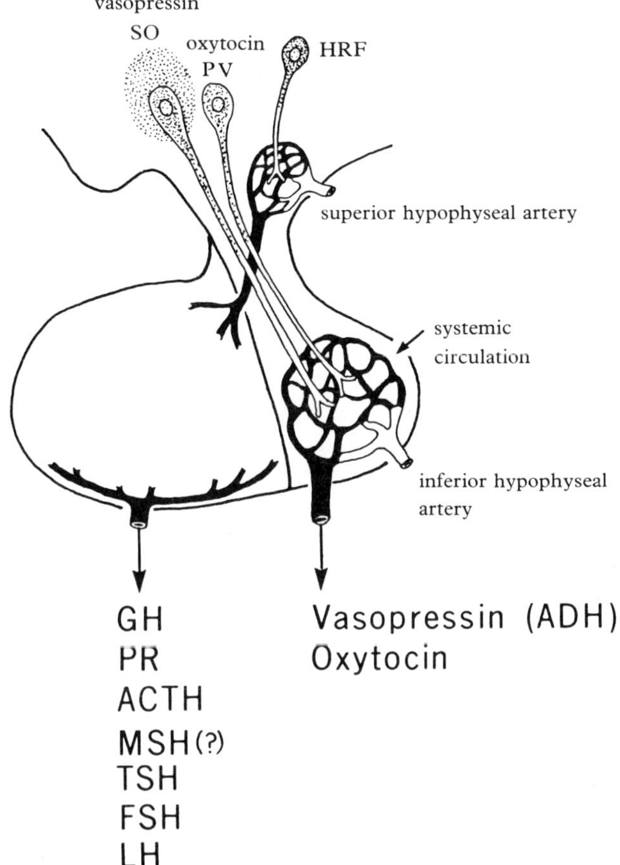

Fig. 39.1 The relationship between the hypothalmus and the pituitary gland. Vasopressin (antidiuretic hormone, or ADH) and oxytocin are manufactured in nerve cells in the supraoptic (SO) and paraventricular (PV) nuclei of the hypothalamus. These hormones are not released into the circulation until they have reached the neurohypophysis. The shaded area surrounding the SO cell body represents the 'osmoreceptor' that is responsive to changes in osmolality of the fluid perfusing it. HRF represents an ill-defined group of cells that secrete a series of releasing factors into the primary capillary network of a portal vein. This vein passes in the pituitary stalk to the adenohypophysis, where cells manufacture the 7 hormones of this lobe of the pituitary: growth hormone (GH); prolactin (PR); adrenocorticotrophic hormone (ACTH); melanocyte-stimulating hormone (MSH), which is present in some species; thyroid-stimulating hormone (TSH); follicle-stimulating hormone (FSH); and luteinizing hormone (LH). *(Drawn by Margot Mackay, Department of Art as Applied to Medicine, University of Toronto. After a drawing by Blackstock E. In: Ezrin C, Godden J O, Volpe R, Wilson R (eds) 1973 Systematic endocrinology. Harper & Row, New York.)*

hunger, thirst, emotions, sexual drive, and sleep. The hypothalamus controls the body rhythms; a specific cycling centre is responsible for regulating the menstrual cycle.

The hypothalamus may be regarded as an endocrine organ because its cells synthetize two groups of hormones (Fig. 39.1):

1. *Oxytocin and vasopressin.* These are discussed later in this chapter.

2. *Releasing and inhibiting factors or hormones.* These are polypeptides of low molecular weight that pass to the adenohypophysis *via* a short portal vein, and stimulate or inhibit it. The following releasing hormones are recognized:

Corticotrophin-releasing factor (CRF).

Thyrotrophin-releasing factor (TRF); this also acts as a prolactin-releasing factor.

Gonadotrophin-releasing factor (GRF); this causes the release of both follicle-stimulating hormone and luteinizing hormone.

Growth hormone-releasing factor (GHRF).

Prolactin-releasing hormone, which is distinct from TRF.

The action of these hormones can be understood by considering the action of CRF. This hormone leads to the release of corticotrophin (also known as adrenocorticotrophic hormone or ACTH) from the adenohypophysis. ACTH acts on the adrenal cortex to cause the release of cortisol (hydrocortisone). Cortisol inhibits the release of both CRF and ACTH. This inhibition is an example of negative feedback, which is a mechanism encountered in the regulation of other hormone secretions. The releasing factors are produced in picogram (10^{-12} gram) quantities, the pituitary hormones in nanogram (10^{-9} gram) quantities, and the target cells, e.g. the thyroid, produce hormone in microgram (10^{-6} gram) quantities. Thus the chain reaction shows a considerable amplification effect.

In addition to forming release factors, the hypothalamus forms three inhibiting factors:

Gonadotrophin-inhibiting factor.

Prolactin-inhibiting factor.

Growth-hormone-release inhibiting hormone (GRIH or somatostatin). In addition to inhibiting the release of growth hormone by the pituitary, this polypeptide also blocks TRF-stimulated TSH release. It also inhibits insulin and glucagon release by the pancreatic islet cells.

Diseases of the hypothalamus

Many pathological processes affect the hypothalamus; these include meningitis, encephalitis, vascular lesions, head injury, hamartoma, histiocytosis X, and tumour. The effects differ widely depending on which function is predominantly deranged. These effects include the following:

1. Obesity due to overeating
2. Somnolence, or alternatively restless hyperactivity
3. A failure of maintenance of body temperature. There may be hypothermia or alternatively hyperpyrexia
4. Diabetes insipidus due to a deficiency of vasopressin (antidiuretic hormone)
5. Delayed puberty due to a failure of formation of GRF. When combined with obesity the condition is known as *Fröhlich's syndrome*
6. Precocious, or premature, puberty due to a failure of formation of gonadotrophin-inhibiting factor
7. Visual disturbances due to pressure on the optic chiasma
8. Hypothyroidism (rare).

The regulation of hypothalamic-pituitary function is complex, for apart from the gross lesions mentioned above, hypothalamic function can be influenced by impulses emanating from other parts of the brain. For example, stress can inhibit pituitary growth-hormone release in children so that growth is delayed, and there may also be amenorrhoea in young girls.*

THE PITUITARY GLAND (HYPOPHYSIS)

Although small, the pituitary gland, or hypophysis, secretes an amazing variety and number of hormones. The gland and its stalk consist of two parts: the *neurohypophysis*, which develops as an outpouching from the primitive brain, and the *adenohypophysis*, which originates as a diverticulum from the primitive foregut. Both are probably derived entirely from neuroectoderm.[1]

THE NEUROHYPOPHYSIS

The neurohypophysis consists of the posterior lobe of the pituitary, part of the pituitary stalk (the *infundibular stem*), and part of the brain adjacent to the hypothalamus (the *median eminence of the tuber cinereum*). Two peptide hormones, oxytocin and vasopressin, are manufactured by cells in the hypothalamus and pass *via* the cells' axons into the neurohypophysis, where they are stored and subsequently released when needed.

Oxytocin. This hormone causes uterine contraction during labour, and is responsible for milk ejection when an infant is breastfed; the act of suckling initiates a reflex that causes the release of oxytocin.

Vasopressin (antidiuretic hormone or ADH). This hormone acts on the distal and collecting tubules of the kidney, causing water to be retained (see pp. 402 and 423).

Disorders of the neurohypophysis

Diabetes insipidus

This disease is caused by a failure in the development of the neurohypophysis or its destruction by inflammation, ionizing radiation (during pituitary ablation), or a tumour. There is the passage of enormous quantities of very dilute urine (polyuria), with consequent thirst and voracious water drinking (polydipsia).

THE ADENOHYPOPHYSIS

The anterior lobe produces seven hormones:

1. Adrenocorticotrophic hormone—ACTH
2. Melanocyte stimulating hormone—MSH
3. Thyroid stimulating hormone—TSH

* *Amenorrhoea* is the absence of the menses or the menstrual periods. In *primary amenorrhoea* the periods have never commenced, whereas in *secondary amenorrhoea* the menses were at one time normal and have then stopped.

4. Growth hormone—GH
5. Follicle stimulating hormone—FSH
6. Interstitial-cell stimulating hormone—ICSH; in the female this acts as a luteinizing hormone—LH
7. Lactogenic hormone, or prolactin.

Disorders of the pituitary

Hyperplasia or neoplasia of the anterior pituitary may be associated with the hypersecretion of one or several of the pituitary hormones. On the other hand, non-hormone-secreting tumours of the pituitary, or tumours arising in its neighbourhood, may press on and destroy the parenchyma and so lead to a diminished hormonal secretion. This also occurs when the pituitary is destroyed by other lesions, e.g. infarction or inflammation. The clinical picture may therefore be complex, and only the more common types will be outlined. Tumours in the pituitary region give rise to two additional characteristic effects due to their anatomical situation: compression on the optic chiasma causing loss of the temporal fields of both eyes (bitemporal hemianopia) and enlargement of the sella turcica which is detectable radiologically.

Hyperpituitarism

The cells that form growth hormone are usually involved, and the effects of excessive growth hormone are predominant. If the condition arises in childhood the result is *gigantism*: the individual is well proportioned but huge. In addition to excessive skeletal growth there is also an increase in the size of the viscera.

If hypersecretion of growth hormone occurs after closure of the epiphyses, the distal, or acral, parts of the body are affected, and *acromegaly* results. There is a generalized increase in thickness of all the bones of the skeleton due to subperiosteal appositional bone growth. The typical acromegalic appearance is one of overgrowth of the mandible (*prognathism*), prominence of the supraorbital ridges and malar bones, and enlarged hands and feet. The prognathism is a result of further growth in the cartilage in the head of the condyle.

Hyperplasia or an adenoma of the basophil cells may be the primary cause of Cushing's syndrome, which is described on p. 626. The pituitary secretes an excess of ACTH and MSH, and after adrenalectomy this overactivity can be even accentuated, so that generalized hyperpigmentation results, as in Addison's disease (p. 625).

Hypopituitarism

In children the effect is largely related to a lack of growth hormone, and well-proportioned dwarfism is the result. Puberty does not occur in these *Lorain-type*, or Peter Pan, individuals.

The pituitary dwarf is quite different from the achondroplastic dwarf, for the head, body, and limbs are all well proportioned though diminutive. General growth processes are slow, and become arrested at an early age. There is also a delay in the development and eruption of the teeth.

Hypopituitarism with a lack of gonadotrophins impairs gonadal maturation.

Puberty does not take place, and fusion of the epiphyses, normally under the control of the sex hormones, is delayed. If the production of growth hormone is normal, these eunuchoid patients develop abnormally long limbs—their span exceeds their height (normally the two are equal). Gonadotrophin deficiency can also occur in adults: males show testicular atrophy and loss of libido, whereas in females there is amenorrhoea and a regression of the secondary sexual characteristics. In adults insufficiency of the anterior pituitary can manifest itself as hypothyroidism; often this is accompanied by evidence of adrenal cortical and gonadotrophic deficiency.

Hypopituitarism associated with extreme wasting is called *Simmonds's disease*, and is due to the total destruction of the adenohypophysis. The acute onset of hypopituitarism after parturition is thought to be caused by infarction of the gland. The condition is called *Sheehan's syndrome*.

Conditions simulating hypopituitarism. *Anorexia nervosa.* This is encountered usually in emotionally disturbed adolescent girls who develop an obsessional aversion to food. Extreme wasting and amenorrhoea, which are the main features, are due to starvation. The patients are restless and hostile.

Adiposogenital dystrophy. This is the male counterpart of anorexia nervosa. It occurs in emotionally disturbed boys who overeat; they are fat and show delayed onset of puberty. The condition resembles Fröhlich's syndrome, which is also sometimes called adiposogenital dystrophy.

THE THYROID GLAND

The thyroid gland has the unique property of being able to trap iodine from the blood and incorporate it as thyroglobulin in the colloid of its vesicles. By the action of a proteolytic enzyme the iodine-containing thyroid hormones thyroxine and triiodothyronine are released. This occurs when the gland is stimulated by thyroid stimulating hormone (TSH) from the anterior pituitary. TSH secretion is itself stimulated by a low blood level of thyroid hormone.

The inconspicuous C-cells of the thyroid secrete calcitonin, but so far no syndrome has been described in relation to an excess or deficiency of this hormone.

Action of the thyroid hormones. In spite of much research the precise mode of action of the thyroid hormones is not known. However, much has been learned by comparing the normal individual (*euthyroid*) with those who suffer from excessive or diminished secretion (*hyperthyroid* and *hypothyroid*).

Excessive secretion increases the metabolic rate. The effects are described under hyperthyroidism (p. 623).

A deficiency causes:
A reduction in metabolic rate
Impaired mental and physical growth. This is most marked in childhood
Anaemia—this is less constant.

Goitre. Any enlargement of the thyroid is called a goitre, and to a minor extent this occurs at times of stress, e.g. puberty and pregnancy. Indeed, in ancient Egypt the rupture of a thread tied round the neck of a bride was used as an indication of pregnancy. A more potent cause is a diet deficient in iodine, because the thyroid, being unable to manufacture its hormone, cannot check the secretion of TSH which stimulates it to activity. Before iodine was added to table salt, goitres were common in many parts of the world for this reason—in the Great Lakes area of North America, the Andes, the Himalayas, and Derbyshire, England. Repeated phases of hyperplasia followed by involution led to the formation of large nodular goitres containing many colloid-filled areas, some of which showed necrosis and dystrophic calcification (*nodular colloid goitre*).

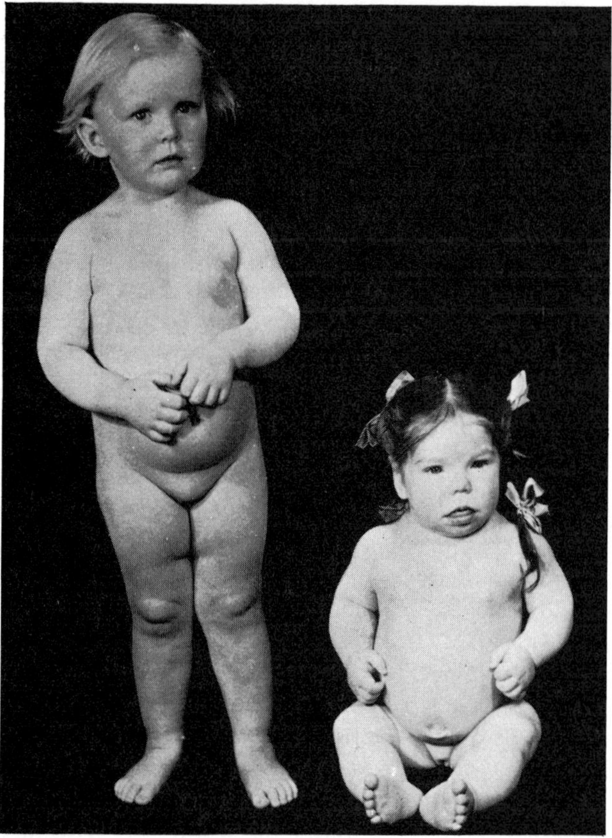

Fig. 39.2 Cretinism. Note the dwarfed appearance of the cretin as compared with a child of like age on her right. Other distinctive features are the torpid expression, round face, eyes set widely apart, enlarged protruding tongue, and the umbilical hernia. *(Photograph by courtesy of Mr G S Hoggins.)*

The goitres associated with hyperthyroidism, Hashimoto's disease, and neoplasia are described later.

Hypothyroidism. Hypothyroidism used to be frequent in areas of endemic goitre, but it may also be due to causes other than iodine lack—for instance, a congenital absence of the thyroid gland. The effects in the child differ from those in the adult.

Cretinism. An insufficiency of thyroid hormone in the infant leads to cretinism. The child has a bloated face, protruding tongue, and vacant expression, and becomes mentally defective (Fig. 39.2). There is a retardation of growth with delayed ossification and delayed epiphyseal union. There is also delay in dental development.

Myxoedema. This is the manifestation of hypothyroidism in the adult. There is a reduction in mental and physical activity, and the patient exhibits a characteristic bloated appearance due to a curious oedema of the skin. There may be an increase in bone density due to a diminution in excretion of calcium and phosphorus.

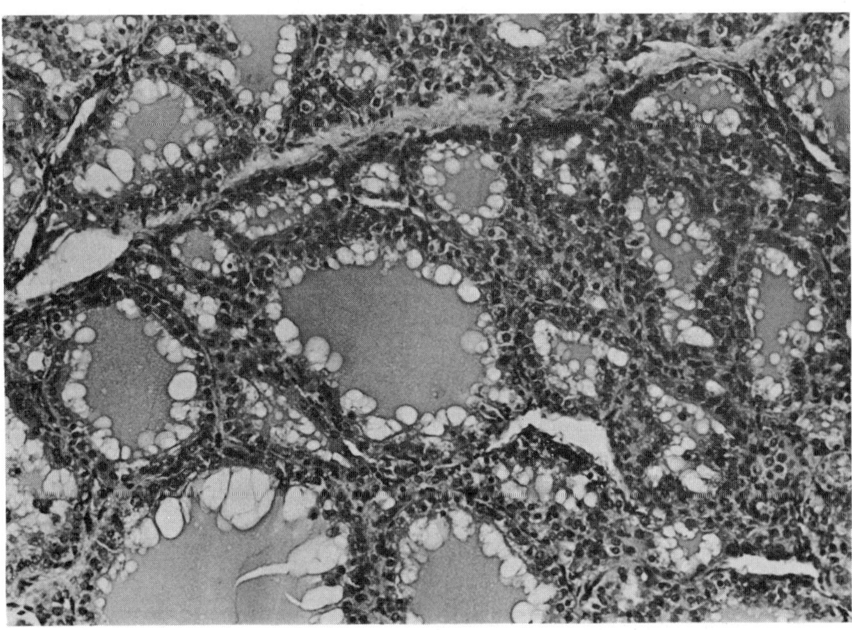

Fig. 39.3 Graves's disease. The thyroid gland is hyperplastic. The epithelium is columnar, and in some small follicles where colloid is deficient, the epithelium encroaches on the acinar spaces. In the large follicles the colloid shows vacuolation where it abuts on the epithelium. × 250.

Hyperthyroidism. This is also known as *thyrotoxicosis*, and occurs in two forms.

Primary hyperthyroidism (Graves's disease). This disease is characterized by a diffuse enlargement of the thyroid gland (goitre) due to a marked hyperplasia of its epithelial elements (Fig. 39.3). There is a raised metabolic rate which manifests itself by a persistent increase of the heart rate, and the individual is typically jumpy and nervous. The hands are warm and sweating; they are seldom at rest, and exhibit a fine tremor when the fingers are stretched out.

Muscular weakness is a common symptom, and can be severe (*thyrotoxic myopathy*). The eyes have a characteristic appearance: the eyelids are retracted, giving the patient a staring expression (Fig. 39.4), while in severe cases the globe is actually pushed forward. If these changes are very severe, the eye muscles can become paralysed and sight can be lost. This is called *malignant exophthalmos*. The skin overlying the tibia may show a focal accumulation of mucopolysaccharide, a condition called *pretibial myxoedema*.

If left untreated, thyrotoxicosis often terminates in heart failure. In long-standing cases osteoporosis may occur. This is due to an increased osteoclastic

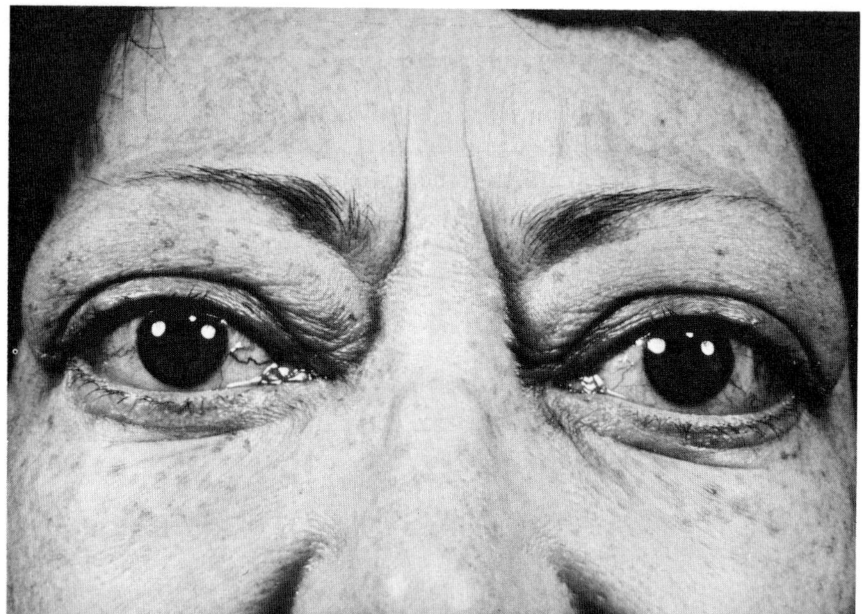

Fig. 39.4 Ocular manifestation of Graves's disease. This patient noted the development of prominence of both eyes at the same time as the appearance of other symptoms of Graves's disease. The eyelids and periorbital tissues are swollen, and the conjunctiva is congested and moist because of excessive lacrimation. The globe itself is pushed forward (*proptosis* or *exophthalmos*) by an accumulation of mucoprotein in the orbital tissues. A similar change is sometimes encountered in the skin of the lower leg, and is called *pretibial myxoedema*. Note that this occurs in Graves's disease. (Photograph by courtesy of Dr. N. Pairaudeau.)

activity which leads to the excessive excretion of calcium and phosphorus in the urine.

The actual stimulus to thyroid hyperplasia is an agent present in the blood. The first thyroid stimulating factor to be isolated differs from TSH in having a much longer stimulating effect on the gland. It is called *LATS (long-acting thyroid stimulator)*, and is an autoantibody; how it acts and the nature of the corresponding antigen are still not clear. Since it is quite often absent in cases of primary thyrotoxicosis and is in highest concentration in cases where there is pretibial myxoedema, LATS is unlikely to be the only factor in the pathogenesis of the disease. A more likely contender for the role is a second IgG which has more recently been discovered. This is called *human thyroid stimulating immunoglobulin (HTSI)*, is present in the serum, of most, and possibly all patients with primary thyrotoxicosis, and appears to displace TSH from its binding site on the human thyroid cell membrane. This suggests that HTSI is capable of binding to the thyrotrophin receptor sites and that the receptor is itself the antigen.[2]

Secondary hyperthyroidism (toxic nodular goitre). This occurs as a secondary phenomenon in a patient who is already suffering from a goitre from some other cause, e.g. iodine deficiency. The disease is less severe than Graves's disease, and exophthalmos does not occur.

Hashimoto's disease. Like most thyroid disease this is more common in women than men. The gland is diffusely enlarged, showing atrophy of its epithelial elements and a massive infiltration with lymphocytes and plasma cells. There are immunoglobulin antibodies to thyroglobulin present in the blood, and their detection is of value in diagnosis. It seems unlikely that these antibodies are destructive to the thyroid tissues, and if Hashimoto's disease is an autoimmune disease it is probably cell-mediated.

Tumours. Benign encapsulated nodules in the thyroid gland are common, but the majority are probably focal areas of hyperplasia. These are usually multiple (nodular colloid goitre).

Carcinoma was apparently not uncommon in goitrous districts, but is nowadays distinctly rare.

THE ADRENAL GLANDS

The adrenal medulla

The cells of the adrenal medulla liberate adrenaline (epinephrine) and noradrenaline (norepinephrine) in response to sympathetic stimulation. These hormones cause a redistribution of blood such that the individual is better adapted to fight or flight. A rare tumour, the *phaeochromocytoma*, derived from the medulla secretes these agents in excess and leads to systemic hypertension.

The adrenal cortex

Three major groups of hormones (corticosteroids) are secreted:

Glucocorticoids, e.g. hydrocortisone (cortisol). In physiological concentrations cortisol accelerates the synthesis of glucose from non-carbohydrate precursors, and inhibits the actions of insulin.

Mineralocorticoids, e.g. aldosterone. This primarily affects electrolyte metabolism. It causes sodium retention and increases potassium loss in the urine.

Sex hormones. These are androgens. Oestrogens are probably not produced in the adrenal cortex, but androgen-precursor steroids produced in the gland can be converted into oestrogens by the liver, fat cells, and the placenta.

Adrenal insufficiency—Addison's disease. Idiopathic atrophy, perhaps by an autoimmune process, or destruction, usually by tuberculosis, is the cause of Addison's disease. A low blood pressure, loss of appetite, loss of weight, weakness, and eventual death are the main features. As would be expected there is hypoglycaemia, a fall in plasma sodium (*hyponatraemia*), and a rise in plasma potassium (*hyperkalaemia*). The skin and mucous membranes, including the oral mucosa, show increased melanin pigmentation. This is because the low plasma hydrocortisone level stimulates the excessive production of pituitary ACTH and MSH. Both these hormones, especially MSH, cause a darkening of the skin by an effect on the melanocytes.

Acute adrenal insufficiency is generally encountered when patients who are unable to increase their corticosteroid production are exposed to sudden stress, such as trauma, haemorrhage, or severe infection. This is seen most often in patients with Addison's disease or panhypopituitarism who are on a maintenance dose of glucocorticoids. Acute adrenal insufficiency is characterized by shock, hypotension, collapse, and sometimes fever.

Adrenal hypersecretion. Idiopathic hyperplasia, adenoma, or rarely carcinoma may be associated with hypersecretion of corticosteroids. The clinical pictures are often mixed, but three main patterns may be discerned.

Adrenogenital syndrome. In boys puberty may occur prematurely, even as early as 4 years ('infantile Hercules'). In girls male characteristics may develop. In adult women this masculinization is called *virilism*, e.g. atrophy of breasts, cessation of menstruation, growth of beard, deepening of the voice, etc.

Conn's syndrome. Excess aldosterone secretion produces a low plasma potassium, sodium and water retention, and hypertension.

Cushing's syndrome. The major features are obesity, hyperglycaemia, osteoporosis, hypertension, and increased body hair growth in women. The syndrome, or mild forms of it, is commonly seen when glucocorticoids (hydrocortisone, prednisone, etc.) are administered in pharmacological doses. Rounding and swelling of the face (moon face) is particularly characteristic.

Glucocorticoid therapy

Replacement glucocorticoid therapy is logical and useful in patients with adrenal insufficiency. However, when used in massive (pharmacological) amounts, the glucocorticoids have two additional actions that can be useful:

Anti-inflammatory action. The glucocorticoids (e.g. prednisone) have a suppressive effect on the inflammatory reaction; for this reason they are used in many diseases, e.g. rheumatic arthritis, zoster, and polyarteritis nodosa. They may be used to advantage when bacterial inflammation might produce serious damage, but antibiotics must also be administered, so that the infection does not spread.

Lymphoid atrophy and depression of the immune response. This may be used to advantage in treating acute lymphatic leukaemia, autoimmune diseases, and hypersensitivity states, such as bronchial asthma. The immunosuppressive action of prednisone is of great use in suppressing the graft rejection reaction, such as in patients with kidney grafts.

Complications of glucocorticoid therapy. The administration of large doses of glucocorticoids over a prolonged period can have serious consequences. Indeed, these may be more serious than the disease for which the treatment was initiated. Important complications are:

1. *Cushing's syndrome.* (See above.)
2. *Opportunistic infections.* Overwhelming fungal or viral infections may prove fatal in some patients; this is related to the immunosuppressive effect of glucocorticoids. A quiescent tuberculous focus can be reactivated and can then lead to miliary tuberculosis.
3. *Osteoporosis.* Severe and widespread osteoporosis can lead to fracture lesions after trivial injury. Collapse of vertebrae is common.
4. *Inhibition of wound healing.* Wound contraction, granulation tissue formation, and collagen formation are inhibited.
5. *Peptic ulcer.* Peptic ulcer and its complications, especially bleeding, are most common.
6. *Cataract formation.*
7. *Diabetes mellitus.* (See Ch. 17.)

8. *Mental effects.* An acute mental breakdown (psychosis) may be precipitated. Suicide is an important cause of death.

9. *Systemic hypertension.* The development of hypertension or the accentuation of existing disease appears to be due to the salt-retaining activity of most glucocorticoids.

10. *Acute adrenal insufficiency.* This emergency, characterized by hypotension, shock and sudden death, occurs if steroid therapy is suddenly withdrawn, It may also occur if a patient who is taking a steroid develops a severe infection or is subjected to severe injury such as major surgery and does not have his dose increased. It is vital that all patients on glucocorticoid therapy as well as their medical attendants be aware of this possibility.

THE APUD SYSTEM[1, 3–6]

The concept of a widely dispersed system of cells derived from the neural crest has been recently proposed. The term APUD is derived from the initial letters associated with their 3 most important properties.

1. A high content of **a**mines
2. The capacity for amine **p**recursor **u**ptake
3. The presence of amino acid **d**ecarboxylase.

This enzyme converts amino acids, such as hydroxytryptophan and DOPA, into amines. The associated cells are recognized on electron microscopy by the presence of characteristic granules in their cytoplasm, and they secrete either amines or polypeptides. At present the following cells are included in the group: the chromaffin cells (e.g. of the adrenal medulla), non-chromaffin paraganglia cells (e.g. of the carotid body), the argentaffin cells of the intestine and elsewhere, the pancreatic islet cells, the C cells of the thyroid gland, and some cells of the adenohypophysis. Tumours of APUD cells, called *apudomas*, may secrete an excessive amount of their corresponding hormone, and are then called *orthoendocrine*, or else they may secrete a hormone that is characteristic of some other APUD cells, when they are called *paraendocrine.*

A good example of an orthoendocrine apudoma is a tumour of the beta cells of the islets of Langerhans secreting insulin and causing attacks of hypoglycaemia. But occasionally such a tumour may secrete an ACTH-like hormone and produce Cushing's syndrome. In this case it would be a paraendocrine apudoma, since ACTH is not normally secreted by the pancreatic islets of Langerhans. Other examples of paraendocrine apudomas causing Cushing's syndrome are seen in connection with oat-cell carcinoma of the lung, medullary carcinoma of the thyroid (derived from C cells that secrete calcitonin normally), and bronchial carcinoid tumour. In each case an ACTH-like hormone is produced.

Carcinoid tumours are also derived from APUD cells (p. 554).

GENERAL READING

Ezrin C, Godden J O, Volpe R, 1979 Systematic endocrinology, 2nd ed, 588 pp, Harper and Row, Hagerstown

Catt K J 1970 Lancet 1: 763, 827, 933, 1097, 1275, 1383 and 2: 255, 353. Series of articles entitled ABC of Endocrinology

REFERENCES

1. Tischler A S, Dichter M A, Bailes B, Greene L A 1977 Neuroendocrine neoplasms and their cells of origin. New England Journal of Medicine 296: 919
2. Leading article 1975 Hyperthyroidism and Graves's disease. British Medical Journal 2: 457
3. Pearse A G E 1974 The APUD cell concept and its implications in pathology. Pathology Annual 9: 27
4. Weichert R F 1970 The neural ectodermal origin of the peptide-secreting endocrine glands. American Journal of Medicine 49: 232
5. Bolande R P 1974 The neurocristopathies. Human Pathology 5: 409
6. Welbourn R B 1977 Current status of the apudomas. Annals of Surgery 185: 1

40

Diseases of the skin

Introduction

The number of diseases of the skin which have been described in the literature far exceeds that of any other individual organ. There are many reasons for this: the skin is exposed to the external environment and is a complex, composite organ. It contains hair follicles with associated sebaceous glands, eccrine and apocrine sweat glands, a surface epithelium, and a connective tissue element with a loose papillary dermis between the epithelial elements and the reticular dermis, itself composed of dense collagenous bundles and coarse elastic fibres. The ease with which the skin can be examined and biopsied and the importance that mankind has given to its appearance have further added to the complexity of dermatology. This chapter describes some common skin reactions, particularly those which may also affect the oral mucosa. Some diseases, e.g. pemphigus vulgaris and lichen planus, can affect the mouth either initially or to a major extent. Biopsy of these mucosal lesions is sometimes difficult, and histological interpretation can be unsatisfactory. The finding of more typical lesions on the skin is therefore rewarding, since skin biopsy is easy and pathological interpretation clear-cut.

Terminology

There are few subjects in medicine that can compete with dermatology for hiding truth behind complex names. Nevertheless, with some basic facts and a minimal knowledge of Latin it is possible to master the terminology and gain some glimmer of understanding.

An area of altered skin, usually red (erythematous), whether pigmented or non-pigmented is, if flat and not palpable, called a *macule* if less than 1.0 cm in diameter and a *patch* if larger. Similar areas which are palpable (usually they are raised and indurated, but in atrophic conditions may be depressed) are called *papules* if small and *plaques* if over 1.0 cm in diameter. A lesion containing a visible accumulation of clear fluid is a *vesicle* if small and a *bulla* if large (over 0.5 cm or 1.0 cm according to definition). *Pustules* contain pus. If flakes of keratin are seen obviously adherent to the lesion it is called *squamous.* Since most such lesions can be felt, they are therefore called *papulosquamous.* The presence of visible abnormally dilated vessels is called *telangiectasia.* Shallow ulcers or erosions are called *excoriations* if they are produced by scratching. The observation and description of each individual skin lesion is important, because certain types are characteristic of certain diseases. For example, psoriasis is characteristically papulosquamous, is occasionally pustular, but is never vesicular.

The distribution of the lesions seen in any skin disease is important. A localized rash often indicates a localized cause. Thus, a dermatitis on only one wrist is probably due to sensitivity to a wrist band or a watch strap. Some diseases, e.g. smallpox, characteristically affect the distal parts, such as the hands, feet, and face, whereas others, e.g. chickenpox, tend to affect the trunk rather then the extremities. In a consideration of any skin disease, it is important therefore to include the distribution of the rash and the individual characteristics of its lesions.

The presence of itching is characteristic of certain skin diseases, such as scabies, neurodermatitis, and atopic dermatitis. The term *pruritus*, which is commonly used, is synonymous with itching. Note that the presence or absence of itching is as dependent upon the make-up of the individual as it is on the nature of the lesions. Some people itch easily, others do not.

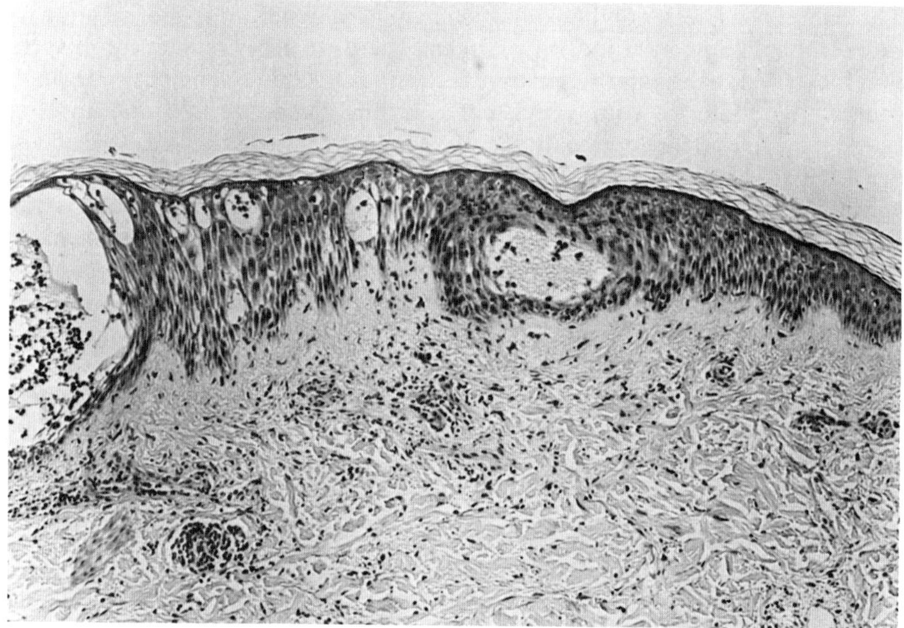

Fig. 40.1 Acute dermatitis. This is an example of acute allergic contact dermatitis due to poison ivy. The epidermis shows spongiosis, and in many places the cells have torn apart to produce intra-epidermal vesicles. The largest of these is on the left-hand side, and contains coagulated exudate and a number of inflammatory cells, mainly lymphocytes. The dermis shows a mild inflammatory reaction, again with a lymphocytic infiltrate. × 120.

Dermatitis and eczema

Dermatitis and *eczema* are synonymous terms used to describe a particular skin reaction pattern that primarily involves the epidermis. Three histological types are recognized: acute, subacute, and chronic.

Histopathological types of dermatitis

Acute dermatitis. The epidermis shows intercellular oedema (*spongiosis*) that terminates in the separation of epidermal cells and in the formation of vesicles or bullae (Fig. 40.1). The dermis shows an acute inflammatory reaction with oedema and, surprisingly enough, a perivascular lymphocytic infiltrate. The sparcity of polymorphs is noteworthy but the explanation is not understood. The spongiotic vesicles formed in the epidermis rupture, and clinically this produces a 'weeping' or crusted surface.

Subacute dermatitis. Spongiosis and vesicle formation are still evident, but the epidermis reacts by increasing mitotic activity so that it becomes thicker (*acanthosis*). Keratinization is disturbed, with the result that in places the keratin layer retains cellular nuclei. This condition is called *parakeratosis*.

Chronic dermatitis. Spongiosis is scanty, and vesicles are not formed. Chronic dermatitis is characterized by acanthosis (thickening of the epidermis)

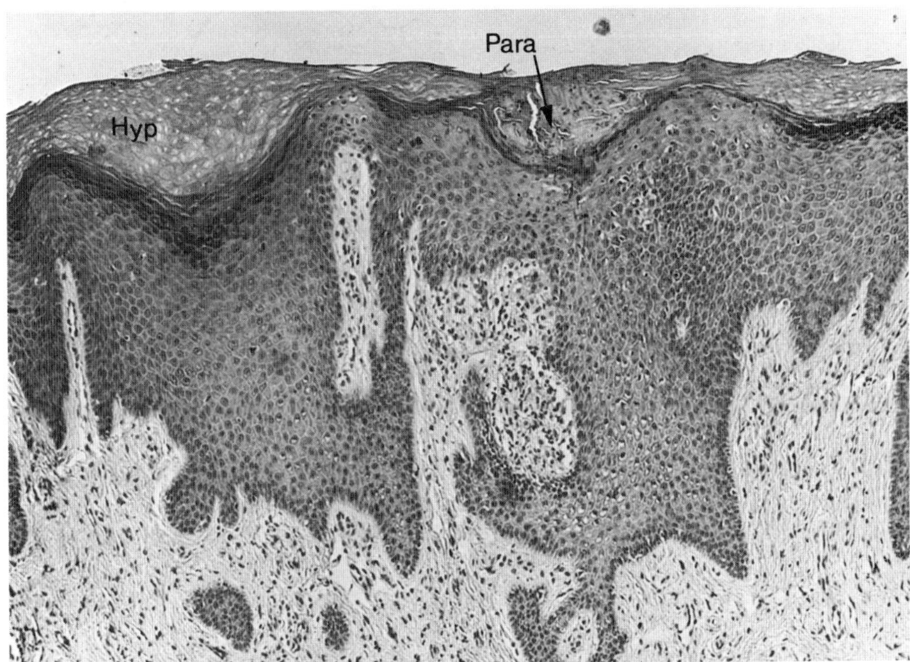

Fig. 40.2 Chronic dermatitis. The epidermis shows marked hyperkeratosis and acanthosis with irregular elongation of the rete ridges. There is a focus of parakeratosis, and the dermis shows a sparse infiltration by lymphocytes. The changes should be compared with normal skin present on the right-hand side of Fig. 40.1 ×120.

together with the formation of excessive keratin (*hyperkeratosis*) and, in places, parakeratosis (Fig. 40.2). Clinically, chronic dermatitis appears as indurated, scaly papules or plaques, and the skin markings tend to be accentuated. This latter feature is known as *lichenification*.

Clinical types of dermatitis

The clinical types of dermatitis are many and various. They cannot be distinguished from each other histologically but differ in their causes and clinical presentation.

Primary irritant dermatitis. Externally applied chemical irritants are a frequent cause of dermatitis (*contact dermatitis*): a common example is the chronic lichenified hand eczema seen in housewives whose hands are brought repeatedly into contact with water, detergents, and other household agents. Alkalis, acids, and many industrial chemicals can act as primary irritants, and if applied over a long period they lead to a refractory chronic dermatitis. Elderly individuals with dry skin may develop a dermatitis that is due to exposure to agents such as water, soap, and detergents that would be harmless in a younger person. Dentists and surgeons who have to wash their hands repeatedly with detergents and antiseptics are also liable to develop contact dermatitis of this type.

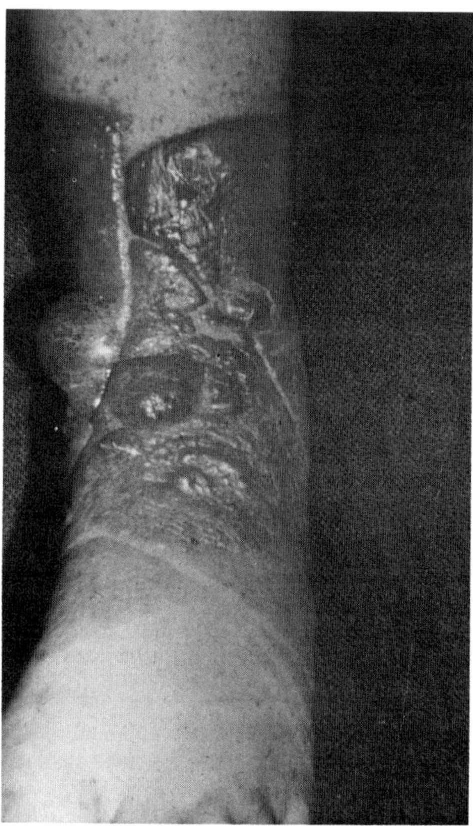

Fig. 40.3 Acute dermatitis. This patient sustained a sprain of the left ankle, and adhesive tape was applied for support. Thirty-six hours later an acute vesicular dermatitis appeared and subsequently became bullous. Note how the eruption is limited to the region previously covered by the tape (lines of demarcation are obvious). Areas where the skin was folded are spared.

Allergic contact dermatitis. The development of cell-mediated hypersensitivity toward chemicals results in the production of *allergic contact dermatitis.* Iodine, formaldehyde, dyes, plants (e.g. poison ivy), and nickel (used in costume jewellery) are among the many agents that can cause this type of allergic dermatitis (Fig. 40.3). It is noteworthy that certain parts of the skin are more sensitive to irritants than others. Thus, allergic contact dermatitis is more common on the backs of the hands than it is on the palms. Likewise, the face is particularly sensitive and may react to agents that elsewhere cause little trouble.

Dermatitis around the eyes can be due to nail polish, which causes little trouble when applied to the hands or feet.

Photodermatitis. Ultraviolet light can act on chemicals (either applied topically or taken systemically) present in the skin and so alter them that direct irritant effects (*phototoxic dermatitis*) or new antigen formation and subsequent sensitization (*photoallergic dermatitis*) results. Agents that are well known to cause this sensitizing effect when applied topically are perfumes, coal-tar derivatives, and halogenated salicylanilides (used in deodorant soap).

The face is commonly affected, and an example of particular interest is the sensitizing effect that the eosin in lipstick has in the production of sun-sensitive cheilitis.

Many drugs taken internally can have a similar effect. Common examples are chemotherapeutic agents such as sulphonamides and tetracyclines, diuretics (e.g. chlorothiazide), and tranquillizers (e.g. chlorpromazine), to name a few.

It is evident that with any patient who has a disease of the skin or mucous membrane, the nature of which is not immediately apparent, it is of great importance to enquire what drugs have been applied locally or used systemically.

Infantile eczema and atopic dermatitis. These two conditions occur in atopic (allergic) individuals, but the pathogenesis is obscure, for although the associated respiratory diseases such as hay-fever and bronchial asthma appear to be caused by IgE sensitization, the skin lesions are more complex and the damage is probably cell-mediated.

Nummular eczema. This condition tends to occur in atropic individuals and is characterized by the formation of localized, coin-shaped plaques of subacute or chronic dermatitis. Itching is usually marked.

Stasis dermatitis. Stasis dermatitis is common on the legs and is related to chronic venous stasis. It occurs following venous thrombosis in the lower limbs and in patients with varicose veins. In addition to the usual features of a dermatitis, stasis dermatitis is characterized by a brown discoloration of the skin. This is produced by haemosiderin secondary to petechial hemorrhages. Chronic ulcers are a common complication and are usually initiated by trauma, caused either accidentally or by scratching. Such *stasis ulcers* are often situated over the medial malleolus and heal slowly because of the poor blood supply to the skin.

Seborrhoeic dermatitis. A type of chronic dermatitis is frequently seen in the scalp and results in the formation of greasy scales or dandruff. This condition is termed *seborrhoeic dermatitis*; although it is extremely common, its precise nature is not understood. The dermatitis can extend beyond the scalp and affect the face Occasionally there is involvement of the trunk, particularly the front of the chest, and the flexural regions such as the axilla or under the breasts. This type of dermatitis can be encountered in all age groups, ranging from infants (cradle cap) to old people.

Neurodermatitis. A feature of some forms of dermatitis, including the atopic variety, is marked itching. This leads to scratching and self-perpetuation because of the continued physical trauma. The condition is then referred to as *chronic neurodermatitis* (Fig. 40.4). Localized plaques of neurodermatitis, which frequently occur on the back of the neck and the front of the ankles, are called *lichen simplex chronicus.*

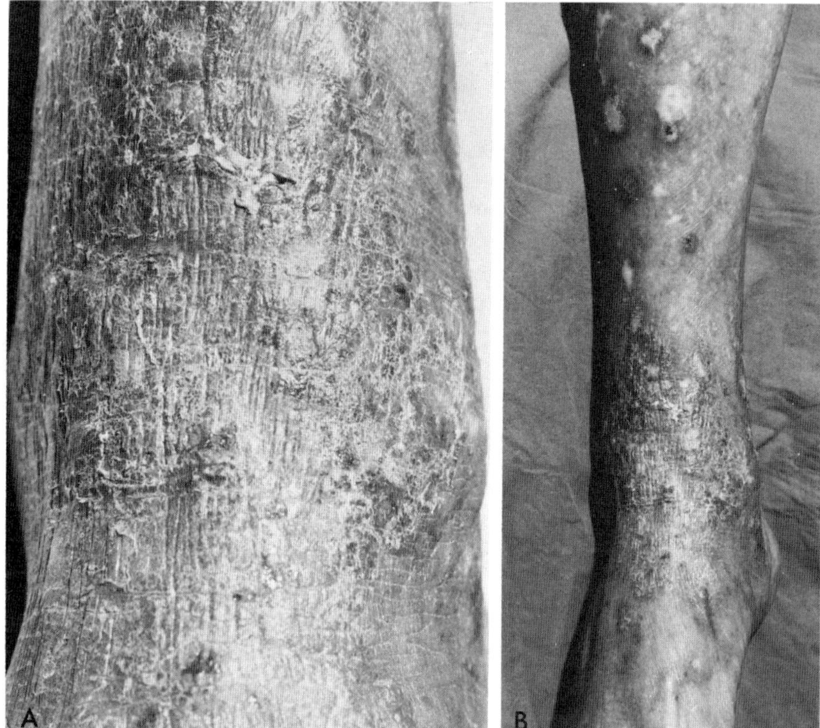

Fig. 40.4 Neurodermatitis. This patient had a chronic lichenified dermatitis on the front of both ankles. *A* shows a close-up of the hyperkeratosis and accentuation of the crease lines that are typical; they are fancifully likened to lichen on a tree trunk. Constant scratching and rubbing, often with the opposite heel, perpetuated the condition. The nodules shown higher on the leg in *B* are also self-induced. They consist of dense scar tissue with over-lying acanthosis and depigmentation. The lesions are called *prurigo nodularis* (from the Latin word prurire, meaning to itch) and are produced by the patient continually picking at them.

Papulosquamous eruptions

The description of this wide group of dissimilar diseases, which includes secondary syphilis and ringworm, will be restricted to two common examples, both of unknown aetiology.

Psoriasis. This is a chronic disease that fluctuates in intensity both spontaneously and under the influence of treatment. It occurs as sharply demarcated erythematous plaques with a dry, silvery scale. Common sites are the elbows, knees, and other extensor surfaces. The palms, soles, and scalp are also frequently affected. Psoriasis is not usually itchy, and vesicles are never formed. This distinguishes it both clinically and histologically from dermatitis.

Histologically, it resembles chronic dermatitis, but the acanthosis involves a regular elongation of the rete ridges, and the intervening papillary dermis is usually oedematous and vascular (Fig. 40.5).

Lichen planus. Lichen planus (Fig. 40.6) occurs as pruritic, somewhat violaceous, flat-topped papules. Any site may be involved but common areas are around the wrists and ankles. The mucous membranes are commonly affected, and in about 15 per cent of cases these are the only areas involved. In the oral

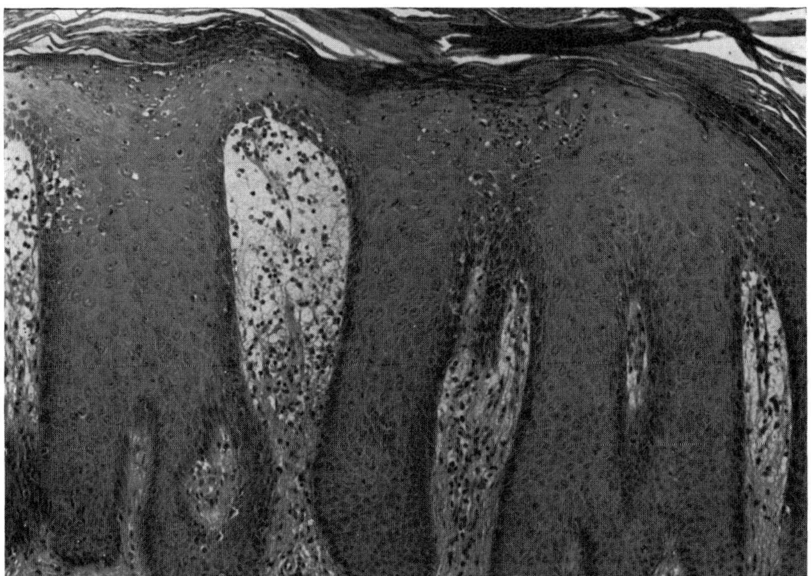

Fig. 40.5 Psoriasis of the skin. The epidermis shows marked hyperkeratosis, parakeratosis, and acanthosis. The elongation of the rete ridges is particularly well shown, and the broad club-shaped processes are seen to anastomose on the right side of the picture. The papillae between the rete ridges exhibit the highly characteristic vasodilatation and oedema. There is a sparse inflammatory infiltrate in this part of the dermis, and cells are seen to be migrating through the epidermis. These cells are for the most part polymorphonuclear leucocytes, and small collections of them appearing in the keratin layer are a characteristic feature of psoriasis. They are called Munro micro-abscesses. × 120.

mucosa the lesions are white and form a lace-like network on the buccal mucosa. Superficial erosions may occur. The glans penis is another common situation. Lichen planus of the oral mucosa is sometimes followed by malignancy, but less frequently so than in dysplastic leukoplakia.

Lichen planus of the skin has a very characteristic histological appearance (Fig. 40.7). There is acanthosis and hyperkeratosis, but three features distinguish typical lesions sharply from those of chronic dermatitis and psoriasis:

1. Parakeratosis is absent.
2. There is hydropic degeneration or loss of the basal-cell layer of the epidermis.
3. The superficial, or papillary, dermis shows a dense well-delineated band of lymphocytic infiltration (Fig. 40.7).

The oral lesions are similar in appearance except that parakeratosis may be present (Fig. 40.8).

Although plasma cells form a conspicuous feature of the inflammatory infiltrate in many oral lesions, they are conspicuously absent in lichen planus.

Diseases characterized by a dermal inflammatory reaction

An inflammatory reaction in the dermis is present in many skin diseases including those which appear primarily to affect the epidermis, e.g. dermatitis and psoriasis. A localized area of dermal inflammation is a feature of many infections, e.g. tuberculosis and erysipelas, but there is a group of conditions in which a

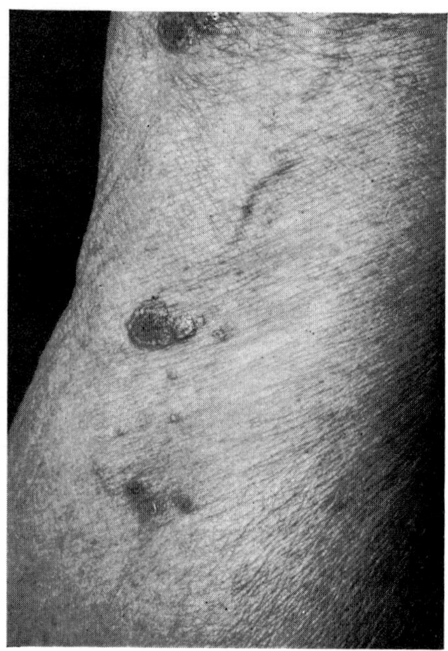

Fig. 40.6 Lichen planus on the anterior aspect of the wrist. The lesions are flat-topped papules and show the diagnostic white lines called Wickham's striae. In this case they are well shown around the periphery of the larger papules. The faint dark circle near the edge of the large central papule indicates the area which is biopsied. It showed the typical appearance of lichen planus, and the changes, particularly the prominent granular layer, were most pronounced in the region of the striae.

widespread vascular reaction occurs for no very apparent reason. The most mild example in this group is urticaria.

Urticaria. In acute urticaria ('hives'), there is an acute inflammatory reaction in the dermis with vasodilatation, mild polymorph accumulation, and marked oedema. Multiple areas of dermal oedema occur, at first red but later becoming pale as a weal develops. The lesions resemble changes seen in a mosquito bite or the triple response of Lewis (p. 83). Acute uticaria may be a type I hypersensitivity reaction mediated by IgE, but is also seen in immune-complex disease. It follows the ingestion of a particular food or drug, and as with other hypersensitivity reactions, small quantities of the agent can be sufficient to induce an attack. Thus, the menthol in a cigarette or toothpaste can precipitate acute urticaria in a sensitized person. Repeated attacks of urticaria may occur over many years (chronic urticaria), and in these patients the cause is rarely found.

Urticaria affects the dermis. When the subcutaneous tissues are also involved, the condition is termed *angio-oedema.* In both urticaria and angio-oedema the mucous membranes, including that of the tongue, can be involved. In one type of hereditary angio-oedema, there is a deficiency of Cl-esterase inhibitor. This is a serious condition, for lesions occur in the intestine causing colic, and in the larynx causing death from asphyxiation.

Toxic erythema. This general term is applied to many conditions in which the epidermis is normal, at least in the early stages, but in which there is a dermal

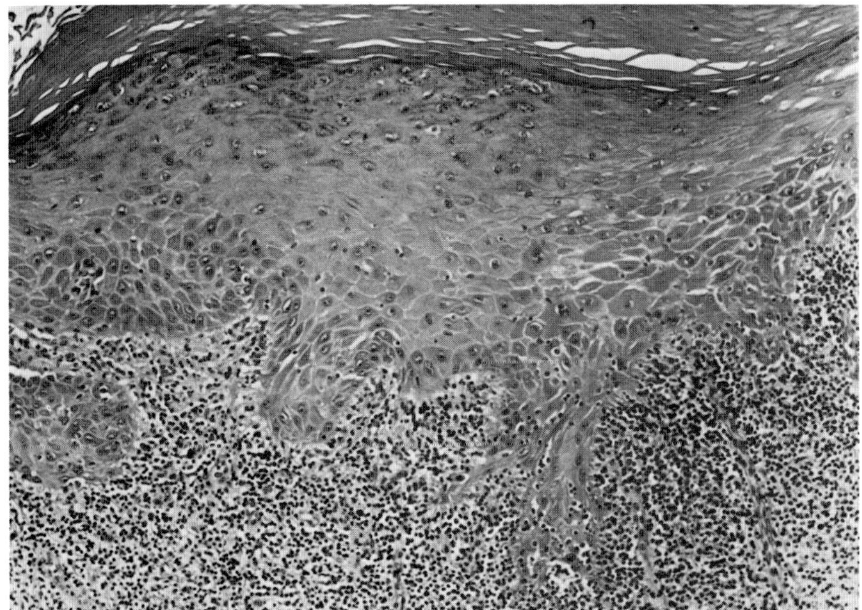

Fig. 40.7 Lichen planus of the skin. The epidermis shows marked hyperkeratosis, but there is a complete absence of parakeratotic nuclei. The granular layer is increased in prominence, and the epidermis shows acanthosis with elongation of some rete ridges. The basal layer of the epidermis has been replaced by flattened cells, and the epidermis has a saw-toothed appearance. The characteristic band of lymphocytic infiltrate in the papillary dermis is well shown. × 120.

inflammatory reaction showing vasodilatation and a perivascular collection of cells, chiefly lymphocytes. As an acute condition toxic erythema accompanies many viral infections (e.g. measles, German measles, and infectious mononucleosis) and the intake of drugs. Damage to blood vessels by immune complexes is the probable pathogenesis.

Erythema multiforme. This may be regarded as a severe variant of toxic erythema. The onset is sudden and the patient rapidly develops symmetrical lesions of varying types—urticarial, erythematous macules and papules, and sometimes vesicles. Target, or iris, lesions are characteristic. The dermal oedema is sometimes so marked that it progresses to form a subepidermal vesicle or bulla. The dermal reaction causes secondary degenerative changes in the epidermis. The severity of the dermal inflammatory reaction and the degenerate appearance of the epidermal roof serve to distinguish these lesions from those of bullous pemphigoid (see below). Erythema multiforme is often idiopathic, but it sometimes appears to be precipitated by a variety of factors, e.g. previous herpes simplex of the lips, drug intake, exposure to sunlight, to mention but a few. Erythema multiforme tends to affect the extremities, and can also cause lesions on the mucosal membranes. Severe cases of erythema multiforme which affect the oral mucosa are termed the *Stevens-Johnson syndrome.*

Vesiculo-bullous disease

The formation of vesicles or bullae is the outstanding feature of this group of diseases, and for accurate diagnosis a biopsy of an *early* lesion is often necessary,

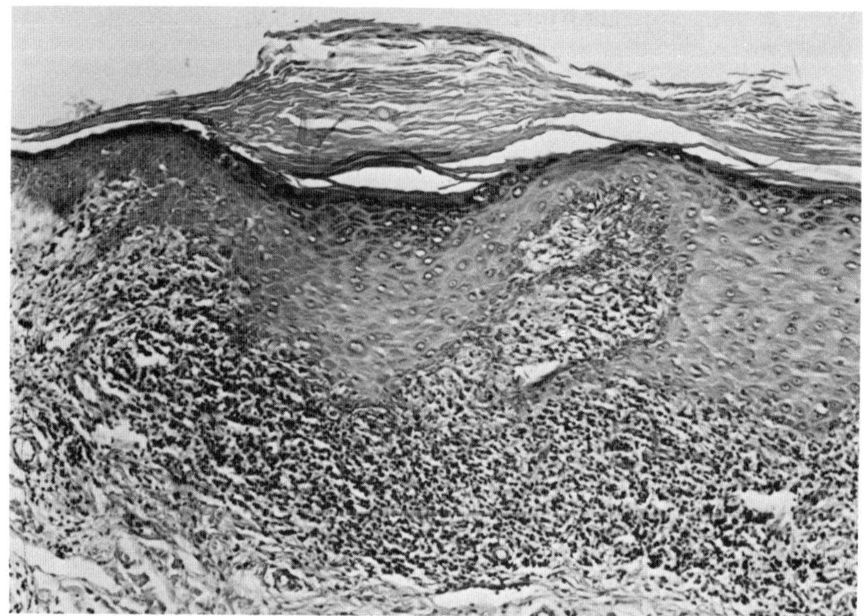

Fig. 40.8 Lichen planus of oral mucosa. The appearances are very similar to those shown in Fig. 40.7. The prominent granular layer is well shown; normally the oral mucosa does not show this. Occasional parakeratotic nuclei are seen in the keratin layer, a feature not seen in lichen planus of the skin. The loss of the basal-cell layer is particularly well shown. The lymphocytic infiltrate is closely applied to the epithelium, and in places cells are migrating between the epithelial cells. × 120.

because the situation of the vesicle is of vital importance in differential diagnosis. Some vesicles are intra-epidermal, while others form beneath the epidermis. It should be noted that a late subepidermal vesicle becomes intra-epidermal as tongues of regenerative epidermis cover the base. This is one of the reasons for biopsying an early lesion.

Subepidermal vesicles

Bullous pemphigoid. A dermal inflammatory reaction is followed by the formation of a subepidermal vesicle. The disease is not uncommon, and is characterized by the occurrence of crops of *tense* vesicles and bullae appearing on the trunk and sometimes on the mucous membranes. The disease is chronic, tends to occur in elderly people, and is sometimes the first manifestation of a tumour of some internal organ. A disease with similar histology, *benign cicatrizing mucosal pemphigoid*, affects the oral mucosa and the conjunctiva. Numerous eosinophils are a feature of the dermal inflammatory infiltrate.

Erythema multiforme. This has already been described.

Dermatitis herpetiformis. In this disease groups of vesicles appear, and are severely pruritic. Histologically, the dermis shows an inflammatory reaction initially restricted to the papillae and characterized by the presence of numerous neutrophils. The mucous membranes are rarely affected.

Porphyria cutanea tarda and **epidermolysis bullosa** are rare causes of subepidermal bulla formation.

Intra-epidermal vesicles

The superficial subcorneal vesicles and pustules of candidiasis and impetigo can generally be diagnosed clinically without the aid of biopsy. So also can the spongiotic vesicles of acute and subacute dermatitis. The fluid in these vesicles contains inflammatory exudate, but a few detached epidermal cells may be present. This contrasts with an important group of blistering diseases in which the vesicles are formed as a result of a loss of adherence between adjacent epidermal cells. The detached cells become rounded off and lie free in the fluid. This process is called *acantholysis*, and is a dominant feature of two groups of diseases.

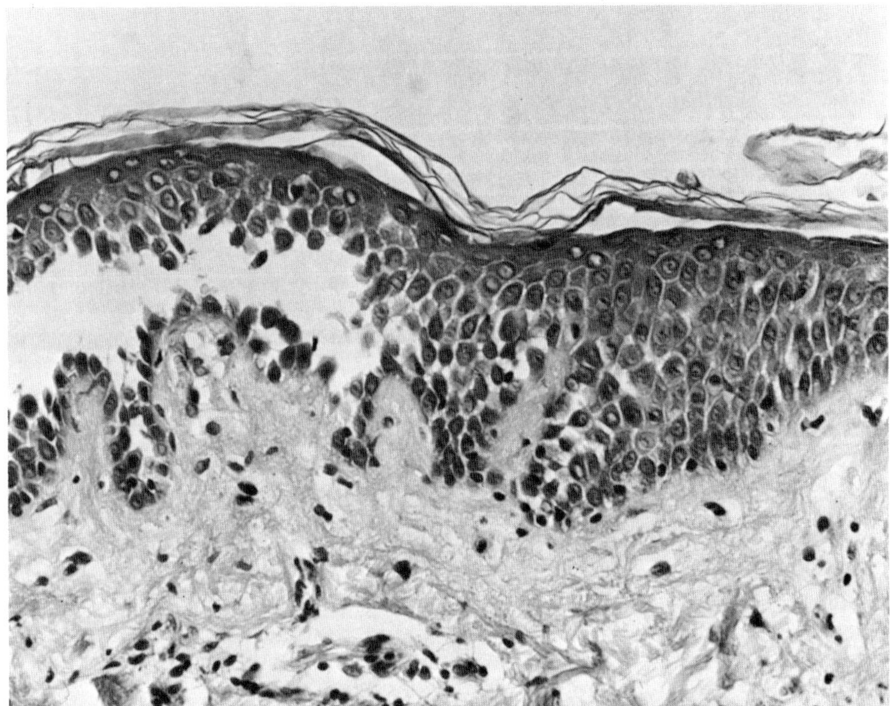

Fig. 40.9 Pemphigus vulgaris. The epidermal cells are seen to lack cohesion, so that an intraepidermal vesicle is formed. Isolated acantholytic cells lie in the cavity. It can be appreciated that the vesicle will be flaccid, and that pressure on it will result in lateral extension. This is known as Nikolsky's sign. The papillae of the dermis are covered by a layer of relatively unaffected basal cells which have been likened to a row of tomb-stones. × 200.

1. **The pemphigus group.** In pemphigus vulgaris the acantholytic process commences immediately above the basal layer of the epidermis, so that a suprabasal acantholytic cleft is formed. The basal layer remains unaffected and resembles a columnar epithelium covering the dermal papillae (Fig. 40.9). The term papillomatosis is applied to this appearance. Clinically, the patient develops *flaccid* vesicles and bullae which rupture leaving extensive raw areas. The distinction from bullous pemphigoid is important, because pemphigus vulgaris is

often fatal and can be kept under control only by heavy immunosuppression. Bullous pemphigoid is chronic and tiresome but rarely fatal. Pemphigus vulgaris often affects the oral mucosa; in about 50 per cent of cases this is the predominant and presenting symptom.

2. **The vesicular viral group.** In zoster, varicella, smallpox, vaccina, and herpes simplex, acantholytic intra-epidermal vesicles are formed. Fusion of epidermal cells may produce multinucleate giant cells; some of these are acantholytic and seem to be floating free within the vesicle. There is a marked dermal inflammatory reaction present in most examples. The distinction between the individual members of this group is difficult to make histologically, but electron microscopy of the vesicle fluid and other virological techniques can be used to identify the cause.

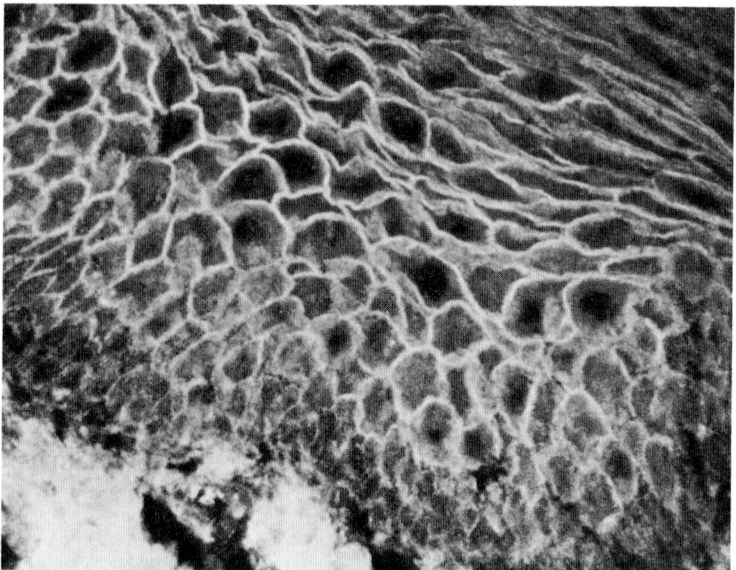

Fig. 40.10a The immunofluorescence pattern of pemphigus vulgaris. A frozen section of a skin biopsy taken from a patient with active pemphigus vulgaris was stained with fluorescein-labelled anti-IgG and examined under ultraviolet light. The staining of the intercellular material of the epidermis is well shown.
(Photograph by courtesy of Dr Susan Ritchie, University of Toronto.)

Immunopathology of the Vesiculo-bullous Diseases. Patients with pemphigus vulgaris commonly have an IgG auto-antibody in their plasma, and its titre reflects the activity of their disease. The antibody is directed against intercellular substance of squamous epithelium. Hence a patient's skin or mouth biopsy treated with fluorescein-labelled anti-human IgG shows brilliant fluorescence around each epidermal cell when examined under ultraviolet light (Fig. 40.10a). This is the *direct test.* The plasma antibody is detected *indirectly* by incubating normal human skin (or monkey oesophagus) with patient's serum; the skin is then washed, and labelled anti-IgG serum is applied.

The relationship of pemphigus antibody to the pathogenesis of the disease is not understood, but detection of the antibody is a useful diagnostic tool. In bullous pemphigoid an antibody directed against skin basement membrane is often found. The direct test shows a linear band of fluorescence in the basement membrane zone (Fig. 40.10b). The indirect test shows antibody to be present in the serum of about 70 per cent of patients. In the cicatricial form of the disease serum antibodies are found less frequently. In dermatitis herpetiformis IgA auto-antibodies are usually found in the dermal papillae, or sometimes in the basement membrane zone.

Hamartoma

The hamartomata of the skin are termed naevi. The common melanotic and angiomatous varieties are considered elsewhere.

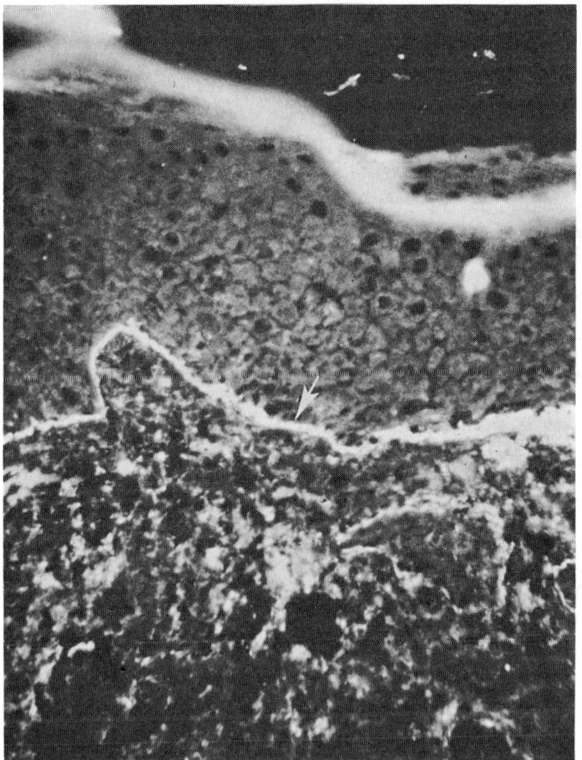

Fig. 40.10b Deposition of IgG antibody in the basement membrane of skin in bullous pemphigoid. A frozen section of skin taken adjacent to a recent vesicle was stained with fluorescein-labelled anti-IgG and examined microscopically under ultraviolet light. The linear staining of the basement membrane is characteristic of this disease. The ill-defined fluorescence on the surface of the skin is non-specific staining of the stratum corneum.

Tumours of the skin

Squamous-cell papilloma is generally used as a descriptive term which covers a number of separate entities. One variety is present at birth and is a type of hamartoma termed an *epithelial naevus.* Although non-neoplastic and benign, it often recurs after simple removal by curettage. The common wart (*verruca vulgaris*) is a type of papilloma due to an infection by one of the papovaviruses. In elderly people it is very common to find multiple *seborrhoeic keratoses* on the backs of the hands, trunk, and face.They are papillomata often with considerable acanthosis and melanin pigmentation. Clinically they appear to be 'stuck on' the surface of the skin either as elevated warty papillomata or as flat, roughened, pigmented plaques. Curettage effects an easy cure. They are not premalignant, but when heavily pigmented are liable to be confused with other pigmented lesions—melanotic naevi, pigmented basal-cell carcinoma, Hutchinson's freckle, or malignant melanoma.

Other benign tumours are not uncommon: fibroma, lipoma, neurofibroma, etc. These will not be further considered.

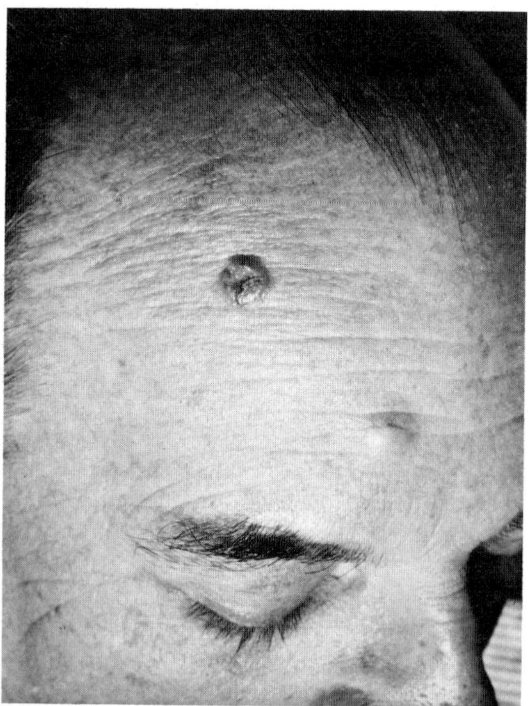

Fig. 40.11 Basal-cell carcinoma on the right side of the forehead of a 56-year-old man. The lesion has the typical appearance with a depressed centre and a raised, rolled edge over which dilated blood vessels can be seen traversing. The dome-shaped swelling just above the medial aspect of the eyebrow has the features of an epidermoid cyst, commonly called a sebaceous cyst, or wen.

Malignant tumours of the skin

The most common malignant tumour of the skin in white races is the basal-cell carcinoma (p. 350). See Fig. 40.11.

Squamous-cell carcinoma. This tumour commonly arises on the sun-exposed skin in a pre-existing *actinic keratosis* (Fig. 40.12). Actinic keratoses are areas of epidermal dysplasia caused by prolonged, repeated exposure to sunlight. They appear as scaly erythematous areas on the face or hands, and in contradistinction to seborrhoeic keratoses, they must be regarded as precancerous. Squamous-cell carcinoma arising in an actinic keratosis is invasive, but metastasis is late and the prognosis is good. Squamous-cell carcinoma may also arise in normal skin or in a chronic erythematous lesion called *Bowen's disease*. This is a type of *carcinoma-in-situ*, and can occur on any part of the body. This type of squamous-cell carcinoma is more malignant than that arising in an actinic keratosis. Squamous-cell carcinoma must be differentiated both clinically and pathologically from a keratoacanthoma, which it closely resembles and which also occurs on a sun-exposed area (see p. 313).

Melanoma. Malignant melanoma of the skin can arise in three ways:

1. In *normal skin*. Some tumours invade the dermis early (*nodular melanoma*), and also metastasize early so that the prognosis is very bad. Other tumours have a much better prognosis, for although they involve the epidermis and papillary dermis over an area, there is no early deep invasion (*superficial spreading melanoma*).

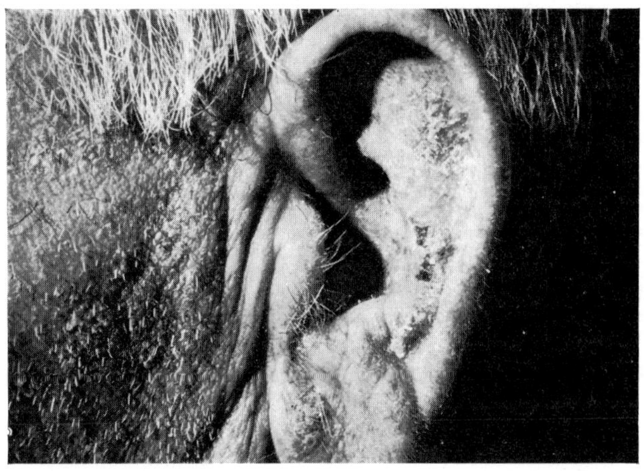

Fig. 40.12 Actinic keratoses on the left ear of an elderly man who had spent much of his working life out of doors. The lesions are erythematous and hyperkeratotic. The epidermal dysplasia is a precursor of carcinoma, and an area of crusting in the centre was regarded as suspicious. Biopsy at this site revealed no evidence of squamous-cell carcinoma.

2. In *pre-existing naevocellar naevi* the incidence of malignancy is unknown, but considering the number of naevi in the average person, it must be very uncommon. Danger signals which suggest malignancy are a recent increase in size, ulceration, bleeding, and change in colour.

3. In *Hutchinson's freckle*. Hutchinson's freckle is a pigmented patch or plaque usually on the face, which microscopically shows atypical proliferation of melanocytes in the basal layer of the epidermis. It may be regarded as a *melanoma-in-situ*. After many years the melanocytic cells invade the dermis, and malignant melanoma develops. Even then the prognosis is good, in contradistinction to malignant melanoma which arises on normal skin.

Other malignant tumours of the skin, for example lymphomata (*mycosis fungoides*) and sarcomata, occur but are very uncommon.

The management of skin tumours is beyond the scope of the book, but it should be emphasized that before radical treatment is undertaken a positive biopsy must be obtained. The hypothetical possibility of disseminating tumour by biopsy, even in the case of malignant melanoma, is more than offset by the tragedy of treating a benign lesion by radical means. The study of skin tumours has highlighted several curious pseudomalignant lesions. Thus, keratoacanthoma closely mimics carcinoma, nodular fasciitis resembles sarcoma, and before diagnosing malignant lymphoma of the skin it is necessary to exclude certain pseudolymphomatous lesions which may arise spontaneously (pseudolymphoma of Spiegler-Fendt) or as a result of trauma such as an insect or tick bite.

GENERAL READING

Behrman H T, Labow T A, Rosen J H 1971 Common Skin Diseases, 2nd edn. Grune and Stratten, New York

Fitzpatrick T B, Eisen A Z, Wolff K, Freedberg I M, Austen K F, Edrs 1979 Dermatology in General Practice. McGraw-Hill: New York, 1884 pp

Harrist T T, and Mihm M C, 1979 Cutaneous Immunopathology. Human Pathology 10 625

Lever F W, Schaumburg-Lever G 1975 The Histopathology of the Skin, 5th edn. Lippincott, Philadelphia, 793 pp

Milne J A 1972 An Introduction to the Diagnostic Histopathology of the Skin. Arnold, London, 363 pp

Rook A, Wilkinson D S, Ebling F J G (eds) 1972 Textbook of Dermatology, 2nd edn. Blackwell, Oxford, 2118 pp. An exhaustive standard English text in two volumes

Index

Main references are indicated by bold numerals. Illustrations are referred to by italic numerals.

Histopathology

White tissue in specimen signifies
(a) fibrous tissue
(b) necrotic tissue
(c) Carcinoma/malignancy
(d) pus.

Brain specimen
Look at meninges
Look at blood vessels - atheroma
Look for absess.

steroids inhibit phospholipase A.